ATLAS OF
SPINAL DISEASES

A **Slide Atlas of Spinal Diseases,** based on the material presented in this book, is also available. The Slide Atlas is organized into seven topic-based units, each of which corresponds to a chapter or chapters in the book. Each unit consists of superbly illustrated text, with 35mm color slides corresponding to the photographs in the text. In this unique format, all of the slides are labeled, numbered, and indexed for easy reference. Each unit is presented in a durable vinyl binder, with the complete collection housed in an attractive and sturdy slip case.

For further information, please contact:
Gower Medical Publishing
101 Fifth Avenue
New York, NY 10003

ATLAS OF SPINAL DISEASES

Peter G. Bullough,
M.B., Ch.B.

Professor of Pathology
Cornell University Medical College
Director of Laboratories
Hospital for Special Surgery
New York, NY

Oheneba Boachie-Adjei,
M.D.

Assistant Professor of
Orthopaedic Surgery
University of Minnesota
Attending Orthopaedic Surgeon
Abbott Northwestern
Hospital and Twin Cities
Scoliosis Center
Minneapolis

- **J.B. Lippincott Company**
  Philadelphia
- **Gower Medical Publishing**
  New York • London

Distributed in the USA and Canada by:

J.B. Lippincott Company
East Washington Square
Philadelphia, PA 19105

Distributed in all countries except the USA and Canada by:

Harper & Row International
East Washington Square
Philadelphia, PA 19105

Library of Congress Cataloging-in-Publication Data

Bullough, Peter G., 1932–
Atlas of spinal diseases.

Includes bibliographies and index.
1. Spine—Diseases—Atlases. I. Boachie-Adjei, Oheneba, 1950– II. Title. [DNLM: 1. Spinal Diseases—atlases. WE 17 B938ab]
RD768.B84 1988 616.7'3 87-45847
ISBN 0-397-44654-3 (Lippincott)

British Library Cataloguing in Publication Data

Bullough, Peter G.
Atlas of spinal diseases.
1. Man. Spine. Diseases
I. Title II. Boachie-Adjei, Oheneba
616.7'3
ISBN 0-397-44654-3

Project Editor: Joy Noel Travalino
Art Director and Interior Design: Jill Feltham
Layout and Cover Design: Romi Dorsey
Illustration: Susan C. Tilberry
Production Assistant: Indi J. Bowden

Printed in Singapore by Imago Productions (FE) PTE Ltd

Print No. 9 8 7 6 5 4 3 2 1

This work is dedicated to the memory of

CHRISTIAN GEORG SCHMORL
1861–1932

Prosector and Director of the
Pathological Institute of the
Stadtkrankenhaus Friedrichstadt Dresden
1884–1932
who by the systematic examination of all vertebral columns in that institute made this subject his own. It was in his seventy-second year, while preparing a vertebral column for examination, that he contracted the septicemia that was to prove fatal to him.

The greatest thing a human soul ever does in this world is to *see* something, and tell what it *saw* in a plain way. Hundreds of people can talk for one who can think, but thousands can think for one who can see. To see clearly is poetry, prophecy, and religion, all in one.

John Ruskin in
Modern Painters
Vol. 3, Part IV
Chapter 16, Section 28

PREFACE

Our purpose in this Atlas is to provide an anatomical basis to the clinical diagnosis and management of spinal disease.

A number of excellent texts address diseases of the spine from the clinical point of view. Few, however, have stressed the morbid anatomy of the spine. Georg Schmorl's monumental autopsy study of the spine eventually led to publication in 1932 of his classic text, *The Human Spine in Health and Disease*. Schmorl's studies of the pathologic anatomy of the intervertebral disc, and in particular of the displacement of disc tissue, revolutionized the treatment and surgical approach to lumbar disc disease.

In preparing our *Atlas of Spinal Diseases*, we have been encouraged by improved methods of imaging as well as by the availability of color printing. Using noninvasive images of clinical cases and those obtained in the course of autopsy studies, we have compared these images to photographs of the dissected specimens and to photomicrographs of the tissues involved in the disease process. Since the clinician must visualize pathology via imaging techniques, it is important that these images be correlated with the actual anatomy of the spine. It is our hope that through these correlations, the Atlas will provide a sound basis in both normal and morbid anatomy, while providing some insight into the pathophysiology, diagnosis, and management of spinal diseases.

We have organized the book into three sections, each approximately equal in length. The first section deals with normal anatomy, physiology and development, with a short introduction on methods of examination and dissection. We have grouped our discussion of spinal diseases into the remaining two sections: diseases of the articulations and diseases of the bony elements. While diseases beginning in the joints will eventually come to involve the bone and vice versa, it is our aim, in separating the two classes, to stress the *primary* etiology of the disease.

It is our opinion that since most diseases of the spine are accompanied by some deformity, i.e., a deviation from the normal attitude, a discussion of scoliosis and of kyphosis properly belongs in a clinical text of spinal disease. However, where deformity is a prominent feature of a particular disease under discussion, it will be mentioned with respect to that disease. Furthermore, in a separate chapter, we discuss developmental and acquired malformations of the spine.

The majority of the anatomical specimens presented in this Atlas were prepared by Dr. Boachie-Adjei during a fellowship year in pathology and a subsequent residency in orthopedic surgery at the Hospital for Special Surgery in New York. Other specimens have been collected by the senior author over several years, or have been contributed by colleagues throughout the world.

The images presented in this book are printed as large as possible to enhance their clarity. Line drawings are used liberally to indicate specific features in a photograph, be it a radiograph, a gross photograph, or a photomicrograph. In cases where the three-dimensional and/or temporal aspects of structure must be communicated, color schematic and anatomical drawings are provided. Although this book primarily is an Atlas, we have attempted to include adequate and up-to-date textual material. The format is didactic. The bibliography at the end of the book is arranged topically, with general and specific references corresponding to major headings in the book.

It is our hope that this Atlas will provide sufficient basic material on spinal diseases to be included in the armamentarium of the orthopedic surgeon, the radiologist, the pathologist, and the student of medicine, in general.

P.G.B.
O.B.
New York, 1987

Acknowledgments

This Atlas reflects the accumulated efforts and contributions of many people. We should like to begin by thanking those members of the Gower Medical Publishing production staff, through whose untiring efforts we are able to bring the materials in this book together.

Jill Feltham, the designer and art director, and Romi Dorsey, the layout artist and cover designer, are to be congratulated for the excellence of their work, which significantly contributes to our purpose.

We are very fortunate that Susan Tilberry was available to illustrate our book and we believe that her clear drawings help considerably in the comprehension of certain difficult concepts.

A clearly flowing and unambiguous text depends largely upon the editor, and we feel privileged in having had Joy Travalino as our editor. Joy has not only contributed to the clarity of the text but also has been responsible for the overall management of the text and illustrations and the marriage of the two.

We want to thank the following students, who assisted with dissections, photography, and library research:

Brooklyn College (National Black Science Students Organization): Lorna Blair, Dale Campbell, Janet Dyer, Colville Gibbs, Jennifer Gomes, Ruth Hylton, Christopher Jones, Carlton Laing, Colin Ottey, Margaret White, and Beverly Yearwood.

Cornell University Medical College: Jonathan Blank, Class of '85; Judith A. Rovno, Jonathan H. Wheeler, William F. Flynn, Jr., Tom Fahey, Class of '86; Felix Raymond Ortega, Class of '87.

Cornell University Medical College Graduate School of Medical Sciences: John Matyas.

Georgetown University School of Medicine: Peter Rizzo, Class of '86.

Vanderbilt University School of Medicine: Theodore Miller, Class of '87; Adam Abrams, Class of '88.

Albany Medical College: Joseph Feinberg, Class of '85.

We are particularly grateful to our colleagues at the Hospital for Special Surgery, to the members of the International Skeletal Society and to our colleagues throughout the world, who have so generously contributed their cases: Alberto G. Ayala, David S. Bradford, Mario Campanacci, H.V. Crock, Francis Denis, Howard Dorfman, David Eyre, V. Fornasier, R. Lagier, David Levine, Rikuo Machinami, Zdenek Matejovsky, James W. Milgram, James W. Ogilvie, Donald J. Ortner, The Royal College of Surgeons of England, Vorachai Sirikulchayanonta, Professor Terayama, Krishnan K. Unni.

To the technical and clerical staff of the Pathology Department at the Hospital for Special Surgery, we are forever grateful for all their efforts on our behalf.

To our families and friends, who have been sometimes neglected and frequently bored by our monomania, we humbly ask of them pardon.

CONTENTS

1 SECTION

NORMAL ANATOMY AND DEVELOPMENT

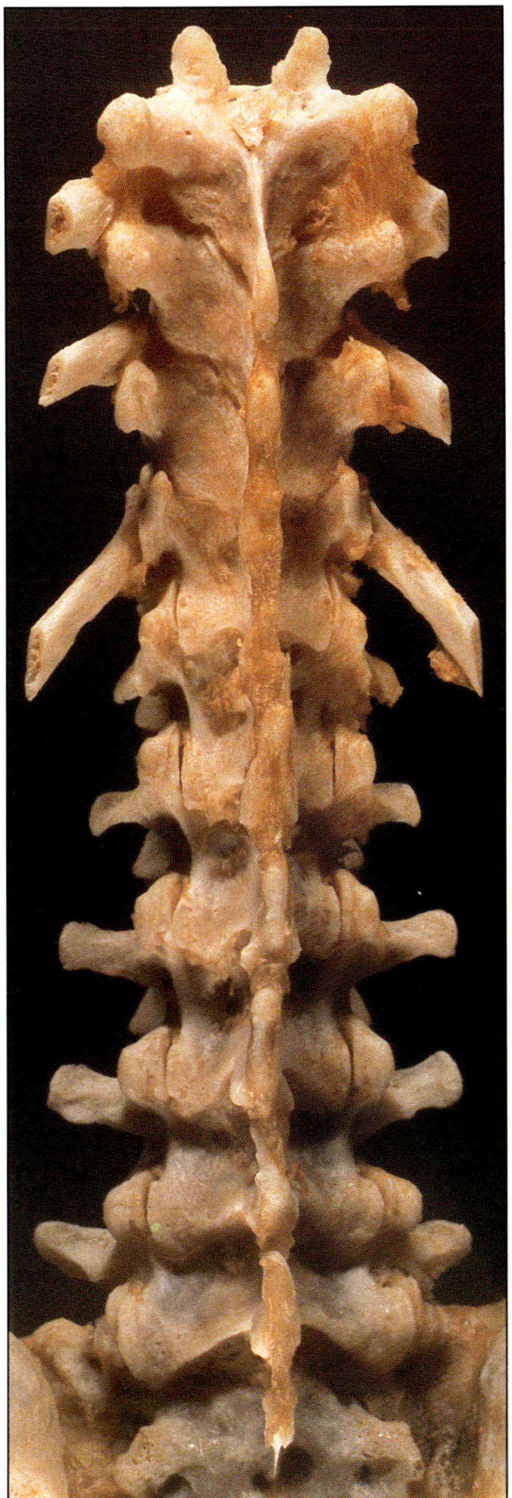

This book is intended to illustrate the common deformities and diseases of the vertebral column. In order that the student might have some standards of comparison, as well as an appreciation of those elements of developmental anatomy necessary to an understanding of many diseases of the spine, the first section of this book is devoted to normal anatomy and development. It is not intended to be an exhaustive review, but rather a highlight of those features that we believe to be important to a study of spinal pathology.

Because we are convinced of the importance of making one's own anatomical studies, we begin with a brief chapter on methods of examination.

1 CHAPTER

METHODS OF EXAMINATION

INTRODUCTION

The spinal column, like all other organs, should be completely removed from the body to facilitate a detailed examination. To slice open a few of the vertebral bodies, as is done on many autopsy services, may be adequate for the examination of some hematologic conditions, but it is inadequate for the study of most other problems. The intervertebral discs for example cannot be evaluated in this way.

Frequently it is presumed that removal of the spine is time consuming or even impossible. However, the results of our own investigations are in agreement with those of Schmorl, that the entire spinal column and adjacent soft tissues, after some practice, can be removed within 10 to 20 minutes, with restoration of body rigidity and form afforded (see below).

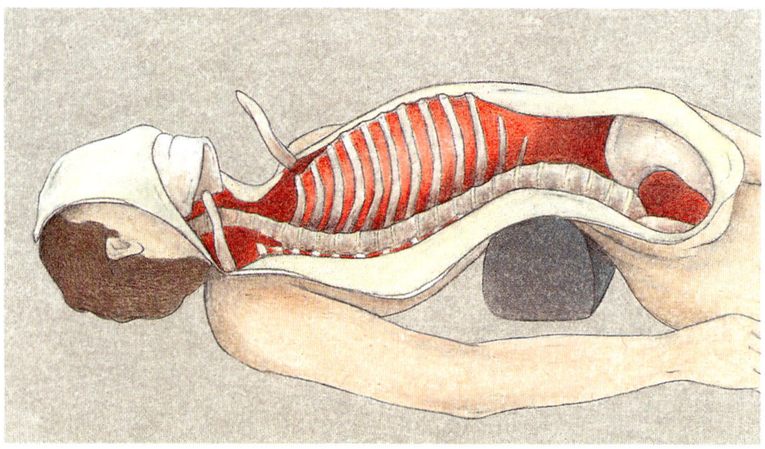

Figure 1.1 Schematic drawing of spine removal to show how following evisceration of the body initial dissection of the spine is facilitated by placement of a block under the thoracolumbar junction.

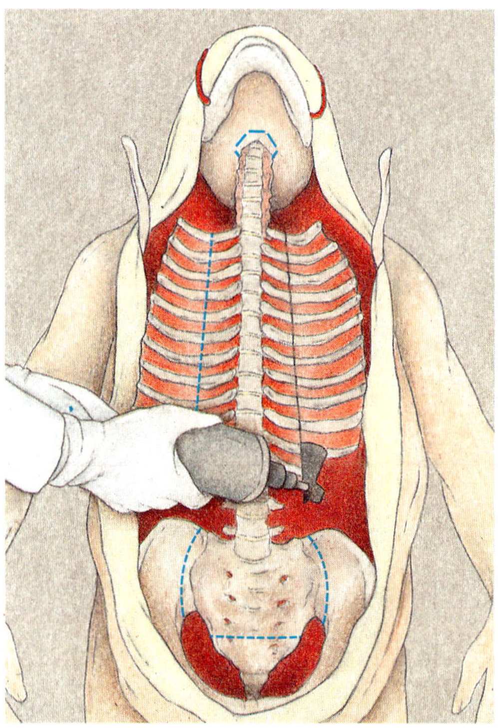

Figure 1.2 Schematic drawing of spine removal to show how the ribs on either side of the spine must be sectioned near the costovertebral articulations, using a Stryker saw, before dissection can proceed. The ilium then is sectioned just beyond the sacroiliac joints, followed by sectioning of the distal sacrum if that portion of the spine and coccyx is not wanted.

DISSECTION

In the dissection of the body, after all the visceral organs have been removed, the spine should be studied in situ, with special attention given to protuberances and to the various curvatures, the conditions of which can be reproduced by a plaster cast. However, if vascular studies of the spine are desired, one must inject either the aorta or the vena cava with barium sulfate (a 50% dilution of the concentration normally available in a hospital radiology department is suitable) before undertaking any evisceration of abdominal organs. Furthermore, prior to injection, one must attempt to ligate those vessels not involved in the supply of the vertebral column.

SPINE REMOVAL

Removal of the spine is facilitated by placement of a block under the lower thoracic spine to maximize the lumbar lordosis (Fig. 1.1). Using a Stryker saw, the ribs are sectioned close to the spine and the pelvis then is sectioned on both sides, just beyond the sacroiliac joints and across the distal sacrum (Fig. 1.2). If so desired, the entire pelvis along with the upper end of the femur may be dissected without too much difficulty, although in such a case reconstruction of the body may be quite difficult.

Hyperextension of the head now should be obtained by moving the block from under the thoracic spine up to the cervical region. This will allow easy dislocation of the cervical spine. If the brain has been removed, the occipital bone around the foramen magnum should be sectioned from within the skull, using a chisel. If the brain has not been removed, this maneuver may be undertaken from the neck (Fig. 1.3).

Once the bone has been divided, dissection with a long pointed knife will free the soft tissues around the base of the skull. The spine then is elevated from the cervical end, while the soft tissues are dissected from the posterior elements (Fig. 1.4). Care should be taken to maintain the integrity of the carotid arteries for embalming purposes.

After removal of the spine from the body (Fig. 1.5), a wooden rod, two by two inches in width and cut to an appropriate length, is inserted into the base of the occiput and nailed to the clavicles and to the remaining portion of the sacrum or to the iliac wings, thus stabilizing the body (Fig. 1.6). The body then is closed in a routine postmortem fashion.

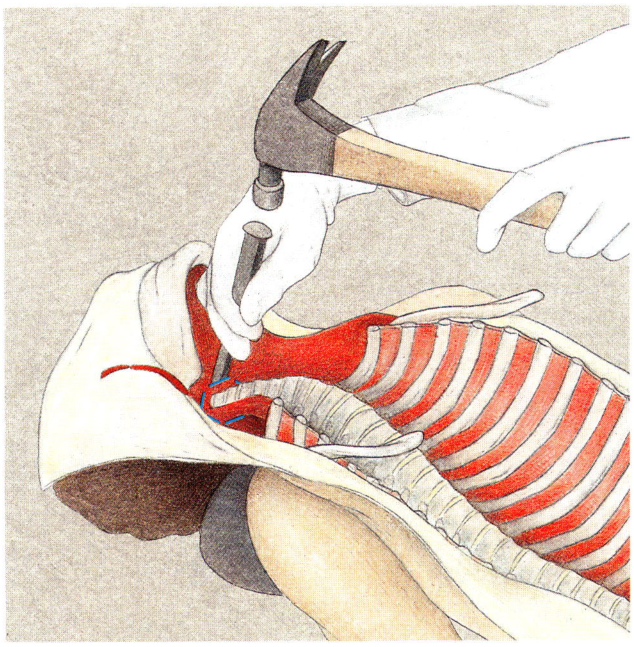

Figure 1.3 Schematic drawing of spine removal to show how dissection of the cervical spine is facilitated by removing the block from under the thoracolumbar junction and placing it under the shoulders, to hyperextend the cervical spine. The base of the skull then is osteotomized anteriorly, the soft-tissue attachments to the lateral masses and posterior arch of C-1 are dissected sharply, and the cervical spine is freed from the foramen magnum by manual dislocation with forward flexion.

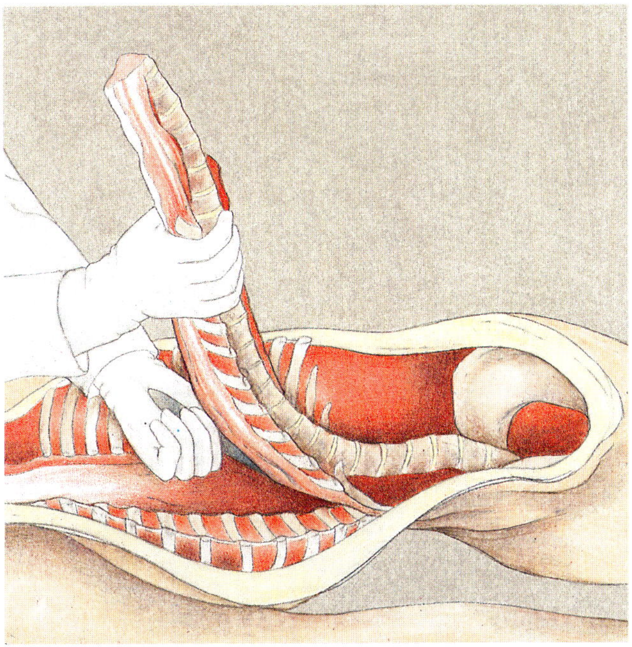

Figure 1.4 Schematic drawing of spine removal to show how with the upper cervical spine freed, the remainder is dissected by peeling in a craniocaudal direction from the posterior soft-tissue attachments with care taken not to buttonhole the skin posteriorly.

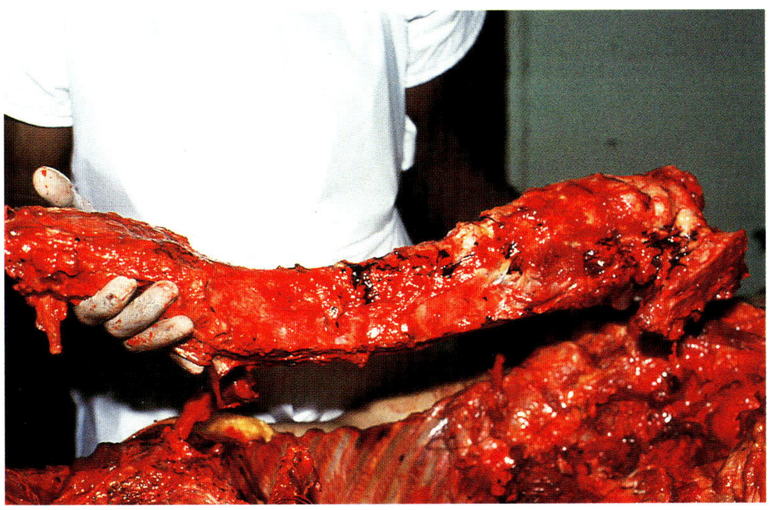

Figure 1.5 Photograph of the dissected spine after removal from the body.

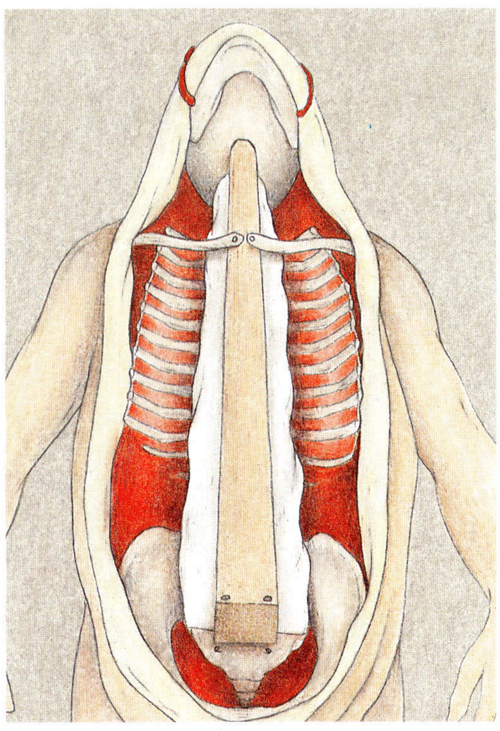

Figure 1.6 Schematic drawing to show reconstruction of the back following spine removal. A wooden rod is cut proximally to secure the foramen magnum while two long nails are driven laterally into the sacrum or wings of the ilium to secure the wood distally.

Specimen Radiographic Studies

Before sectioning of the spine, radiographs should be taken to obtain anteroposterior, lateral, and oblique views of the entire spine. The AP view is best for assessing any lateral curvature or rotation and for evaluation of the vertebral bodies, pedicles, and transverse and spinous processes (Fig. 1.7). The lateral view is useful for evaluation of spinal curvature, the height and shape of the vertebral bodies, and the disc spaces (Fig. 1.8). The oblique projection is useful in visualizing the lumbar facet joints and pars interarticularis, and the cervical intervertebral foramina (Fig. 1.9).

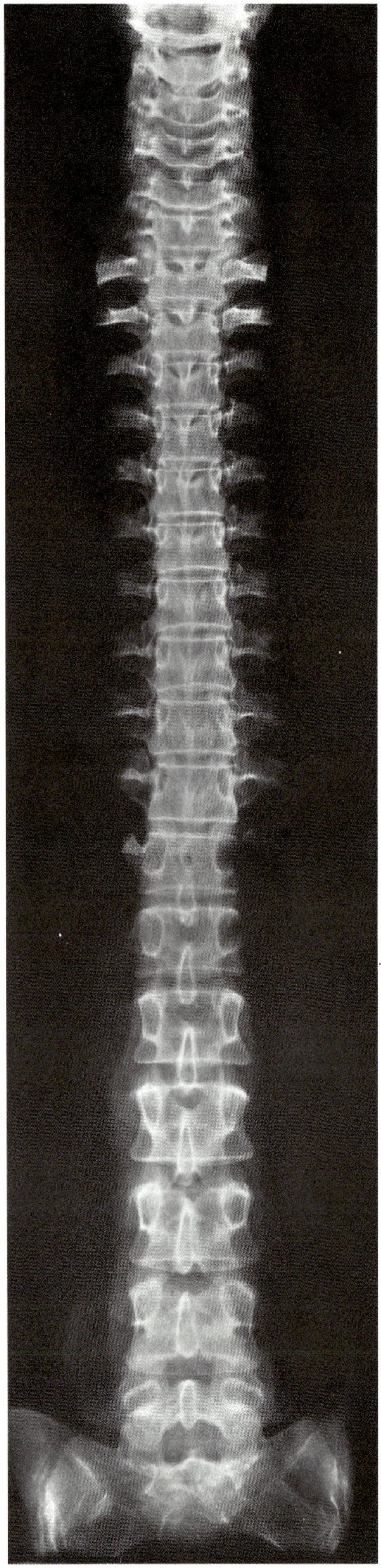

Figure 1.7 AP radiograph of the spine. Note that in this view each vertebral body presents as a face with two eyes (the pedicles) and a nose (the spinous process). Scanning the film for these features will facilitate the recognition of pathology involving these structures. Note also that the interpedicular distance is widest in the cervical and lumbar regions and narrowest at T-4. Note that the end plates are most clearly visualized in the thoracic region where the x-ray beam is normal to the spine while at the upper and lower ends, where the beam is oblique, there is distortion.

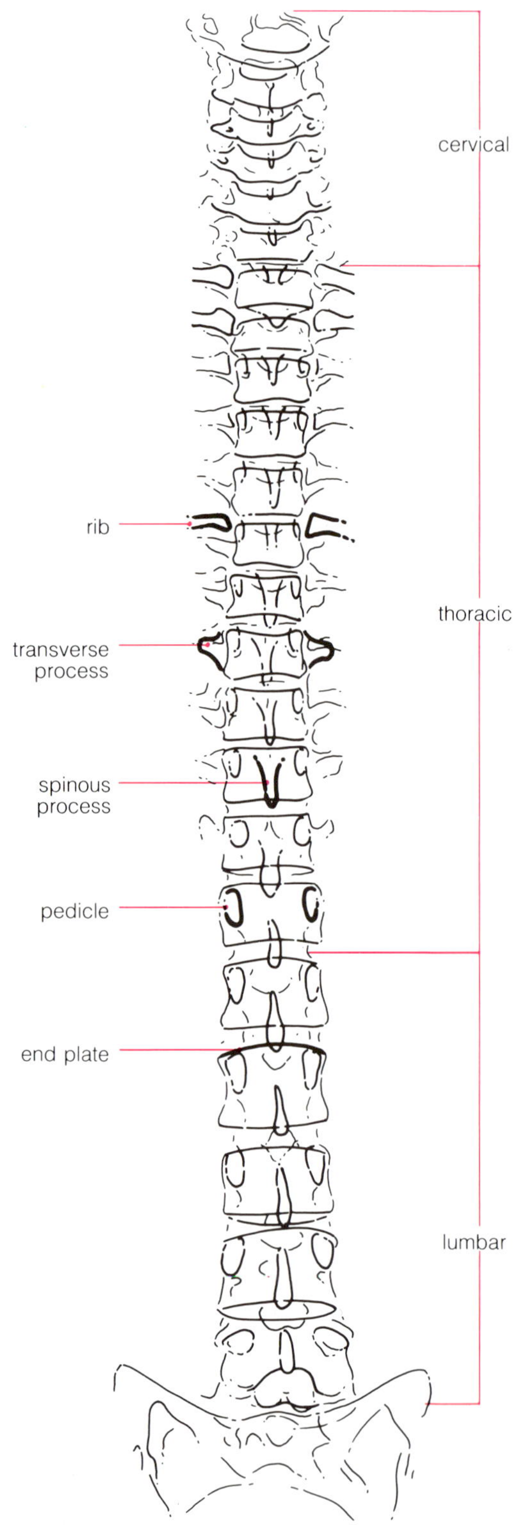

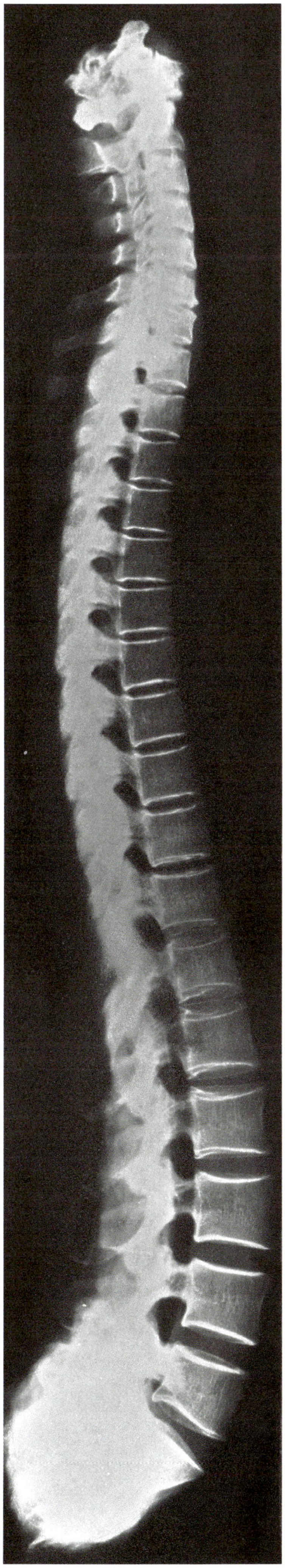

Figure 1.8 Lateral radiograph of the spine. In this view note the spinal curvature, the height and shape of the vertebral bodies, and the height of the disc spaces. The intervertebral foramina are well visualized in the thoracic and lumbar spine while the facet joints are seen clearly in the cervical and thoracic regions.

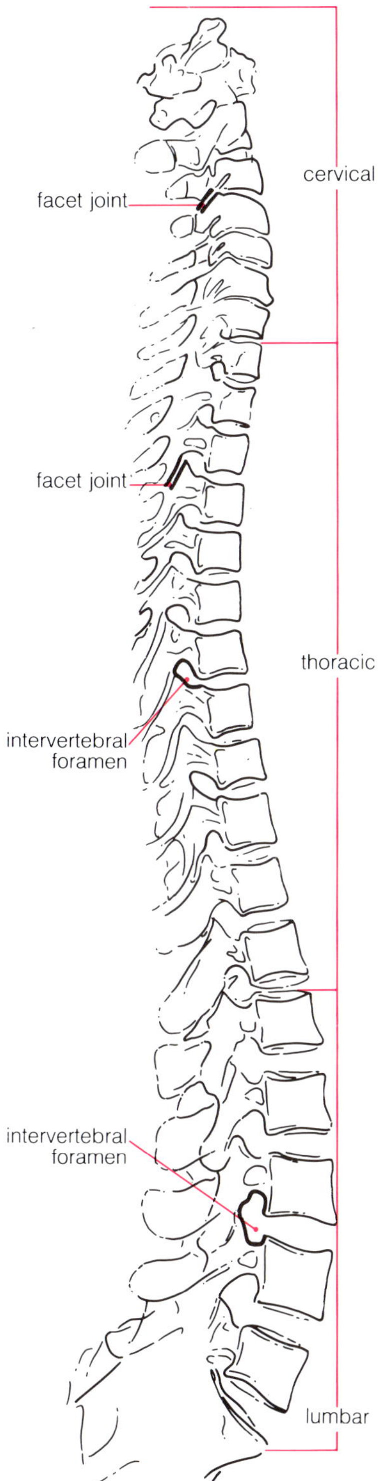

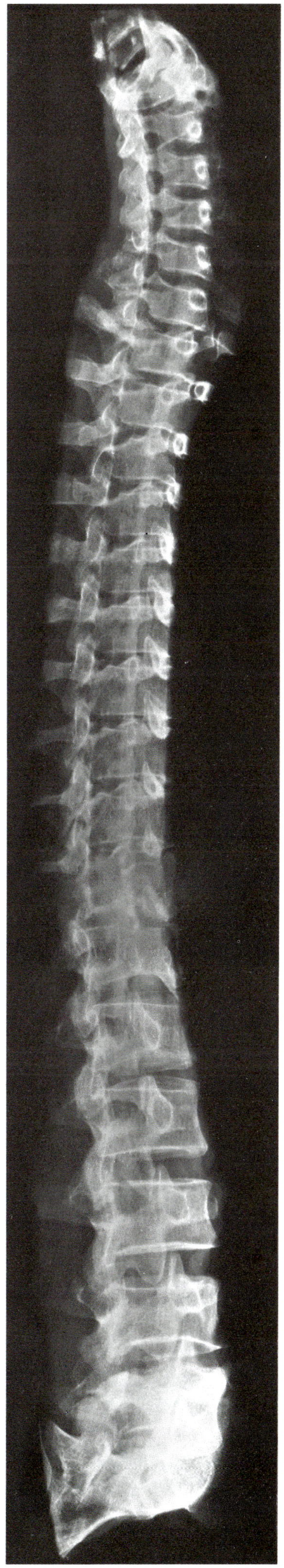

Figure 1.9 Oblique radiograph of the spine. This view is particularly useful for visualizing the facet joints and the pars interarticularis in the lumbar spine, and the intervertebral foramina in the cervical spine.

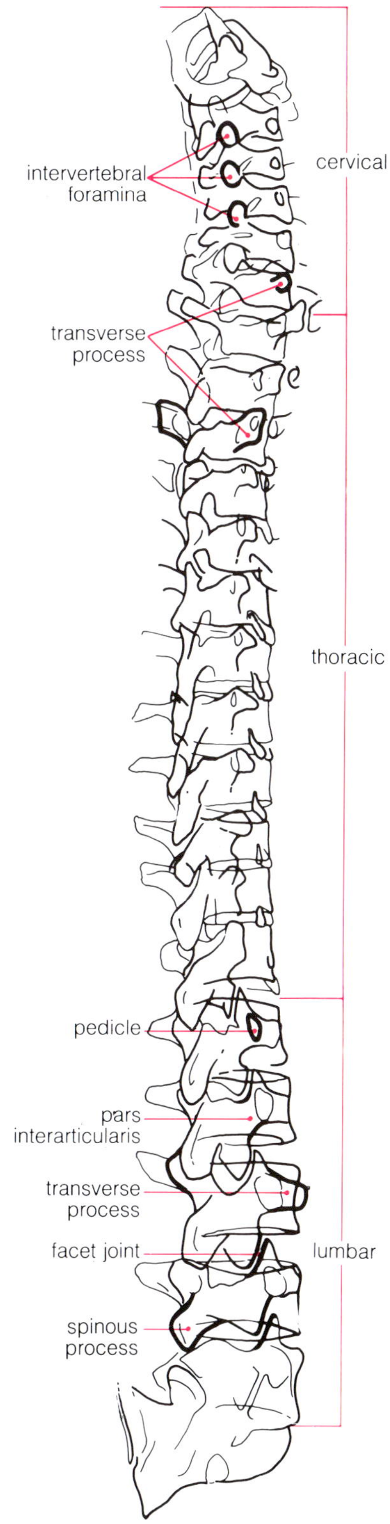

It is important to realize that in all radiographic views of the spine distortion of the image will occur, depending on the distance between the bone surface and the x-ray film and also on the angle at which the x-ray beam approaches the object. The size of each image will be distorted as well as the relative position of the images created by the anterior and posterior surfaces of the elements (Fig. 1.10). For these reasons, visualization of the spine with minimal distortion requires multiple coned-down views. (With the exception of the spines of newborns, all of the whole-spine radiographs presented in this book were created from two films spliced together to form one continuous image.)

Special Imaging Techniques

Computed tomography (CT) scanning may be used to facilitate the visualization of spinal lesions, which normally are obscured by the overlay and distortion inherent in a conventional radiographic image. Magnetic resonance imaging (MRI) studies, which are not good for visualizing bone, may however prove valuable in the visualization of disc, spinal cord, and nerve root pathology (Fig. 1.11).

To assess spinal canal size or to evaluate for intraspinal pathology, myelograms may be prepared by first plugging the distal end of the canal and then infiltrating the proximal end with a fixed quantity of contrast medium (30 mL of 30% Renografin) as shown in Figure 1.12. Normally the contrast agent rises to the level of L1-2 (Fig. 1.13). The narrower the canal, however, the higher the contrast material will rise.

Following myelographic studies and drainage, discograms are prepared using 1 mL of 30% Renografin mixed with methylene blue dye. The contrast medium is injected into the disc space with a 22-gauge needle, using the anterior approach (Fig. 1.14). Radiographs then are taken in AP and lateral

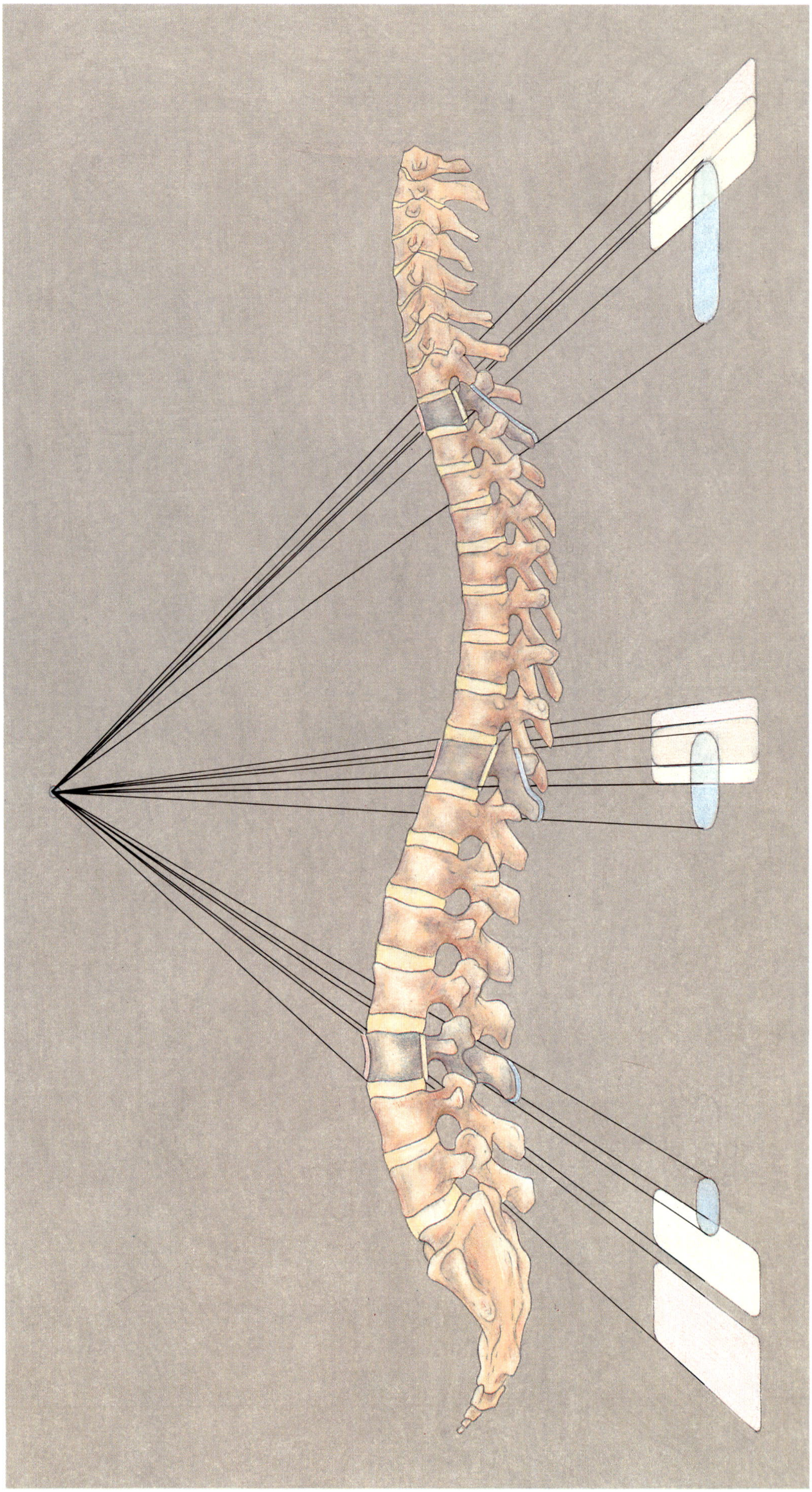

Figure 1.10 Schematic drawing to illustrate the distortions inherent in clinical and specimen radiographs. Note that the vertebral body surface closest to the x-ray source will appear longer than the surface closest to the film; however, because of the cylindrical shape of the vertebral body, the width will remain the same.

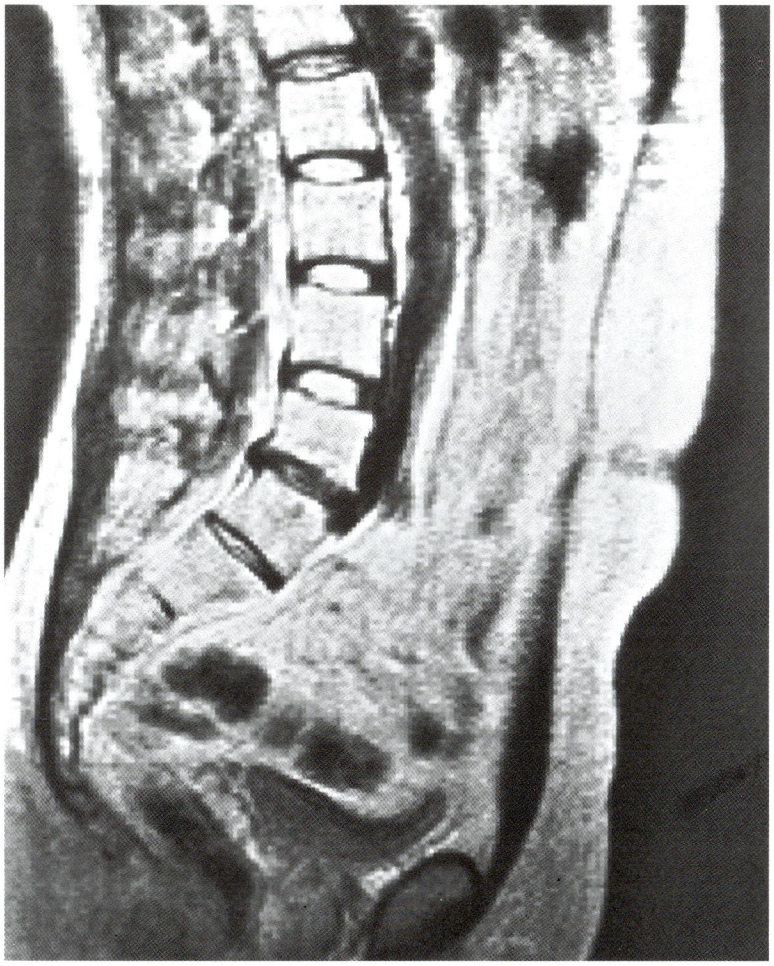

Figure 1.11 Sagittal MRI of the lumbar spine. Because of their high hydrogen content, the nucleus pulposus of the intervertebral disc, the spinal cord, and the nerve roots are well visualized.

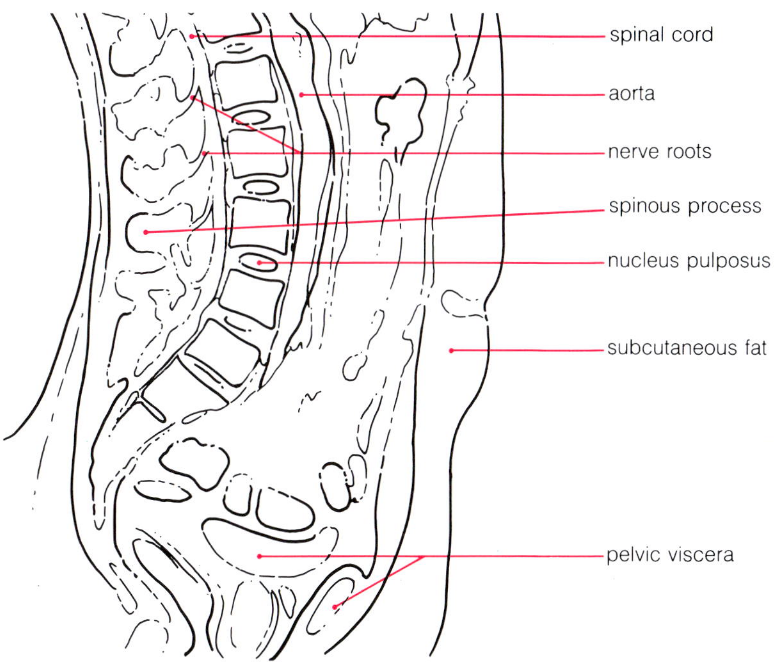

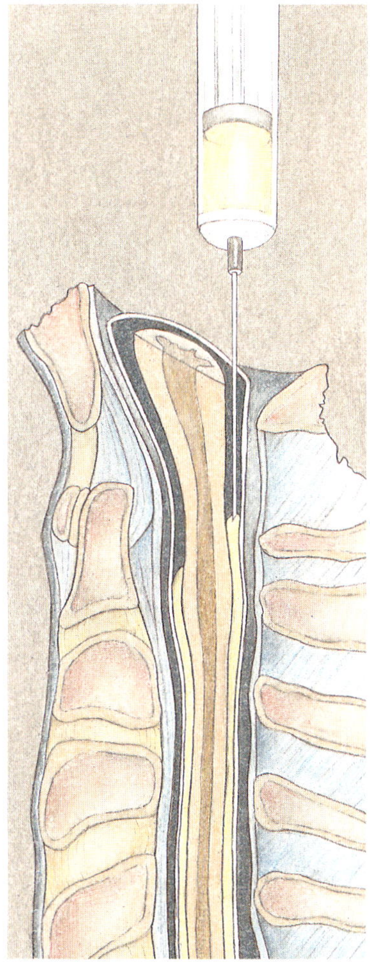

Figure 1.12 Schematic drawing to demonstrate the preparation of a myelogram. After plugging up the opening at the distal end of the spine with a plastic clay or modeling compound, 30 mL of 30% Renografin is introduced into the subarachnoid space at the C-1 level with the spine in the erect position. AP, lateral, and oblique radiographs of the spine then are taken to evaluate the spinal canal and nerve roots.

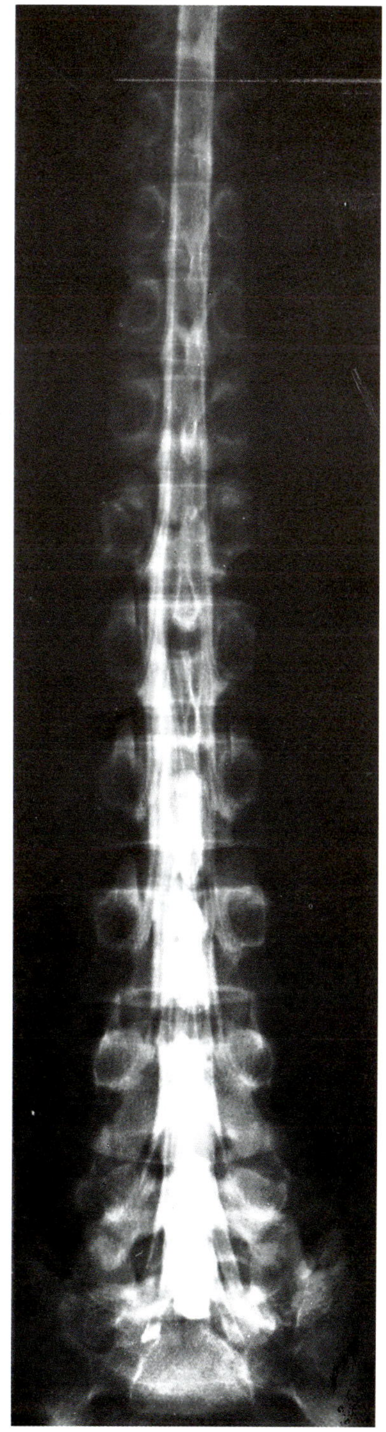

Figure 1.13 AP myelogram of the thoracolumbar spine showing normal spinal canal and normal lumbar nerve roots.

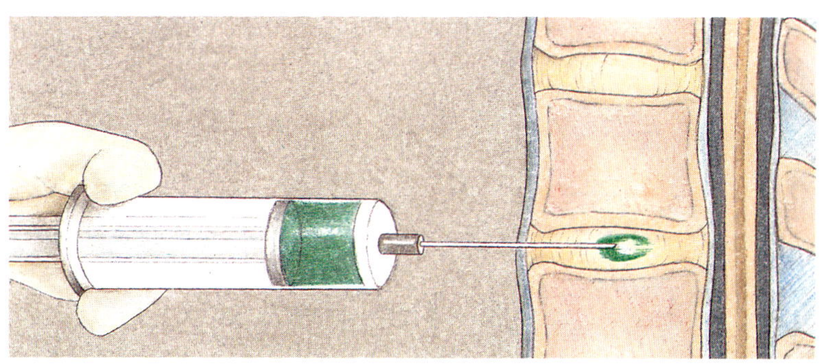

Figure 1.14 Schematic diagram to show how a discogram is prepared by inserting the needle approximately 2 cm into the disc space and injecting 1 mL of 30% Renografin mixed with methylene blue dye.

views (Fig. 1.15). CT scans of the disc spaces also are performed (Fig. 1.16). (These studies should be performed as quickly as possible following the injection of contrast agent.)

Sectioning of the Spine

Following radiographic examination, the spine may be dissected further by:

1. Sagittal section or
2. Separation of the posterior and frontal elements.

The first approach allows for an excellent view of disc pathology along with an assessment of intraspinal pathology and displacement of one vertebra upon the next; the second approach allows for dissection of the spinal cord while providing an excellent view of the anterior and posterior longitudinal ligaments and the ligamenta flava. In both approaches, sections are made by using a commercially available butcher's band saw. Radiographs of sagittal and parasagittal sections now are made for further study.

The importance of radiographic examination as an essential component in the study of the pathologic anatomy of the spine and of bone in general cannot be overemphasized.

Tissue Studies Including Maceration

In order to perform gross studies of the bone texture, the blood should be washed away from the cut surface of the bone. Fine-grain low-voltage radiographs prepared from a thin slice of cut bone can prove to be highly instructive (Fig. 1.17). These radiographs provide an excellent picture of bone texture and are extremely valuable in the interpretation of bone histology.

As a final step, after appropriate histologic material has been taken for microscopic sections, the specimen may be macerated in either of the following ways:

1. In the case of formalin-fixed tissue, first dehydrate the specimen by immersing it in absolute alcohol for at least 24 hours; then defat it by submerging in xylene for 24 hours or longer. Transfer back to absolute alcohol for 24 hours, following which the specimen should be rinsed under running water for 30 minutes. Transfer and immerse it in sodium hypochlorite (household bleach), gently agitating for 30 to 60 minutes, with periodic inspection of the specimen as to the desired level of maceration. Place under running water overnight, and then bathe it in hydrogen peroxide to whiten it. Set the specimen under sunlight for the final drying stage (Fig. 1.18).

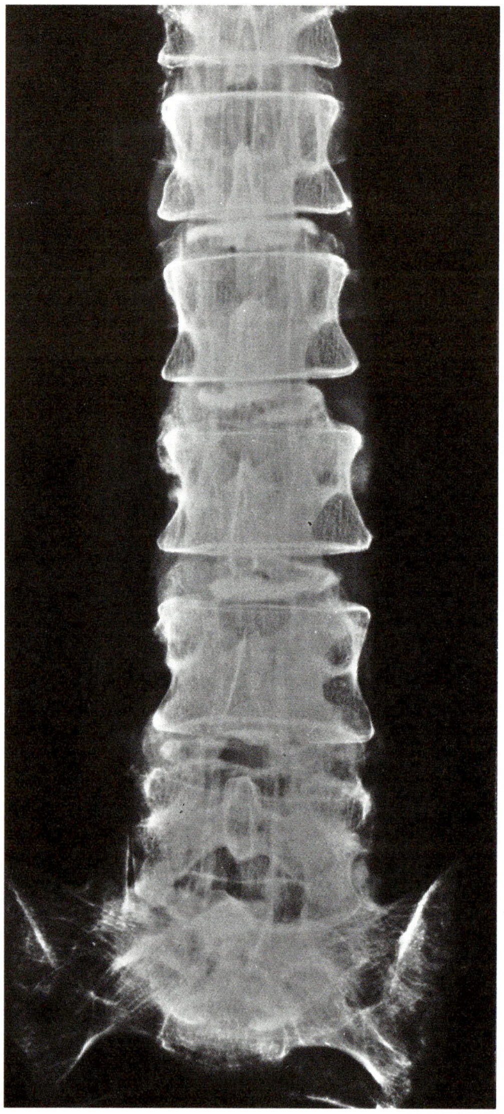

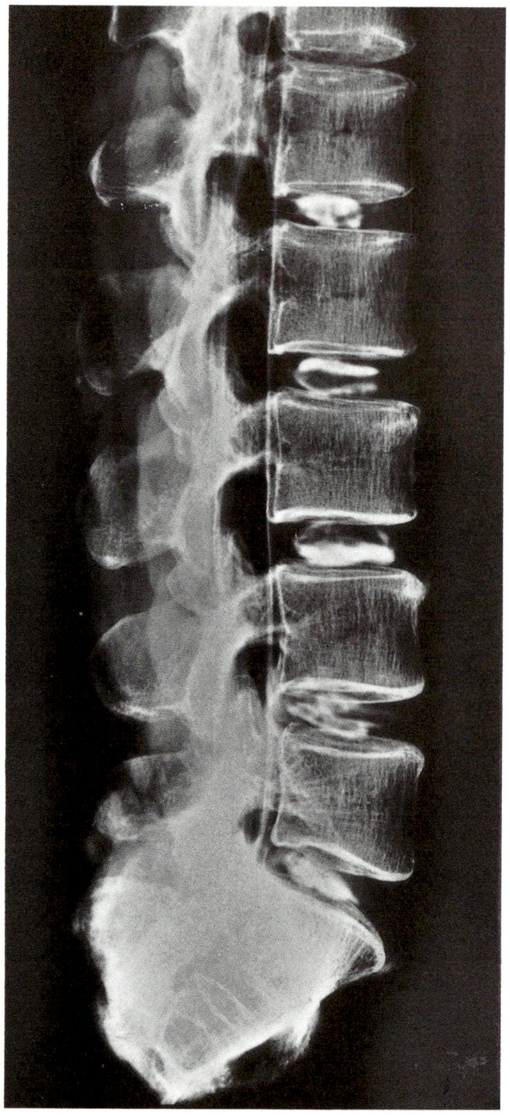

Figure 1.15 AP radiograph of the spine (*left*) shows normal discograms in the lower five disc spaces. A better view of the discograms may be obtained in the lateral projection (*right*), in which variations are seen at different levels in the normal discogram. Note also the meninges, here outlined by contrast material following evacuation of the Renografin used for the myelograms.

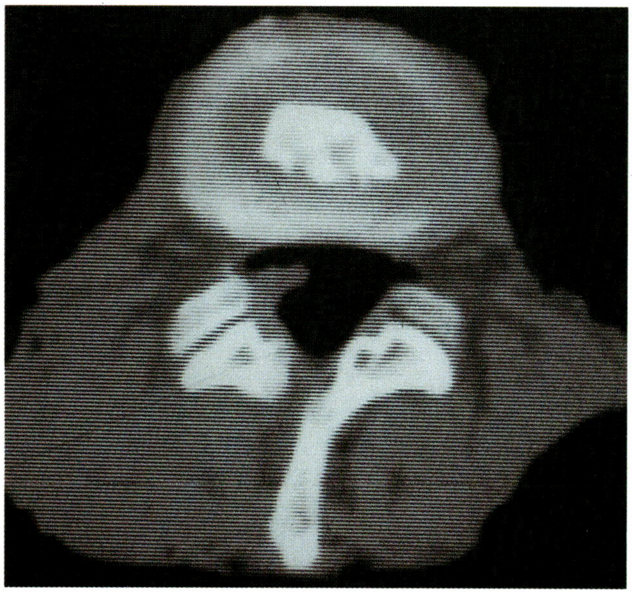

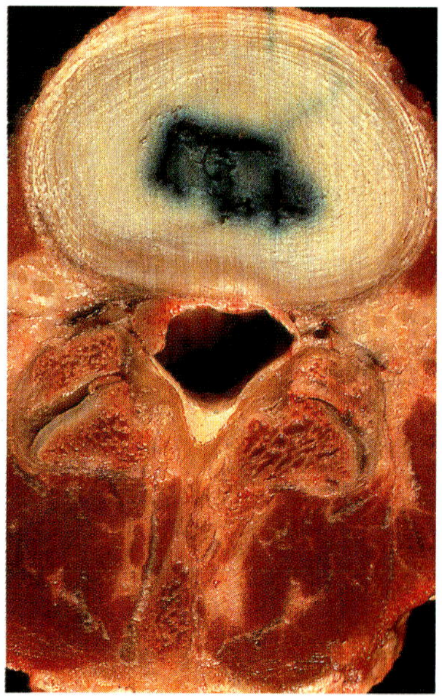

Figure 1.16 CT discogram of a normal disc (*left*) shows the contrast material confined to the region of the nucleus pulposus. Photograph of the same disc (*right*), which following the discogram was sliced to show how the area of tissue stained by methylene blue corresponds to the image produced by the Renografin.

2. In the case of a fresh specimen or one that has been stored in a frozen state, first defrost it under warm running water and dissect it free of soft tissue. Submerge the spine in sodium hypochlorite for one or two hours depending upon the size of the specimen. Inspect every 15 to 20 minutes to assess the state of maceration. Rinse the specimen under running water for 10 minutes, and immerse it in absolute alcohol overnight. Bathe it in hydrogen peroxide for two hours, then dry it in sunlight.

SUMMARY

Presented in Figure 1.19 is a flowchart summarizing the methods of examination discussed in this chapter, given in their proper sequence for a study of the spinal column.

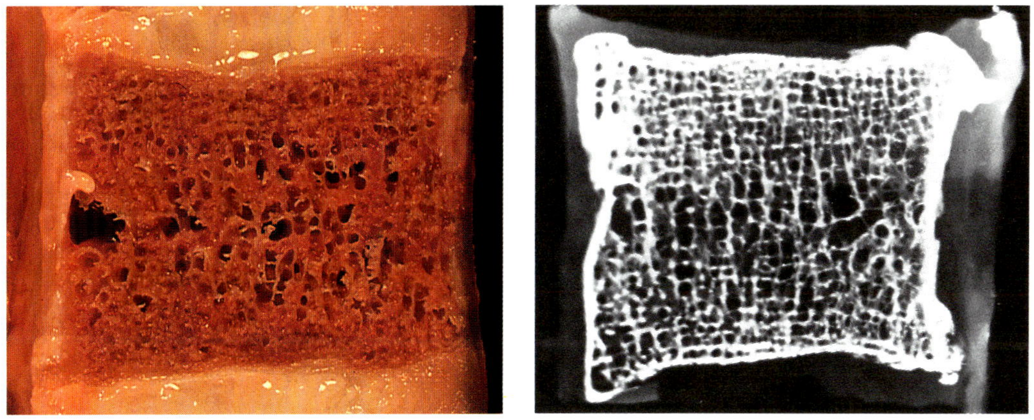

Figure 1.17 Photograph (*left*) of the sectioned surface of a vertebral body from which a 2-mm section was taken for radiographic study. The fine-grain radiograph obtained from this section (*right*) was taken with a low-voltage x-ray machine (Faxitron, Field Emission Corporation, McMinnville, Oregon 97128, USA) and industrial film (Kodalith Ortho film, Type 3). In this radiograph, note the detail of the cancellous bone distribution.

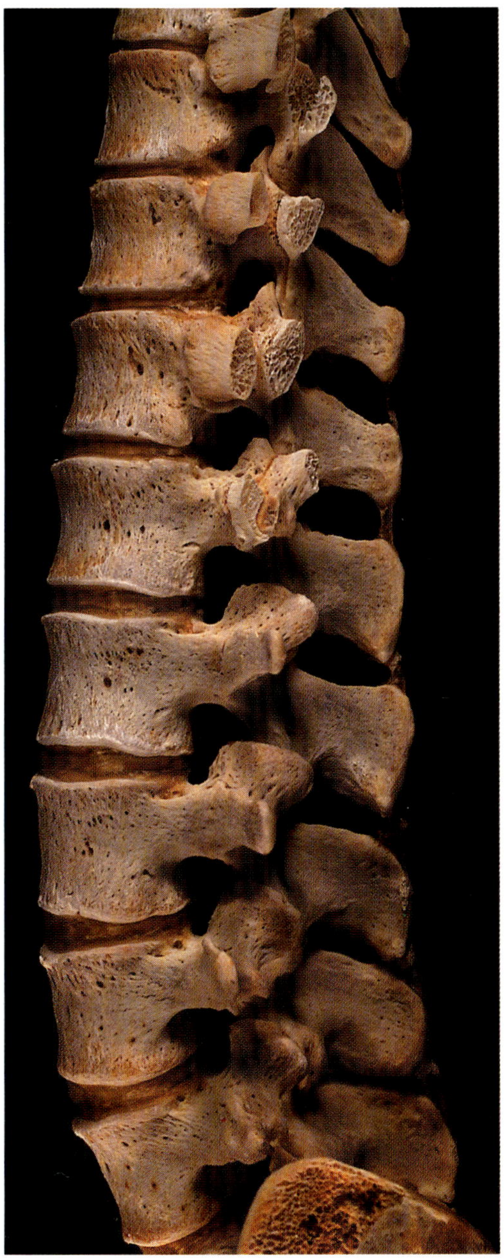

Figure 1.18 Photograph of the thoracolumbar spine with a portion of the sacrum. This specimen was macerated using one of the techniques described in the text.

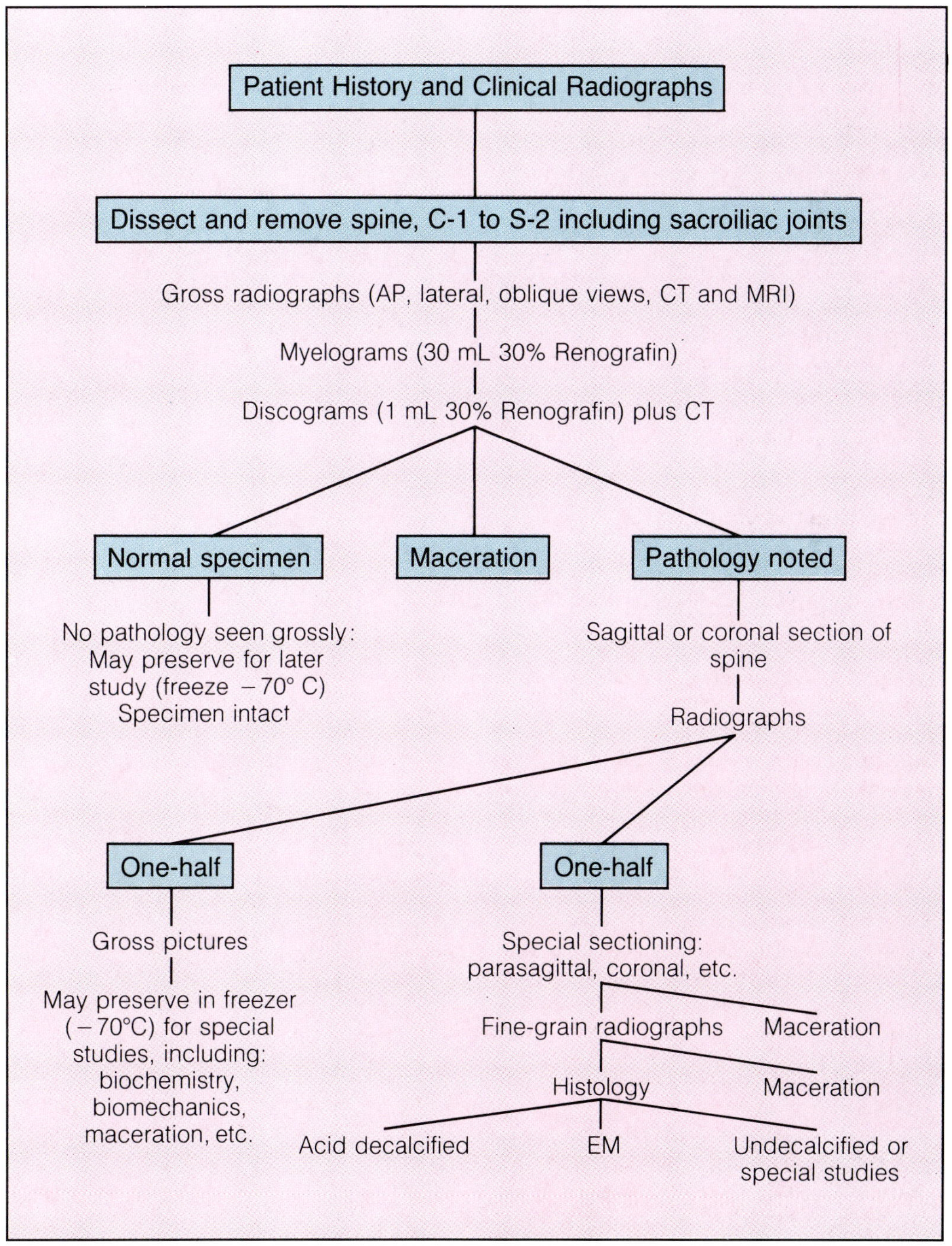

Figure 1.19 Flowchart of the investigative methodology used in our studies of spinal morphology and pathology.

2 CHAPTER

DESCRIPTIVE ANATOMY: GROSS AND MICROSCOPIC

THE SPINAL COLUMN AND THE VERTEBRAL CANAL

The spinal column is a system that provides for movement of the body, support of the viscera and ribs, and protection of the spinal cord. It is part of the axial skeleton (cranium, vertebral column, ribs, and sternum), which, from an evolutionary standpoint, constitutes the primary skeleton.

GENERAL FEATURES

The normal human spine is about 70 cm long in the male and 60 cm long in the female and it is composed of approximately 33 vertebrae: seven cervical, 12 thoracic, five lumbar, and five fused sacral elements; the vestigial coccyx normally contains four elements although the number may vary from three to five (Fig. 2.1). Joining the vertebrae and limiting their movement are the intervertebral discs, the diarthrodial joints between the vertebral arches, and numerous ligaments and paravertebral muscles.

When the spine is viewed from the side, each of its segments is seen to be curved. The thoracic and sacral curves, which are part of a primary structural curve, are dorsally convex, or *kyphotic,* whereas the cervical and lumbar curves, which are the secondary compensatory curves allowing for the upright position, are ventrally convex, or *lordotic* (Fig. 2.2). (Note that lumbar lordosis tends to be more pronounced in the female than in the male.)

In most individuals a slight lateral curve to the left is found in the cervical and lumbar regions of the spine with a compensatory curve to the right found in the lower thoracic region. These curves, not considered to be

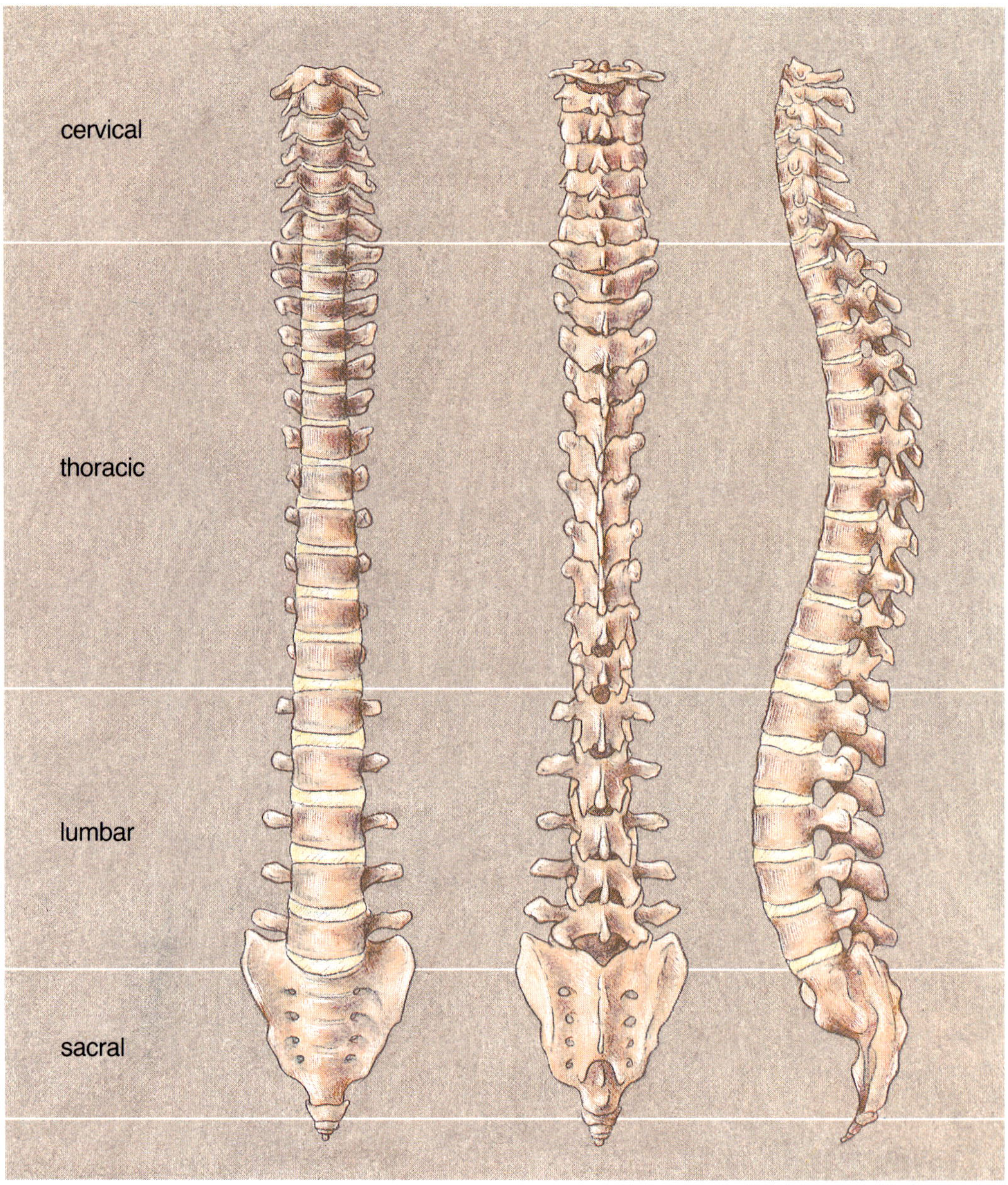

Figure 2.1 Schematic drawing of the normal human spine in anterior, posterior, and lateral views. Note the five main spinal segments and the natural curvatures.

clinically significant, differ from clinically significant scoliotic curves not only by their magnitude but also by their lack of a rotatory element.

The Vertebrae

The typical vertebra consists of two main components: the body, a cylindrical ventral mass of bone, and the arch, which is formed by paired pedicles united dorsally by a pair of flat laminae joined posteriorly to the spinous process (Fig. 2.3).

The vertebral bodies increase in width from the second cervical vertebra to the fifth lumbar vertebra but decrease rapidly from the first sacral vertebra to the tip of the coccyx. The shape and position of the dorsovertebral arches also change at each level of the spinal column, as will be discussed later in greater detail.

THE VERTEBRAL CANAL

The vertebral body and the dorsovertebral arch unite to enclose the vertebral foramen, and, when the vertebrae are articulated, the vertebral canal is formed by the foramina of successive vertebrae. The canal is large and triangular in cross section in the cervical and lumbar regions and small and circular in the thoracic region. In those regions where the canal is triangular, the increase in size occurs in the transverse diameter of the canal—a difference that is reflected in an AP view of the spine but not on the lateral projection. Along with these variations in diameter of

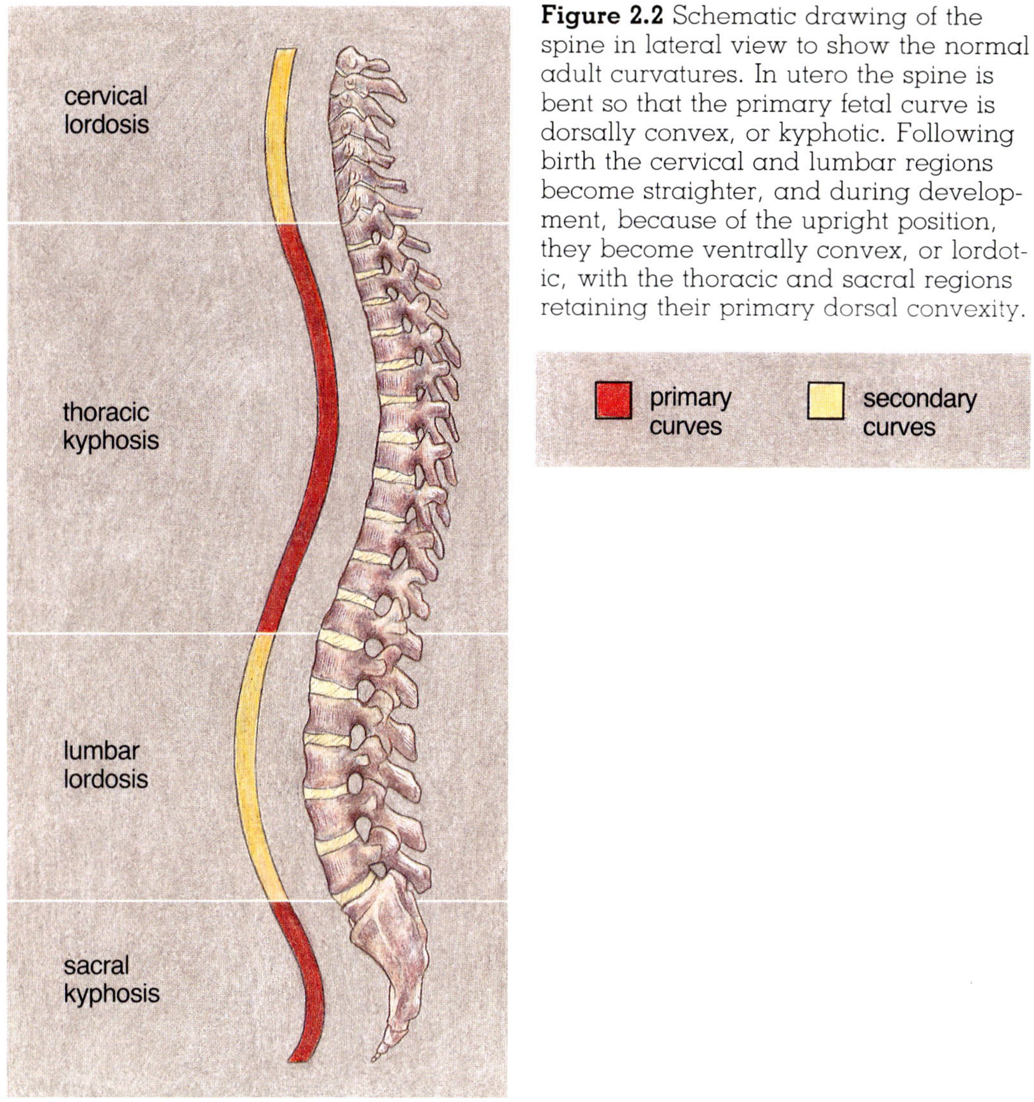

Figure 2.2 Schematic drawing of the spine in lateral view to show the normal adult curvatures. In utero the spine is bent so that the primary fetal curve is dorsally convex, or kyphotic. Following birth the cervical and lumbar regions become straighter, and during development, because of the upright position, they become ventrally convex, or lordotic, with the thoracic and sacral regions retaining their primary dorsal convexity.

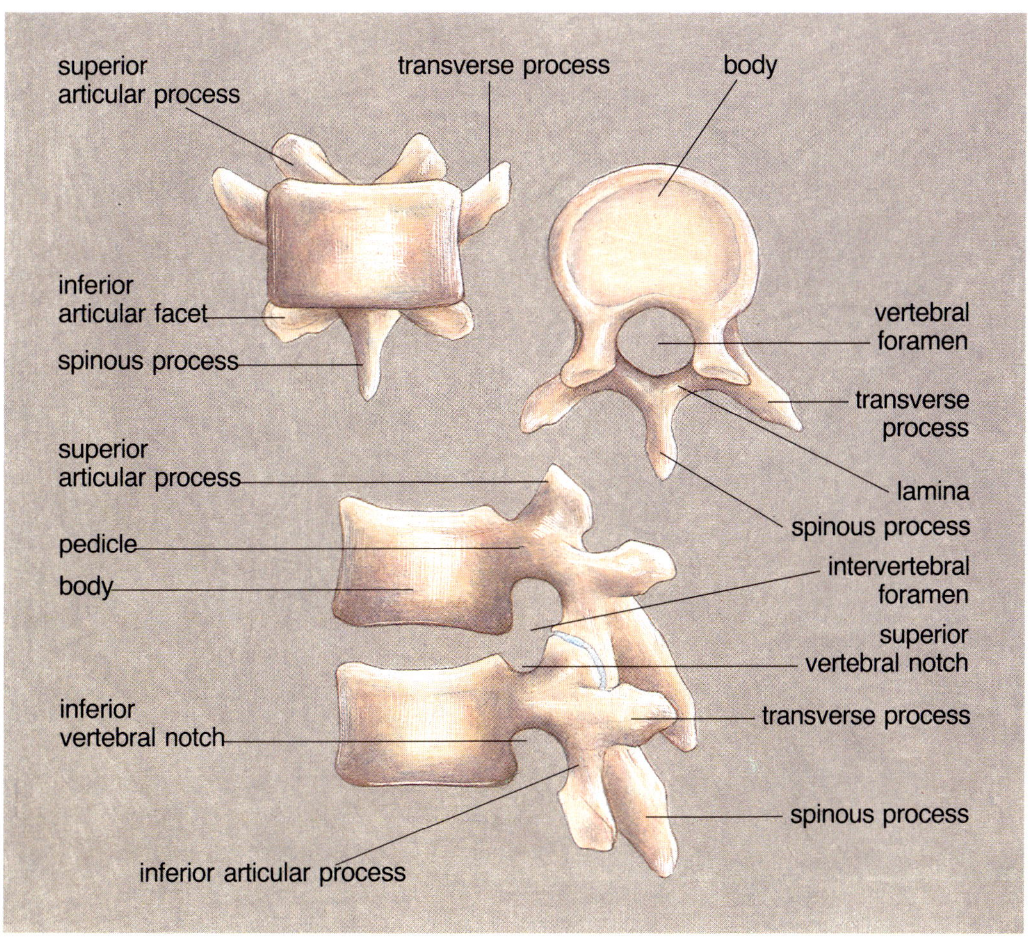

Figure 2.3 Schematic drawing of a stylized vertebra in anterior, superior, and lateral views to show the various vertebral components.

the canal occur variations in the diameter of the cord, associated with the large spinal nerves of the limbs (Figs. 2.4 and 2.5).

The Intervertebral Foramina

The intervertebral foramina are of considerable importance because of their protective function to the segmental nerve roots. They are located behind the vertebral bodies between the pedicles of adjacent vertebrae, and they are bordered posteriorly by the ligamenta flava and the facet joints. The foramina are oval and gradually increase in size from the smallest in the cervical and upper thoracic spine to the largest in the lumbar region.

Each of the intervertebral foramina is bounded superiorly by the inferior vertebral notch, which, because the pedicles of the vertebral arch project from the superoposterior aspect of the vertebral bodies, is much deeper than is the superior notch, which generally is very shallow.

In the cervical region the intervertebral foramina are inclined vertically at about 45 degrees to the sagittal plane (Fig. 2.6), so that radiologic demonstration depends upon use of the anterior oblique projection, as in Figure 1.9.

In the thoracic region the intervertebral foramina lie more behind the vertebral bodies than the intervertebral discs, in the sagittal plane (Fig. 2.7), and a lateral projection provides the best view as shown in Figure 1.8.

In the lumbar region however, the intervertebral foramina are located equally behind the intervertebral discs and the vertebral bodies, though still in the sagittal plane (Fig. 2.8). The presacral intervertebral foramen is always narrower than are the rest of the foramina of the lumbar spine.

As will become apparent in subsequent chapters, considerable tension and pressure on the nerve roots can occur with deformity of the spine, or with displacement of disc tissue or vertebral slippage.

The Vertebrae and Their Articulations

A typical vertebra consists of the vertebral body, composed mostly of cancellous bone with only a thin shell of cortical bone, and the dorsovertebral arch and its processes, composed of compact cortical bone that is relatively thick. As shown in Figure 2.3, three paired processes project from the vertebral arch: the superior articular processes, the inferior articular processes, and the transverse processes. Posteriorly there is a single spinous process.

The transverse and spinous processes serve as levers for the muscles and ligaments concerned with spinal rotation and bending. In the thoracic region the transverse processes also articulate with the ribs. The ar-

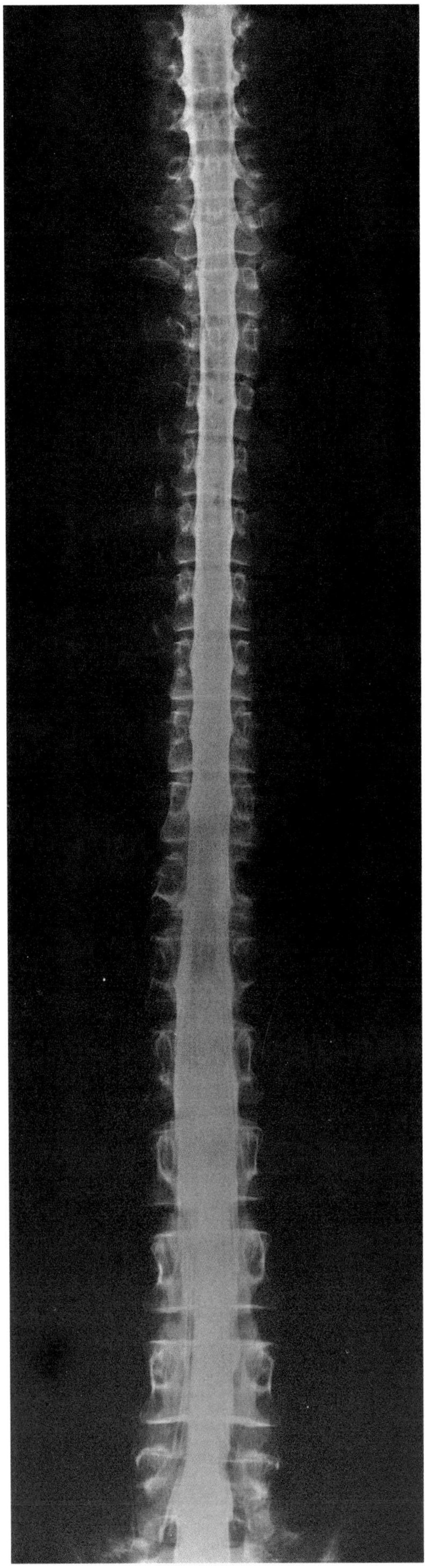

Figure 2.4 Specimen AP myelogram of the spine. Note variation in the transverse diameter of the spinal canal, which is widest in the cervical and lumbar regions due to the large spinal nerves of the limbs.

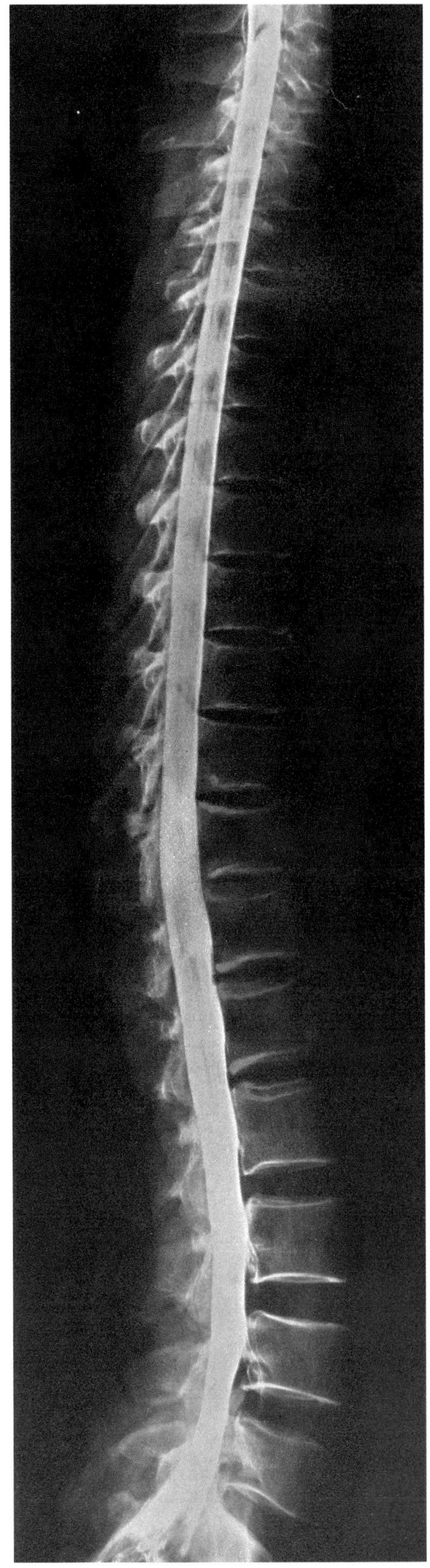

Figure 2.5 Specimen lateral myelogram of the spine. Note how the spinal canal appears narrower than in the previous AP projection and the diameter appears to be much more regular from top to bottom.

ticular processes provide for restricted lateral bending and rotation as well as for flexion and extension.

THE TRANSVERSE PROCESSES

Close to the junction of the pedicles with the laminae are the transverse processes. In the cervical spine the transverse processes are characterized by the transverse foramina, which carry the vertebral arteries (Fig. 2.9). The cervical transverse processes are slightly anterior to the articular processes and lateral to the pedicles and they provide a notch or sulcus for the spinal nerves. In the thoracic region the transverse processes are slightly

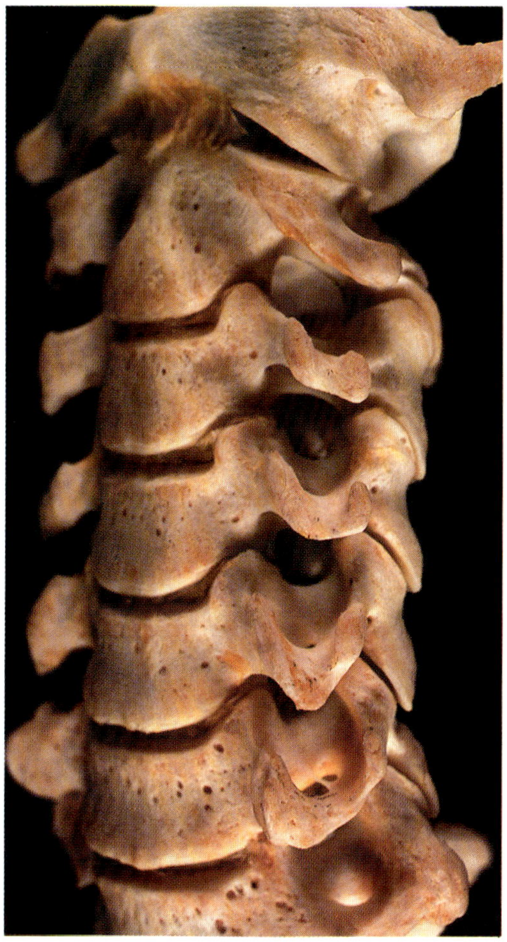

Figure 2.6 Photograph showing anterior oblique view of the cervical spine. Note the intervertebral foramina, which are seen to be inclined somewhat anteriorly and caudally.

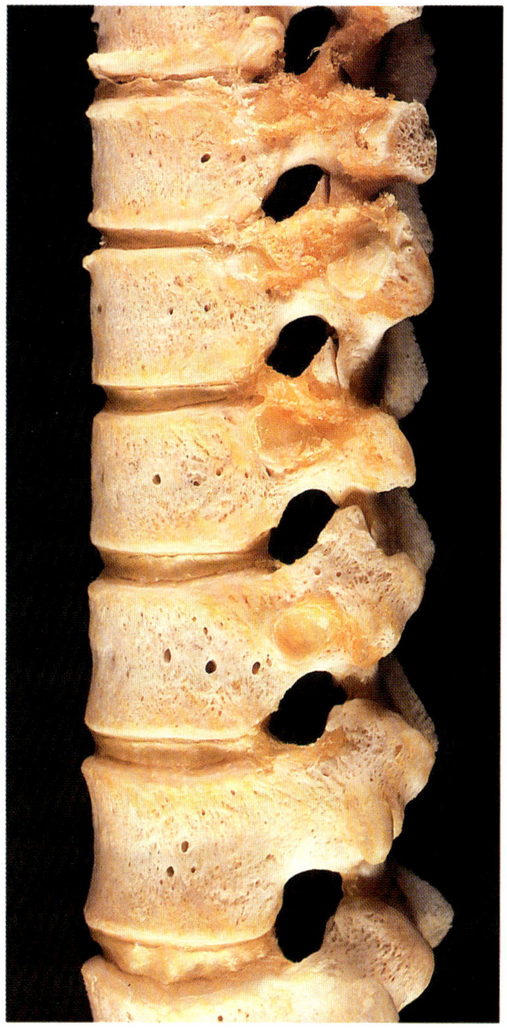

Figure 2.7 Photograph showing a lateral view of a thoracic spinal segment with the ribs removed. Note the disposition of the thoracic foramina as well as their location mostly behind the vertebral bodies.

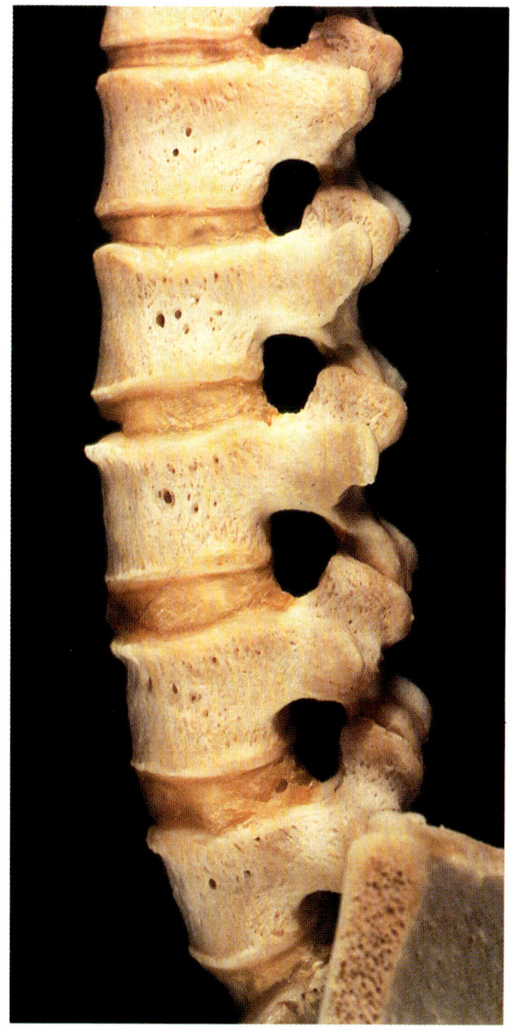

Figure 2.8 Photograph of a lumbar spine in lateral view. Note the disposition of the foramina, which, in contrast to those of the thoracic spine, are bordered anteriorly by both the vertebral bodies and the intervertebral discs.

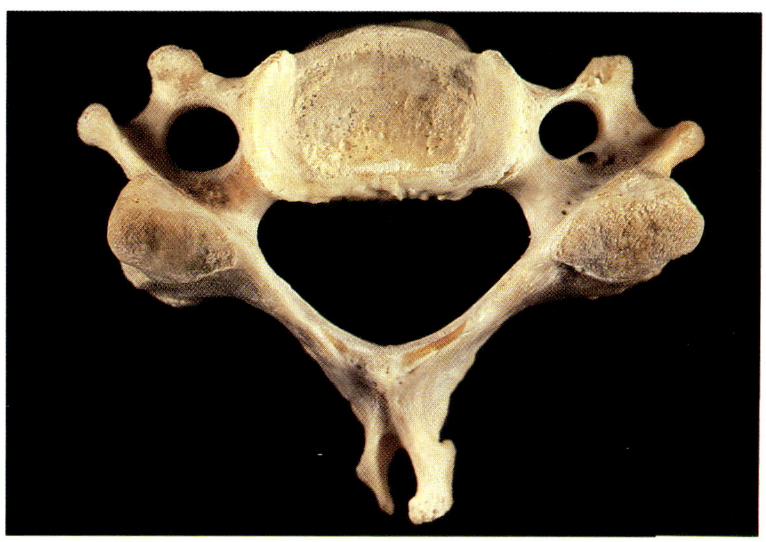

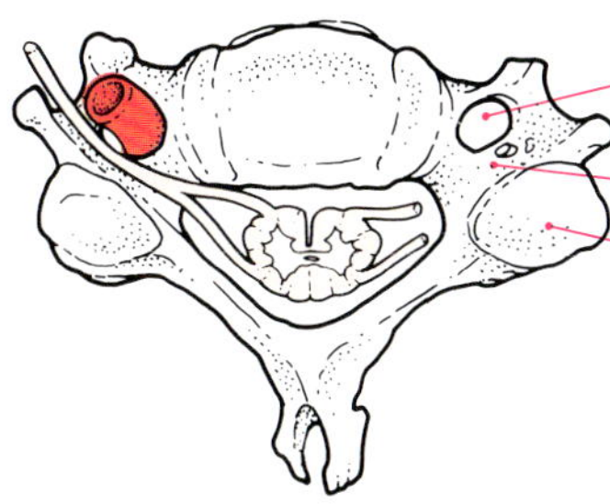

Figure 2.9 Photograph of a cervical vertebra. Note how the transverse processes are located lateral to the pedicles and anterior to the articular facets. The vertebral artery is carried through the transverse foramina, and on the superior surface of the transverse processes is a groove or sulcus for the spinal nerve, which runs posterior to the vertebral artery.

posterior to the articular processes, the pedicles, and the intervertebral foramina (Fig. 2.10), whereas, in the lumbar region, they are anterior to the articular processes although still posterior to the pedicles and the intervertebral foramina (Fig. 2.11).

THE ARTICULAR PROCESSES

The articular processes provide the joint facets for the paired diarthrodial joints between the vertebral arches. The orientation as well as the configuration of these facet joints (sometimes called the apophysial or zygapophysial joints) changes from the cervical to the lumbar regions of the spine so that in C-1 and C-2 the joints are nearly horizontal in the coronal plane (Fig. 2.12), whereas in the thoracic region they are increasingly posterior still in the coronal plane (Figs. 2.13 and 2.14) and in the upper lumbar region they are almost vertical in the sagittal plane (Fig. 2.15). Facet tropism, an asymmetry in the orientation of the facet joints (usually the lumbosacral facets), may result in abnormal and unequal stresses on the anular fibers of the intervertebral disc, thus leading to accelerated disc degeneration.

That portion of the vertebral arch which lies between the superior and inferior articular processes generally is known as the *pars interarticularis*. A defect in the pars, either congenital or acquired, may result in vertebral slippage.

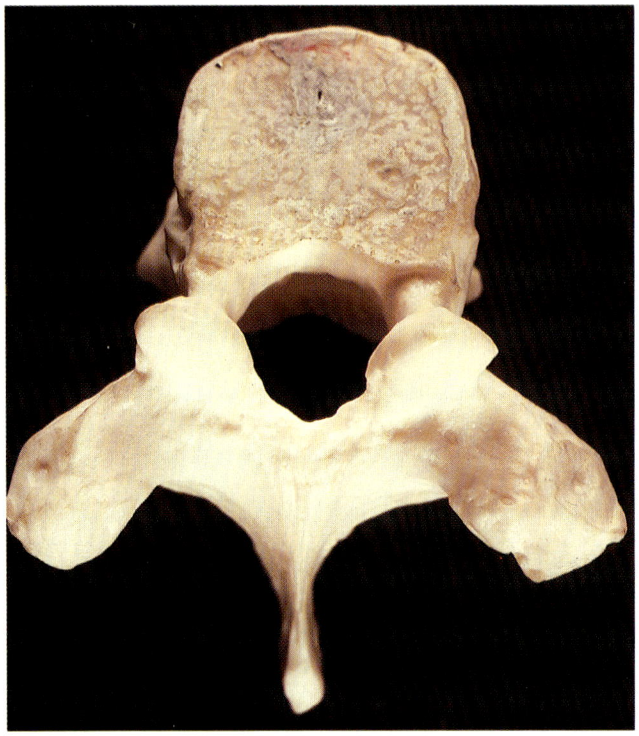

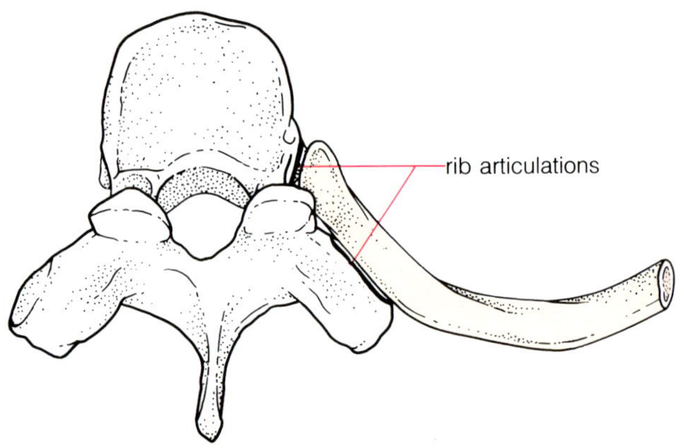

Figure 2.10 Photograph of a thoracic vertebra. Note how the thoracic transverse processes are located posterior to the articular facets. The facets for articulation with the ribs also are seen on the transverse process and on the vertebral body.

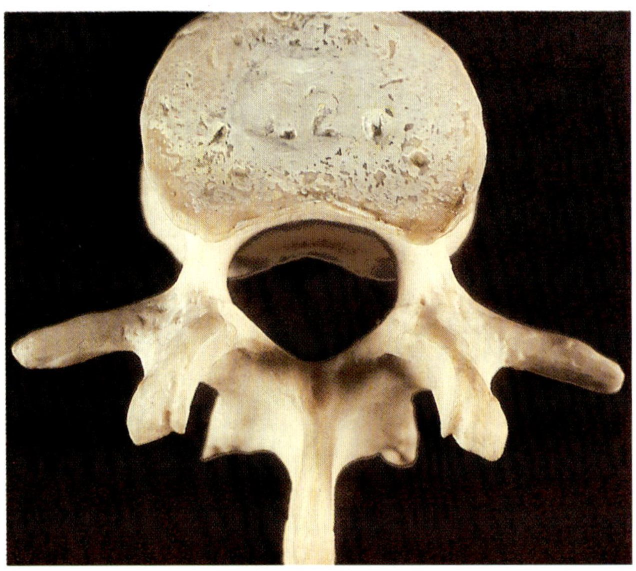

Figure 2.11 Photograph of a lumbar vertebra showing how in the lumbar spine the transverse processes are posterior to the pedicles and anterior to the superior articular facets.

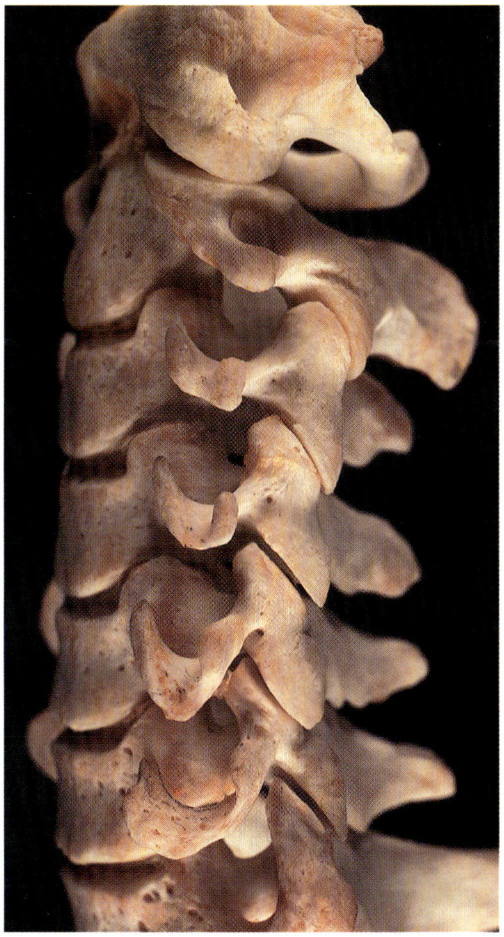

Figure 2.12 Photograph of the cervical spine in lateral view to show how the facet joints between C-1 and C-2 are anterior to the intervertebral and transverse foramina and are almost horizontal, whereas from C2-7 the facets lie behind the transverse and intervertebral foramina (facing their posterior wall) and are inclined posteriorly at about 45 degrees. Note also the prominent spinous process of C-7.

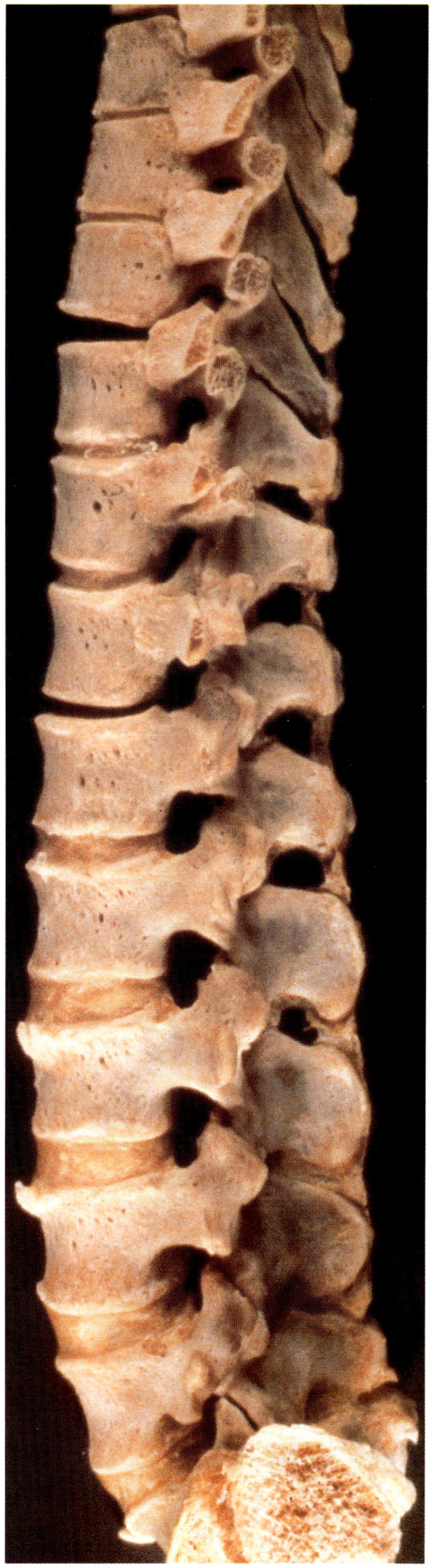

Figure 2.13 Photograph of the lower thoracic and lumbar spine in lateral view with the thoracic facet joints obscured by the costovertebral joints. Note that the spinous processes are almost horizontal in the lower thoracic and lumbar spine.

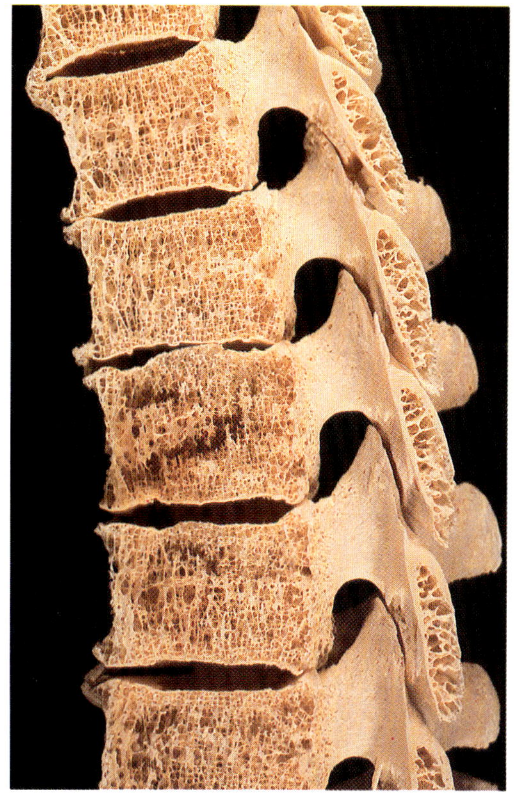

Figure 2.14 Photograph of a sagittal section of the thoracic spine with the facet joints well visualized. Note how they form part of the posterior wall of the intervertebral foramina and are almost vertical in the frontal plane.

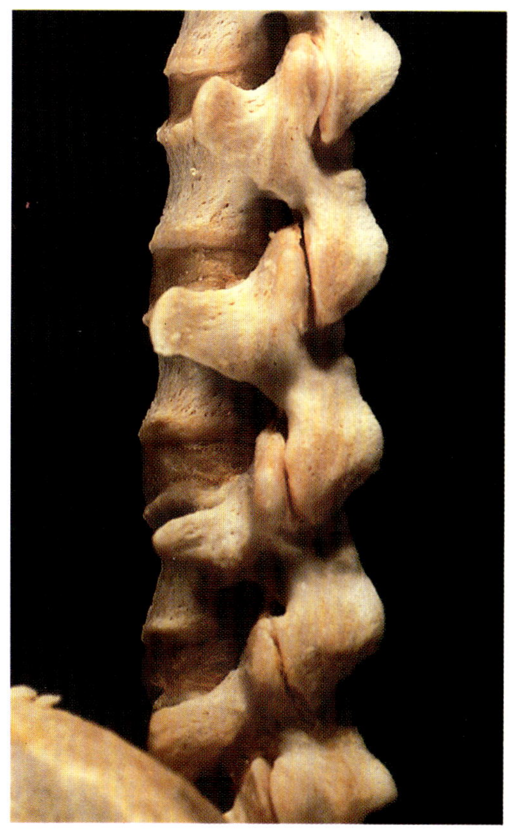

Figure 2.15 Photograph showing a posterior oblique view of the lumbar spine with the facet joints of the upper lumbar spine oriented vertically in the sagittal plane. Note the increasingly coronal orientation in the lower lumbar and lumbosacral spine.

THE SPINOUS PROCESSES

In the cervical spine the spinous processes of C3-6 generally are short, horizontal and bifid, with two knobs terminating each process. The processes of C-1, C-2 and C-7, however, are atypical. C-1 has no spinous process, and the process of C-2 is rather prominent and obviously bifid. The C-7 process is even longer and usually is referred to as the *vertebral prominence*. These processes can be seen in the lateral view of the cervical spine shown above in Figure 2.12. It is important to note here that normally, in a lateral radiograph of the cervical spine in a neutral position, if a line is drawn through each of the spinous processes of C-2 and C-7, the lines will be convergent, and if such lines are not convergent then an injury to one of the cervical vertebrae may be suspected.

In the upper thoracic region, the spinous processes generally face obliquely downward; in the midthoracic region they are long, overlapping, and almost vertically disposed; in the lower thoracic and lumbar region, they are nearly horizontal as seen in the lateral view of the lower thoracic spine shown previously in Figure 2.13.

THE CERVICAL VERTEBRAE

The first two cervical vertebrae are considerably modified for support and rotation of the head.

The first cervical vertebra—the atlas—differs from all other vertebrae in that it lacks a body. Essentially it is formed from two dense lateral masses joined by an anterior and a posterior arch. On the anterior arch there is a prominent tubercle for attachment of the anterior longitudinal ligament while on the posterior arch there is a tubercle that receives the insertion of the posterior rectus capitus muscle. On the inner medial aspect of each of the lateral masses is found a small rough tubercle to which is attached the transverse ligament that passes behind the odontoid process of C-2 and maintains it in place. Between the odontoid process and the transverse ligament, as well as between the odontoid process and the anterior arch of C-1, are found small synovial-lined joints. If these joints are involved in rheumatoid arthritis, then very significant clinical instability may ensue (see Section 2, Chapter 9).

Both the superior and inferior articular processes of C-1 are concave with the superior process facing upward and medially to receive the occipital condyles of the skull (Fig. 2.16). The inferior process faces downward and slightly internally to rotate on the inclined superior articular process of C-2 (Fig.

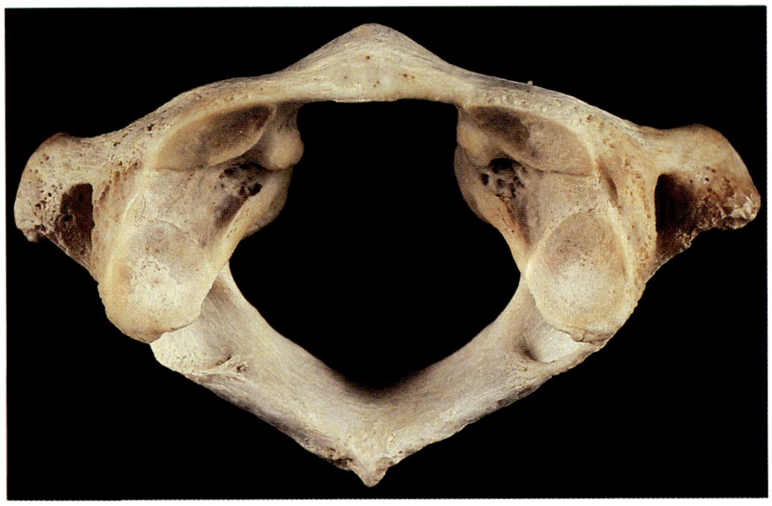

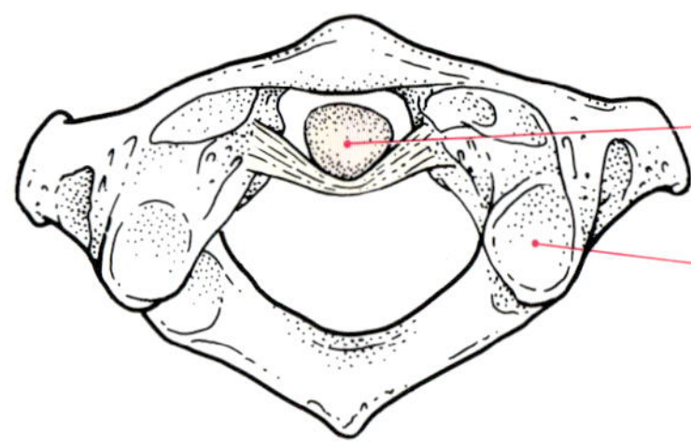

Figure 2.16 Photograph of C-1 viewed superiorly to show its three components: the anterior arch, the posterior arch, and the heavy lateral masses. Note the elongated articular facets for articulation with the skull, as well as the medial tubercles for attachment of the transverse ligament that holds the odontoid process of C-2 in place.

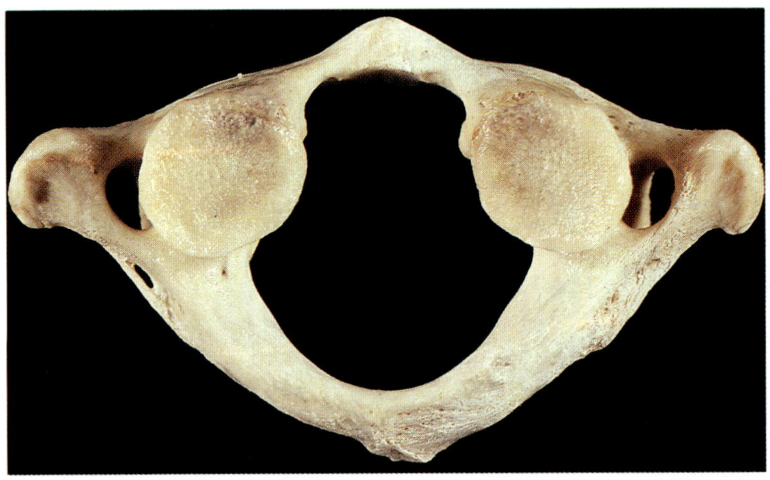

Figure 2.17 Photograph of C-1 shown inferiorly. Note the prominent articular facets for articulation with C-2.

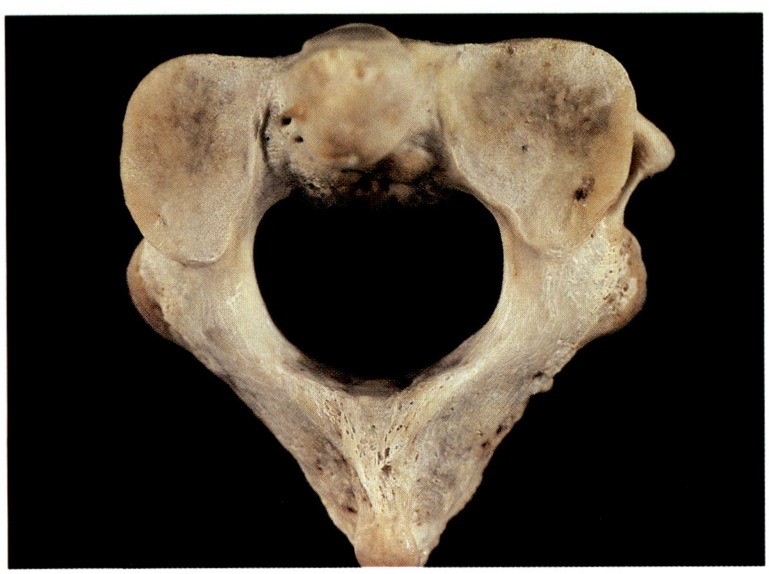

Figure 2.18 Photograph showing a superior view of C-2 with the prominent articular facets lying on either side of the odontoid and with the posterior spinous process.

2.17). The transverse foramina are placed more laterally here than in the rest of the cervical spine and consequently the cervical vertebral artery also is placed more laterally at this level.

The second cervical vertebra—the axis—forms the pivot on which the atlas, and hence the head, rotates. It is distinguished by the odontoid process (the dens), which extends vertically upward from the body (Figs. 2.18 through 2.20). The odontoid process is about 1.5 cm long, with a small oval articular facet in front, which articulates with the back of the anterior arch of the atlas. The posterior surface of the odontoid process is grooved by the transverse ligament, which passes behind it and holds it in place. Both the anterior and posterior articulations of the odontoid process are synovial-lined joints.

The apex of the dens is pointed and its apical ligament is attached to the anterior margin of the foramen magnum. On the upper lateral aspects of the odontoid process are the paired alar ligaments, which attach to the base of the skull to limit lateral rotation of the head.

The bodies of the lower five cervical vertebrae are distinguished by the uncinate or lunate processes—bony ridges that extend superiorly from each side of the vertebral body, giving its superior surface a saddle

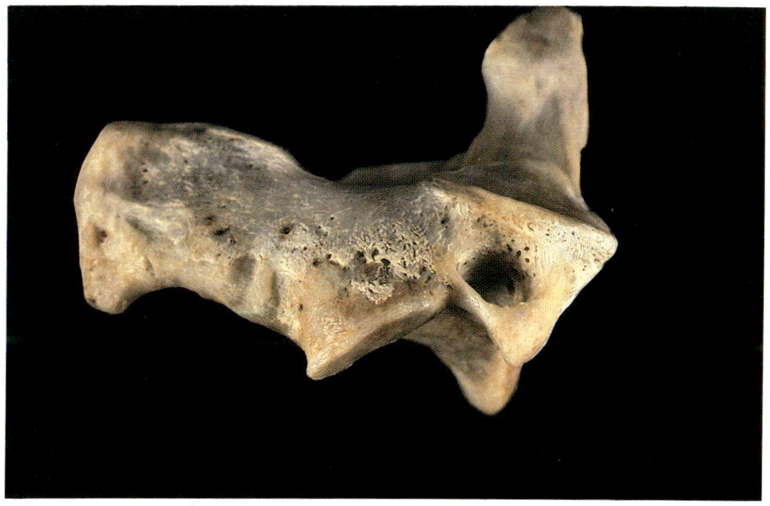

Figure 2.19 Photograph of C-2 in lateral view to show the odontoid process. Note how the facet for C-1 is horizontal while that for C-3 is inclined anteriorly. Also seen is a groove on the posterior surface of the odontoid, resulting from the impression of the transverse ligament.

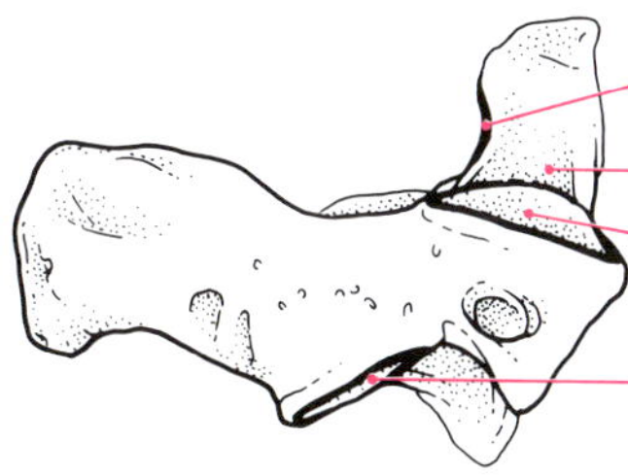

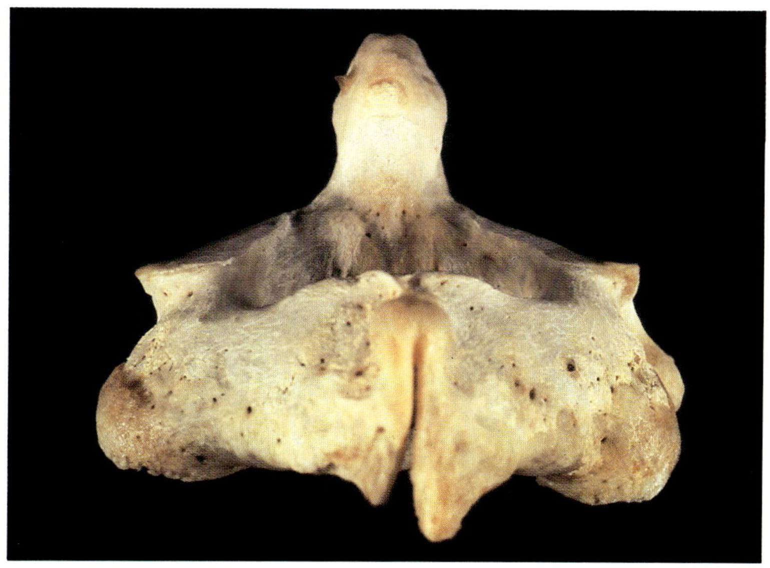

Figure 2.20 Photograph of C-2 in posterior view to show the smooth groove on the back of the odontoid, where the transverse ligament crosses it. Also seen are the flat superior articular facets, somewhat laterally inclined, and the bifid spinous process, seen posteriorly.

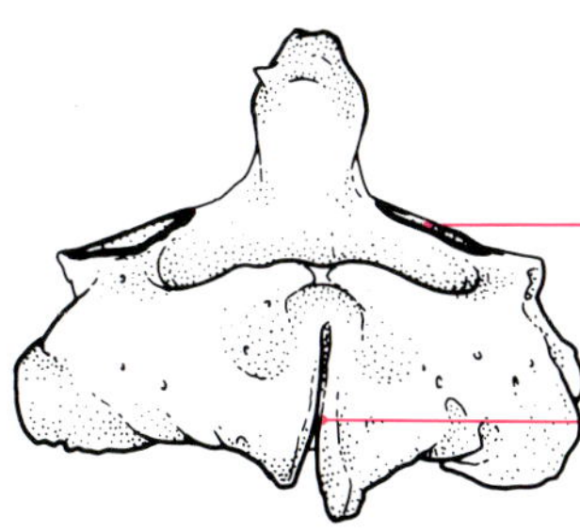

shape that decreases gradually in the caudal direction (Fig. 2.21). Because of these ridges, an additional articulation—called the lateral uncovertebral articulation—forms between the lateral edges of the vertebrae. Collectively these articulations are known as the *joints of Luschka* (Fig. 2.22). Note that they are not synovial joints.

THE THORACIC AND LUMBAR VERTEBRAE

The typical thoracic vertebral body is heart-shaped in cross section and on its lateral surface has both superior and inferior articular facets for articulation with the ribs (Figs. 2.10 and 2.23). The last two thoracic vertebrae, however, show transitional lumbar features, with diminution of the transverse processes and an increasingly horizontal orientation of the spinous processes. Note that T-11, T-12, and in some cases T-10 lack inferior articular facets for rib articulations (see Fig. 2.13 above).

The lumbar vertebrae are characterized by their large vertebral bodies and by the mamillary bodies—dorsal projections of the superior articular facets thought to represent rudimentary ribs. The vertical sagittal disposition of the facet joints restricts rotation of the lumbar spine while allowing flexion and extension (Figs. 2.11 and 2.24).

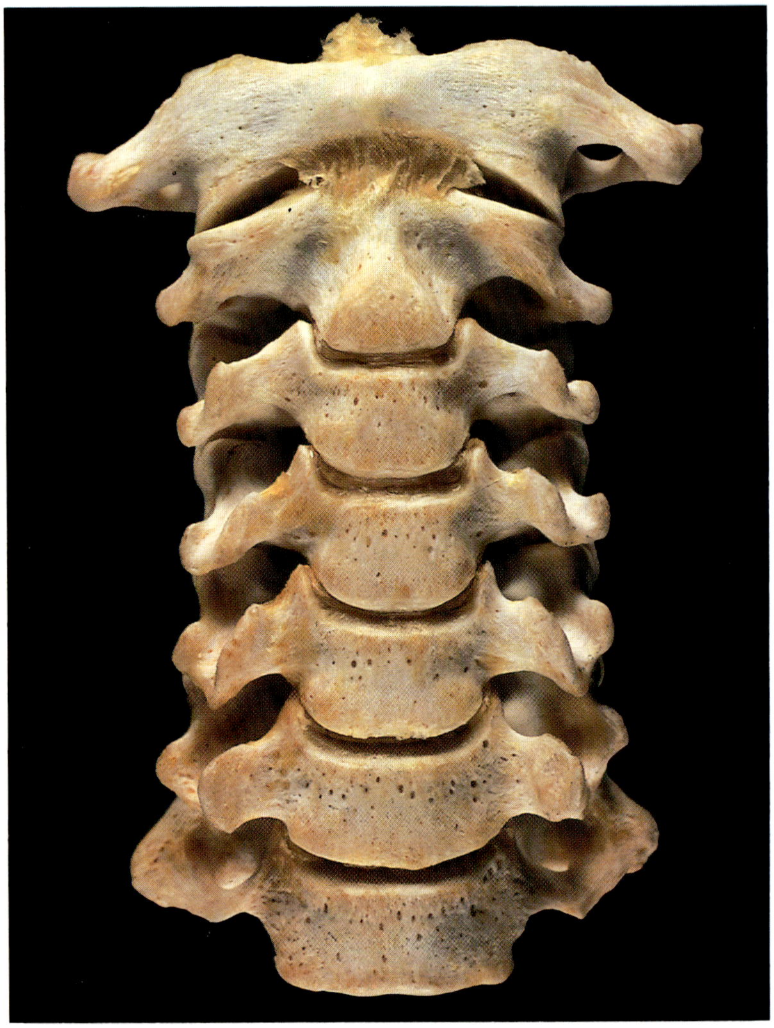

Figure 2.21 Photograph of the cervical spine in AP view to show the superior lateral bony ridges (the uncinate processes) that give a saddle-shaped profile to the intervertebral disc spaces.

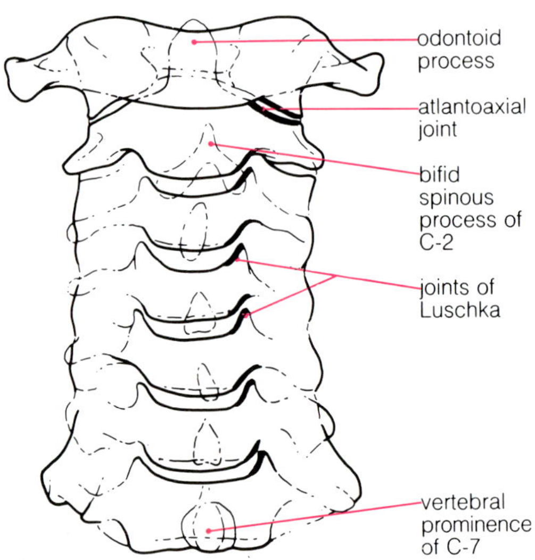

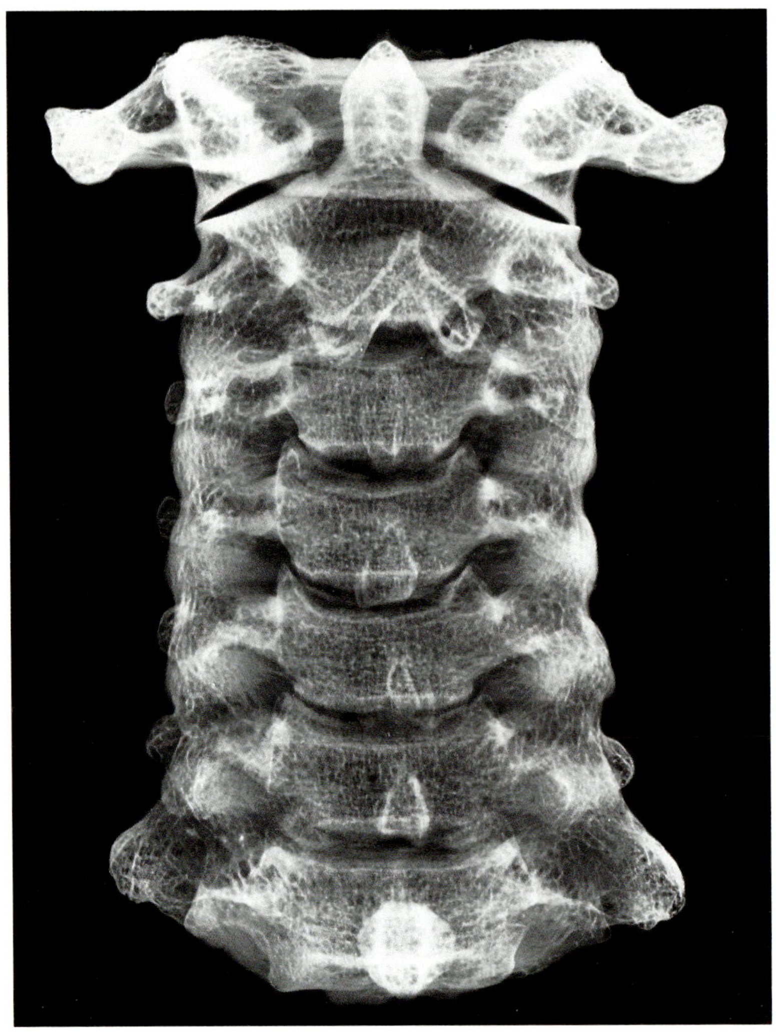

Figure 2.22 PA radiograph of the specimen shown in Figure 2.21. Note the lateral uncovertebral articulations (the joints of Luschka), the large atlantoaxial joints and the bifid spinous process of C-2, and the vertebral prominence of C-7.

THE SACRUM AND THE COCCYX

The sacrum is triangular and is formed by the fusion of the five sacral vertebrae. It articulates with the fifth lumbar vertebra superiorly, with the pelvis through the sacroiliac joints, and with the coccyx inferiorly. The anterior pelvic surface of the sacrum is concave and has four foramina on each side for transmission of the ventral rami of the sacral nerves (Fig. 2.25). The posterior sacral surface also has four paired foramina for transmission of the dorsal rami of the sacral nerves (Fig. 2.26). The terminal posterior midline opening into the sacral canal is called the sacral hiatus and it results from failure of the dorsal laminae of the fifth sacral vertebra to

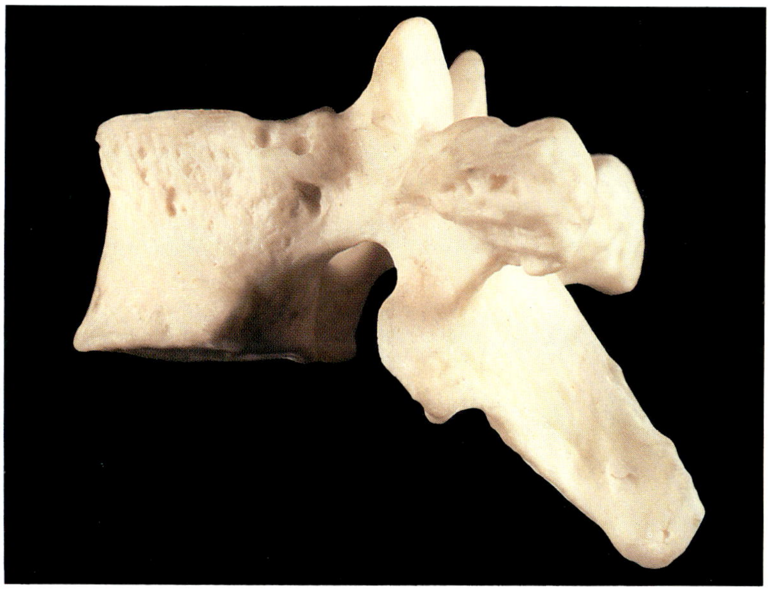

Figure 2.23 Photograph showing lateral oblique view of a thoracic vertebra. Note the deep inferior vertebral notch and the long spinous process typical of thoracic vertebrae.

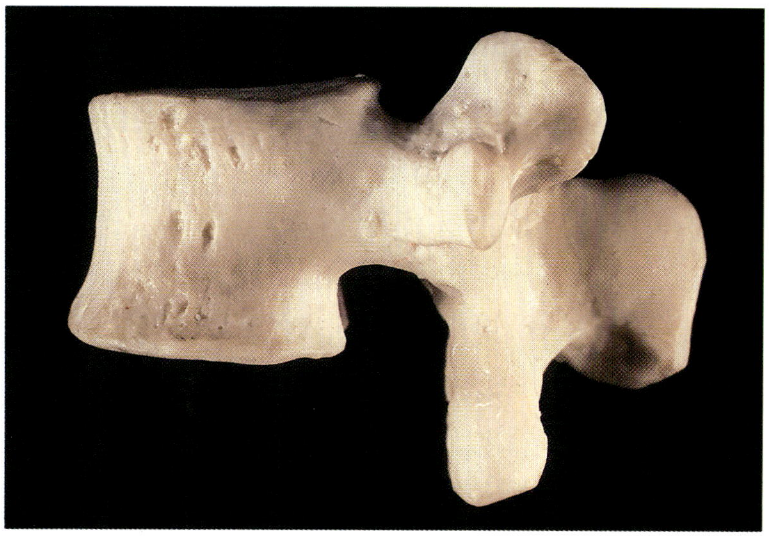

Figure 2.24 Photograph showing lateral view of a lumbar vertebra. Note that, in comparison to the thoracic vertebra shown in Figure 2.23, the superior vertebral notch is deeper indicating that the intervertebral foramina now lie more posterior to the intervertebral disc.

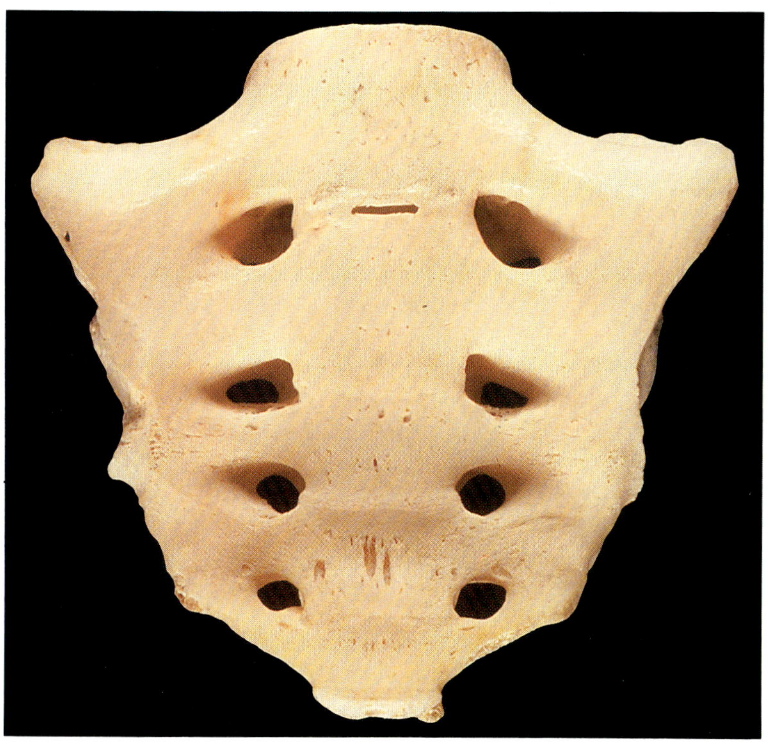

Figure 2.25 Photograph showing an anterior view of the sacrum. Note the four pelvic foramina on each side, which transmit the ventral branches of the sacral nerves.

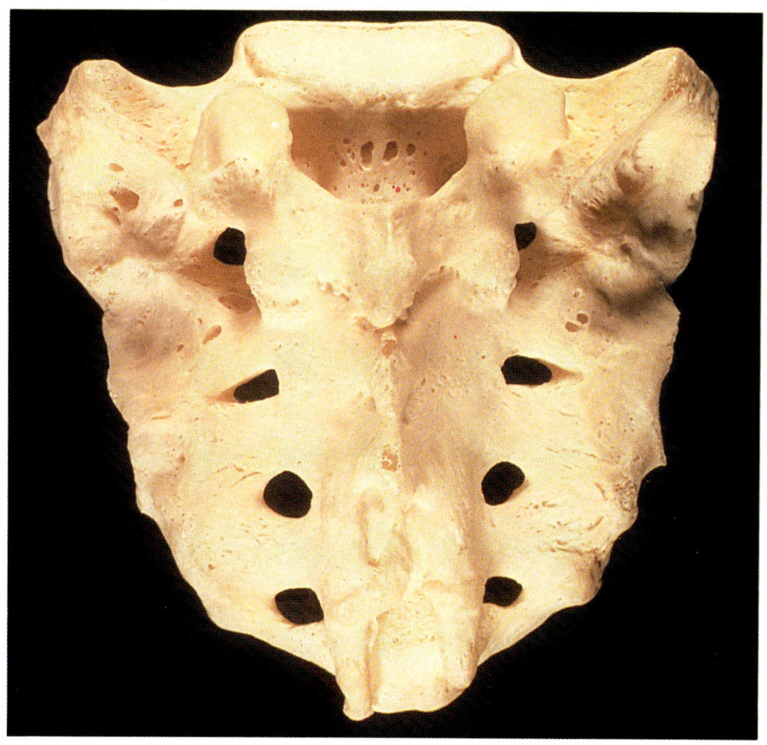

Figure 2.26 Photograph showing a posterior view of the sacrum. At the lower end of the specimen, note the midline sacral hiatus caused by failure of the dorsal laminae of S-5 to fuse. Note also the dorsal sacral foramina through which pass the dorsal branches of the sacral nerves.

fuse. In some cases sacralization of the fifth lumbar vertebra will occur, in which L-5 is fused (usually incompletely) to the sacrum (Fig. 2.27). In lumbarization of the first sacral vertebra, occurring less frequently, S-1 fails to fuse to the remaining sacrum.

The coccyx is composed of from three to five vertebral rudiments including a body and transverse processes but no components of the arch. Although the coccyx does not contribute any supportive function to the spine, it serves as a point of origin posteriorly for the gluteus maximus, and anteriorly for the muscles of the pelvic diaphragm.

The Intervertebral Disc

The intervertebral disc is a fibrocartilaginous complex that forms the articulation between the vertebral bodies. It contributes to the mobility and stability of the spine as well as to the transmission of load through it.

Radiographically in the newborn, the disc-space height in the lumbar region approximately is equal to the height of the ossification centers of the lumbar vertebral bodies (Fig. 2.28), whereas in a child the height of the disc space is approximately 40% the height of the vertebral body (Fig. 2.29) and in a healthy young adult it is approximately 25% that of the vertebral body (Fig. 2.30). This diminution in height results in part from the progressive ossification of the vertebral bodies but it also may reflect the decreasing hydration of the disc tissue.

In general it should be noted that disc height is not the same in all segments of the spine with the cervical and thoracic discs being narrower than those of the lumbar region. Disc height varies also from front to back, relative to the curvature of the spine.

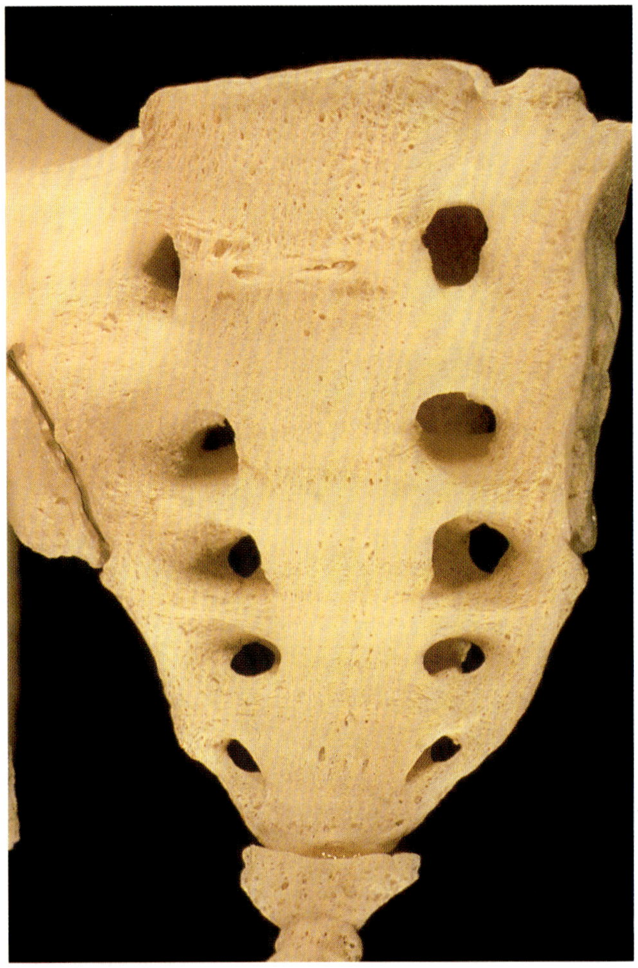

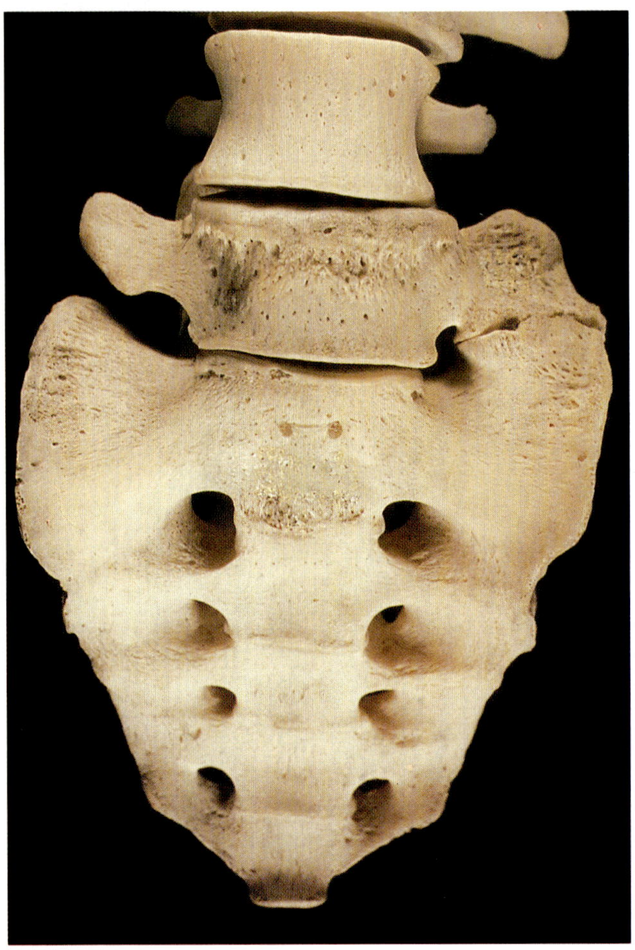

Figure 2.27 Photograph (*top*) showing bilateral sacralization of L-5. In this example the fifth lumbar vertebra is fused with the sacrum completely and on both sides. Photograph (*bottom*) showing unilateral incomplete fusion of L-5 to the sacrum.

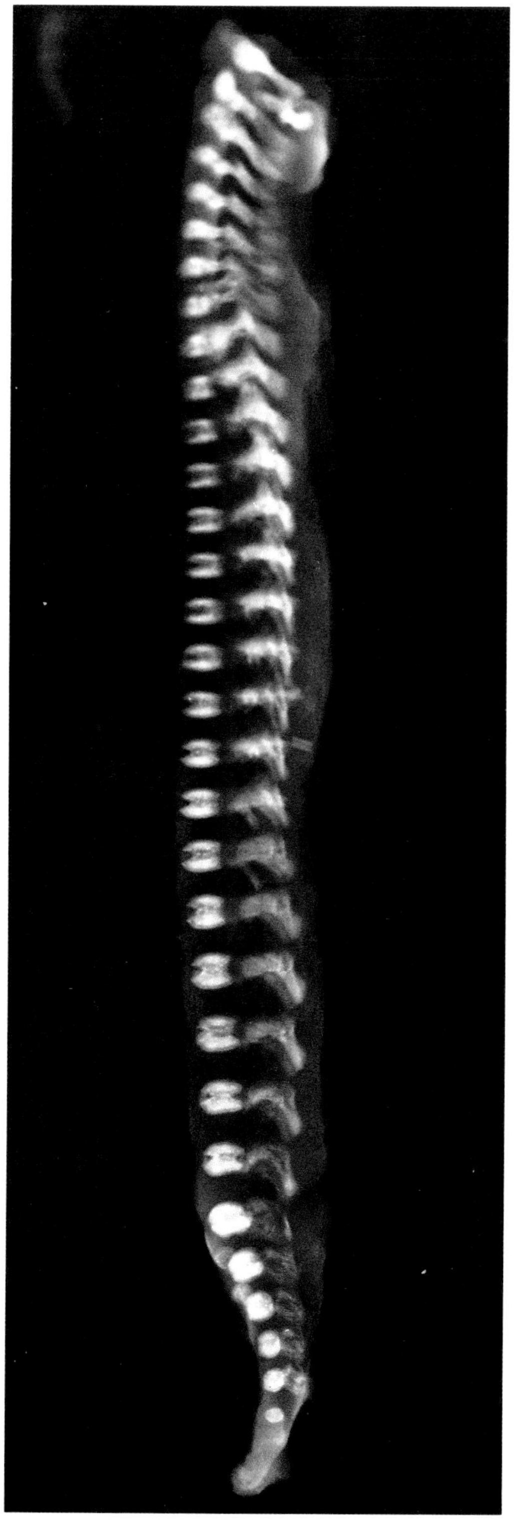

Figure 2.28 Specimen radiograph of the spine from a newborn. Note that the disc space (especially in the lumbar spine) is approximately equal to the height of the vertebral body. Note also the relative lack of curvature of the spine.

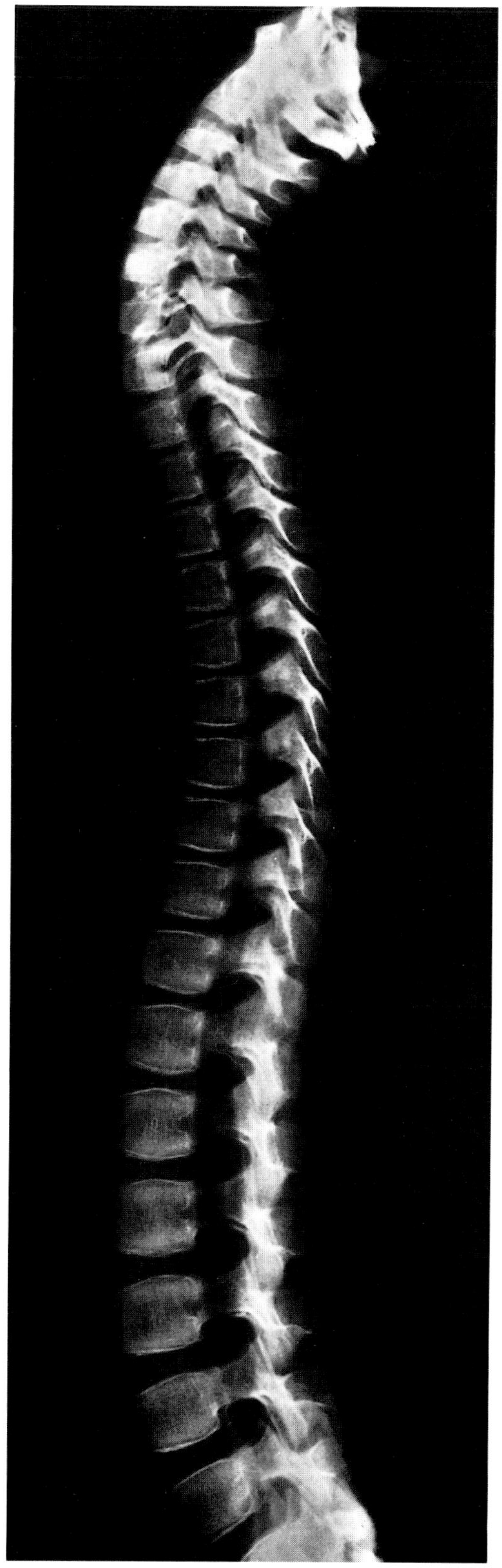

Figure 2.29 Specimen radiograph from a 4-year-old child shows the disc space in the lumbar spine to be approximately 40% the height of the vertebral body. Note the development of the spinal "double S-curve" as compared to the spine shown in Figure 2.28.

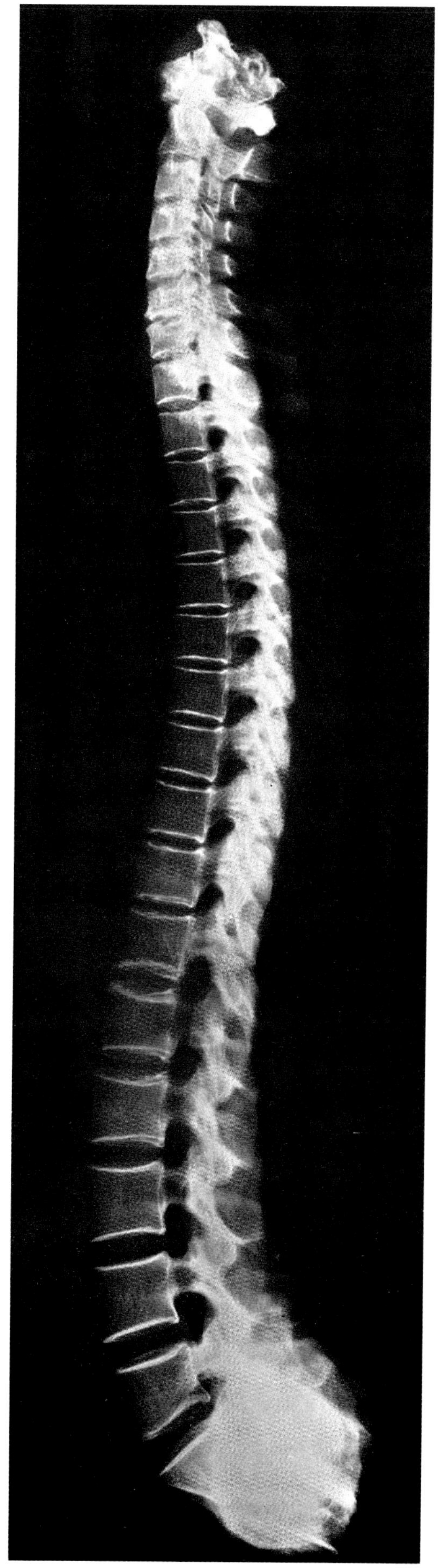

Figure 2.30 Specimen radiograph from a 25-year-old. The disc space is seen to be approximately 25% the height of the vertebral body. Note that the disc space is biconvex, in contrast to the biconcavity of the space shown in Figure 2.29.

THE ANULUS FIBROSUS

The intervertebral disc can be divided into two components, as seen in Figure 2.31:

1. The outermost fibrous ring, or anulus fibrosus
2. The innermost gelatinous core, or nucleus pulposus

The anulus, when viewed from above, is seen to contain fibrous tissue layers that are arranged in concentric circles. Each layer extends obliquely from vertebral body to vertebral body, with the fibers of one layer running in a direction opposite to that of the adjacent layer. These alternating layers provide for motion that is universal in direction but restricted in degree (Figs. 2.32 and 2.33). The fibers of the anulus are attached by Sharpey's fibers to the bony end plates of the adjacent vertebral bodies (Fig. 2.34). The fibrous lamellae are stronger and more numerous in the anterior and lateral aspects of the disc than in the posterior aspect where they are sparser and thinner and thus the anterior anulus is almost twice the thickness of the posterior anulus.

Although the disc is an avascular structure, some blood vessels are seen to extend into the cartilage of the developing vertebral body, adjacent to the disc proper, although these vessels usually are obliterated by the age of 4 (Fig. 2.35). Since there are no blood vessels present in adult disc tissue (Fig. 2.36), nutrients must diffuse from capillary beds at the disc margins. The restricted flow of nutrients to the nucleus and inner anulus may contribute to or even underlie disc degeneration in the adult.

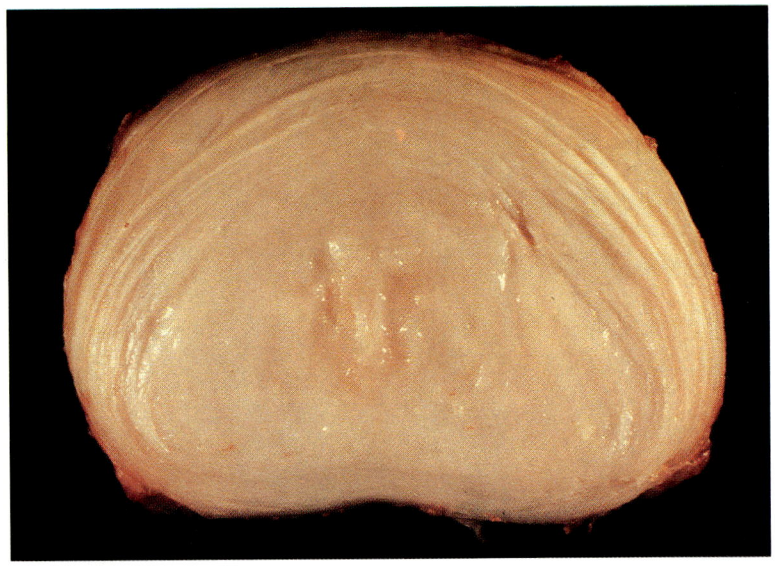

Figure 2.31 Photograph of an intervertebral disc seen from above. Note the layers of circumferential fibers that make up the anulus fibrosus in comparison to the bulging central mass of the nucleus pulposus.

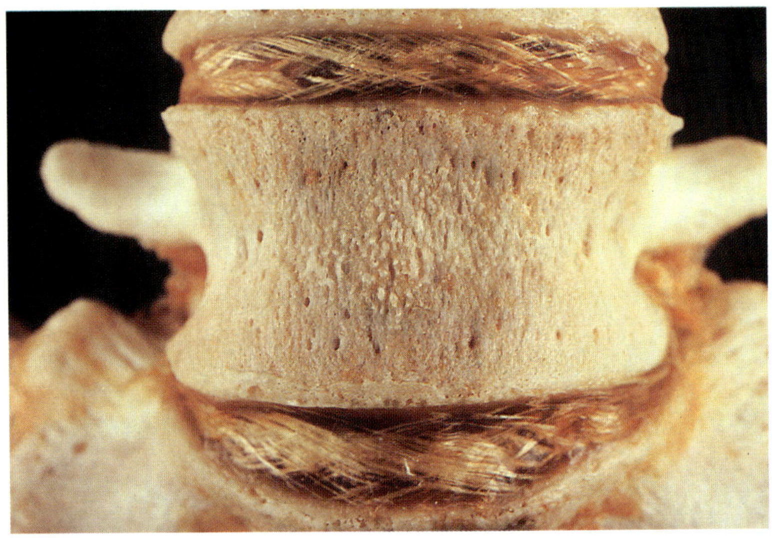

Figure 2.32 Photograph showing frontal view of L-5 with the adjacent intervertebral discs. Note the oblique disposition of the collagen fibers of the anulus fibrosus in this macerated specimen.

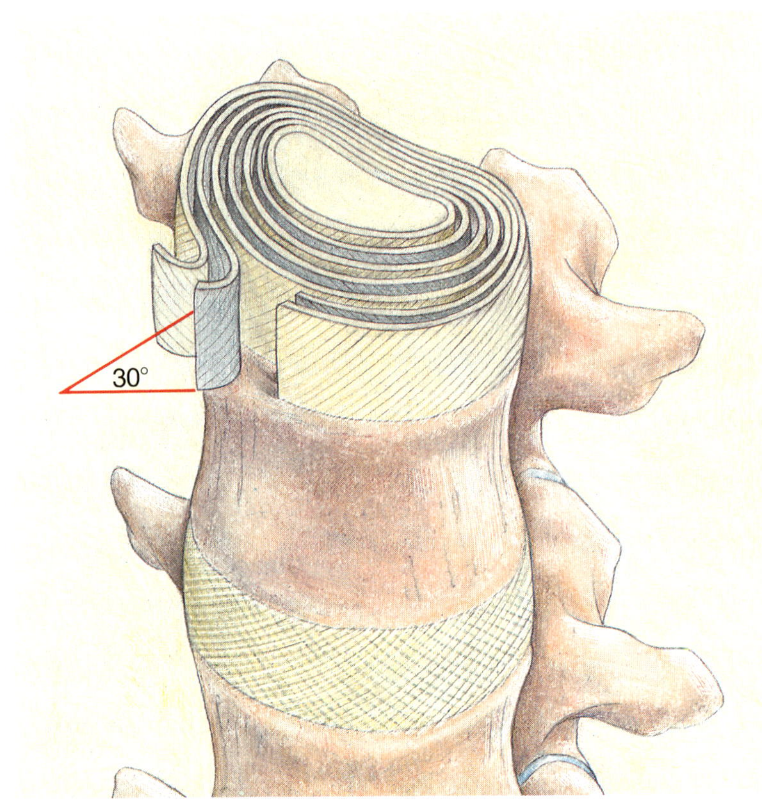

Figure 2.33 Schematic drawing of the intervertebral disc to demonstrate the layered arrangement of collagen fibers in the anulus. The fibers of each layer run at an approximately 30-degree angle to the surface of the vertebral body and in a direction opposite that of the adjacent layer.

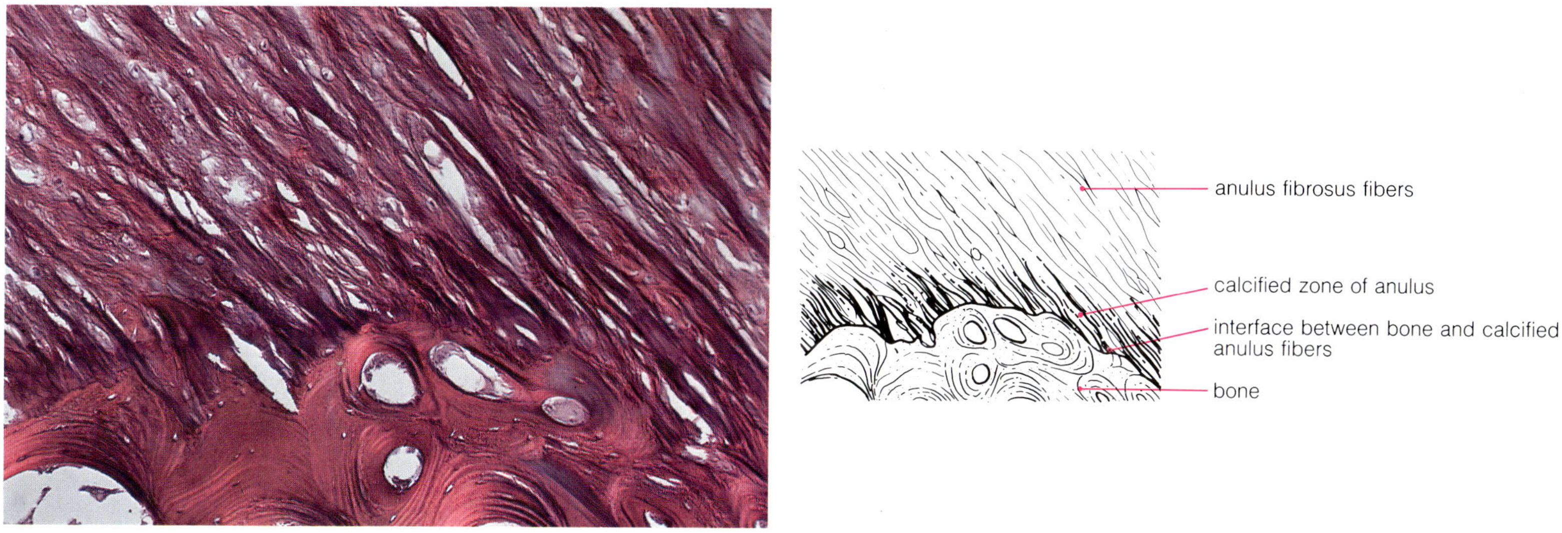

Figure 2.34 Photomicrograph to demonstrate the insertion of the fibers of the anulus fibrosus into the bone of the margins of the articular surface of the vertebral body. Where the collagen fibers of the anulus enter the bone, *Sharpey's* fibers, they are calcified. (Hematoxylin and eosin stain, partially polarized light, × 4 objective, approximately 100 magnifications)

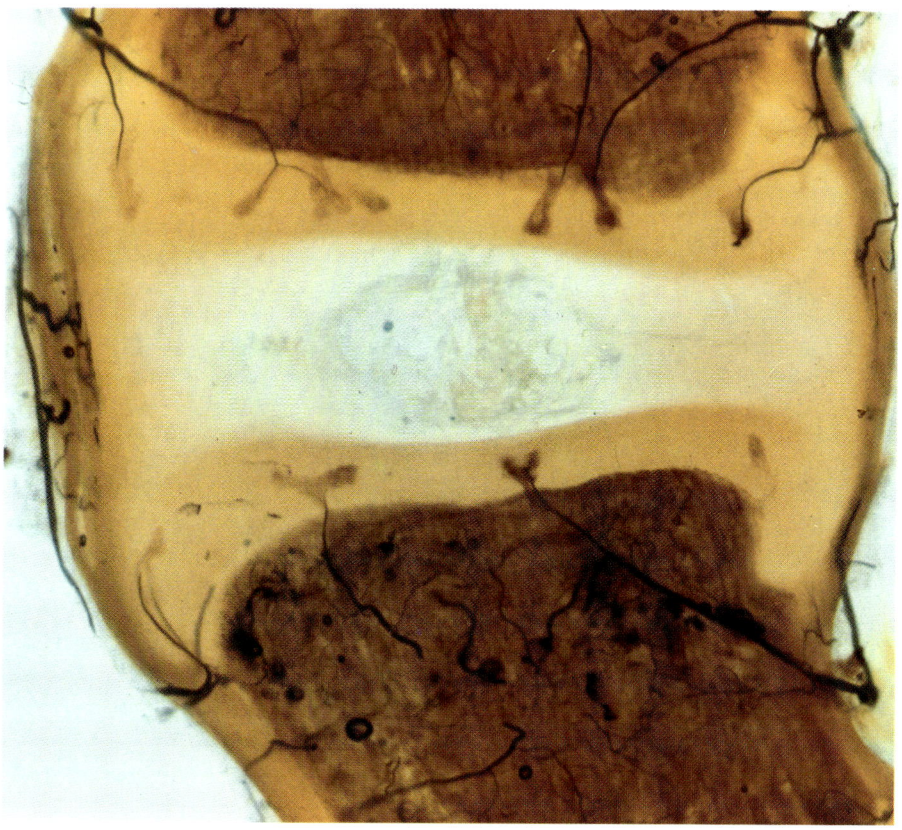

Figure 2.35 Photograph of a thin medial sagittal section of a specimen (injected with barium sulfate and cleared by the *Spalteholz* technique) from a newborn, showing portions of L-5 and S-1 vertebral bodies. Note the basic pattern of distribution of the interosseous arteries with some of the vessels terminating in cartilage. Note that the disc is avascular although it is said that there may be some vascularization of the periphery of the anulus. (From Crock HV, Yoshizawa H: *The Blood Supply of the Vertebral Column and Spinal Cord in Man*. New York, Springer-Verlag, 1977, with permission)

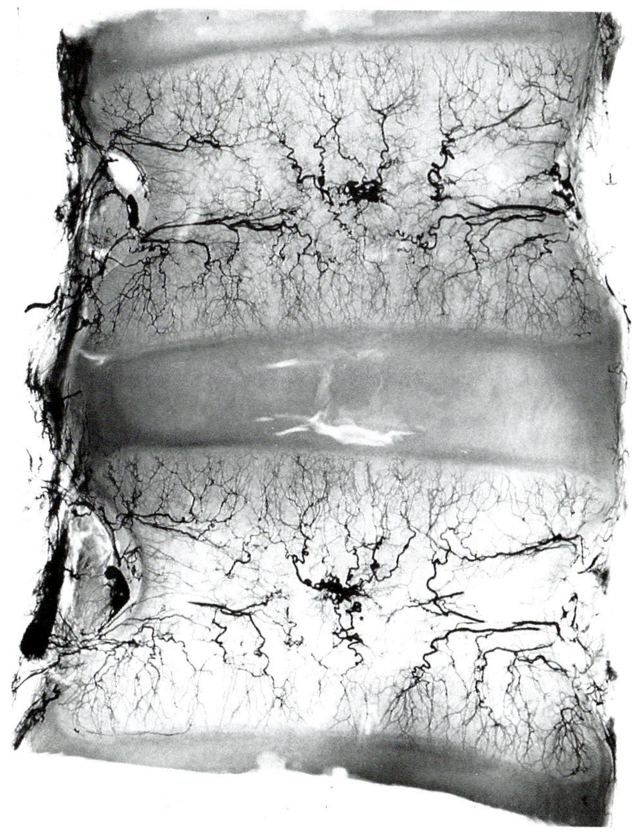

Figure 2.36 Photograph of a thin coronal section through the center of adjacent lumbar vertebral bodies (injected with barium sulfate and cleared by the *Spalteholz* technique) from a 65-year-old male. Note the intraosseous distribution of arteries and the absence of vessels in the intervertebral discs. (From Crock HV, Yoshizawa H: The blood supply of the lumbar vertebral column. *Clin Orthop* 115:6, 1976, with permission)

THE NUCLEUS PULPOSUS

Typically the nucleus pulposus occupies an eccentric position within the disc space, usually being closer to the posterior margin. The tissue of the nucleus is separated from that of the bone by a clearly defined layer of hyaline cartilage that extends to the inner margins of the insertion of the anulus (Fig. 2.37). In the sectioned disc of a young person, the nucleus pulposus is seen to protrude from the surrounding anulus although the nuclear margin is difficult to establish precisely; injection of a colored solution into the disc, however, generally will produce a fairly well demarcated nucleus (Fig. 2.38).

On microscopic examination the nucleus pulposus shows a large number of cells suspended in a loose fibrous matrix. Many of these cells are fusiform and resemble typical fibrocytes; also interspersed in the matrix are chondrocytes within lacunae (Fig. 2.39).

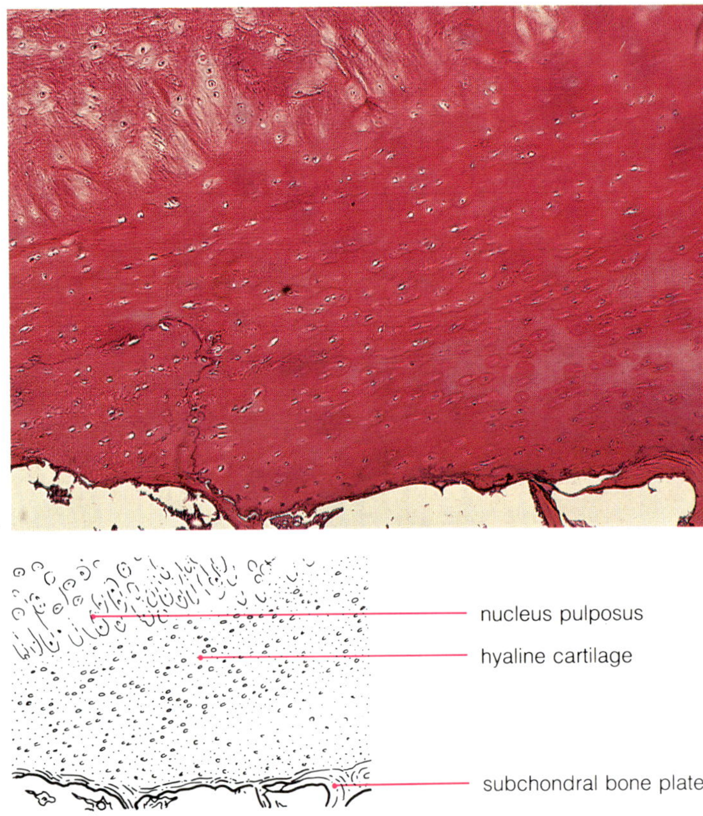

Figure 2.37 Photomicrograph to demonstrate the location of the cartilaginous end plate and its relation to the nucleus pulposus. The nucleus is separated from the bone by a dense layer of hyaline cartilage. (H & E stain, × 4 objective, approximately 100 magnifications)

BIOCHEMICAL FEATURES

The intervertebral disc is neither fibrocartilage nor hyaline cartilage yet it has the biochemical features of both. The main matrix constituents of both the anulus and the nucleus are collagen (types I and II), proteoglycans, and water. These constituents are dispersed within the disc matrix in varying concentrations. The anulus contains mainly type I collagen with some type II collagen whereas the nucleus contains mainly type II collagen. Also within the nucleus is an abundance of nonaggregated proteoglycan molecules (Fig. 2.40).

In terms of load bearing, the most important constituent of the intervertebral disc is the water. In the newborn the water content of the disc is approximately 88% of its total weight, whereas by age 12 it has fallen to approximately 80%, and by age 72 to approximately 70%. Normally the water content of the anulus is roughly 10% less than that of the nucleus (Fig. 2.41) although this difference decreases with increasing age, as seen when the disc of an elderly person is sectioned; the nucleus in the disc of an older person does not protrude from the anulus as it does in the disc of a younger person (Fig. 2.42).

In addition to water loss, other age-related changes in disc-matrix composition include the loss of chondroitin sulfate and the build-up of noncollagenous protein.

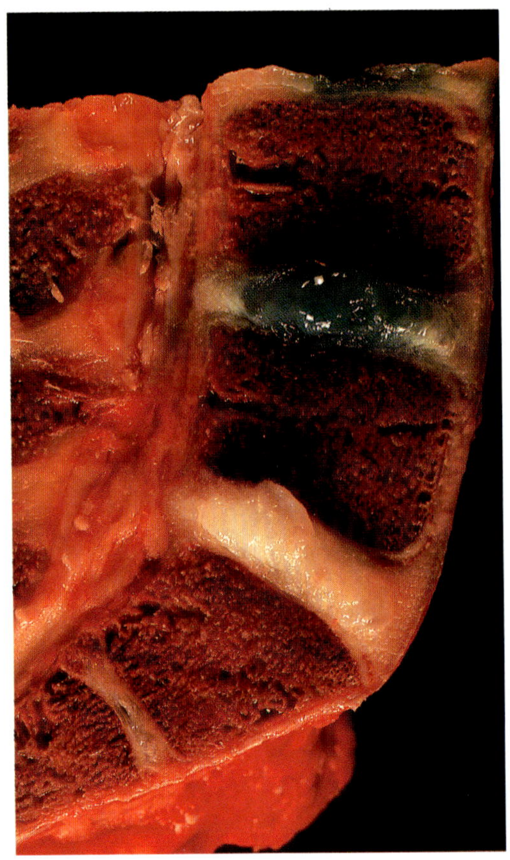

Figure 2.38 Photograph showing sagittal section of the lumbosacral spine of a 12-year-old to demonstrate the bulging discs. Prior to sectioning the L4-5 disc was injected with methylene blue dye to demonstrate demarcation of the nucleus from the surrounding anulus.

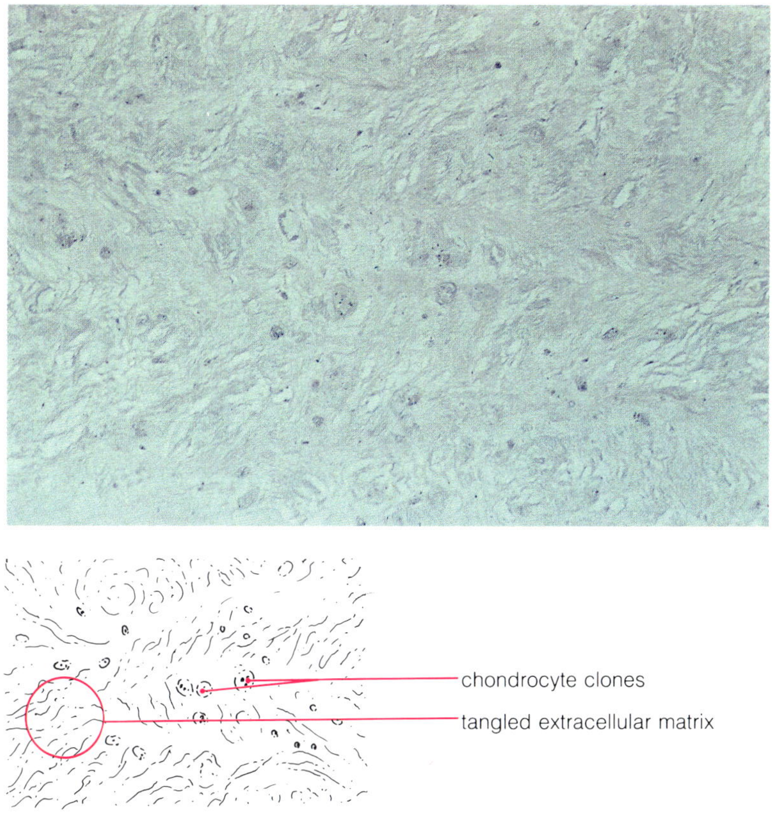

Figure 2.39 Photomicrograph of the normal nucleus pulposus. The matrix is loose and fibrous with scattered small stellate cells and occasional chondrocytes in clumps. (H & E stain, × 4 objective, approximately 100 magnifications)

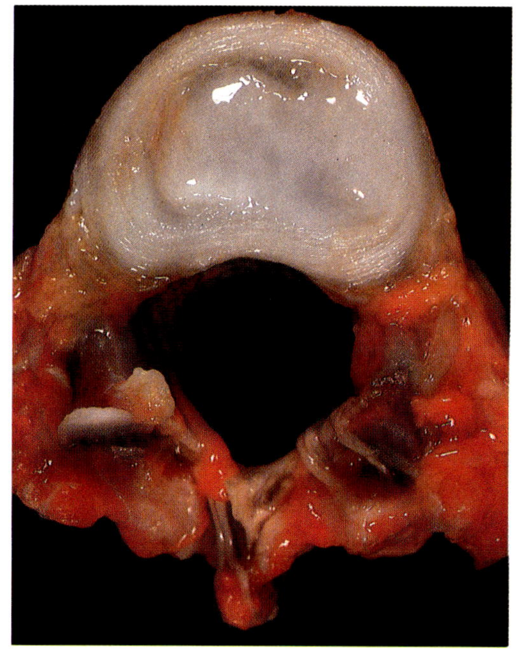

Figure 2.41 Photograph of a transverse section of a lumbar disc from a 7-year-old child to demonstrate the bulging gelatinous nucleus that is well demarcated from the surrounding anulus.

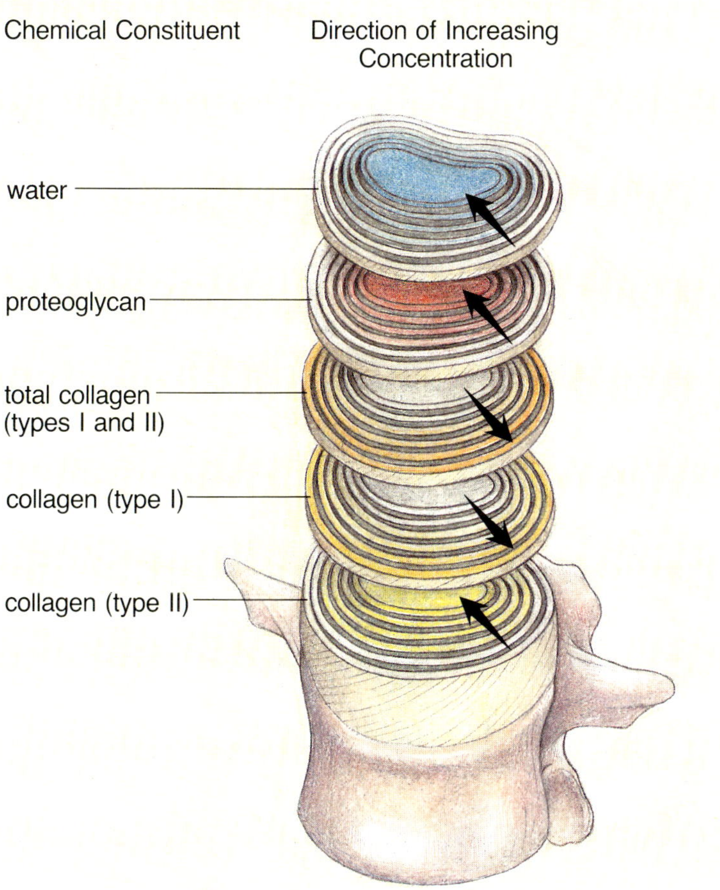

Figure 2.40 Schematic drawing to show the principal chemical constituents of the intervertebral disc and their relative distribution throughout the disc matrix.

The following approximate percentage weights (except for those of water content) were obtained from measurements of disc dry weight: *Proteoglycan*—Inner disc: 60% for young adult, 30% for old adult; outer disc: 10% for both young and old adults. *Collagen type I*—Inner disc: 0% for both young and old adults; outer disc: 40–60% for both young and old adults. *Collagen type II*—Inner disc: 10–25%; outer disc: <5% for both young and old adults. *Water*—Inner disc: 80% for young adult, 70% for old adult; outer disc: 70% for both young and old adults. Note that the values for proteoglycan content represent rough approximations. (Data courtesy of Dr. David Eyre)

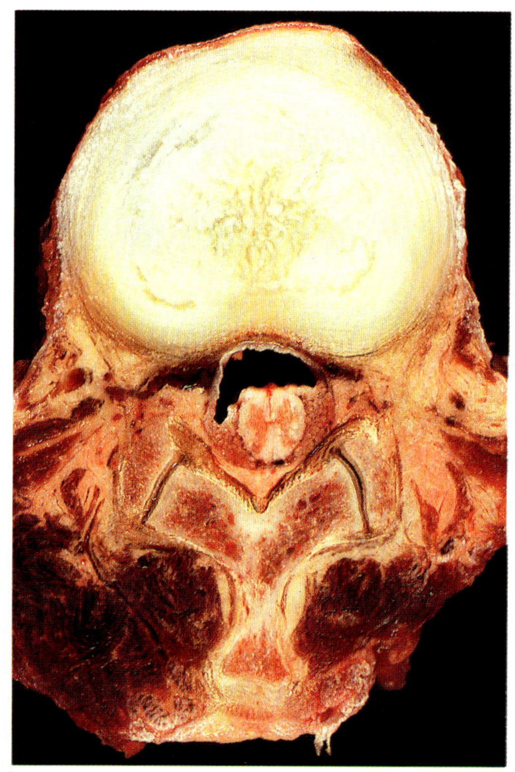

Figure 2.42 Photograph of a transverse section of a lumbar disc from a 30-year-old for comparison with the disc shown in Figure 2.41. Here the nucleus is less well demarcated and does not protrude as much from the surrounding anulus.

The Spinal Ligaments

The components of the spinal column are attached to one another by the following ligaments shown schematically in Figure 2.43:

1. The anterior longitudinal ligament
2. The posterior longitudinal ligament
3. The paired ligamenta flava
4. The interspinous ligaments
5. The supraspinous ligaments
6. The paired intertransverse ligaments
7. The paired costotransverse ligaments (medial, superior, and lateral)

Both the anterior and posterior longitudinal ligaments develop from a membrane surrounding the vertebral bodies and intervertebral discs of the developing spine. The anterior longitudinal ligament is a broad strong band of fibers that extends from the base of the skull to the anterior surface of the sacrum (Fig. 2.44). It covers and is firmly attached to the anterior and lateral surfaces of the vertebral bodies yet it is only loosely connected to the intervertebral discs.

In contrast the posterior longitudinal ligament consists of a strong central band of fibers that broadens in a fanlike fashion behind each intervertebral disc but narrows in the area behind each vertebral body (Fig. 2.45). It also is narrower than the anterior longitudinal ligament, contains more elastic fibers, and is attached firmly to the intervertebral discs, spanning the slightly concave posterior surfaces of the vertebrae.

In the cervical region the posterior longitudinal ligament is known as the tectorial membrane, which attaches the axis to the occiput and covers the posterior surface of the odontoid process and the transverse ligament (Fig. 2.46).

Differences in structure and form between the strong central band of the posterior longitudinal ligament and its thin lateral expansions are pertinent to problems involving central-posterior and posterolateral prolapse of the nucleus pulposus. Whereas central prolapse is restrained by the strong midline band, posterolateral protrusion can dissect more easily the thin lateral expansions of the ligament. Attached to the lateral expansions are numerous nerve fibers that may be of clinical significance in disc disease.

Between the posterior longitudinal ligament and the posterior surface of the vertebral body lies a venous network that communicates with the vertebral veins. Thus the posterior longitudinal ligament also may serve to protect the spinal cord from pressure variations in this venous network.

The ligamenta flava, which are paired, cover the posterior wall of the vertebral canal and connect the laminae of adjacent arches

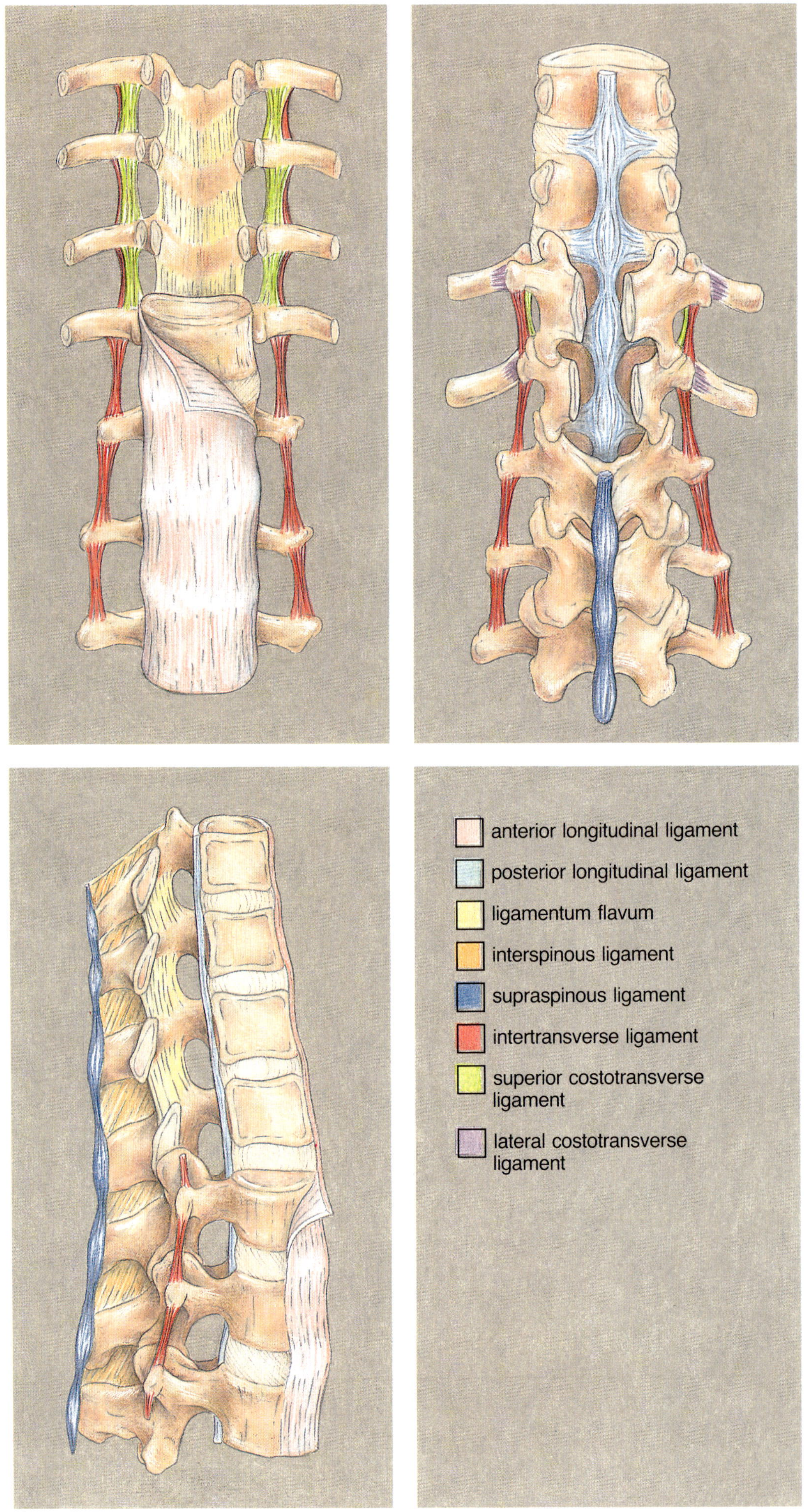

Figure 2.43 Schematic drawings of the lower thoracic and upper lumbar spine showing the ligaments in anterior (*top left*), posterior (*top right*), and lateral (*bottom left*) views.

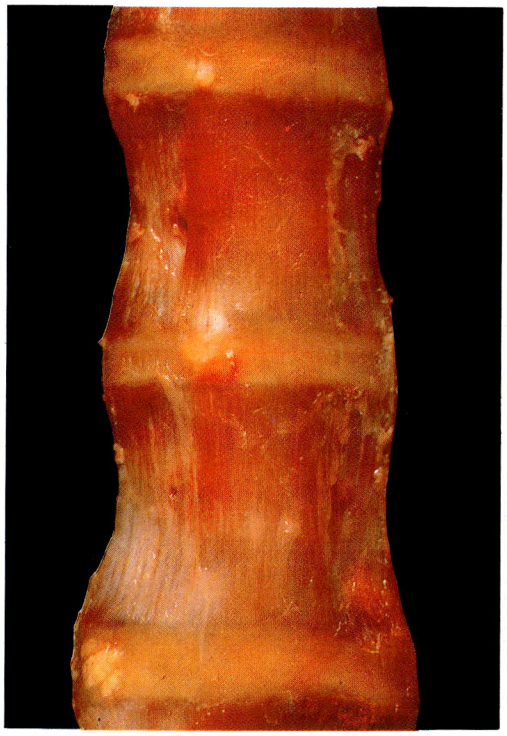

Figure 2.44 Photograph of the anterior longitudinal ligament which is seen covering all of the anterior and some of the lateral surface of the vertebral bodies. It is firmly attached to the periosteum though only loosely attached to the intervertebral discs.

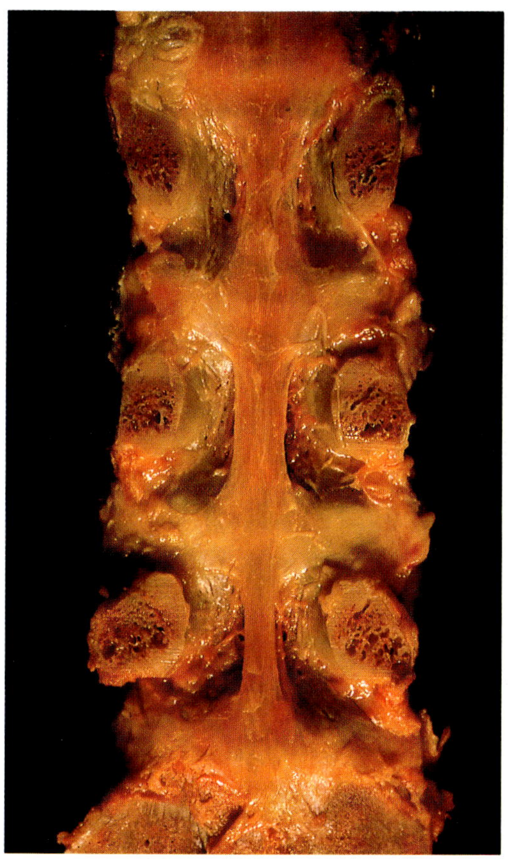

Figure 2.45 Photograph of the posterior longitudinal ligament, which is narrower and more clearly defined than the anterior longitudinal ligament but which, at its lateral expansions, attaches firmly to the disc anulus. It is attached only loosely to the bone.

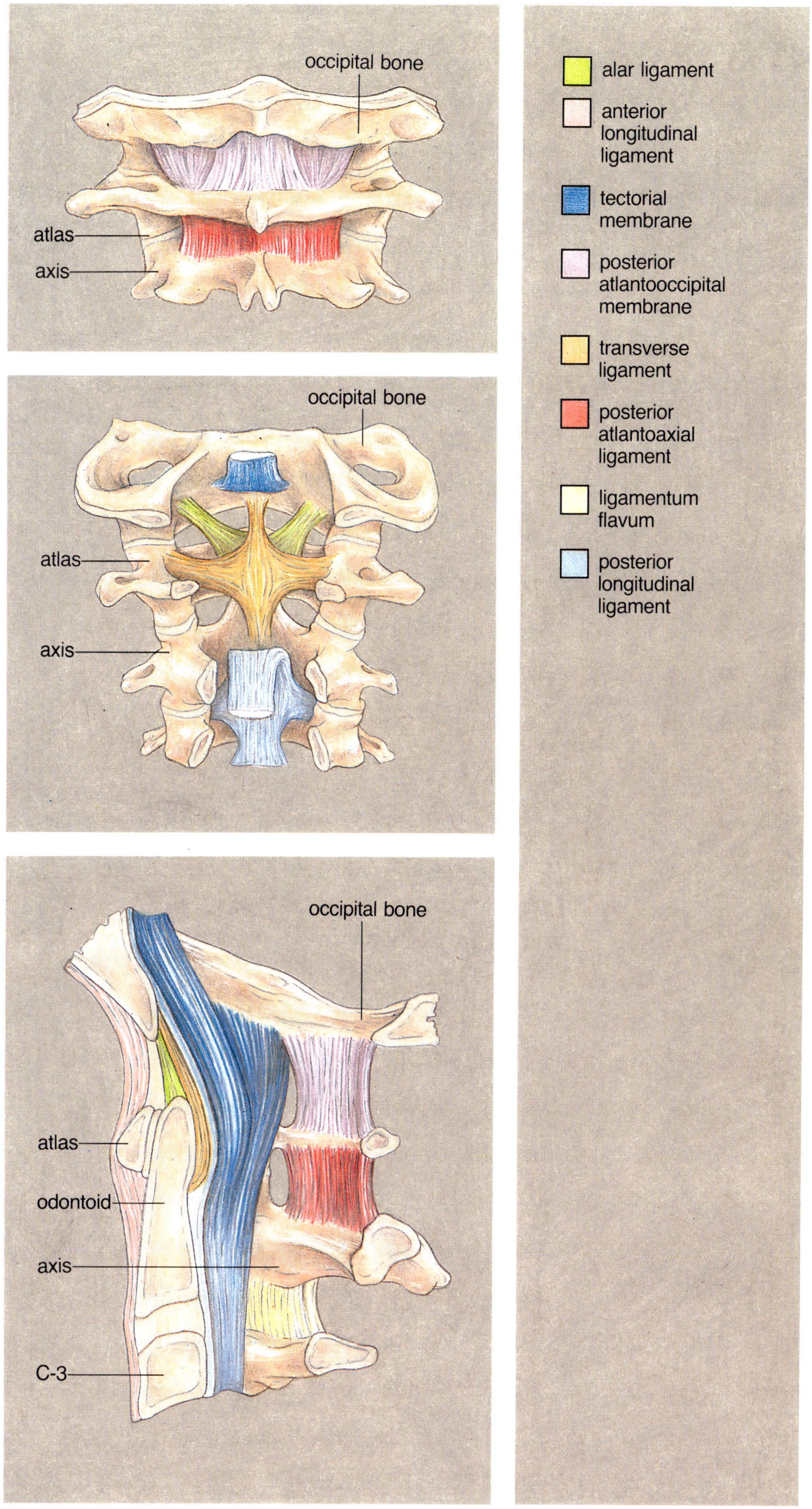

Figure 2.46 Schematic drawing of the cervical spine in lateral and posterior views to show the relationship of the posterior longitudinal ligament to the cervical vertebrae and to the occiput. In the lower posterior view, the posterior elements have been removed.

(Fig. 2.47). They are highly elastic and protect against flexion injuries while restraining the mobility of the apophysial joints; they are yellow because of their high elastin content (Figs. 2.48 and 2.49). In the lumbar region these ligaments are quite broad and also are particularly thick.

Extending between the superior and inferior borders of adjacent spinous processes is the interspinous ligament. The supraspinous ligament extends between and covers the tips and posterior borders of adjacent spinous processes; in the cervical region this ligament becomes the broad expansion known as the ligamentum nuchae (Fig. 2.50). The intertransverse ligament runs between adjacent transverse processes. The medial costotransverse ligament, together with the superior and lateral costotransverse ligaments, restrains the gliding costotransverse articulation (Fig. 2.51).

THE SACRAL LIGAMENTS

The sacrum articulates with the ilium through an irregularly shaped synovial joint that is relatively immobile and which, in an elderly person, may be partially fused. It is covered ventrally and dorsally by strong ligaments (the ventral and dorsal sacroiliac ligaments) that attach to the joint margins (Fig. 2.52). Superiorly the sacrum and the il-

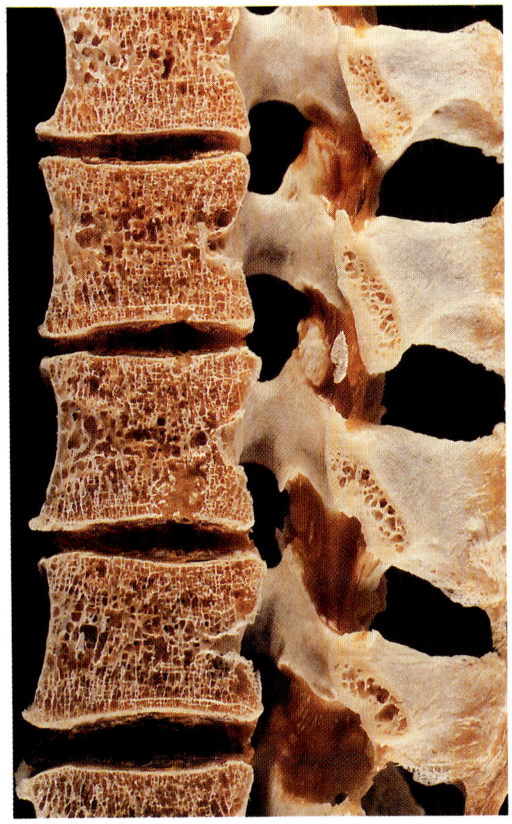

Figure 2.47 Photograph showing the relationships of the ligamentum flavum. Note how it attaches superiorly and inferiorly to the adjacent laminae, forming a significant portion of the posterior wall of the spinal canal. (Anteriorly it is separated partially from the posterior wall of the intervertebral foramen by the capsule of the facet joint.)

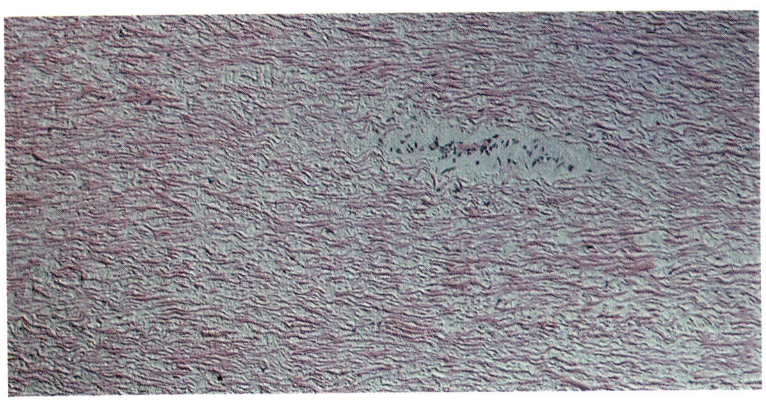

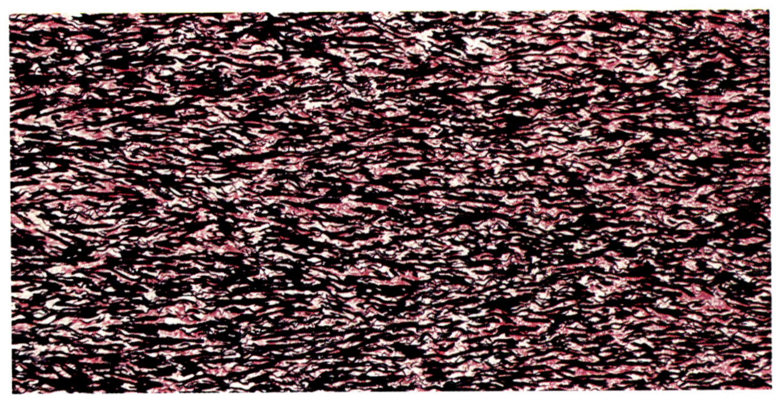

Figure 2.48 Photomicrograph (*left*) of a longitudinal section of the ligamentum flavum to show the parallel well-oriented fiber structure. (H & E stain) Photomicrograph (*right*) of a section of the ligamentum flavum similar to that shown at left, but stained with an elastic tissue stain. Note the presence of collagen (stained red) in between the elastic fibers (stained black). (Verhoeff-van Gieson elastic tissue stain, × 10 objective, approximately 100 magnifications)

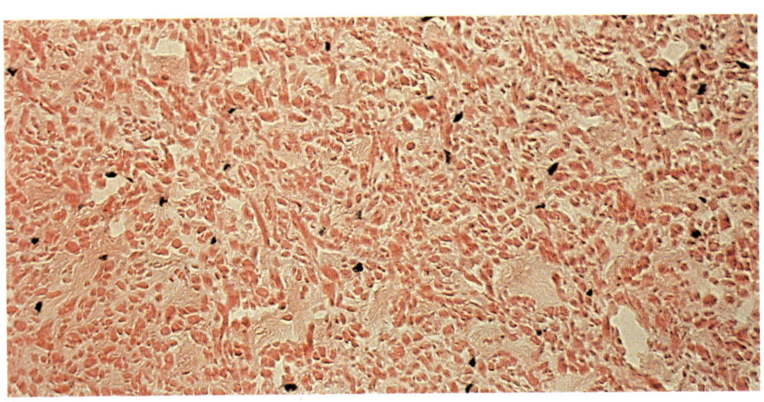

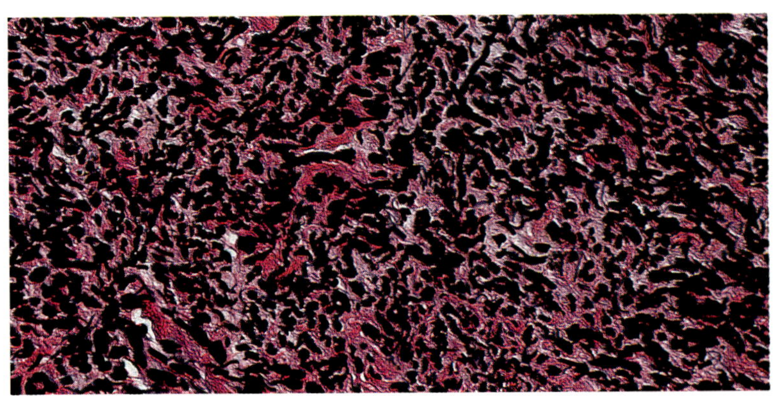

Figure 2.49 Photomicrograph (*left*) to show the elastic fibers of the ligamentum flavum in cross section. (H & E stain, × 25 objective, approximately 200 magnifications) Photomicrograph (*right*) of a cross section through the ligamentum flavum, stained with an elastic tissue stain to show the normal relationship of the collagen to the elastic fibers. (Verhoeff-van Gieson elastic tissue stain, × 25 objective, approximately 200 magnifications)

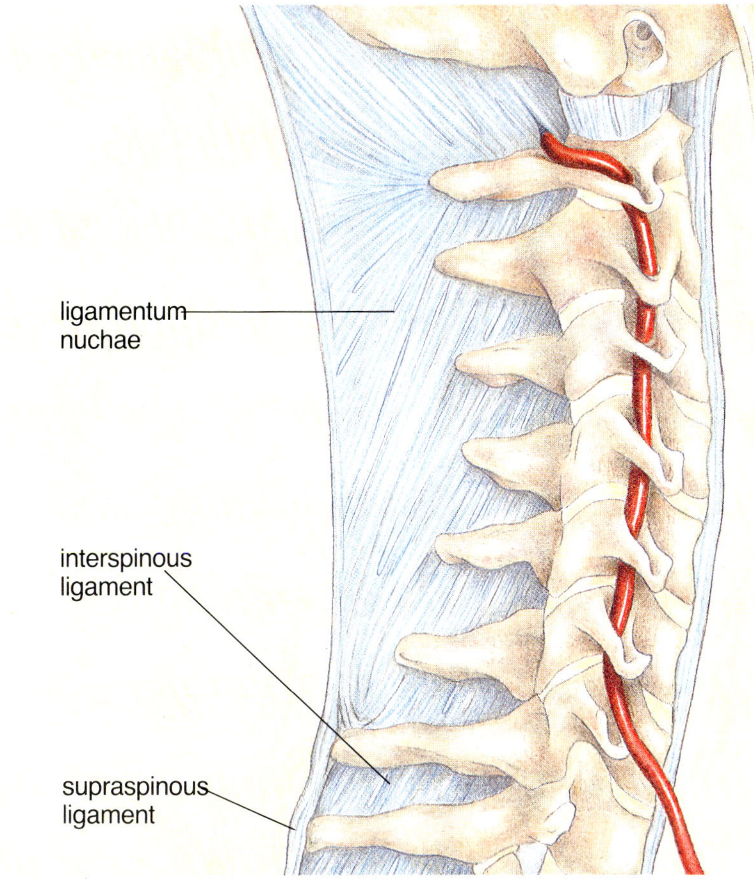

Figure 2.50 Schematic drawing of the upper thoracic and cervical vertebrae to show the interspinous ligament and the supraspinous ligament which, in the cervical region, becomes the ligamentum nuchae. Note the course of the vertebral artery.

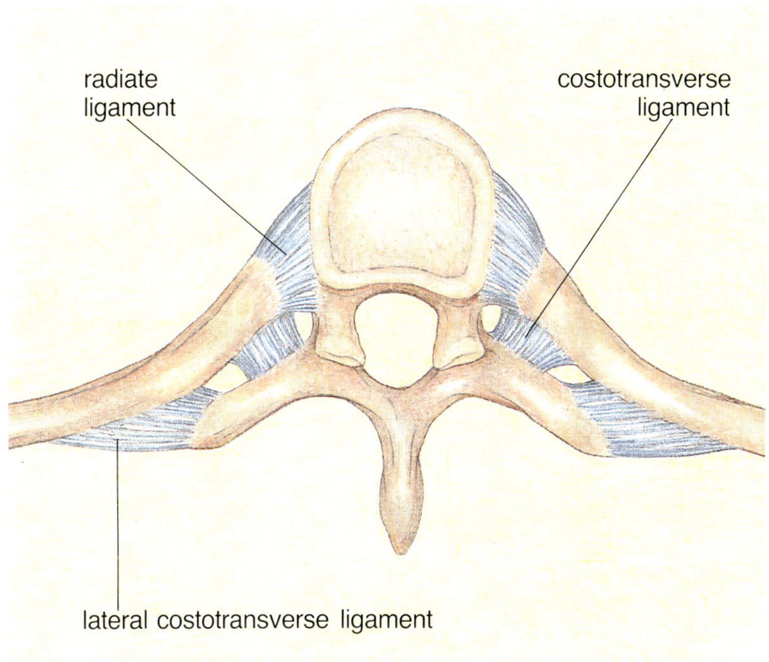

Figure 2.51 Schematic drawing of a thoracic vertebra to show the paired costotransverse ligaments, which extend from the anterior surface of an adjacent transverse process to the rough surface of the back of the neck of a rib, the paired lateral costotransverse ligaments, which extend from the apex of a transverse process to the rough nonarticular portion of the tubercle of the adjacent rib, and the radiate ligaments. The superior costotransverse ligament is illustrated in Figure 2.43.

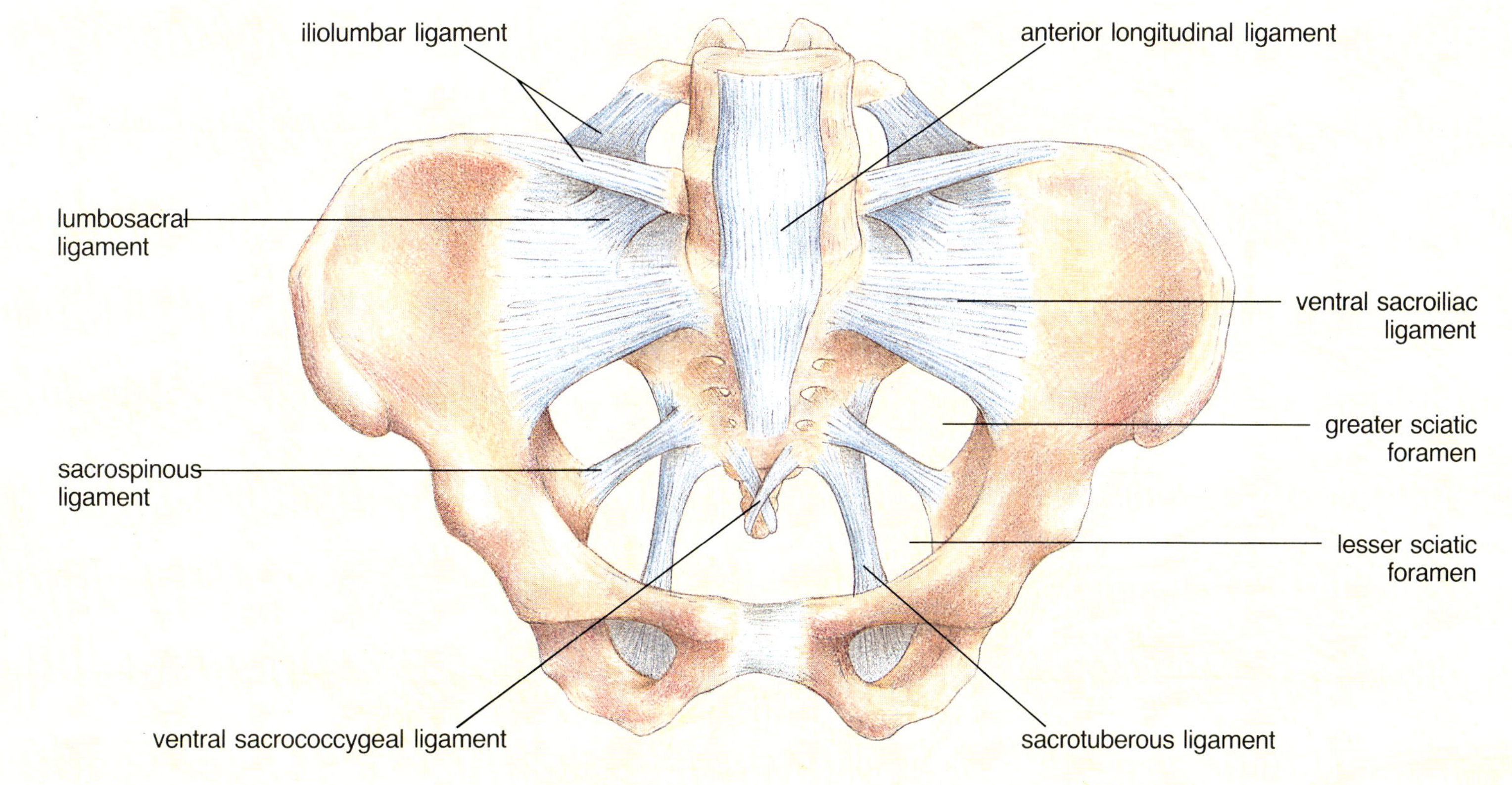

Figure 2.52 Schematic drawing showing a ventral view of the pelvis. The ventral sacroiliac ligament covers the joint and lies in front of the interosseous ligament (not seen in this drawing).

ium are joined by a dense interosseous ligament that forms the major connection between these two bones (Fig. 2.53).

The spine and the pelvis also are connected through a number of vertebropelvic ligaments, with the iliolumbar ligament connecting the ilium to the fifth lumbar vertebra, and the sacrotuberous and sacrospinous ligaments connecting the sacrum to the ischium. The sacrotuberous ligament attaches at one end to the posterior iliac spines, to the lower transverse tubercles of the sacrum and to the lateral margins of the lower sacrum and upper coccyx, and at the other end to the medial margin of the ischial tuberosity.

The sacrospinous ligament attaches to the spine of the ischium, medially to the lateral margin of the sacrum and coccyx, and anteriorly to the sacrotuberous ligament. The iliolumbar, sacrotuberous, and sacrospinous ligaments are seen best in posterior view (Fig. 2.54).

The greater sciatic foramen (transmitting the superior gluteal neurovascular bundle, the piriform muscle, the inferior gluteal neurovascular bundle, the sciatic and posterior femoral cutaneous nerves, and the nerve supply of the short external rotators of the hip) is bounded superiorly by the upper part of the pelvic brim (the sciatic notch), posteriorly by the sacrotuberous ligament, and inferiorly by the spine of the ischium and by the sacrospinous ligament.

The lesser sciatic foramen (transmitting the tendon of the obturator internis together with its nerve and the reentering pudendal nerve) is bounded above by the spine of the ischium and by the sacrospinous ligament, in front by the body of the ischium, and behind by the sacrotuberous ligament.

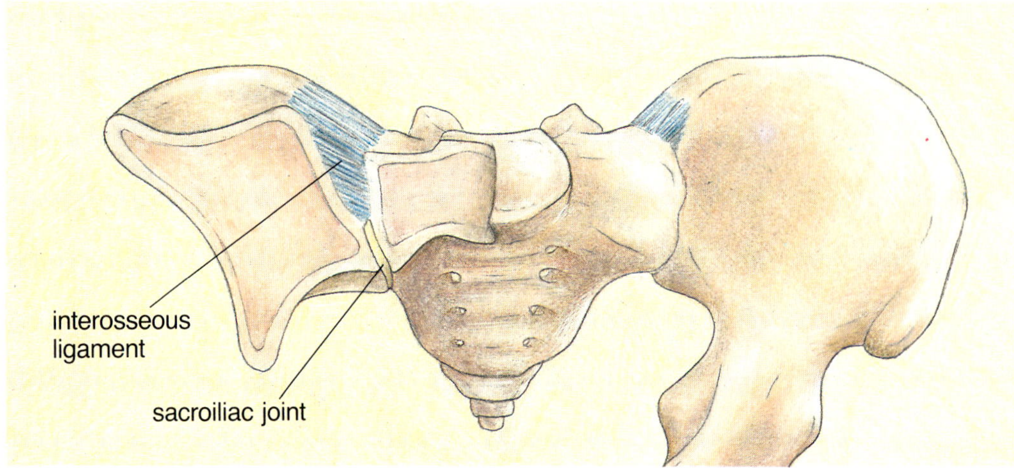

Figure 2.53 Schematic drawing of a section through the sacroiliac joint to show its relationship to the interosseous ligament.

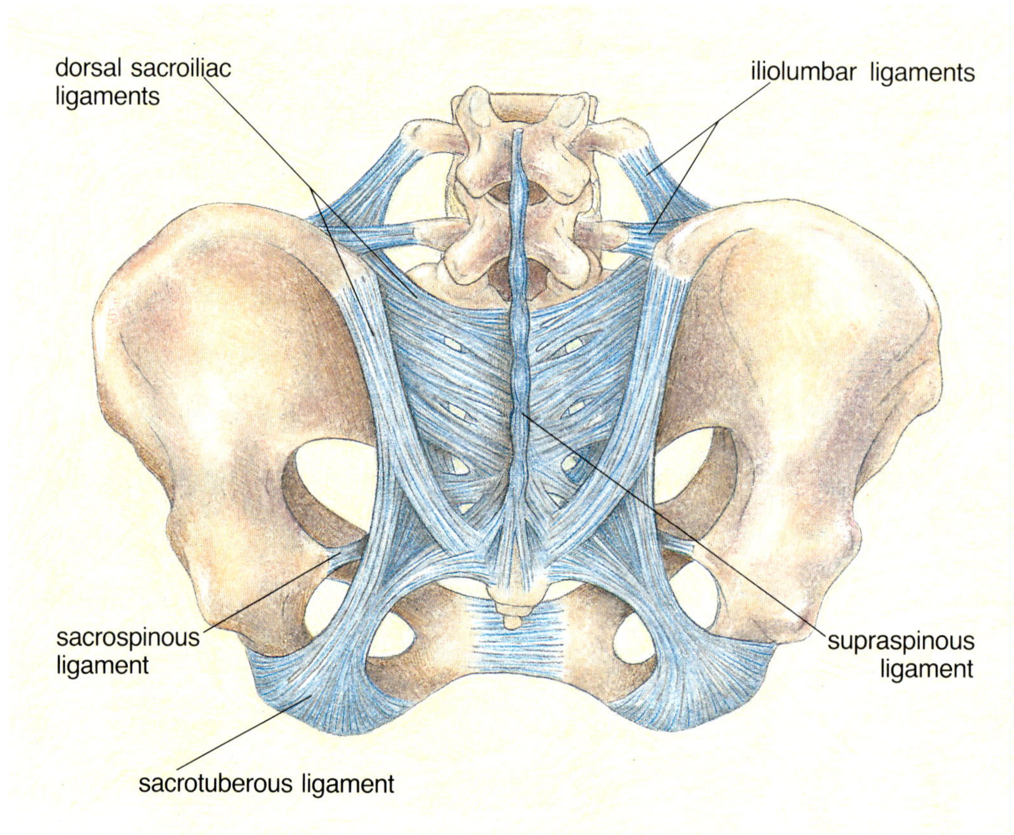

Figure 2.54 Schematic drawing of a posterior view of the pelvis showing the ilium connected to the fifth lumbar vertebra by the iliolumbar ligaments, and the sacrum connected to the ischium by the sacrotuberous and sacrospinous ligaments.

Vascular Supply of the Vertebral Column

The vertebral bodies and arches have an extensive vascular system that is closely connected to that of the spinal canal and spinal cord.

ARTERIAL SUPPLY

The arteries of the spinal column are segmented in the cervical spine from the paired dorsal vertebral arteries, and from the thoracic intercostal arteries and from the lumbar arteries.

The dorsal vertebral arteries originate from the subclavian arch. Beginning at the caudal end with the transverse process of C-6, each artery extends through the transverse foramina of the cervical transverse processes, in close proximity to the uncovertebral joints. The artery also is related closely to the lateral exits of the intervertebral foramina. At the cephalic end it perforates the posterior atlantooccipital membrane above the posterior arch of C-1, continuing through the foramen magnum into the interior of the skull (Fig. 2.55). Shortly before the right and left dorsal vertebral arteries unite to form the basilar artery, they give origin to the posterior and anterior spinal arteries, which eventually fuse to form a longitudinal channel along the spinal cord, with branches that connect with the spinal branches of the vertebral arteries.

The first two thoracic vertebrae are fed by the superior intercostal and deep cervical branches of the costocervical trunk arising from the subclavian arteries. The remaining thoracic vertebrae are supplied by vertebral branches that arise from the posterior intercostal branches of the thoracic aorta (Fig. 2.56).

The lumbar spine gets its blood supply from the paired lumbar arteries, which arise

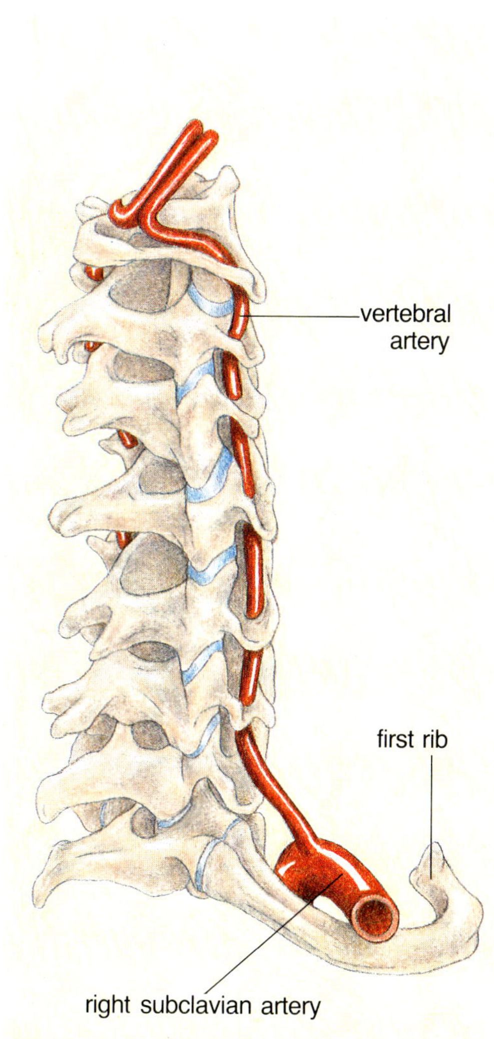

Figure 2.55 Schematic drawing of a posterolateral view of the cervical spine to show the right vertebral artery arising from the subclavian artery and its ascent through the transverse foramina to the axis, where it turns laterally to ascend through the transverse foramen of the atlas. At the atlas the artery bends posteromedially to enter the cranium through the foramen magnum, where at the border of the pons it anastomoses with the left vertebral artery to form the basilar artery.

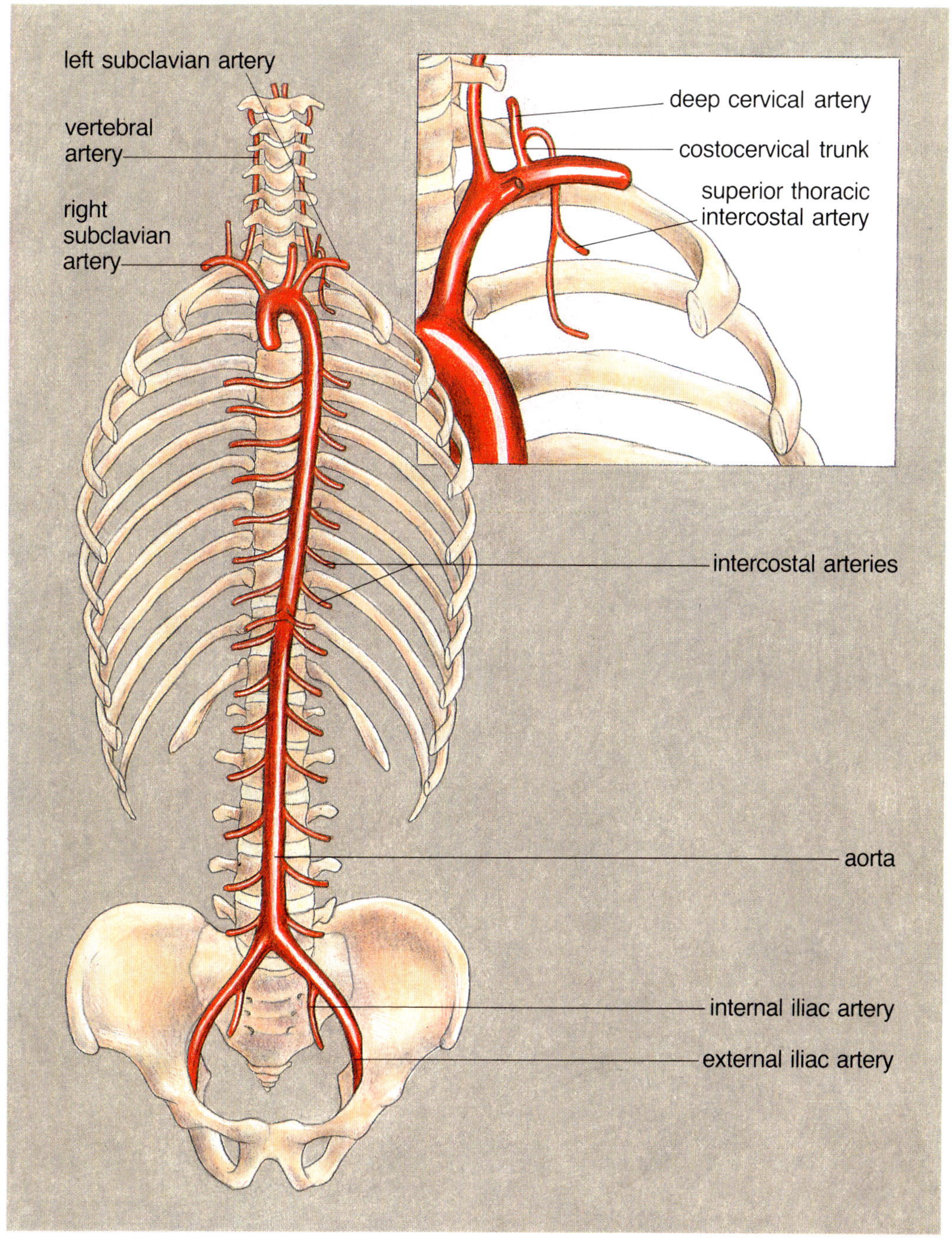

Figure 2.56 Schematic drawing to show the origins of the blood supply to the thoracic spine as well as to the rest of the vertebral column.

from the posterior wall of the lumbar aorta (Fig. 2.57). The median sacral artery (arising at the aortic bifurcation) and the lateral sacral arteries (arising from the posterior trunk of the internal iliac arteries) supply the sacral vertebrae and the contents of the sacral canal.

The vascular supply of each of the vertebral bodies develops through branches that grow into the ossification center anteriorly, anterolaterally, and posteriorly (Fig. 2.58). The posterior branch enters through the intervertebral foramina and contributes to the supply of the spinal cord, the spinal nerves, and the dura mater (Fig. 2.59).

VENOUS DRAINAGE

Venous blood drains from the vertebral bodies through numerous openings on the anterior and lateral aspects of the bodies as well as through broad openings on the posterior surfaces of the bodies, thus forming the internal and external vertebral venous plexuses (Fig. 2.60).

The internal vertebral venous plexus extends from the sphenoidal clivus above to the sacrum below. It has anterior and posterior components, which follow the arterial arcades. These veins exit segmentally through the intervertebral foramina and fuse with the segmental veins of the external vertebral venous plexus.

The external vertebral venous plexus runs the entire length of the spine and is segmented like the arterial supply. The anterior portion of the external venous plexus in the neck drains largely into the venae comitantes of the vertebral arteries, and the posterior portion of the plexus drains into the deep cervical veins on each side. These two venous systems in turn drain into the brachiocephalic veins. In the thoracic region the intercostal veins join the azygous system. The upper lumbar veins drain into the lumbar azygous veins and the lower lumbar veins drain directly into the inferior vena cava (Fig. 2.61).

The vertebral venous system, which consists of veins without valves, acts as a collateral system *(Batson's plexus)* in the event of an obstruction of the superior or inferior vena cava. The absence of valves along with the possibility of retrograde flow may provide an explanation for the extension of inflammatory or metastatic disease from the pelvic organs into the spinal column, or even into the skull.

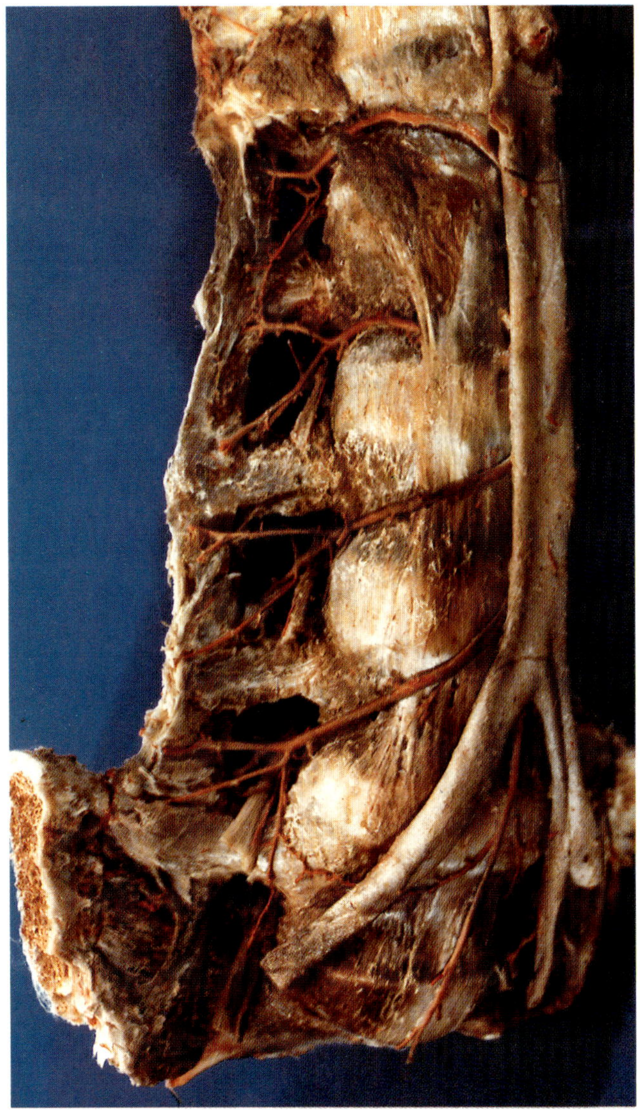

Figure 2.57 Photograph showing the dissected lumbar vertebral column of an adult, viewed from the right side. Note the origins and distribution of the lumbar arteries from the aorta as well as the medial sacral artery. (From Crock HV, Yoshizawa H: *The Blood Supply of the Vertebral Column and Spinal Cord in Man.* New York, Springer-Verlag, 1977)

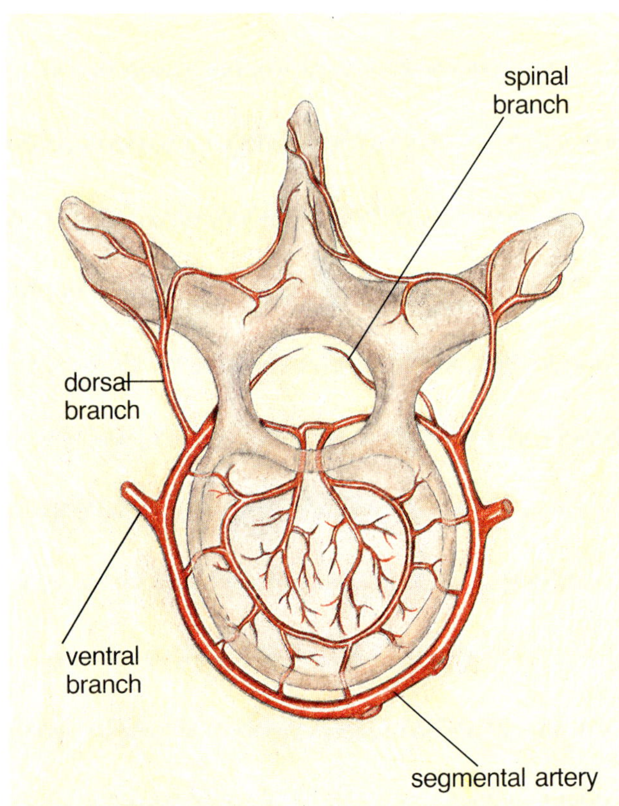

Figure 2.58 Schematic drawing to show the anastomosing arterial supply of a vertebral body, spinal canal, and posterior elements.

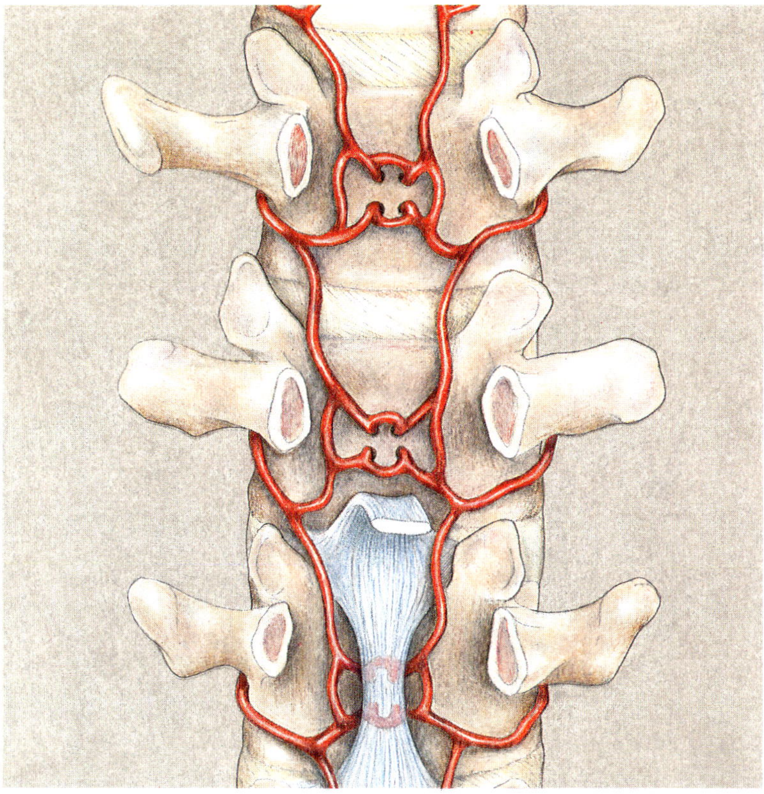

Figure 2.59 Schematic drawing of the vertebral blood supply, seen from behind with the laminae removed, to show the anastomosing spinal branches of the segmental arteries.

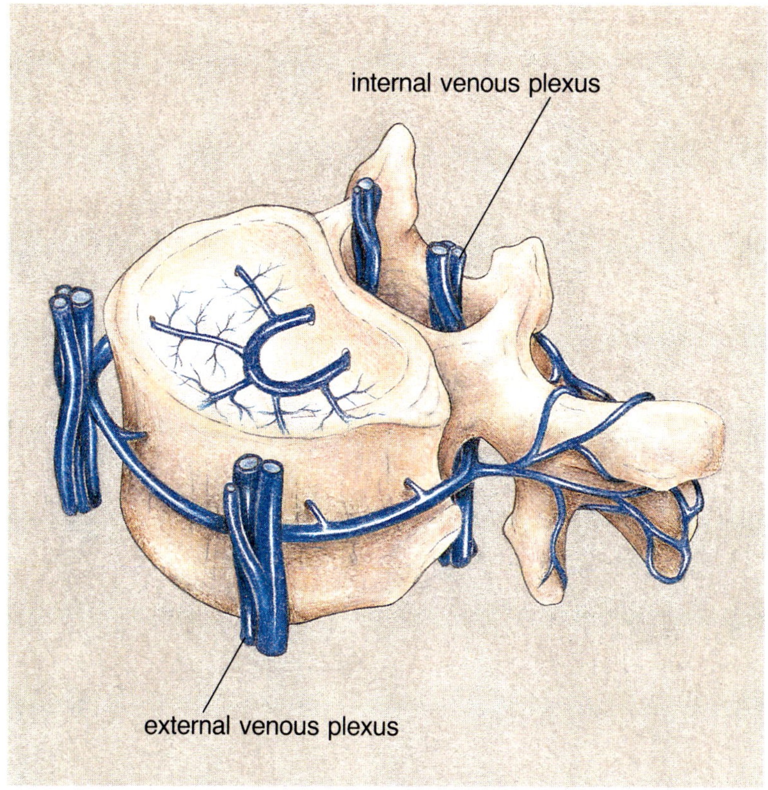

Figure 2.60 Schematic drawing to show the venous drainage of the vertebral bodies and the formation of the internal and external vertebral venous plexuses.

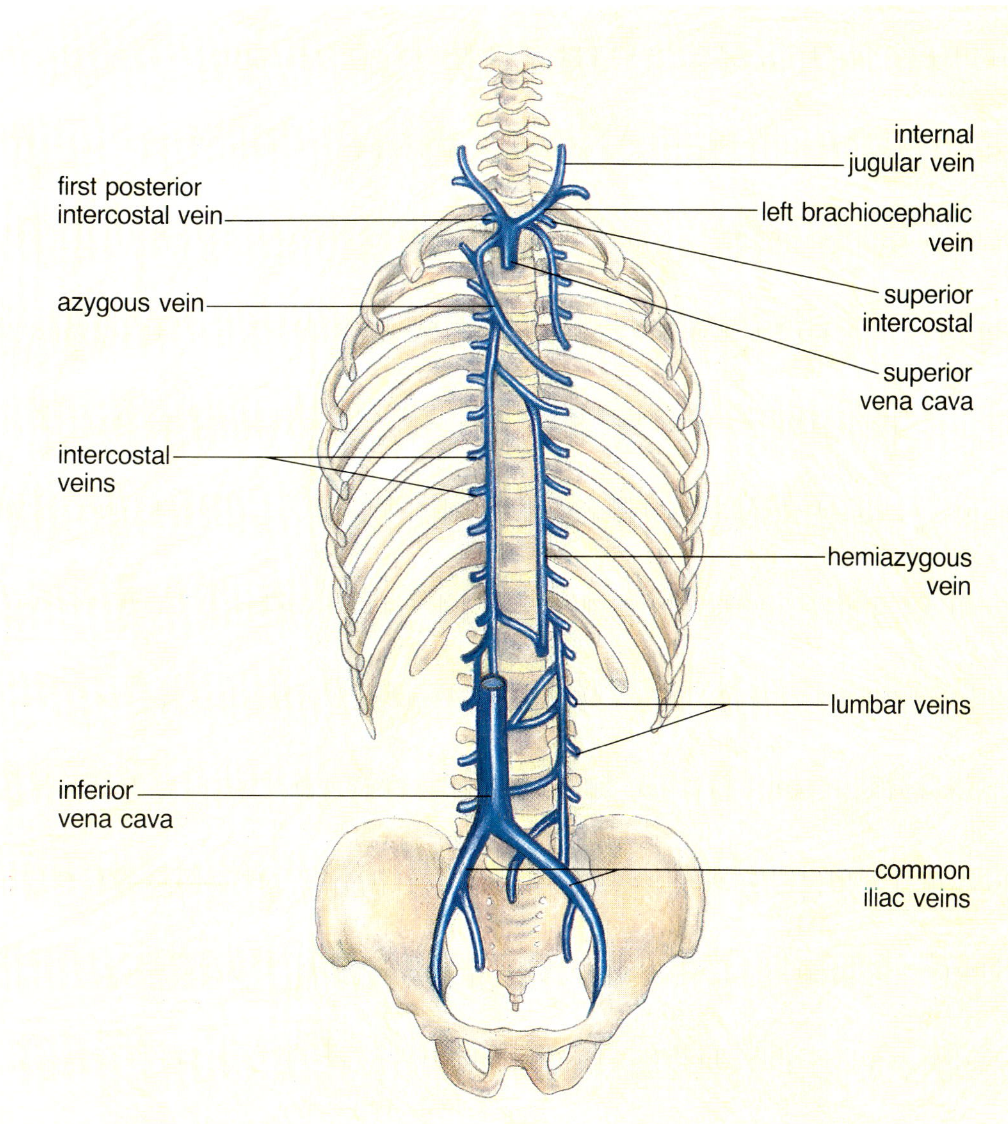

Figure 2.61 Schematic overview of the venous drainage of the vertebral column showing its connection to the vena cava.

3 CHAPTER

FUNCTIONAL ANATOMY AND BIOMECHANICS

GENERAL FEATURES

The spinal column plays a central role in the motor system of the body, possessing a number of both static and kinetic functions. It participates in the locomotion of the entire body while also providing for sensory physiologic orientation. Arising above the pelvis, it carries the head, shoulders, upper extremities, thoracic cage and abdominal contents, and it transmits their weight to the pelvis. Serving as a protective organ for both the spinal cord and the originating spinal nerves, it also provides a point of attachment for the thoracic and abdominal organs.

In general, the various components of the spinal column contribute in different ways to its biomechanical functioning. The vertebral bodies, collectively, through their bony mass provide support. The dorsovertebral arches protect the spinal cord while also participating in weight bearing, and, with their articular facets, they contribute to spinal column mobility. The spinous and transverse processes provide attachments for muscles and ligaments, allowing for controlled movement. The intervertebral discs are important in load distribution and for motion between vertebrae. The spinal curves, as a unit, provide for shock absorption as well as for increased flexibility and balanced stability.

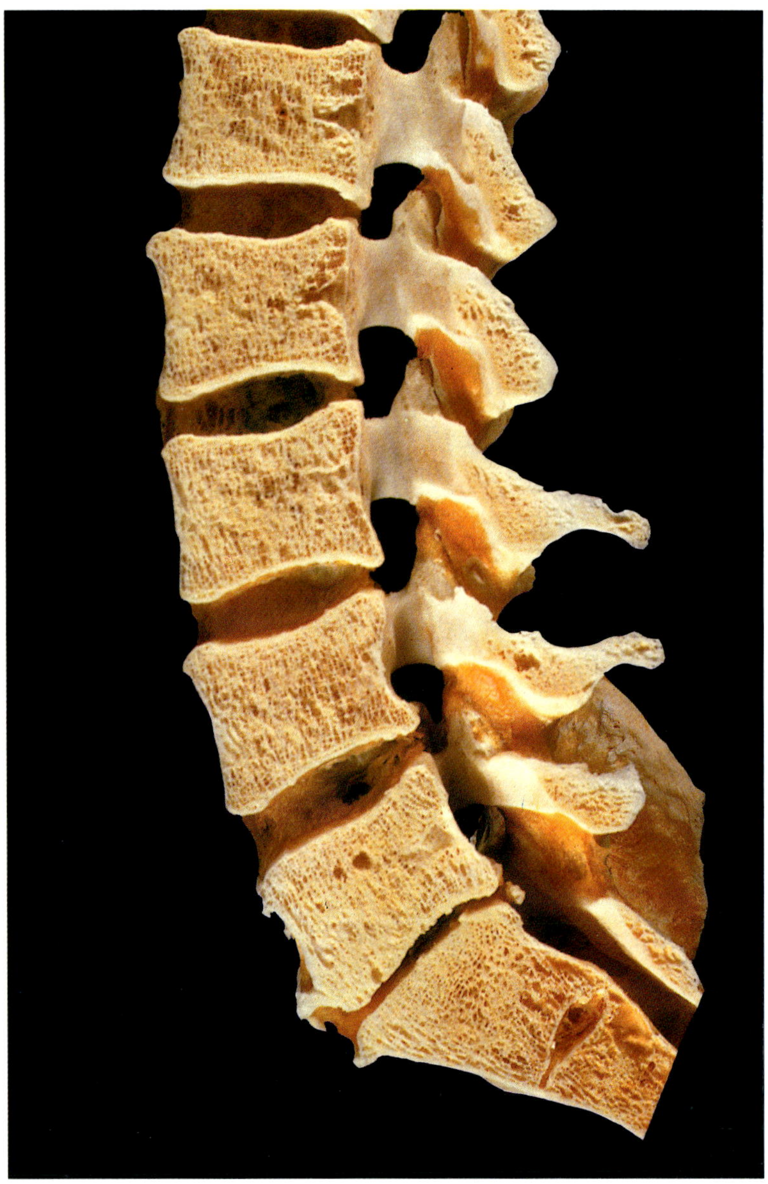

Figure 3.1 Photograph of a macerated spine with severe narrowing of the L-5 to S-1 disc space and subchondral bone sclerosis of the adjacent vertebrae. Three factors contribute to this predilection for L-5 to S-1: (1) transition from the mobile lumbar spine to the fixed sacrum; (2) increased angulation; (3) the line of gravity extending anteriorly.

The Vertebral Column

THE SPINAL CURVES

The spinal column contains four normal curves in the lateral or sagittal plane: two are convex anteriorly in the cervical and lumbar regions, and two are convex posteriorly in the thoracic and sacral regions.

The thoracic and sacral curves form the midline portion of the posterior walls of the thoracic and pelvic cavities and allow for accommodation and support of the visceral organs within. The thoracic and sacral curves are referred to as "structural" and are due to the slightly diminished vertical height of the anterior thoracic and sacral vertebral bodies in contrast to their posterior bony height. The "compensatory" anterior curves of the cervical and lumbar regions are due largely to wedge-shaped intervertebral discs. In particular, the height of the intervertebral disc between L-5 and S-1, because of its position along the sloping upper surface of the sacrum, is even shorter posteriorly than the others. Because this area is exposed to a high degree of shear stress, early disc degeneration frequently is found here, along with varying degrees of angulation and slippage (Fig. 3.1).

The mechanical basis for the spinal curves is that they give the spinal column increased flexibility and augmented shock-absorbing capacity while at the same time still providing for adequate stiffness and stability at the intervertebral joint level. Just as a bent position of the knee, in jumping, helps to absorb the shock of landing, so the S-like bending of the spine contributes favorably to the elastic absorption of vertical forces.

The double S-curve means that the line of gravity intersects the column at various points, producing a variety of mechanical environments that result in different patterns of injury at different levels (Fig. 3.2).

The spine, when viewed in the frontal plane, generally appears to be straight and symmetrical although a physiologic scoliosis, characterized by a slight left-lower cervical and upper thoracic curve and a slight right-middle thoracic curve, may be found in the spines of most people. The origin of these curves is unclear, although they have been attributed to the handedness of the individual.

VERTEBRAL COLUMN STRENGTH

From the top of the spinal column to the body of L-5 there is an increase in both the size and mass of the individual vertebral bodies—an increase that is no doubt directly related to the increasing loads to which the vertebrae are subjected.

Studies have shown that vertebral end-plate fracture will occur when an excessive compression load is applied gradually to the spinal column. In contrast, when an excessive load is applied rapidly, disc injury may result.

In the case of end-plate compression fractures, when the adjacent disc is healthy and intact, fractures will tend to be central with the anulus containing the increased pressure of the nucleus and the bone under the end plate giving way. However, when disc degeneration is present, the bony injuries will be diffuse.

With advancing age, particularly in women beyond age 50, there occurs a decrease in bone mass (to be discussed at length in Section 3). It should be noted, however, that a 25% decrease in bone mass may result in a 50% loss of vertebral bone strength, and it is the loss of cancellous bone that is the major contributor to the loss of bone strength.

In general, to obtain realistic figures of vertebral column strength, biomechanical studies of the spine should be conducted with testing done on segmental spine (including both bone and soft-tissue elements) rather than on individual bony units.

It is important to realize that the spinal column, with its surrounding muscles and ligaments, is probably that part of the locomotive apparatus that is the least relaxed. Even in the bedridden patient or during the nightly rest of healthy individuals, the spine constantly is subjected to stress from repeated turning or from uneven support. In the course of a day, the spine may be subjected to multiple injuries of variable magnitude, a situation that probably is compounded by the mechanical age in which we live.

The Intervertebral Disc

The intervertebral disc is subjected not only to compression but to other types of loads as well. Since rotation and bending in general are known to be coupled, the stresses in the disc are thus a combination of tension, compression, and shear.

As discussed previously, the intervertebral disc is organized into an outer fibrous anulus containing several layers of obliquely oriented collagen and an inner nucleus that contains more water and proteoglycan than does the outer anulus. The hydrodynamic mechanical properties of the disc are the result of this anatomical arrangement, and they are of considerable importance to spinal motion and to load distribution throughout the vertebral column.

The water in the nucleus is incompressible and it serves to transmit applied compres-

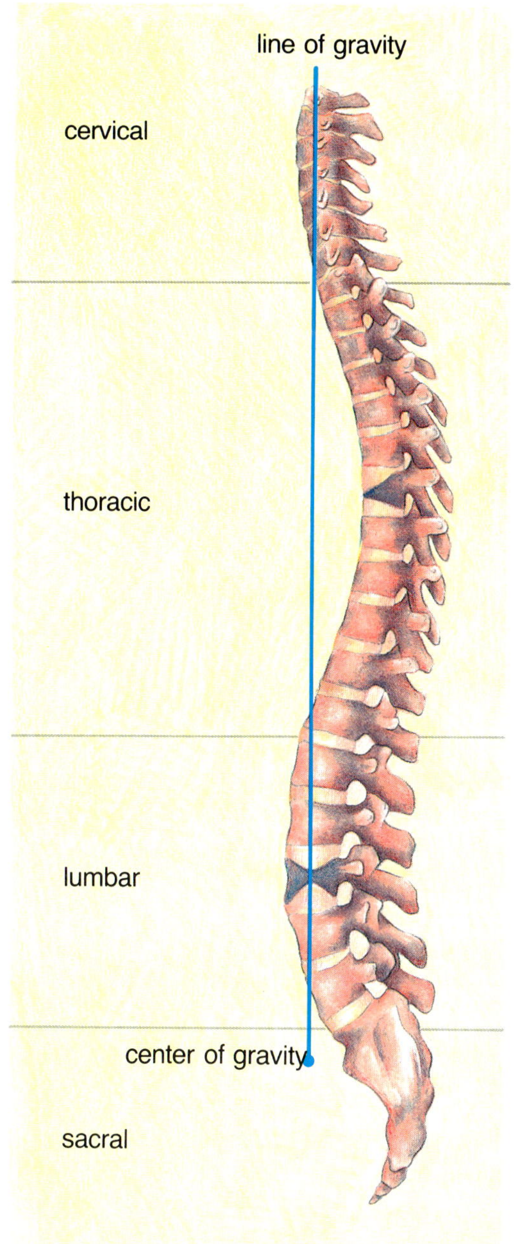

Figure 3.2 Schematic drawing to illustrate the line of gravity in relation to the spinal column. Fractures in the thoracic spine will tend to be wedge shaped anteriorly while fractures in the lumbar spine will tend to be biconcave. Fracture incidence also will be influenced by the degree of mobility and by abrupt changes in mobility, as occur at the thoracolumbar junction. The direction and degree of slippage of one vertebral body on the next also will be affected by the line of gravity.

sion forces radially, to be resisted as tension in the anular fibers, and to the vertebral body through the cartilaginous and bony end plates (Fig. 3.3). Taking the upright standing intradiscal pressure as the norm, it should be noted that a five-degree tilt will increase the pressure by 25%, unsupported sitting will increase it by 40%, and lying supine decreases the pressure by 50%. By marked forward flexion and rotation, the intradiscal pressure may increase by as much as 400% (Fig. 3.4). For these reasons, one can see how it is best to lift weights with a straight spine and bent knees thereby avoiding excessive forward spinal flexion (Fig. 3.5). The hydrodynamic properties of the disc also are present to some extent in partially degenerated discs, but not in those discs that are more severely affected.

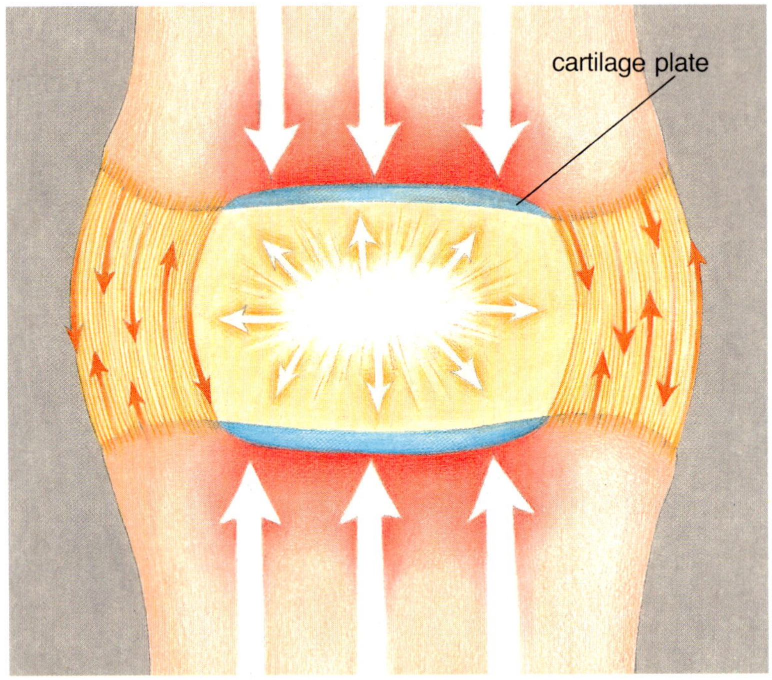

Figure 3.3 Schematic drawing of the forces acting through the area of the vertebral body and intervertebral disc. Compressive forces are transmitted through a central layer of hyaline cartilage interposed between the nucleus and bone, whereas tensional forces generated in the anulus are transmitted to the bone through Sharpey's fibers attached around the periphery.

DISC INJURY

In vitro experiments have shown that when segments of the spinal column are subjected to very high compressive loads, applied gradually, there is no injury to the fibers of the anulus. Instead, there is a tendency for the vertebral end plates to fracture with subsequent herniation of the nucleus pulposus into the adjacent vertebral body (Schmorl's node). In other words, the tensile strength of the normal anulus is greater than is the compressive strength of the vertebral bodies and their end plates. This may explain why excessive static loading of the spine results commonly in fractures of the vertebral body rather than in disc herniation.

Experimental findings suggest that the loads most damaging to disc tissue are bending and torsional loads, especially those applied suddenly, and, in marked contrast to discs subjected to compressive loads, it is those subjected to torsional loads that will demonstrate failure of the anular fibers.

With bending, the disc bulges on the concave side (Fig. 3.6). Forward flexion reduces the posterior bulge and may explain why flattening the back to reduce lumbar lordosis, and hence reduce pressure on neural tissue, is of benefit to patients with low-back pain or radicular symptoms.

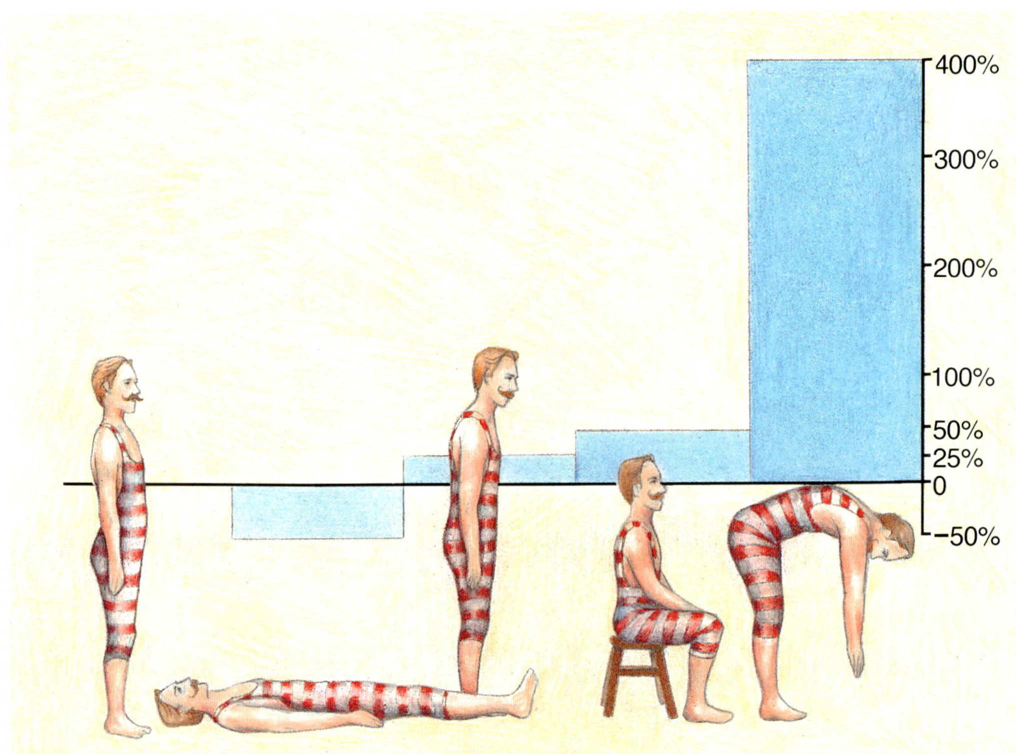

Figure 3.4 Schematic drawing to show the percentage change in load acting on the lower lumbar discs, with various positions of the body. The standing position is taken as the reference point. (Based in part on the original work of Dr. Alf Nachemson)

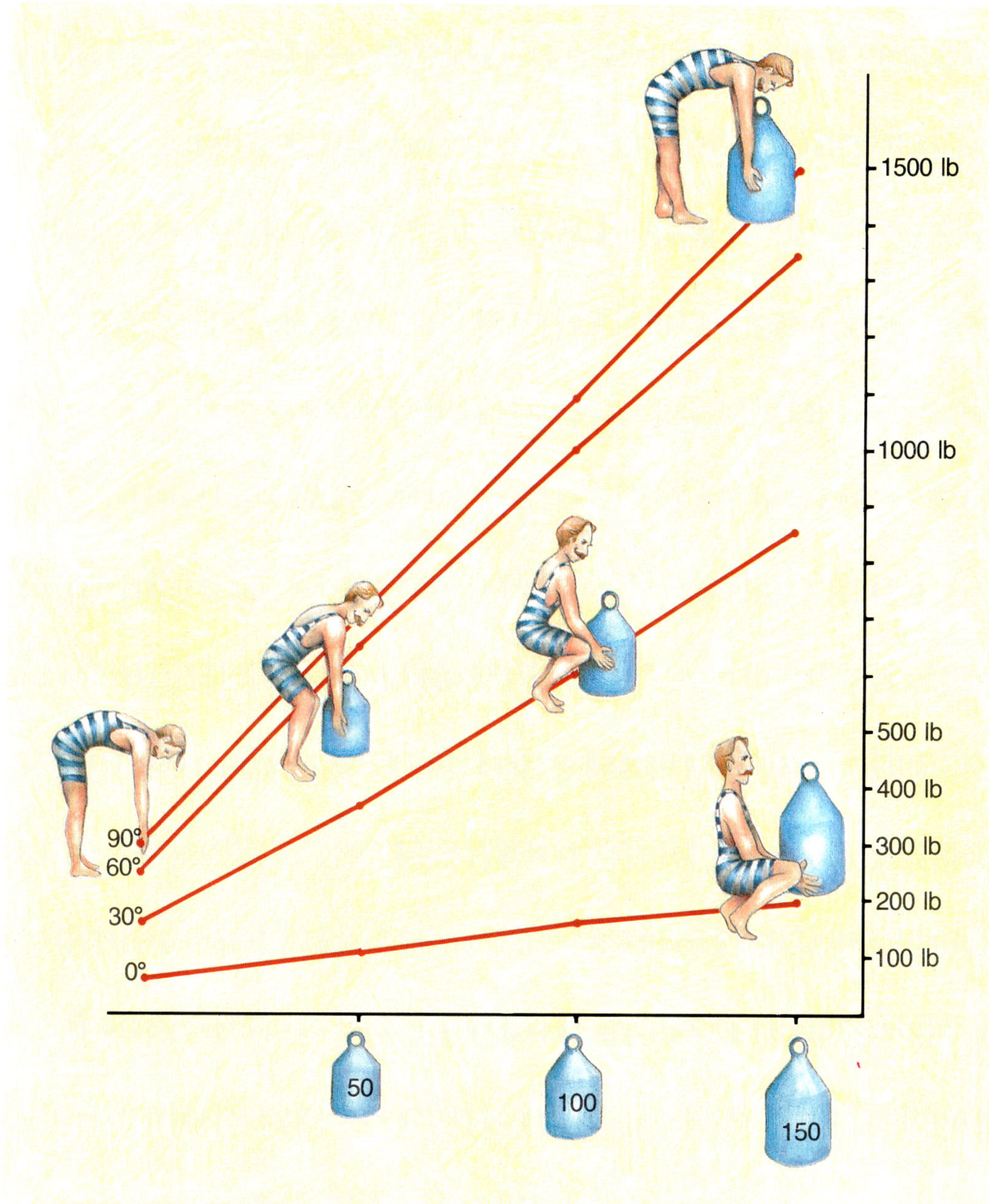

Figure 3.5 Schematic drawing to show the forces acting on the lower lumbar spine when a different-sized weight is lifted with different degrees of knee bending and spine flexion. Note that the load on the discs of the man without a weight but with forward flexion is greater than the load on the discs of the man with a 150-lb weight and a straight back. (Adapted from Schmorl, according to Münchinger)

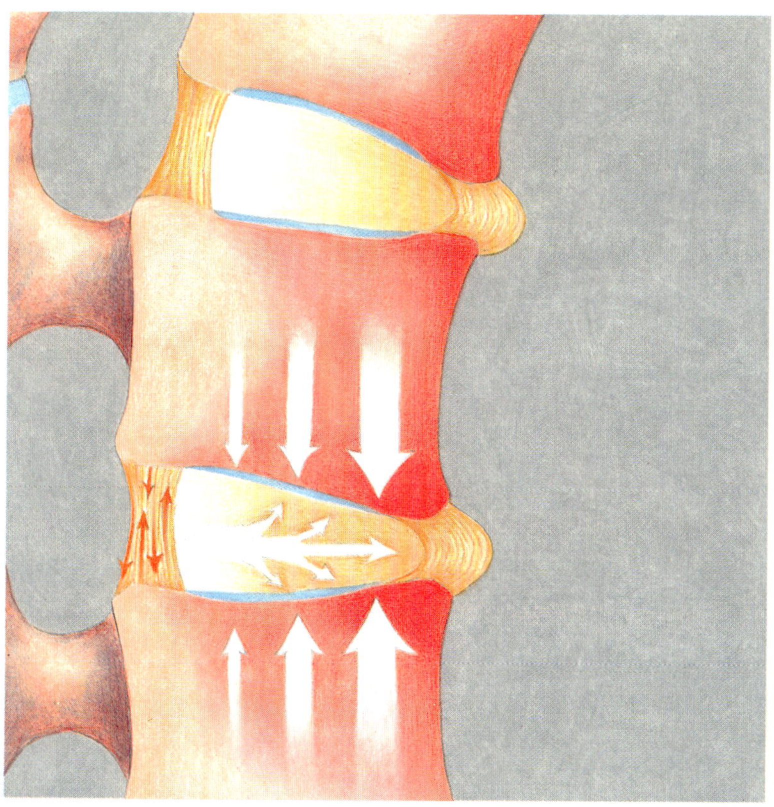

Figure 3.6 Schematic drawing to show how flexion causes the intervertebral disc to bulge in the direction of the bend.

The Facet Joints

The diarthrodial joints between the individual segments of the spine provide for both mobility and stability, and, by their arrangement, help to provide for an equitable distribution of load from the top of the spine to the bottom. These articulations (usually called apophysial joints, zygapophysial joints, or facet joints) limit the mobility between two vertebrae to a predetermined degree and direction.

The joint facets are found on the articular processes of the vertebral arches. The articular surfaces of these facets are covered by hyaline cartilage, and, at the periphery, there is an intervening fibrous meniscus interposed between the articular surfaces of the facets, similar to that found in a phalangeal joint. The joint capsules are richly supplied by nerves probably important in proprioception, and these may contribute significantly to the sensation of back pain following injury. Biomechanical studies have shown that with combined compression and bending loads, the facet joints carry from 12 to 25% of the total intervertebral load. However, Adams and Hutton (1983) have shown that disc narrowing can result in as much as 70% of the intervertebral load being transmitted across the facet joints. Therefore, excessive loads across the facet joints also can result in initiation of the osteoarthritic process and in back pain.

FACET ORIENTATION

The inclination of the apophysial joints with respect to the midline varies among individual vertebral segments (Fig. 3.7). In the cervical region the joints are relatively horizontal, the inferior facets are medially inclined, and the superior facets are laterally inclined at about 45 degrees. The nearly horizontal plane provides good support for the head through the articular pillars on either side of the vertebral bodies. When the neck is rotated, however, the supportive function of the lateral columns is weakened and in this position hyperextension injuries are more severe. In the thoracic region, the facets are more vertically inclined in the frontal plane and also are slightly medially inclined by 20 degrees. In the lumbar region, they are almost vertical and in the sagittal plane. Because of these differences in orientation, different radiographic projections are required for adequate visualization of the apophysial joints of different spinal segments. To visualize the joints in the lumbar region, an oblique projection is necessary, whereas, in the cervical and thoracic regions, a lateral projection is satisfactory.

FACET JOINT MOBILITY

Individually, the mobility of each of the spinal joints (both the discs and the apophysial joints) is not great, although, in combination, they provide the spine itself with a great range of motion. The degree of flexion-extension, lateral bending, and axial rotation varies at each level of the spinal column, as is graphically demonstrated in Figure 3.8. However, it is important to note that because of the muscular envelope surrounding the spine of a living person, the actual range of motion is substantially smaller than that of a dissected bony specimen.

In the cervical spine, about 50% of flexion and extension takes place at the atlanto-occipital joint; approximately half of the rotation takes place between the atlas and the axis with the other 50% distributed among the subaxial joints. The degree of axial rotation that is possible at C-2 can sometimes result in obstruction or kinking of the vertebral artery (especially in the presence of degenerative arthritis of the spine), with consequent cerebral hypotension and transient neurologic symptoms. These include nausea, dizziness, and occasional loss of consciousness.

In the lower cervical spine, the greatest range of motion is found at the C5-6 interspace, which might account for the high degree of cervical disc disease found at this level. Cervical lateral flexion is limited by the articular pillars and the intertransverse ligaments.

In the thoracic spine, flexion-extension is minimal at T1-2 and maximal at T-12 to L-1, whereas axial rotation is maximal at T1-2 and minimal in the lower three levels.

The orientation of the facet joints in the lumbar spine permits forward flexion and lateral flexion and extension, but limits rotation.

The synovial articulations of the lumbosacral junction are unique in that the facets of the inferior articular process of L-5 face forward and downward to engage the backward- and upward-facing sacral facet (Fig. 3.9). Because of this orientation, some rotation is permitted at the lumbosacral junction, in contrast to the lack of rotation at the more superior lumbar joints. The lumbosacral ar-

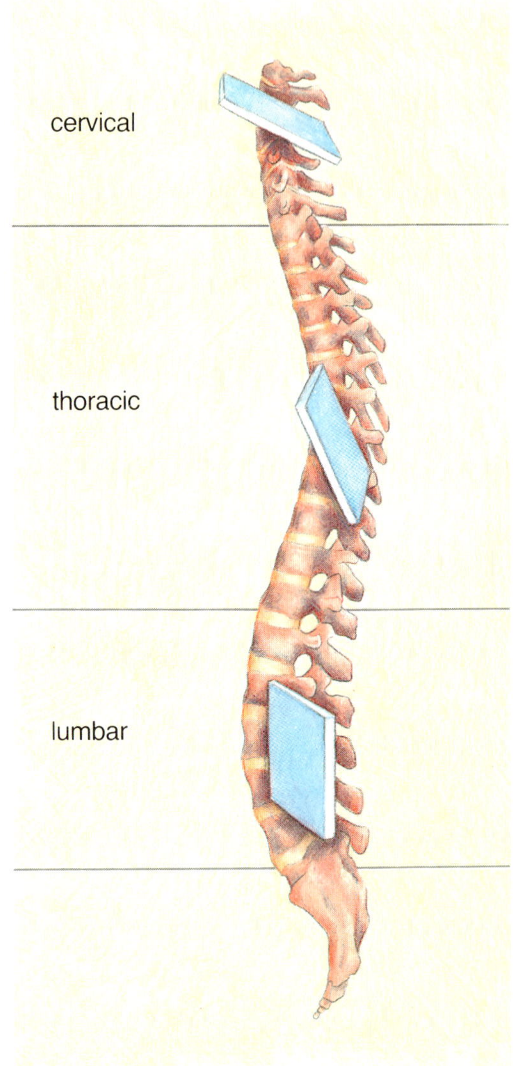

Figure 3.7 Schematic drawing to illustrate the principal orientation of the facet joints at different levels of the spinal column. These differences affect both load bearing and motion between vertebral bodies.

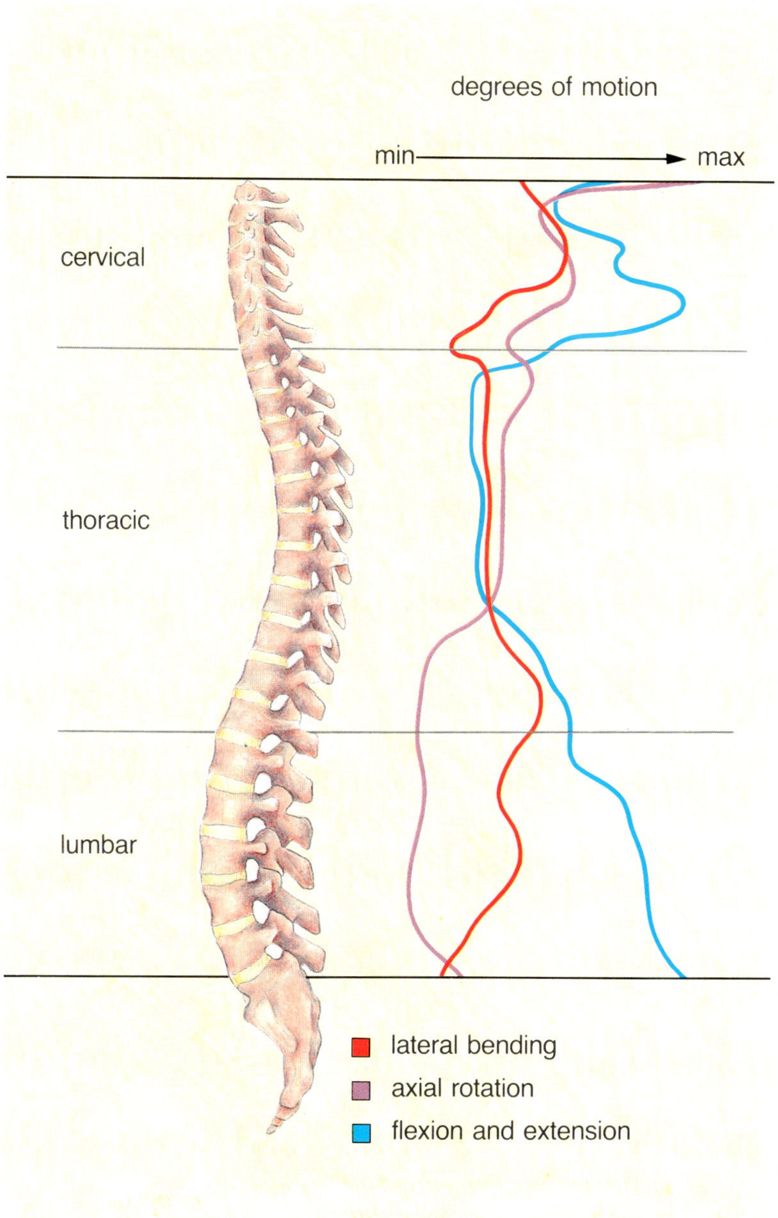

Figure 3.8 Schematic drawing to illustrate estimated degrees of spinal mobility at each level of the vertebral column of a living person (as derived from dissected specimens). The degree of motion is affected by ligaments and other attachments, as well as by facet joint orientation.

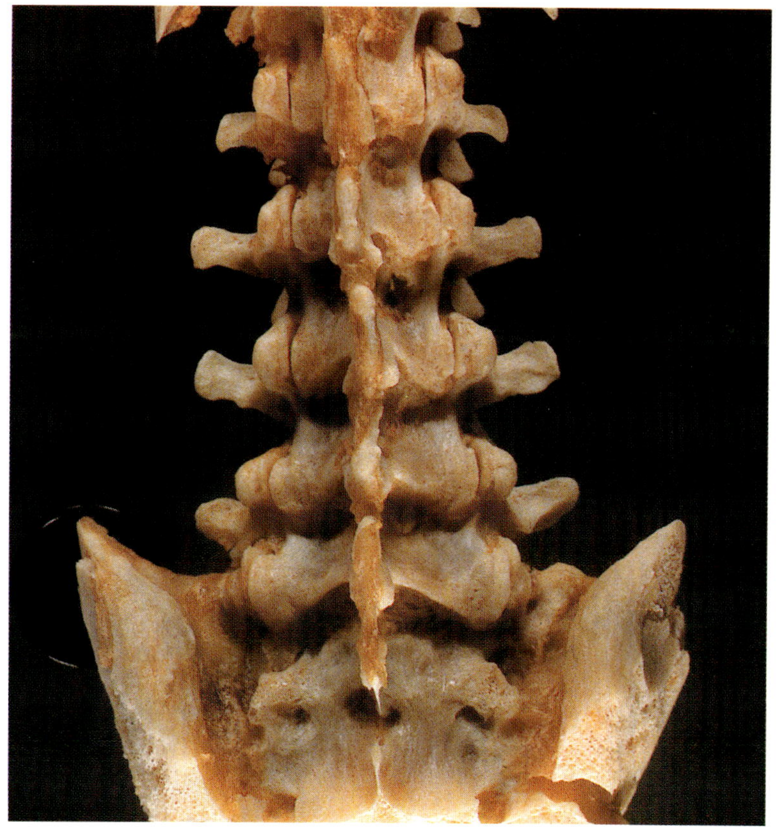

Figure 3.9 Photograph showing a posterior view of a macerated lumbosacral spine. Note the sagittal orientation of the lumbar facets as compared to the more anteriorly inclined lumbosacral facet.

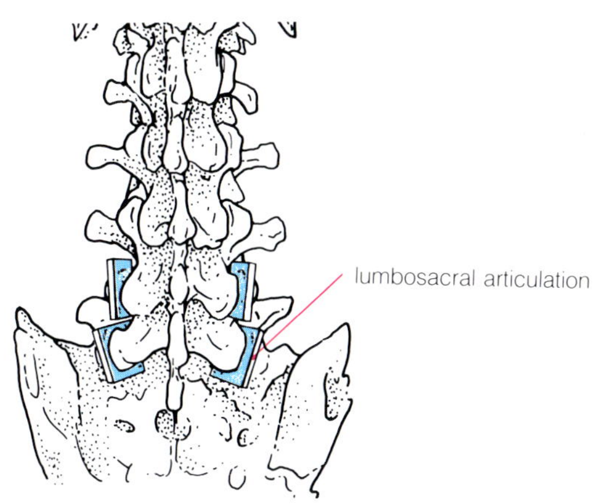

ticulations serve also as buttresses against forward and downward displacement of L-5 in relation to the sacrum.

It is not unreasonable to speculate that the high incidence of clinical disc disease found in the lower lumbar spine is related to the fact that L4-5 and L-5 to S-1 bear the greatest loads and tend to undergo the most motion.

The Sacroiliac Joints

The connection between the sacrum and the ilium occurs through the wedge-shaped sacroiliac joint, which locks the spine into the pelvis. The surfaces of this joint are covered by cartilage that is thicker on the sacral side than it is on the ilial side, and the facing surfaces are so irregular as to be secured against shearing. The support of the sacrum and the ilium is maintained by the posterior ligamentous mass, which connects the sacrum to the pelvis.

A small amount of anteroposterior rotatory movement occurs at the sacroiliac joint during flexion and extension, and this movement undergoes a slight temporary increase during pregnancy. The largest change in position of the sacrum relative to the ilium occurs in the standing position, when the sacral promontory moves as much as 5–6 mm forward as the weight of the body is taken upon the sacrum and transferred to the ilium. The sacrotuberous and sacrospinous ligaments oppose upward motion of the sacrum while tilting the lower portion of the sacrum under the downward thrust that is imparted to the upper portions of the sacrum by the body weight.

The Spinal Ligaments

The ligaments of the spine must allow for adequate motion while providing for fixed postural attitudes between vertebrae. The ligaments must protect the spinal cord by restricting motion during daily activities, and, in addition, must protect against the fast application of high loads.

Ligaments resist only tensile forces and buckle when subject to compression, and since ligaments transfer their tensile loads to the bone, a traumatic load may result in injury to either the bone or the ligament. In general, when an excess load is applied slowly, it is the bone that fails; when it is applied rapidly, it is the ligament that fails (Fig. 3.10). At laminectomy, for example, one frequently sees histologic evidence of tearing and scarring in the ligamentum flavum, and

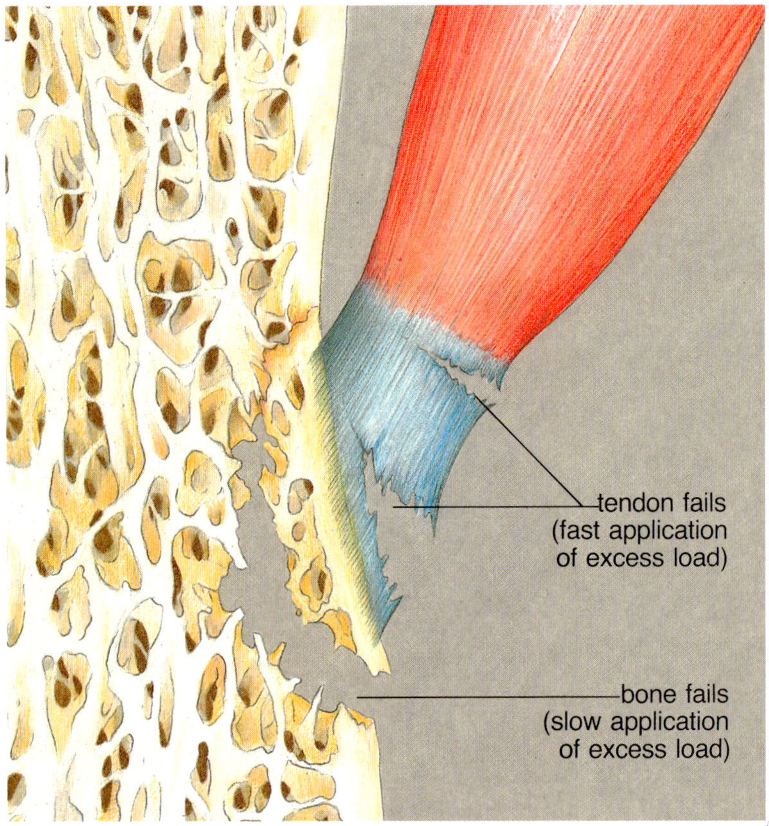

Figure 3.10 Schematic drawing to show the transfer of traumatic load from a tendon to a bone. An excess load applied slowly will result in bone failure while an excess load applied rapidly will tear the ligament, typically in one of two places: either close to the bone or close to the muscle junction. The tendon is attached to the bone by fibers that upon entering the bone form a calcified mass of interlocking fibers and bone.

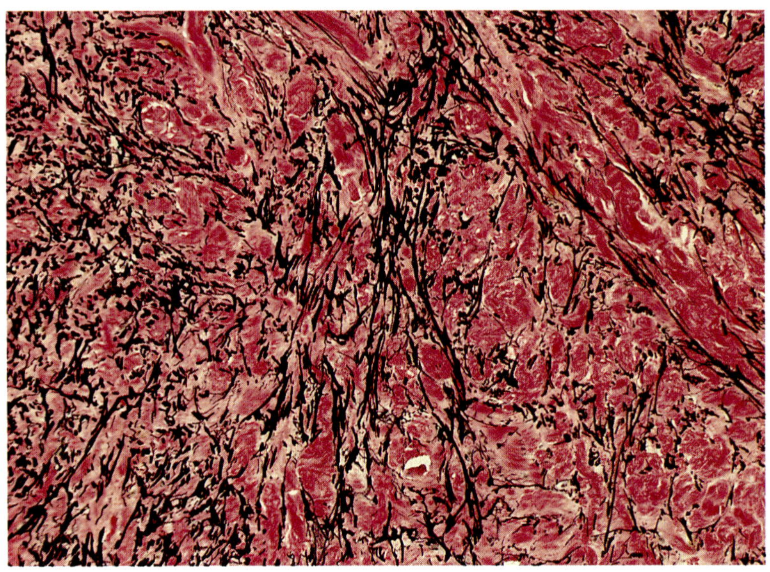

Figure 3.11 Photomicrograph of scarred ligamentum flavum tissue obtained at laminectomy. Note the elastic fibers in disarray and the increased amount of collagenous tissue, in comparison to the sample presented in Figure 2.48. (Verhoeff-van Gieson elastic tissue stain, ×4 objective, approximately 100 magnifications)

such scarring may be an important source of pain in this region (Fig. 3.11).

Biomechanical studies have led to a number of conclusions regarding the spinal ligaments. In the physiologic range of motion, a relatively small force is required to move the spine and not much energy is expended. This ease of movement with low ligamentous stiffness, however, is limited by the relatively stiff behavior of the ligaments outside of the physiologic range. In the traumatic range of loads to the spine, the stiffness values in the ligaments are perhaps 75 times greater than those of the physiologic range of loading, and nearly seven times more energy is absorbed by the ligaments in moving the spine.

In general, flexion is the most pronounced movement of the vertebral column as a whole. It results in anterior compression of the disc and in sliding separation of the articular facets. This movement is checked by the posterior ligaments (the posterior longitudinal ligament, the ligamentum flavum, and the supraspinous and interspinous ligaments) and by the paraspinal muscles. Extension is checked by the anterior longitudinal ligament, by the intervertebral discs and ventral muscles, and by the laminae and spinous processes. Lateral flexion is accompanied by some rotation with sliding separation of the facet joints, and is checked mainly by the intertransverse ligaments, and, in the thoracic segments, by the rib margins.

Protection of the Spinal Cord

Protection of the spinal cord is crucial to survival. In general, the spinal canal is lengthened during flexion and shortened during extension. To accommodate for these changes in length, a corresponding change in spinal cord length is provided by a folding and unfolding of the cord in a fashion similar to that of an accordian. However, at the limits of flexion and extension, some actual elastic deformation of the cord occurs.

The spinal cord is fixed caudally by the filum terminale and is suspended from the dura mater by the dentate ligaments (Fig. 3.12). During flexion, the cord, its nerve roots, and the dentate ligaments are under tension. However, because the dentate ligaments are inclined laterally and caudally from the cord to the dura, they maintain the central position of the cord within the canal with flexion and extension, and, moreover, in flexion they limit the extension of the cord. With movement of the spine also occur changes in the dimensions of the intervertebral foramina—changes that may result in entrapment of the nerve roots and their associated structures in the intervertebral canal.

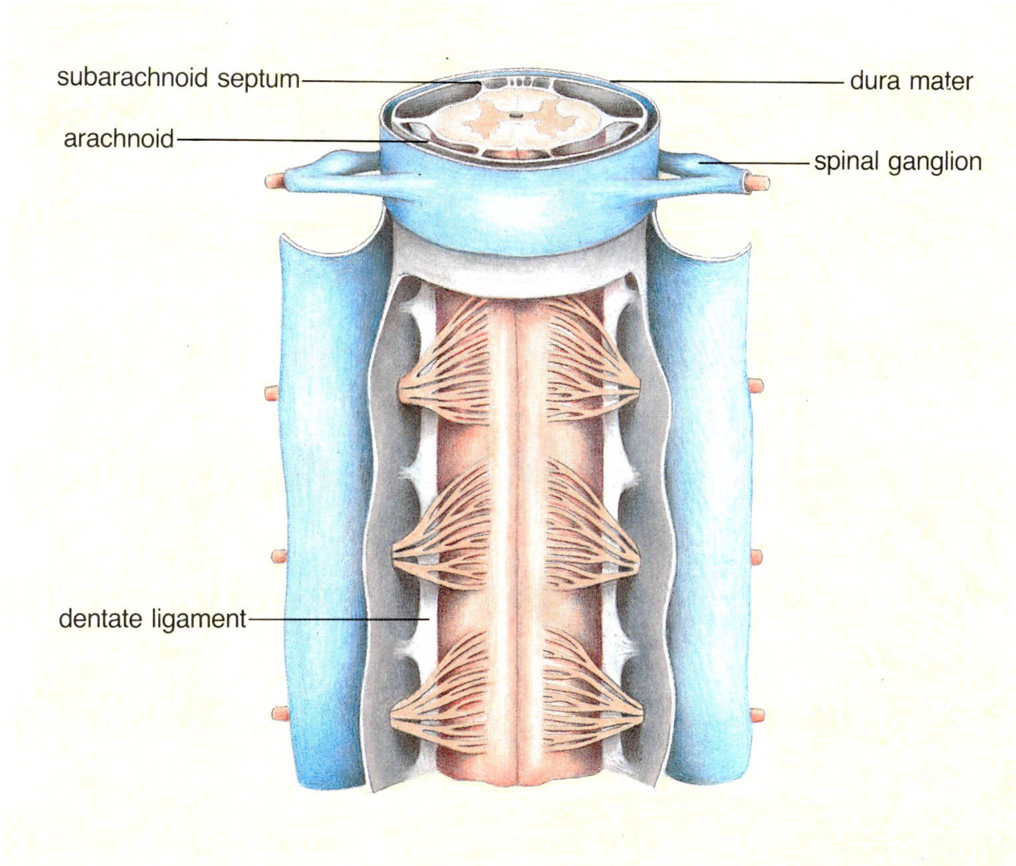

Figure 3.12 Schematic drawing to show the dentate ligaments as they appear in the spinal canal. They are notched to allow fusion of the ventral and dorsal nerve roots, and, together with the subarachnoid septa, they maintain the central position of the spinal cord in the canal during movement.

4 CHAPTER

DEVELOPMENTAL ANATOMY

The Notochord and Segmental Origins of the Spine

The notochord forms between the second and third weeks of gestation, when the neurenteric canal fuses with the adjacent endoderm. The notochord provides for the axial orientation of the early embryo, and it plays a decisive role in the development and segmentation of the vertebral column in that it is responsible for induction of the mesoderm and neuroectoderm.

Mesenchymal cells from the most medial portion of the mesodermal somites migrate ventrally to surround the notochord and dorsally to surround the neural tube, thus providing for the future vertebral column and posterior neural arches. These mesenchymal cells eventually fuse anteriorly and posteriorly to form segmented blocks of cells that completely surround the notochord and from which the segmented cartilaginous model of the vertebral column will develop (Fig. 4.1).

Through mitotic divisions, the cells of the primordial vertebral segments around the notochord (the *sclerotomes*) proliferate, with the caudal half of one primordial vertebral segment growing to meet the cranial half of the subjacent one. The vertebral bodies, intersegmental in origin, are formed from adjacent primordial vertebral segments (the top half of one and the bottom half of another) that fuse and undergo chondrification at about the fifth or sixth week of gestation. Thus, the intervertebral disc is a segmental structure that develops from the middle portion of the condensed primordial vertebral segment. This is why the segmented spinal nerves generally are on a level with the intervertebral discs (Fig. 4.2).

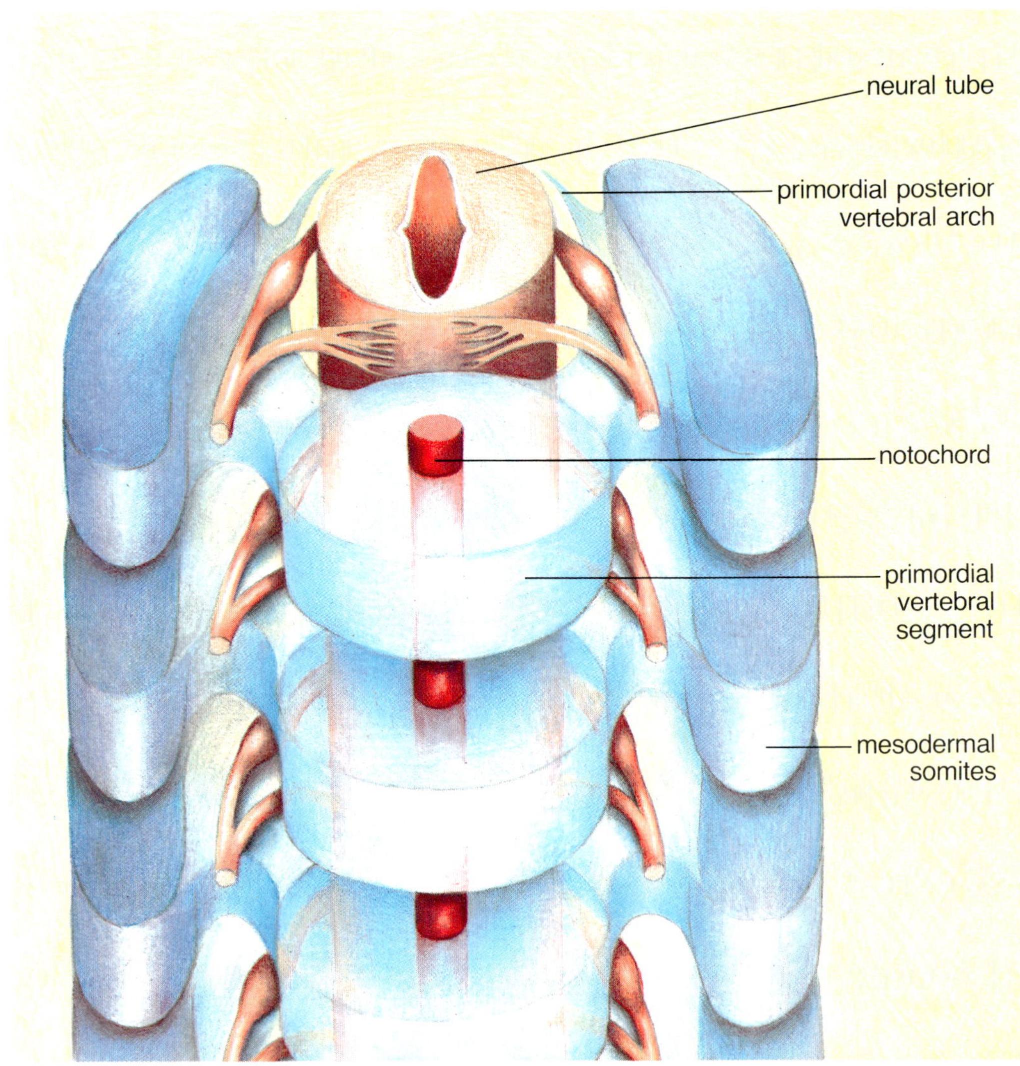

Figure 4.1 Schematic drawing to show the formation of the segmented precartilaginous anlagen of the vertebral column and posterior vertebral arches from the segmented mesodermal somites.

The Growth and Ossification of the Spine

NOTOCHORDAL REGRESSION

In the precartilaginous and early cartilaginous development of the vertebral column, the notochord is an undivided rod that passes through the developing vertebral bodies and intervertebral discs (Fig. 4.3). At approximately the same time as when ossification

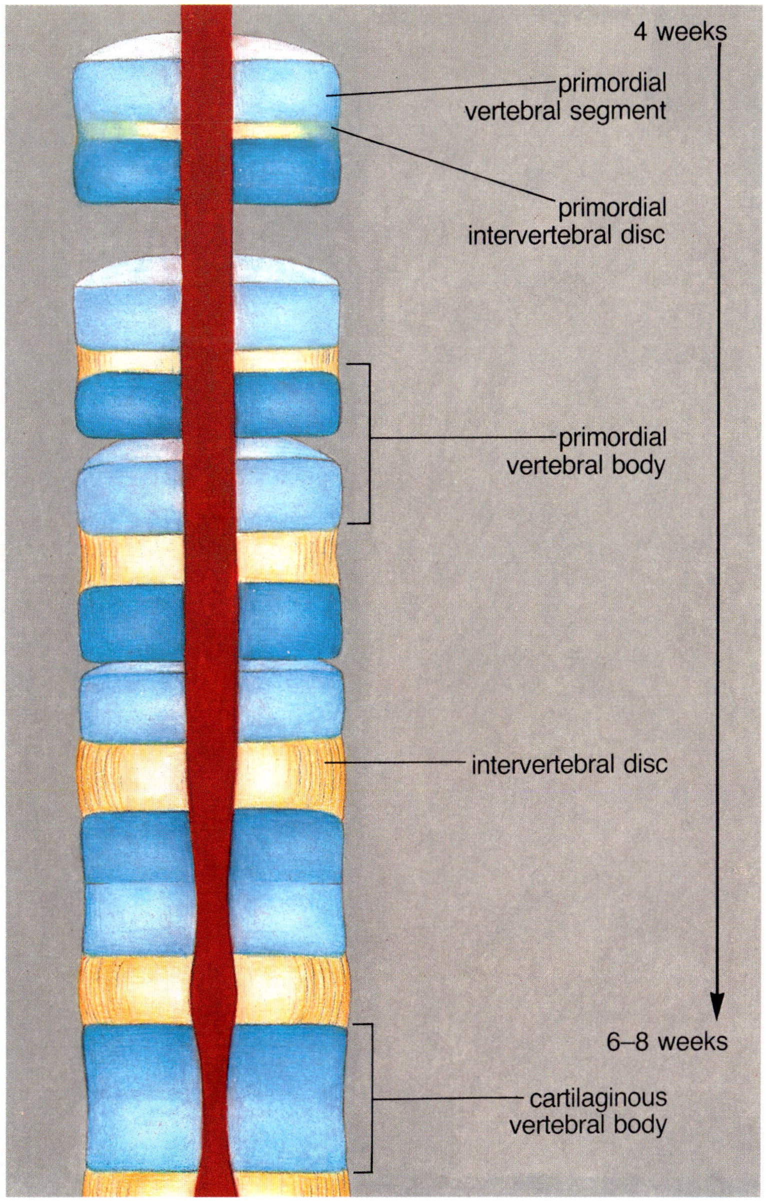

Figure 4.2 Schematic drawing to show the segmental origins of the intervertebral discs and the intersegmental origins of the vertebral bodies from the primordial vertebral segments surrounding the notochord.

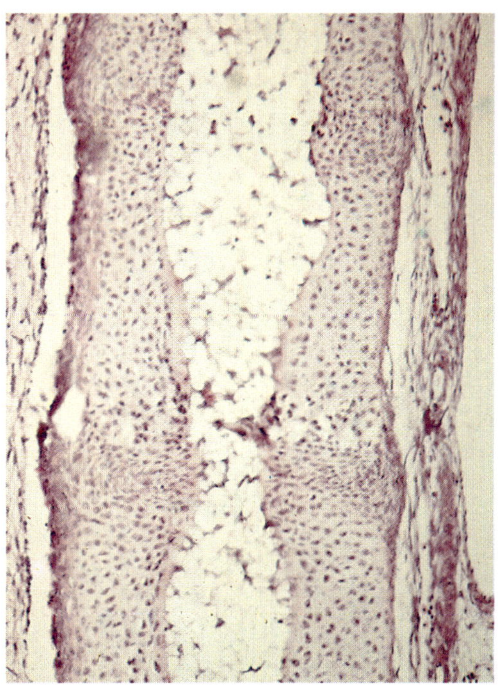

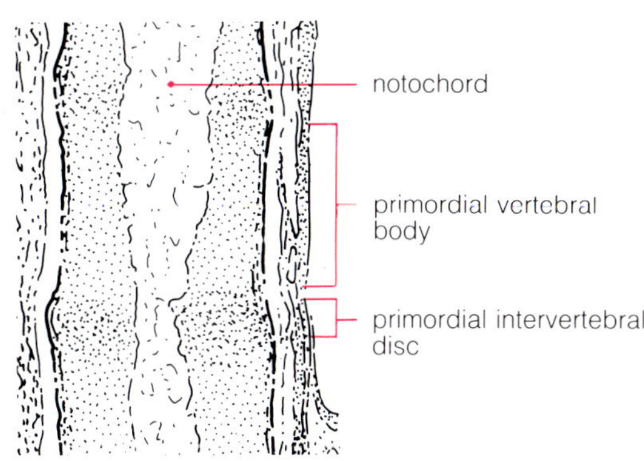

Figure 4.3 Photomicrograph of a sagittal section through the developing vertebral column, showing the notochord and the primordial vertebral bodies and the intervertebral discs. (H & E stain, ×4 objective, approximately 100 magnifications)

appears in the cartilaginous vertebral bodies, so the notochord begins to break up and regress (Fig. 4.4). Portions of the notochord, however, persist longer in the central part of the intervertebral disc and may contribute to the development of the nucleus pulposus (Fig. 4.5).

Small islands of residual notochordal tissue, so-called *ecchordosis physaliphora,* may be found in the intervertebral discs of adults and may eventually give rise to the formation of a neoplasm, or *chordoma*. Although these tumors are found most often in the region of the sacrum or in the clivus, they may appear in the cervical spine and in the thoracic or lumbar spine, though rarely.

DEVELOPMENT OF THE VERTEBRAL BODIES

Ossification of the vertebral bodies occurs first in the lower thoracic and upper lumbar spine, appearing in the third month of embryonic life (Fig. 4.6). By the end of the fourth month, ossification centers have appeared in all the vertebral bodies.

In the newborn, the ossification centers of the vertebral bodies are ovoid, and, on a lateral radiograph, small indentations are present both anteriorly and posteriorly and are associated with a linear radiolucency passing horizontally through the center of each body (Fig. 4.7). These indentations and

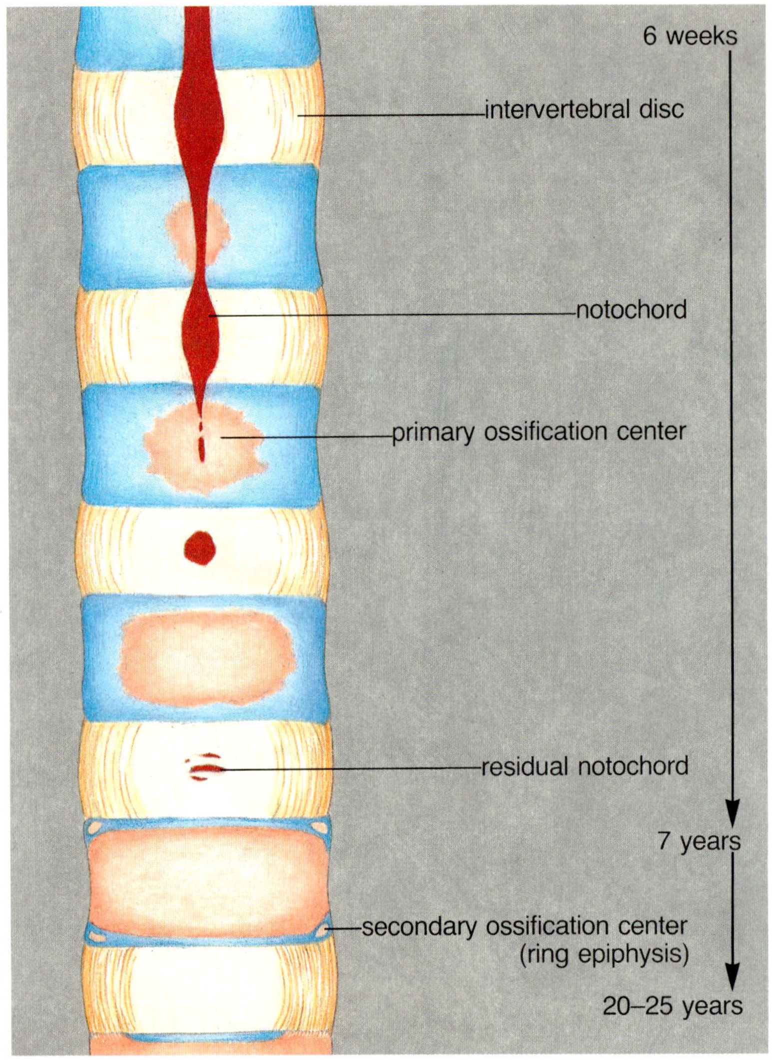

Figure 4.4 Schematic drawing to show regression of the notochord as ossification proceeds. (Adapted from Schmorl G, Junghanns H: *The Human Spine in Health and Disease*. Am. ed. 2. New York, Grune & Stratton Inc., 1971, p. 3)

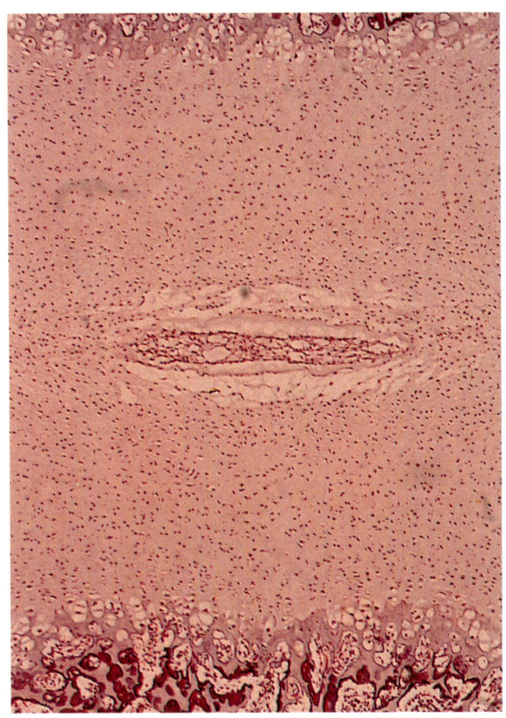

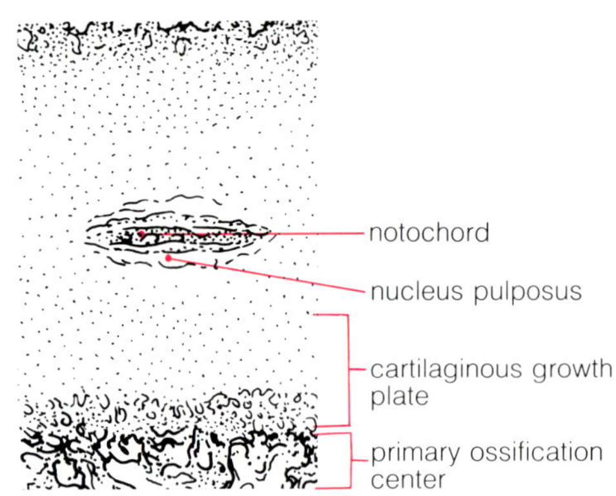

Figure 4.5 Photomicrograph of a sagittal section of a portion of two vertebral bodies from a 28-week-old fetus, with intervening presumptive intervertebral disc. Note the residual notochordal tissue appearing in the position of the future nucleus pulposus. (H & E stain, × 2.5 objective, approximately 30 magnifications)

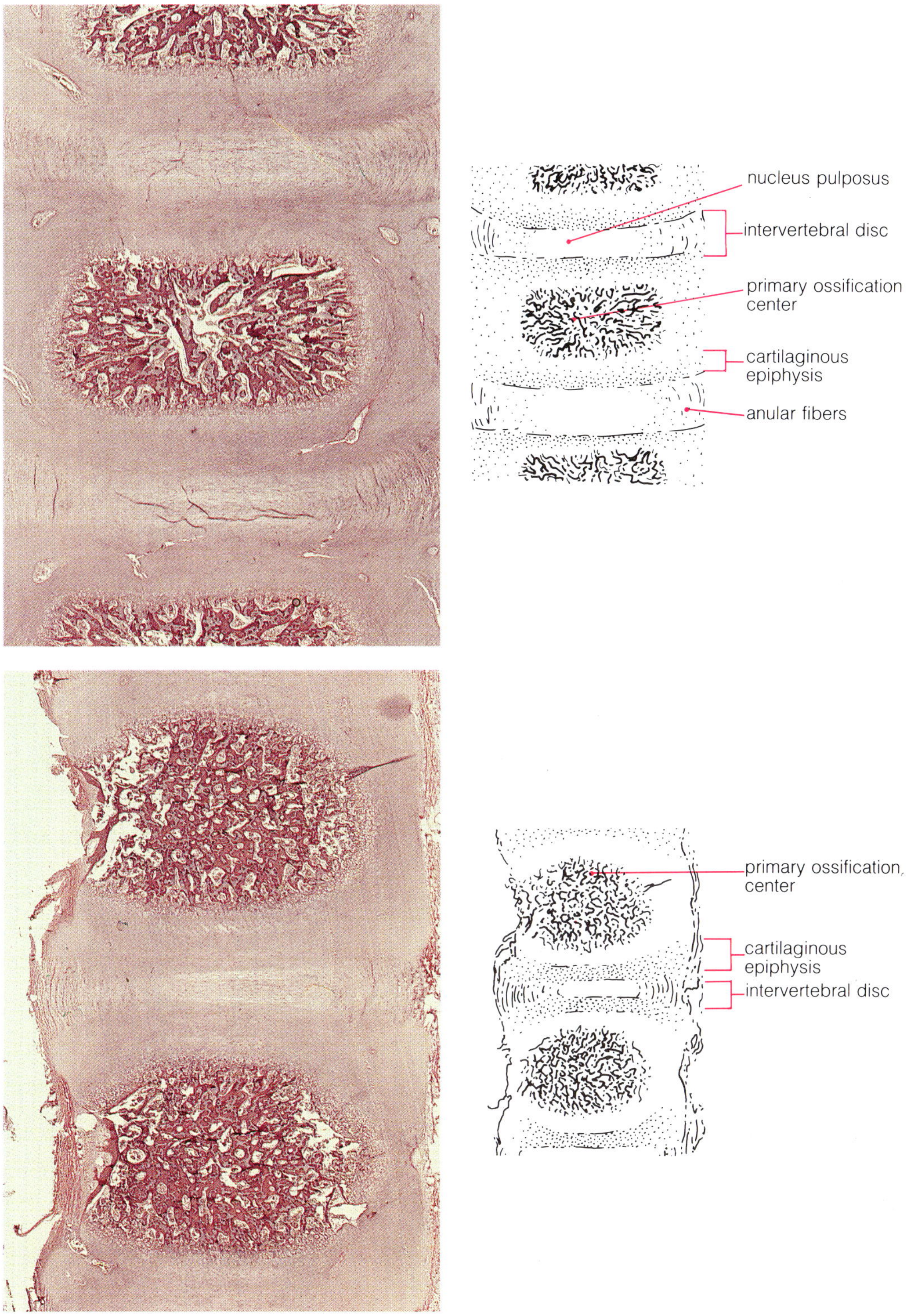

Figure 4.6 Photograph (*top*) of a frontal section through L-1 from a 28-week-old fetus, showing the ossification center. Note that, in this view, endochondral ossification, i.e., growth, appears to be taking place all around the periphery. Photograph (*bottom*) of a sagittal section through the same specimen. In this section note that the ossification centers are not located centrally in the vertebral body, as suggested by the top photograph, but in fact are located anteriorly (to the left in the photograph), with endochondral ossification occurring more on the posterior aspect as well as superiorly and inferiorly. (H & E stain, approximately 20 magnifications)

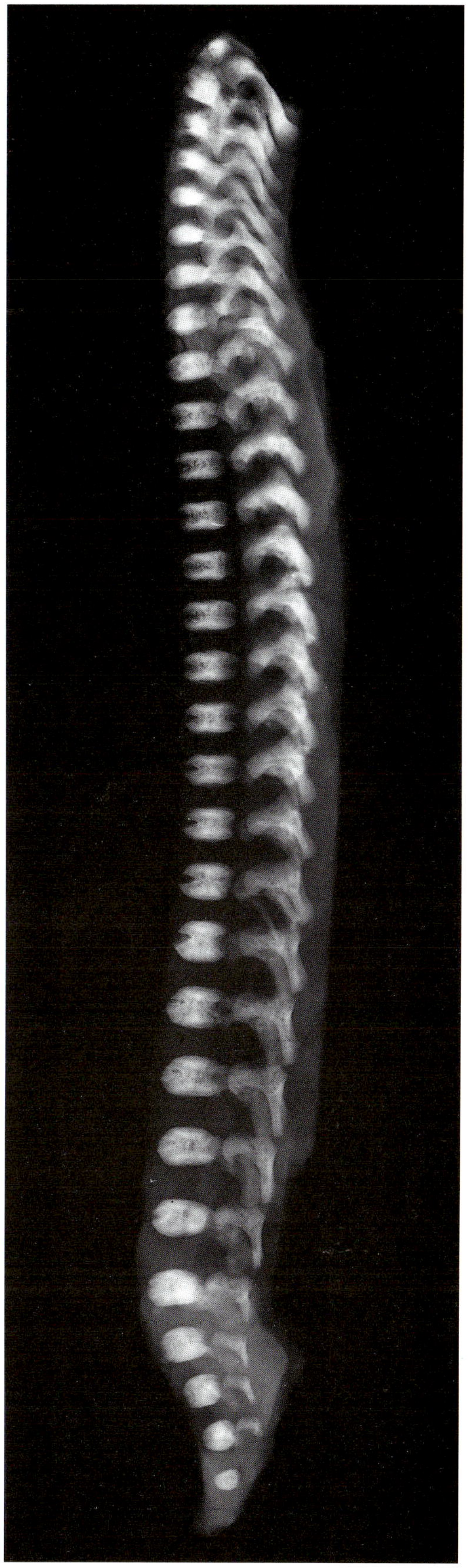

Figure 4.7 Lateral radiograph of the vertebral column of a 30-week-old stillborn. The separate centers of ossification for the vertebral bodies and posterior elements are seen clearly. Note the presence of a notch on the anterior and posterior surfaces of each vertebral body, along with a radiolucent line that passes through the bodies and results from the vascular penetration of the developing bodies.

radiolucencies are the result of the vascular channels passing through the ossification centers (Fig. 4.8).

At birth, the lumbar vertebral body is approximately equal in thickness to the intervening intervertebral space, which is formed not only of intervertebral disc tissue but also of the as yet unossified cartilage of the vertebral bodies (Fig. 4.9). This can be seen in Figure 4.7 above, where the intervertebral spaces (comprised of both disc tissue and growth cartilage) are almost equal in thickness to the ovoid vertebral bodies.

On the upper and lower surfaces of the vertebral body is a layer of hyaline cartilage interposed between the vertebral body and the intervertebral disc. Like the lid on a jam pot, this layer fits into the vertebral body to provide a firm lock between the disc and the body (Fig. 4.10).

As the vertebral bodies grow, they become more rectangular and their height increases in comparison to that of the disc space, which radiographically appears to narrow. As growth continues, one can see steplike unossified recesses appearing on the anterior edges of the vertebral bodies in both the sagittal section of the gross specimen and in the lateral radiographic projection (Fig. 4.11). These steplike recesses, also seen on AP view, are due to the presence of a cartilaginous rim that is deeper anteriorly than it is posteriorly or laterally.

A macerated vertebral body at about age 8 or 9 will clearly show undulating margins on its superior and inferior surfaces (particularly on the anterior and lateral edges) with the formation of radially disposed grooves (Fig. 4.12). These grooves allow for the interlocking of multiple secondary centers of ossification that now begin to appear in the cartilaginous rim described above. These multiple secondary ossification centers surround the edges of the vertebral body like a

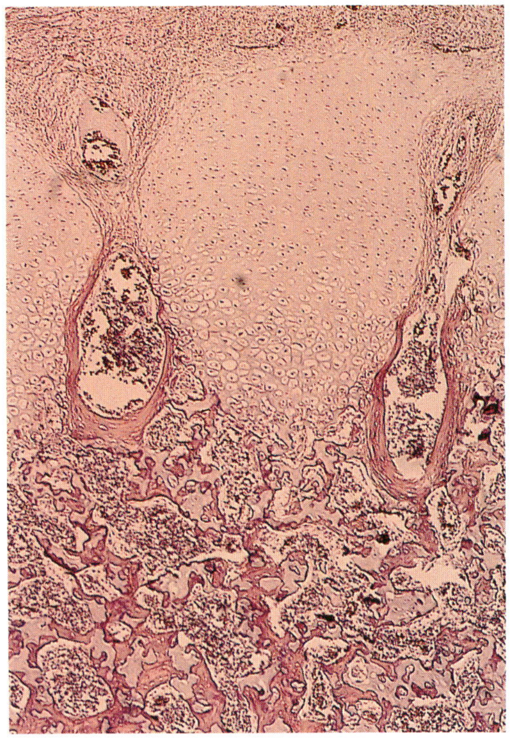

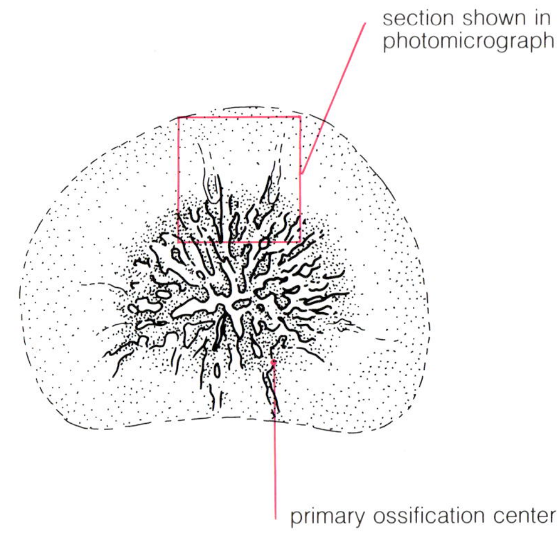

Figure 4.8 Photomicrograph of a transverse section through the mid-portion of the anterior half of a vertebral body, showing the large paired blood vessels that perforate the cartilage to feed the ossification center. (H & E stain, × 4 objective, approximately 100 magnifications)

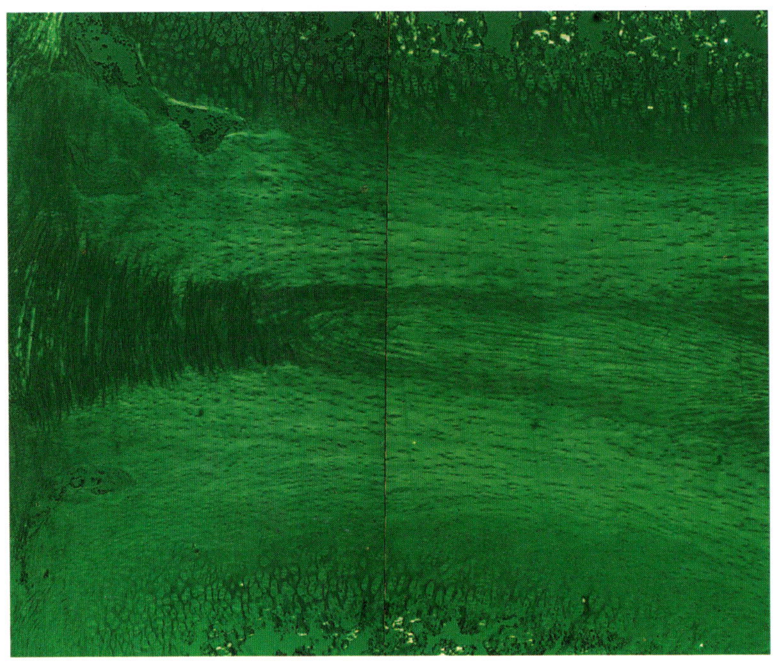

Figure 4.9 Photomicrograph of a frontal section of the intervertebral disc area with the adjacent cartilaginous components of the vertebral bodies on either side. (Polarized light, ×4 objective, approximately 100 magnifications)

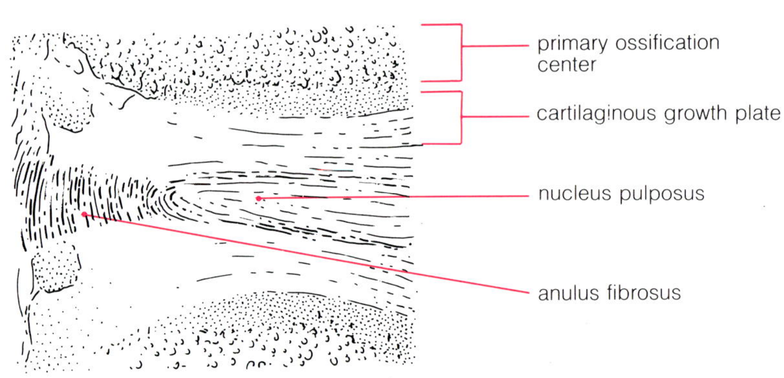

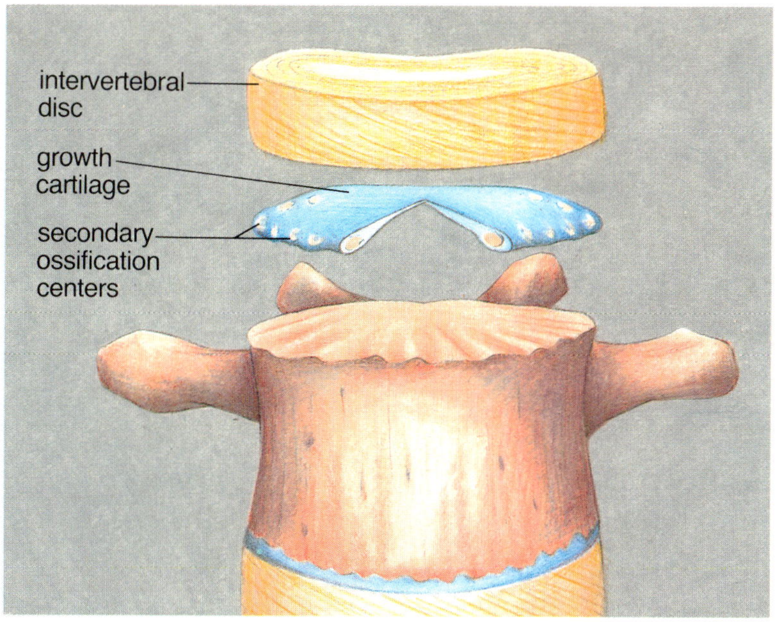

Figure 4.10 Schematic drawing of the vertebral body and intervertebral disc area to show the growth cartilage interposed between the disc and the bony vertebra. Note that the growth cartilage fits onto the bone like a lid top.

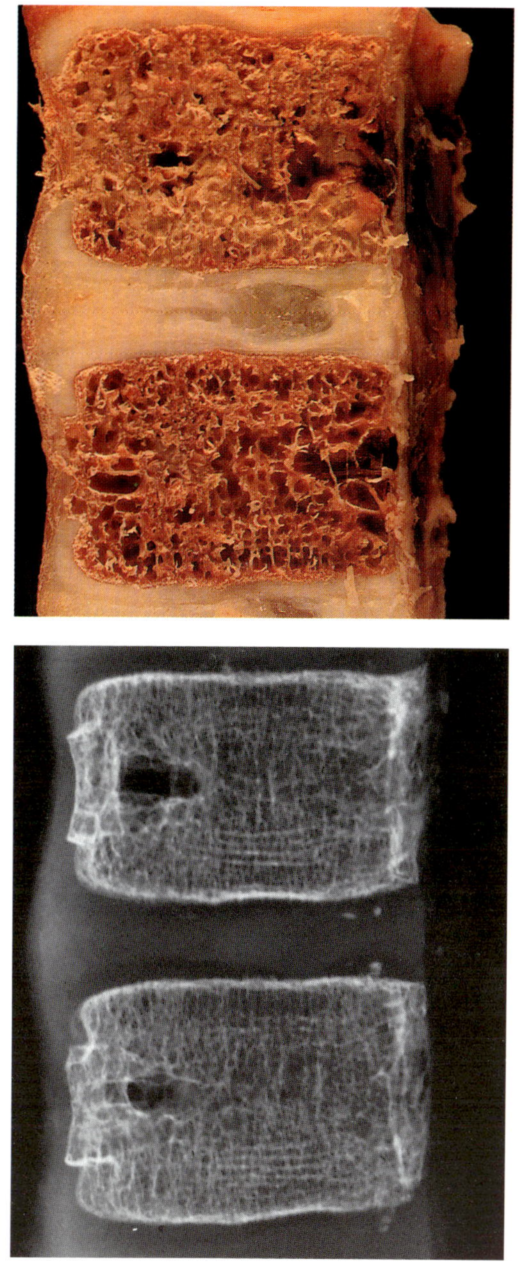

Figure 4.11 Photograph (*top*) of a sagittal section through a segment of thoracic spine from a $7\frac{1}{2}$-year-old female. Note that there is a steplike recess on both the anterosuperior and anteroinferior portions of the vertebral body into which the cartilage of the disc space projects. A radiograph (*bottom*) of the same specimen also shows steplike recesses in the peripheral margins of the vertebral bodies, representing the cartilaginous rim.

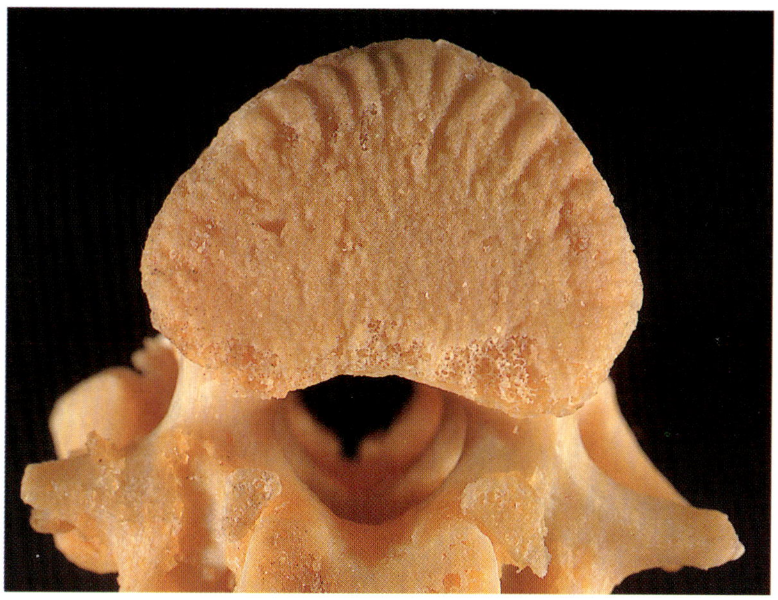

Figure 4.12 Photograph of the superior surface of a vertebral body from a 12-year-old male. Note the appearance of radially disposed grooves (especially along the anterior margin) that serve to lock the growth cartilage, with its peripheral secondary centers of ossification, to the underlying vertebral body.

string of beads and are known as vertebral ring epiphyses (Fig. 4.13).

The vertebral ring epiphyses are initiated, in girls, between the ages of 6 and 8, and, in boys, between ages 7 and 9. By age 12, in both boys and girls, these separate centers of ossification have fused into a unified bony rim (Fig. 4.14). At about age 15, this rim begins to fuse with the underlying vertebral body. Completion of this fusion process may not occur until about age 22 (Fig. 4.15).

DEVELOPMENT OF THE END PLATE

The central part of the cartilaginous epiphysis appears to fuse much earlier than does the ring epiphysis, forming a dense bony end plate that in many specimens from adolescents and young adults appears to form a double line (Fig. 4.16). As discussed in Chapter 3 of this section, it is the central portion of the vertebral surface that is subjected to compressive loads transmitted by the nucleus pulposus while the peripheral portion, in the region of the ring epiphysis, is subjected to tensional forces from the anulus fibrosus. Interruptions in the proper development of the vertebral epiphysis will result in spinal disease, to be discussed in Sections 2 and 3.

(Occasionally, spinal radiographs of the newborn will show bony lines that run along the contour of the vertebral body surface. They are more prominent on the upper and lower surfaces than on the lateral surfaces and give the appearance of a bone within a bone. Illustrated in Figure 4.17, these lines are seen most often in the thoracic spine and may represent growth arrest, or *Harris's* lines.)

DEVELOPMENT OF THE VERTEBRAL ARCHES

The vertebral arches and their processes develop independently, and the ossification centers for the arches are separated from those of the vertebral bodies by a broad band of intervening cartilage (Figs. 4.18 and 4.19). This band of cartilage fuses between the

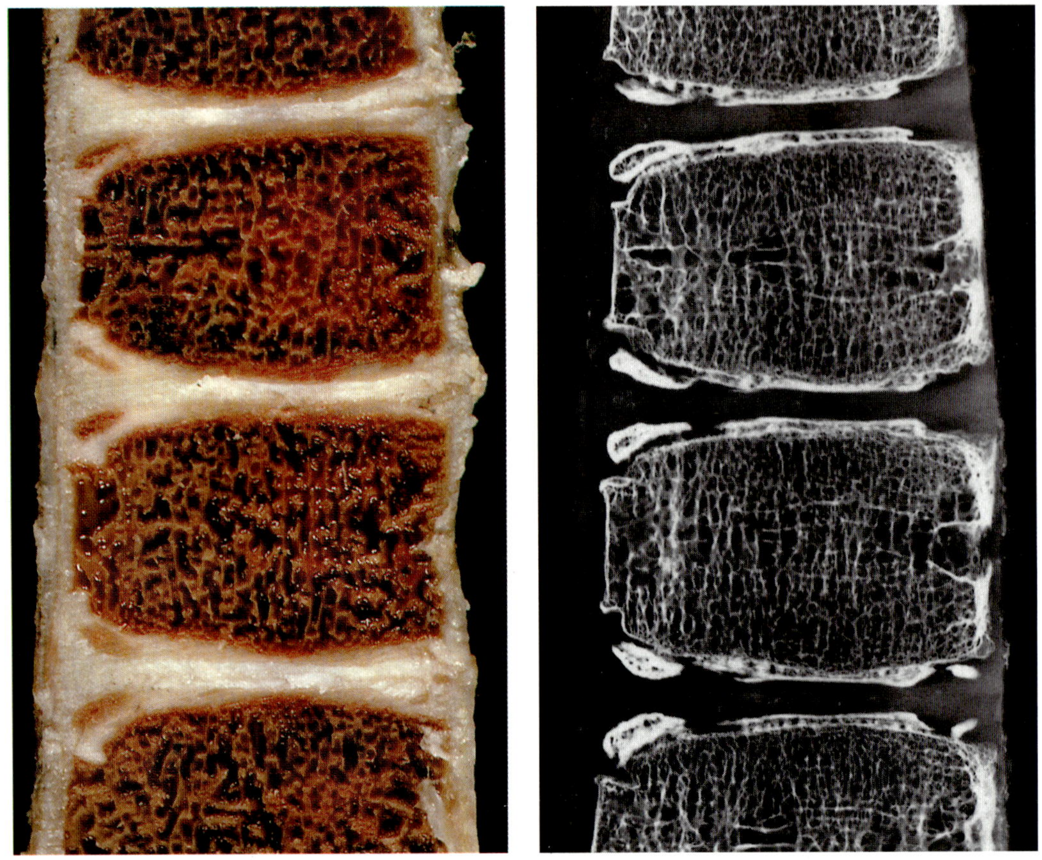

Figure 4.13 Photograph (*left*) of a sagittal section through a segment of the thoracic vertebrae from a 12-year-old male. Note the secondary ossification centers in the cartilaginous rim that comprise the ring epiphyses. A radiograph (*right*) of the same specimen clearly shows the peripheral ossification centers, in addition to the developing subchondral bone end plate that covers the central portion of the vertebral body.

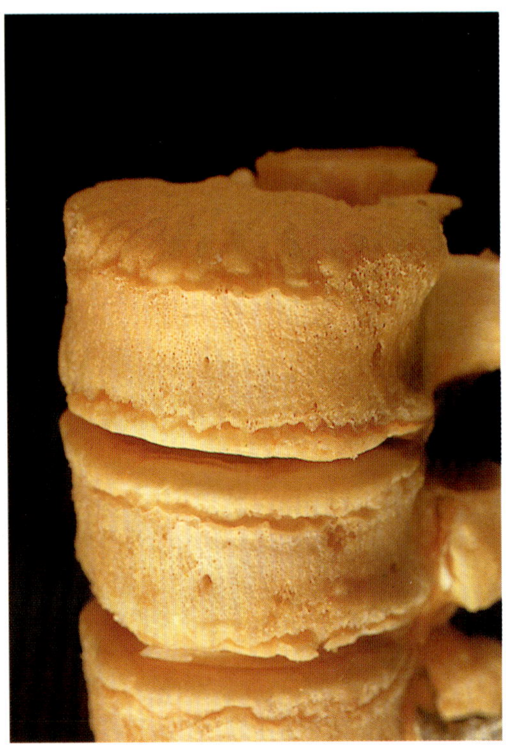

Figure 4.14 Photograph of a macerated segment of vertebral column from a 12-year-old male. Note the fused ossification centers in the ring epiphysis (covering the peripheral margins of the vertebral body), which grow to form the eventual bony rim. The superior ring epiphysis has been removed to uncover the underlying grooves shown previously in Figure 4.12.

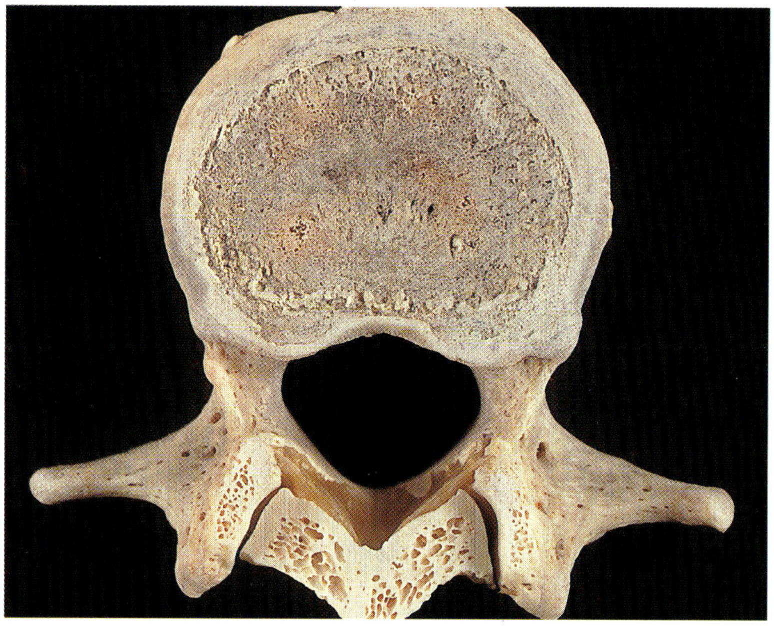

Figure 4.15 Photograph of the superior surface of a macerated vertebral body from a 27-year-old male. Note the fused vertebral ring epiphysis that forms a bony ridge around the periphery of the body. To this ridge are attached the fibers of the anulus fibrosus of the disc (Sharpey's fibers).

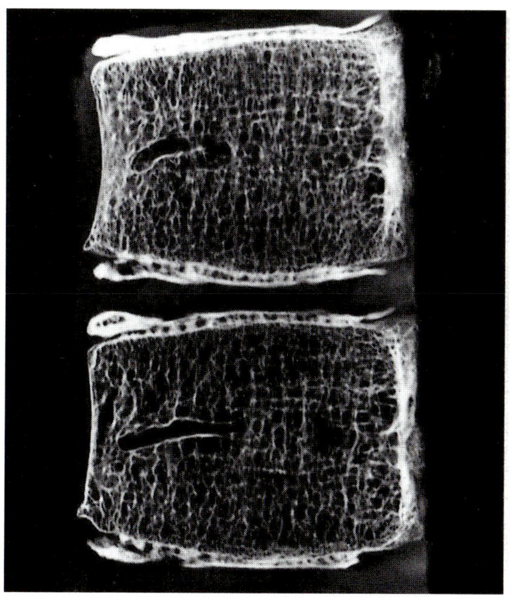

Figure 4.16 Specimen radiograph of the two upper thoracic vertebral bodies of a 12-year-old male. Note the fusion of the central part of the vertebral epiphysis.

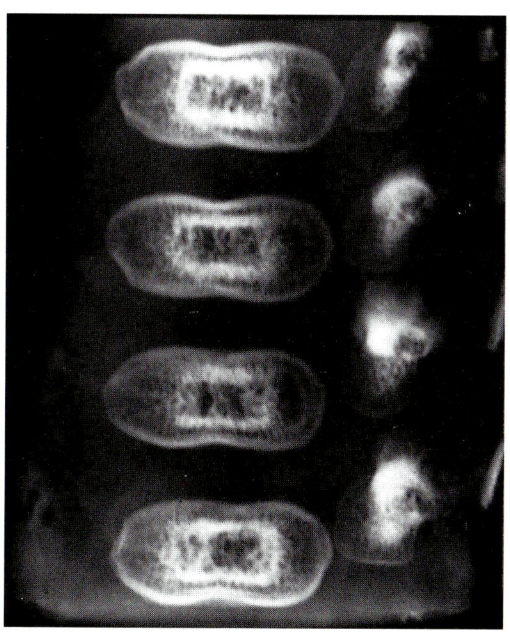

Figure 4.17 Specimen radiograph of a segment of the lower thoracic spine of a newborn to demonstrate the appearance of a bone within a bone. This finding represents growth arrest or perhaps a normal variant.

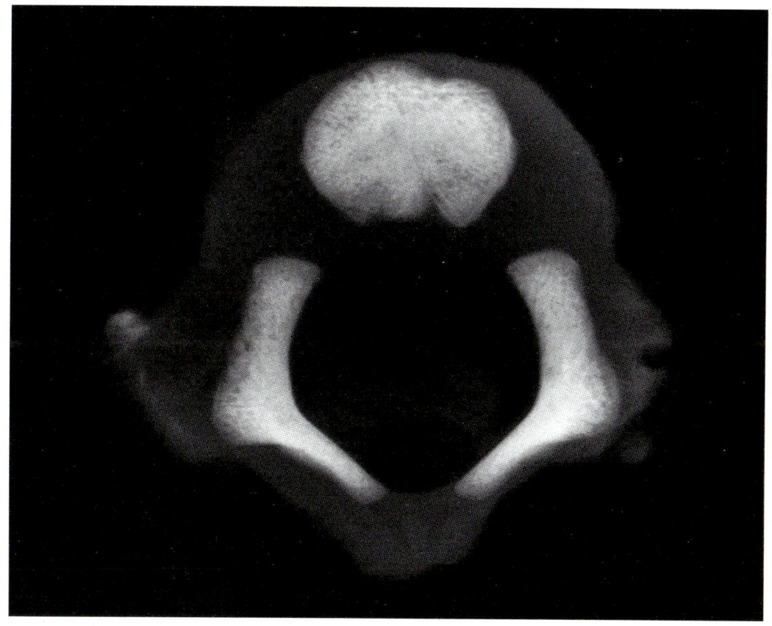

Figure 4.18 Specimen radiograph of a lumbar vertebra from a newborn to show the three separate centers of ossification for the vertebral body and the paired vertebral arches.

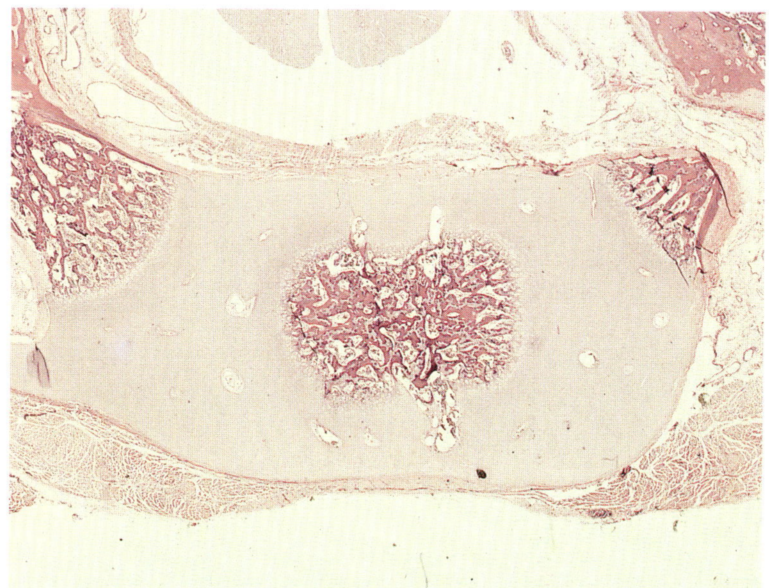

Figure 4.19 Photomicrograph to demonstrate the band of cartilage between the centrum of the vertebral body and the ossification centers of the vertebral arches in a 28-week-old fetus. (H & E stain, approximately 20 magnifications)

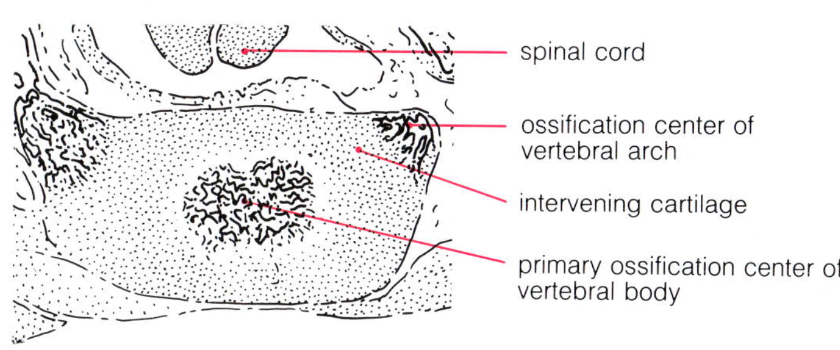

third and eighth year of life, although rarely it may persist to the 14th year or even later (Fig. 4.20).

Each vertebral segment has a pair of dorsal processes that later unite to form an osseous ring enclosing the spinal canal (Fig. 4.21). By the end of the second month of life, ossification can be seen in the arch of the atlas, and gradually, ossification proceeds distally, until, by the end of the fourth month, it has occurred in all the vertebral arches.

The spinous processes do not have their own ossification centers and so are formed during the first year of life by fusion of the posterior extensions of the vertebral arches (Fig. 4.22). Later, apophyses are formed at the tips of the spinous processes, and these fuse between the fourth and sixth years of life.

In general, the growth of the vertebral column is completed by the 25th year, when all the ossification centers have fused (Fig. 4.23).

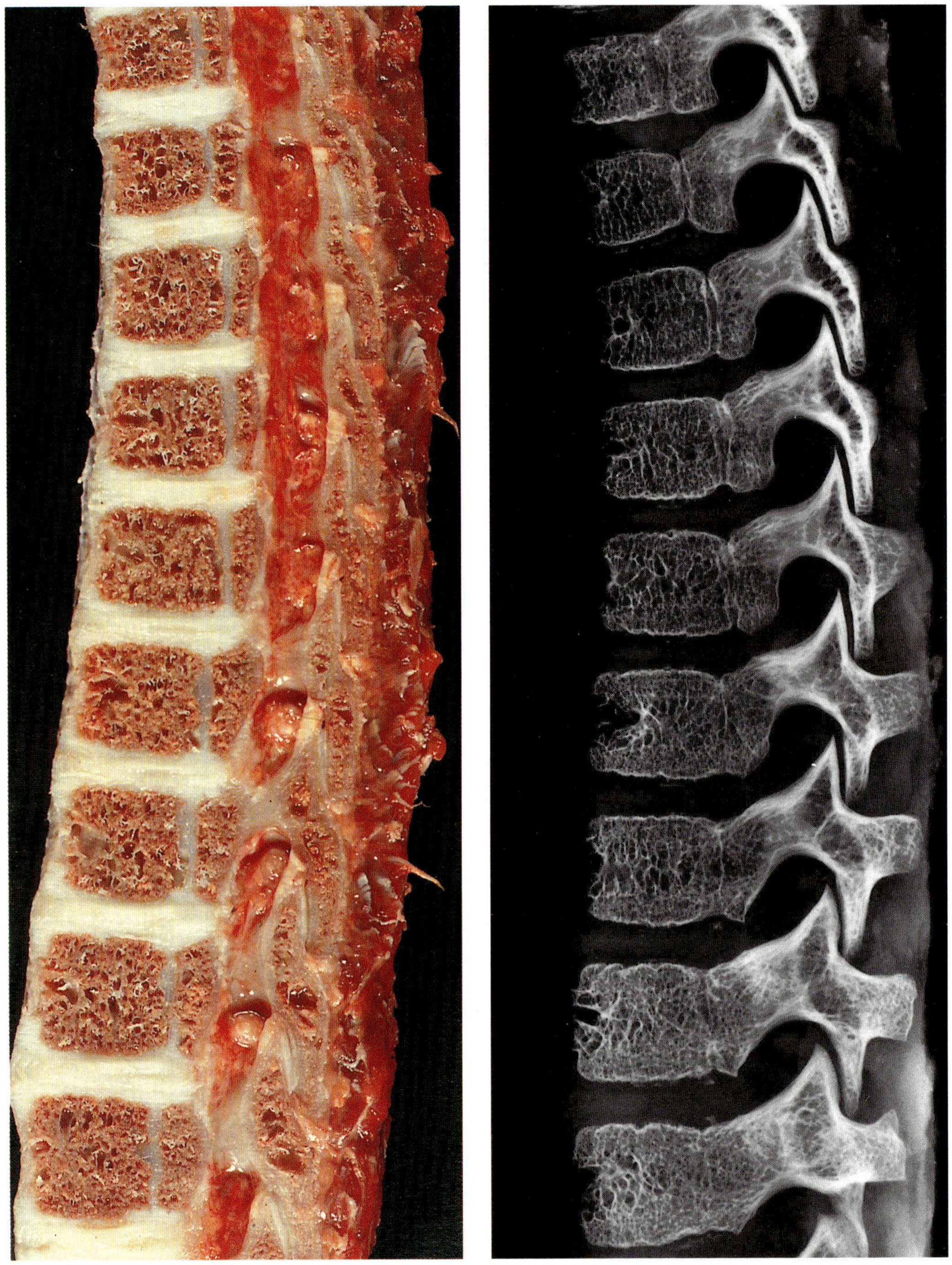

Figure 4.20 Photograph (*left*) of a parasagittal section through the midthoracic spine of a $7\frac{1}{2}$-year-old female. Note the thin band of cartilage between the centrum and the posterolateral portion of the vertebral bodies. There is partial bony fusion. Radiograph (*right*) of the same specimen shows that fusion of the intervening cartilage is more advanced in the lower spinal segments than in the upper segment.

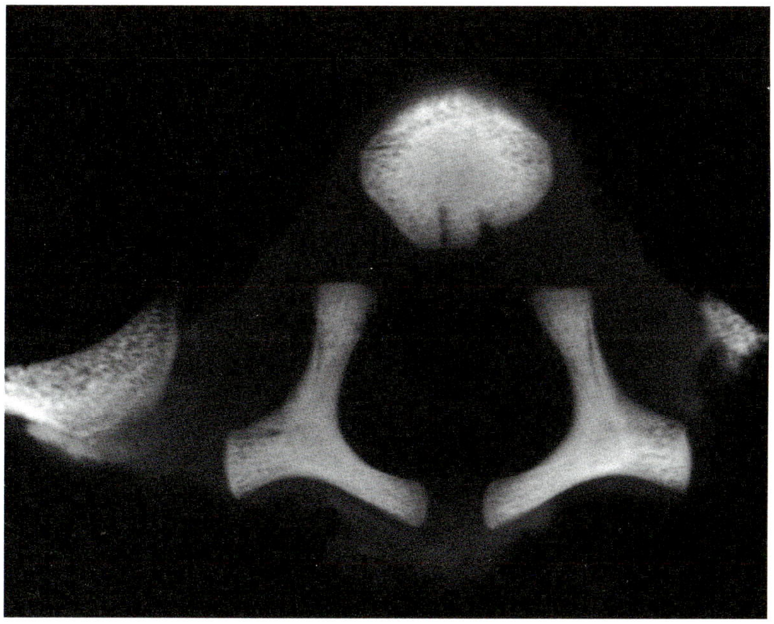

Figure 4.21 Specimen radiograph of a thoracic vertebra from a newborn. Note the transverse processes and the rib fragments on either side of the vertebral body. The posteromedial portions of the arches will fuse to form the spinous process, at the tip of which will form an apophysial center.

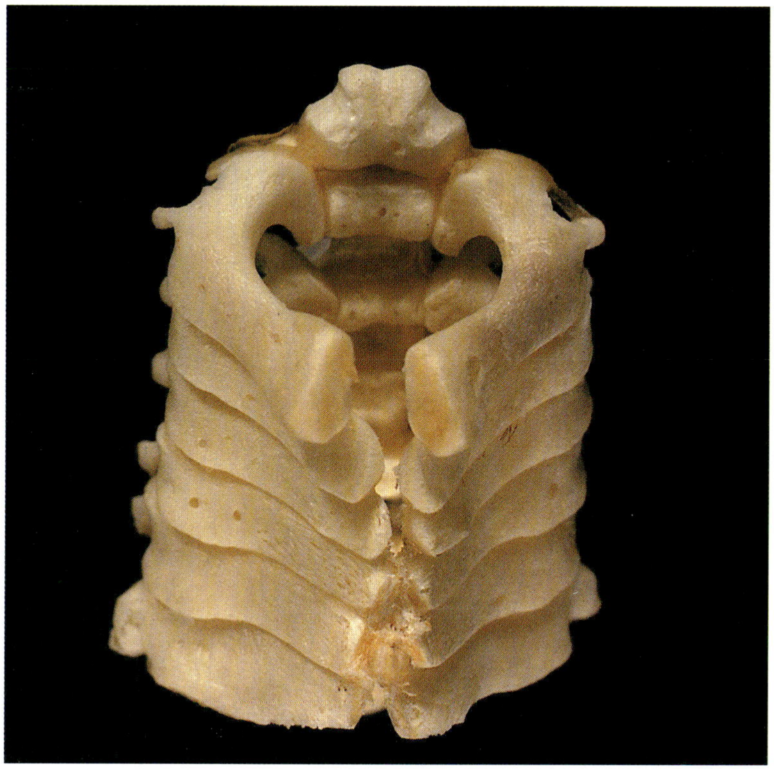

Figure 4.22 Photograph of the cervical spine from a stillborn at 32 weeks gestation. The posteromedial bony components of the arches have not yet fused to form the spinous processes.

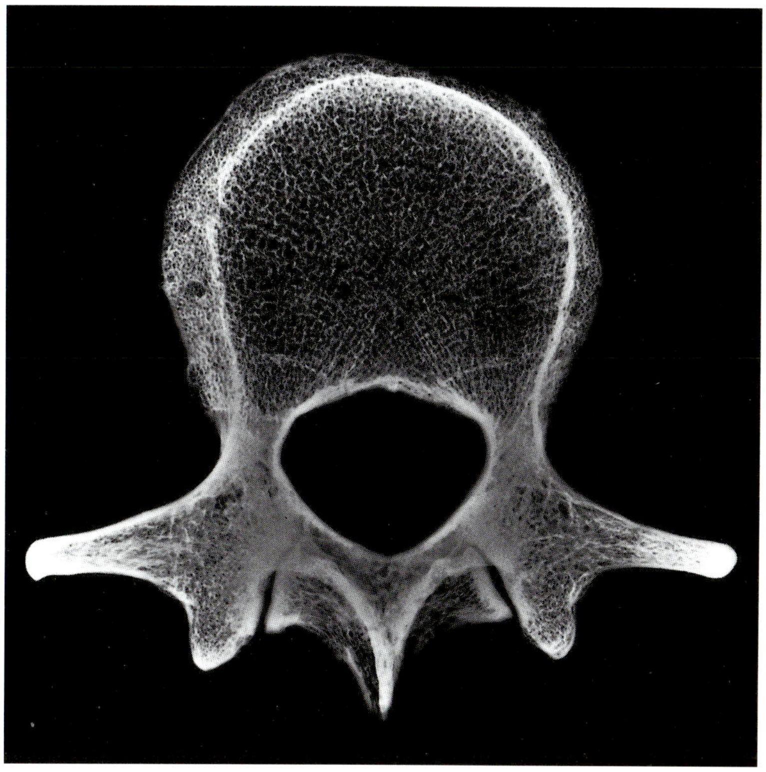

Figure 4.23 Specimen radiograph of the first lumbar vertebra of a young adult. Note how the three ossification centers have fused.

Age	Event
2 wks	Formation of notochord occurs (2–3 wks)
3 wks	
4 wks	
5 wks	Chondrification of primordial vertebral segments (sclerotomes) occurs (5–6 wks)
2 mos	Ossification complete in arch of atlas
3 mos	Ossification first appears in lower thoracic and upper lumbar vertebral bodies Regression of notochord begins (3–4 mos) Ossification complete in all vertebral arches (3–4 mos)
4 mos	Growth of spinal cord slows relative to growth of canal Primary ossification centers appear in all vertebral bodies (4–5 mos)
5 mos	
6 mos	
7 mos	
8 mos	
Birth	Lumbar vertebral body space equals disc-space height
	Formation of spinous processes complete (1 yr)
2 yrs	
3 yrs	
4 yrs	
5 yrs	Fusion of apophyses at tips of spinous processes (4–6 yrs) Fusion of intervening cartilage between bodies and pedicles (3–8 yrs)
6 yrs	
7 yrs	Appearance of secondary ossification centers in girls (6–8 yrs)
8 yrs	Appearance of secondary ossification centers in boys (7–9 yrs)
9 yrs	
10 yrs	
11 yrs	Fusion of secondary ossification centers to form bony rim (12 yrs)
15 yrs	Fusion of bony rim with vertebral body begins
20 yrs	Fusion of bony rim with vertebral body ends (22 yrs)
25 yrs	Fusion of all ossification centers to complete development of vertebral column

 Figure 4.24 Vertebral column growth and development.

To help summarize the progression of growth and development, a table is presented in Figure 4.24.

Development of the Spinal Cord

In early embryonic development, growth of the neural tube (the presumptive spinal cord) is almost exactly even with that of the spinal canal so that the neural tube occupies the entire length of the canal and the nerve roots lie perpendicular to the cord with the spinal nerves emerging between the vertebral bodies through the intervertebral foramina.

At approximately 4 months of gestation, growth of the neural tube slows considerably in relation to the growth of the vertebral canal, so that the cord no longer occupies the entire length of the canal and the nerve roots become more vertically disposed. In particular, the lumbar and sacral nerve roots, which together form the cauda equina, must traverse a considerable distance in the canal before emerging from their respective foramina (Fig. 4.25). Due to continued growth discrepancy, the spinal cord continues to move proximally, and, by the age of 5, comes to lie in its adult position, opposite the upper border of the second lumbar vertebra. Therefore, after birth, relatively little migration of the spinal cord occurs.

In the adult, the spinal cord ends in the conus medullaris around the level of L1-2, where it becomes the *filum terminale,* the atrophied portion of the neural tube that runs down the center of the cauda equina. The filum terminale attaches the spinal cord to the distal end of the sacral canal.

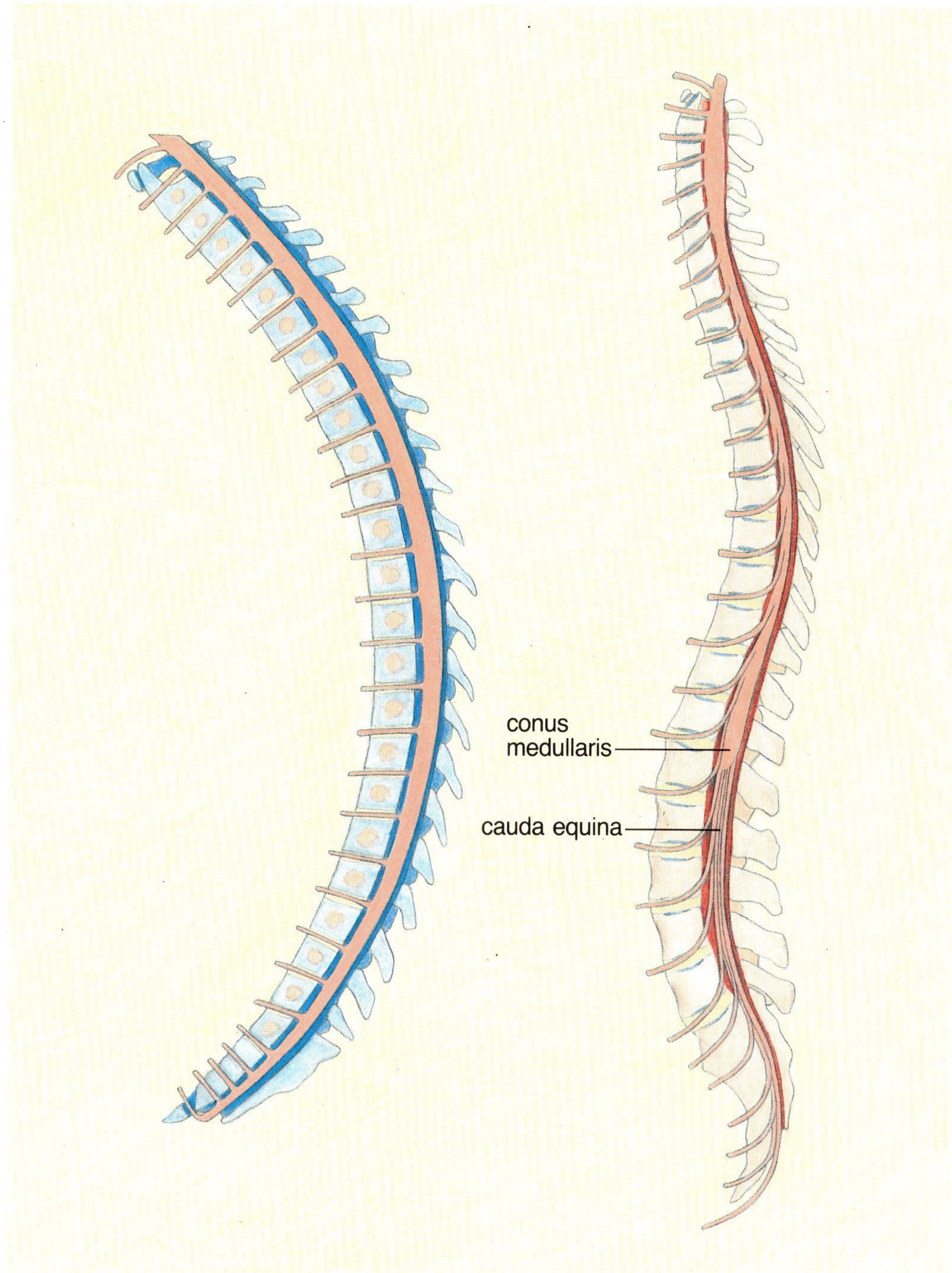

Figure 4.25 Schematic drawing to show the development of the vertebral column in relation to that of the spinal cord.

2 SECTION

DEGENERATIVE DISC DISEASE AND SPINAL ARTHRITIS

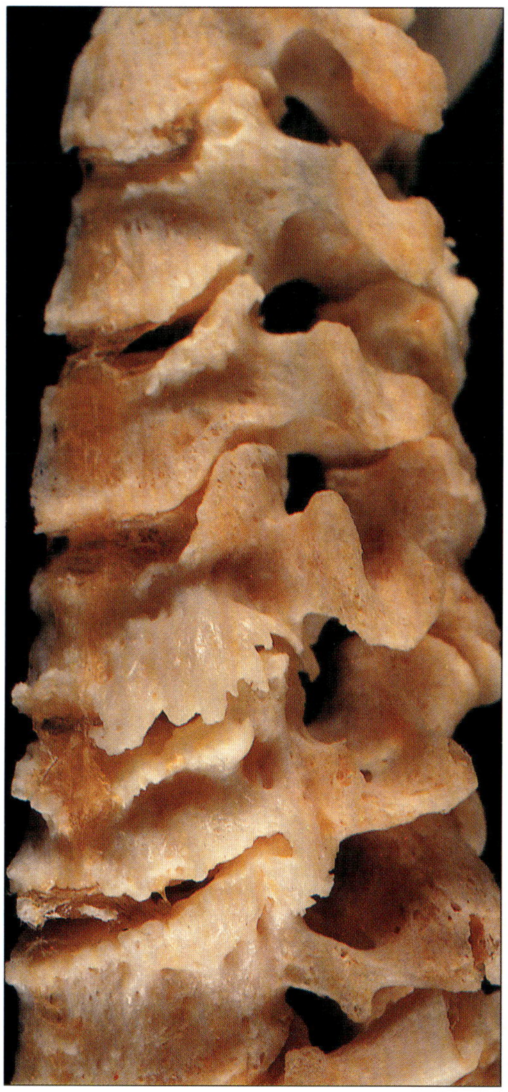

The spinal column contains over 130 articulations, including the solid intervertebral discs and the synovial joints of both the posterior articular processes and the vertebral articulations of the ribs. Certain diseases, such as disc-tissue displacement, initially will affect the discs, while other diseases, such as rheumatoid arthritis, initially will affect the diarthrodial joints. In general however, in the clinical setting, both the joints of the vertebral bodies as well as those of the arches eventually are affected by disease.

In the chapters that follow, we begin with a discussion of the different types of disc-tissue displacement. Secondly, we consider the effects on disc tissue of the deposition of metabolic products, such as calcium apatite and calcium pyrophosphate dihydrate. In the third chapter, we compare the effects of normal aging on disc tissue with those of degenerative disc disease, while in the fourth chapter, we consider degenerative arthritis of the spinal column itself (facet joint arthrosis, spondylosis, degenerative spondylolisthesis and Charcot spine) and spinal stenosis. Lastly, we discuss the effects of inflammatory arthritis (rheumatoid arthritis and sero-negative inflammatory spondylitis) and the ankylosing spondyloarthropathies (ankylosing spondylitis and ankylosing hyperostosis of the spine).

5 CHAPTER

DISC TISSUE DISPLACEMENT

General Features and Pathogenesis

Displacement of disc tissue (generally the nucleus pulposus) from the intervertebral disc space may occur anteriorly, posteriorly, superiorly, or inferiorly (Fig. 5.1). Displacement of disc tissue anteriorly usually produces spondylosis deformans, while displacement posteriorly produces pressure on the nerve roots or encroachment on the contents of the spinal canal. Displacement superiorly or inferiorly, into the adjacent vertebral bodies, will result in the development of Schmorl's nodes.

The different forms that displacement can take include protrusion, prolapse, extrusion, and sequestration (Fig. 5.2). *Protrusion* is a bulging of the nucleus pulposus through a weakened anulus fibrosus, generally in a posterior or posterolateral direction; *prolapse* is a rupture of the nucleus pulposus through the anulus, but not through the posterior or anterior longitudinal ligament; *extrusion* is a rupture of the nucleus pulposus through both the anulus and the ligament, usually the posterior longitudinal ligament; *sequestration* is a fragmentation of the extruded segment, occasionally with displacement of the free fragment into the spinal canal, often to a site far removed from the point of rupture. The term disc herniation is a general one, used to describe either prolapse, protrusion, or extrusion. (Protrusion, extrusion, and sequestration are further illustrated grossly

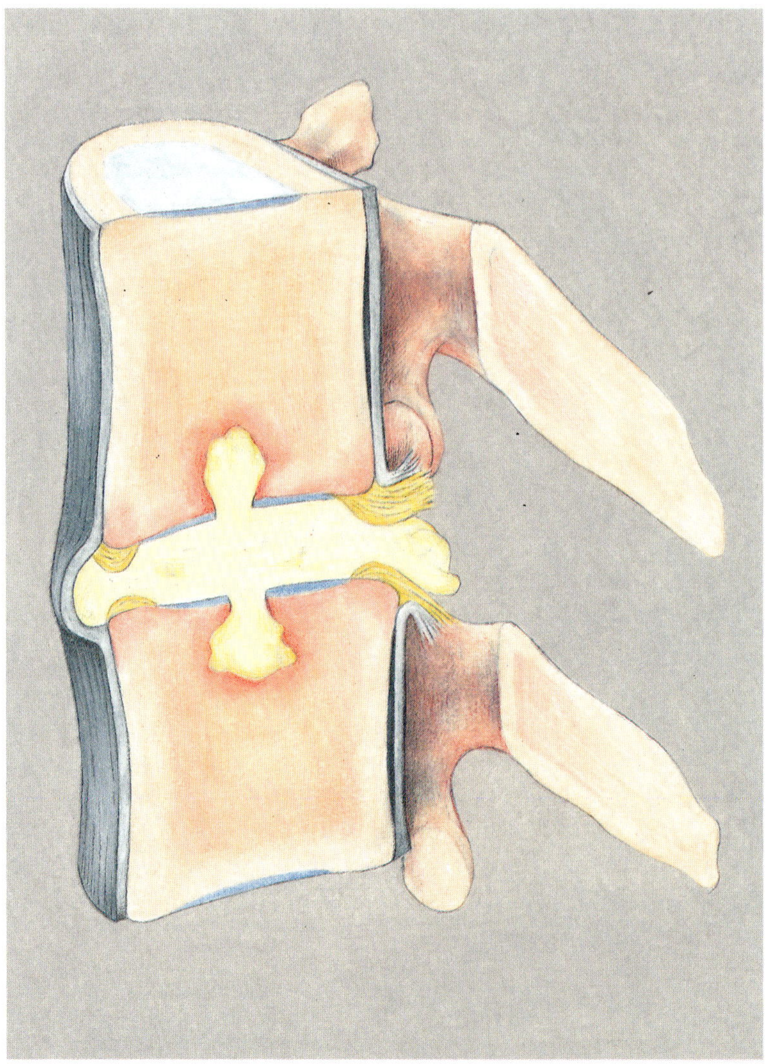

Figure 5.1 Schematic drawing to illustrate the several directions in which disc tissue displacement may occur: anteriorly, posteriorly, superiorly, or inferiorly.

and radiographically in Figures 5.3 through 5.5.) In the case of disc tissue extrusion, the displaced tissue also may include portions of the anulus fibrosus. This occurs when both radial and circumferential tears in the anulus are combined.

The displaced fragment of nucleus pulposus may undergo a number of changes. It may be released from the confines of the disc into the epidural space, where it may begin to grow in a way similar to that of cartilaginous loose bodies in an arthritic joint; it may invoke an inflammatory response and go on to be destroyed subsequently by vascular granulation tissue; or, it may become calcified, and later, ossified. Following disc herniation, the involved disc undergoes degenerative changes, with fibrosis and marked narrowing. Ultimately, bony ankylosis may result.

From the clinical point of view, significant displacement of the nucleus following injury to the anulus is more likely to occur in a young adult. It is less likely to occur or to cause significant compromise of the neural canal or foramen in an older individual, in whom disc tissue, especially the nucleus pulposus, is shrunken and dehydrated. For displacement of nuclear tissue to take place, there must be a tear in the collagen fibers of the anulus fibrosus, either partial (in the case of protrusion) or total (in the case of prolapse). Such tears usually are associated with torsional and compressional injuries that have occurred as a result of the sudden application of force.

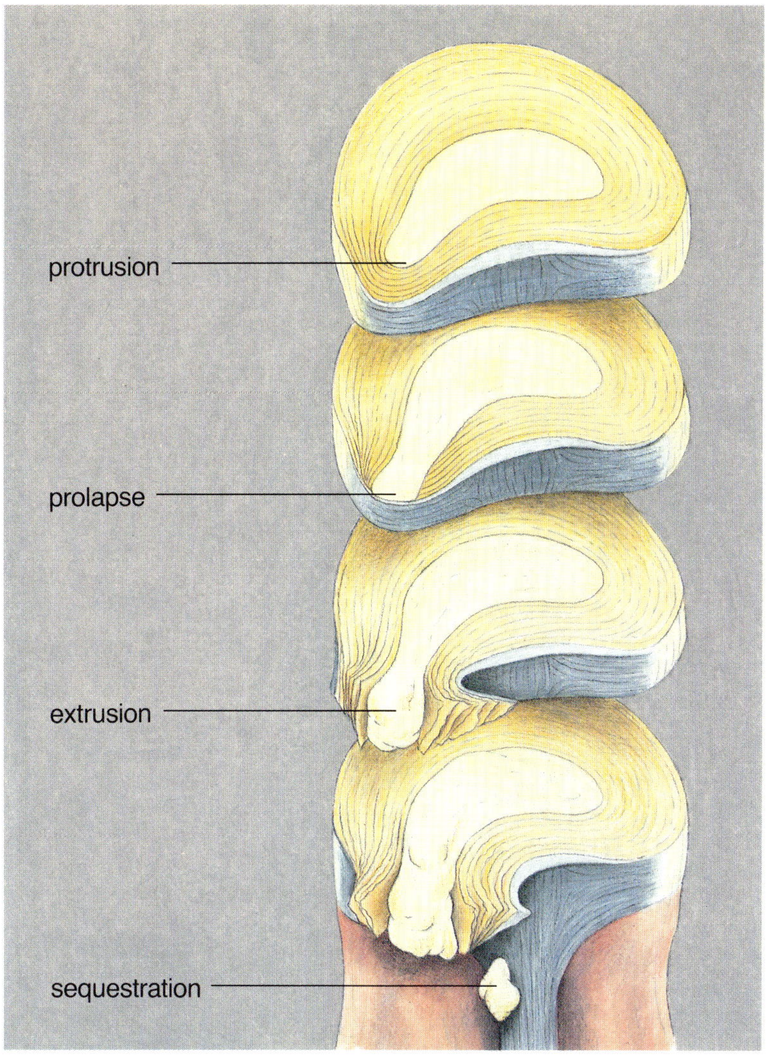

Figure 5.2 Schematic drawing to illustrate the different types of disc tissue displacement: protrusion, prolapse, extrusion, or sequestration.

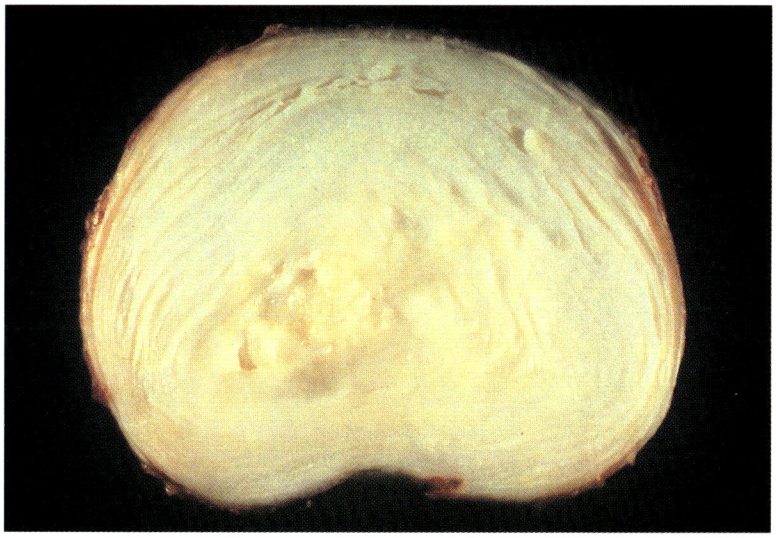

Figure 5.3 Photograph of a cross section through the L3-4 disc, showing protrusion of the nucleus pulposus, or bulging of the nucleus pulposus into the anulus, posterolaterally.

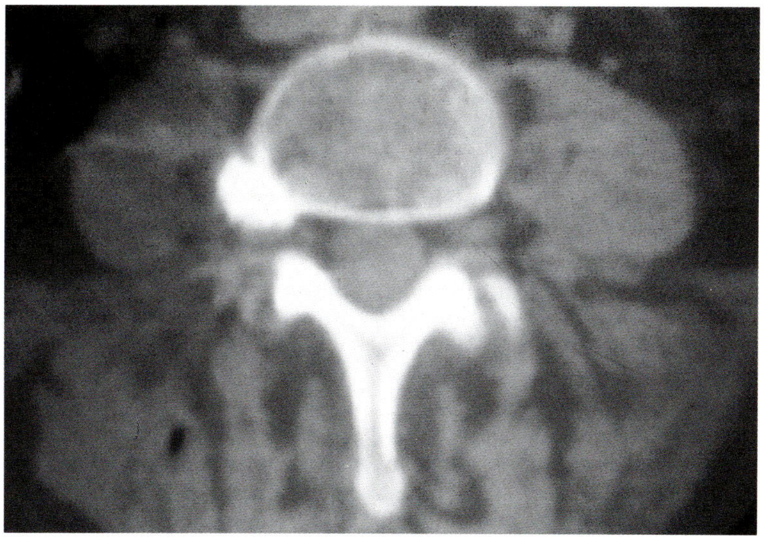

Figure 5.4 CT scan through the upper part of the body of L-5, in a patient who complained of radiating leg pain. Contrast medium has been injected into the intervertebral disc, and a large piece of extruded disc material containing contrast medium can be seen on the posterolateral aspect, encroaching on the intervertebral foramen.

Anterior Displacement and Spondylosis Deformans

Anterior or anterolateral protrusion of intervertebral disc tissue usually leads to spondylosis deformans, which is one of the most common forms of spinal disease seen both radiographically and at autopsy. Based on Schmorl's series of over 4,000 spines obtained at autopsy, Junghanns reported that the incidence of spondylosis deformans increased with advancing age, and that by age 50 it was present in approximately 60% of women and 80% of men—an incidence that is higher than that reported in clinical radiographic studies. The disease appears to occur more frequently in people engaged in occupations requiring heavy physical labor, and while any segment of the vertebral column may be affected, the lumbar spine is the site affected most commonly.

Based upon his studies, Schmorl was the first to propose that spondylosis deformans is initiated by tears that occur anteriorly in the periphery of the anulus, where the collagen bundles attach to the vertebral bodies by Sharpey's fibers (Fig. 5.6). Tears in this area lead to both anterior and anterolateral herniation of nuclear disc tissue, a process that is accentuated when the nucleus pulposus is relatively normal to begin with. Displacement is potentiated by weight bearing and by spinal motion, and it is for this reason that spondylosis deformans is found only rarely in inactive or immobilized individuals.

Once displacement has occurred, dissection of the anterior longitudinal ligament from its bony attachment by the displaced disc tissue permits extension of tissue, cephalad or caudad, between the anterior longitudinal ligament and the vertebral body wall. Because the anterior longitudinal ligament has only weak attachments to the anulus, continuous tearing of these attachments by prolapsed disc material will stimulate the development of bony outgrowths (termed *osteophytes*), particularly along the anterior and lateral aspects of the vertebral

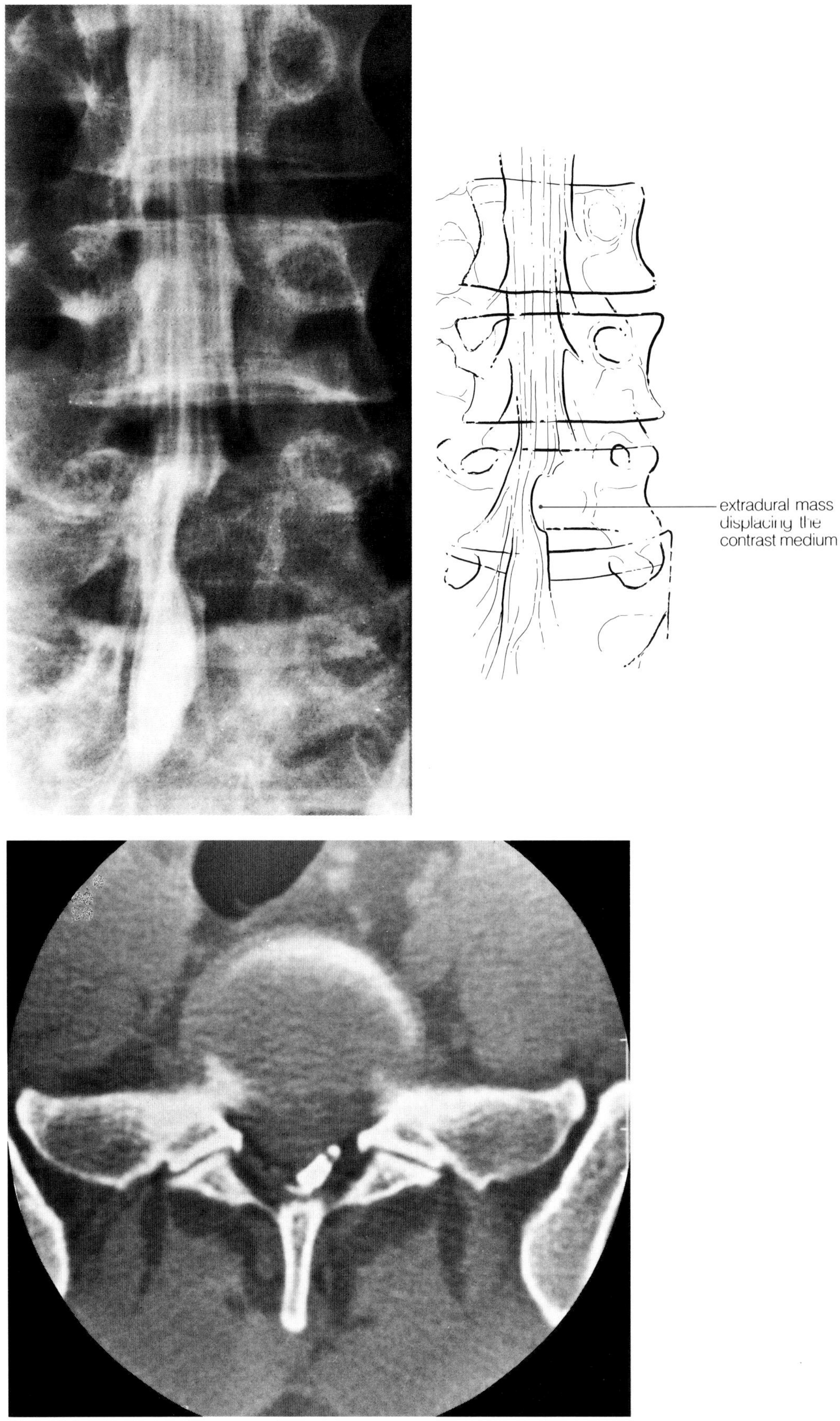

Figure 5.5 AP myelogram (*top*) to demonstrate sequestration. Note the presence of a mass that is overlying the lower two-thirds of L-5, and displacing the cauda equina posteriorly and to the left. The differential diagnosis on this view would include tumor or displaced disc tissue. In the corresponding CT scan (*bottom*) of this patient, the cut goes through the mass seen on the myelogram, demonstrating that the mass is extradural and has the same density as intervertebral disc. At surgery, a large mass of extruded disc tissue was removed.

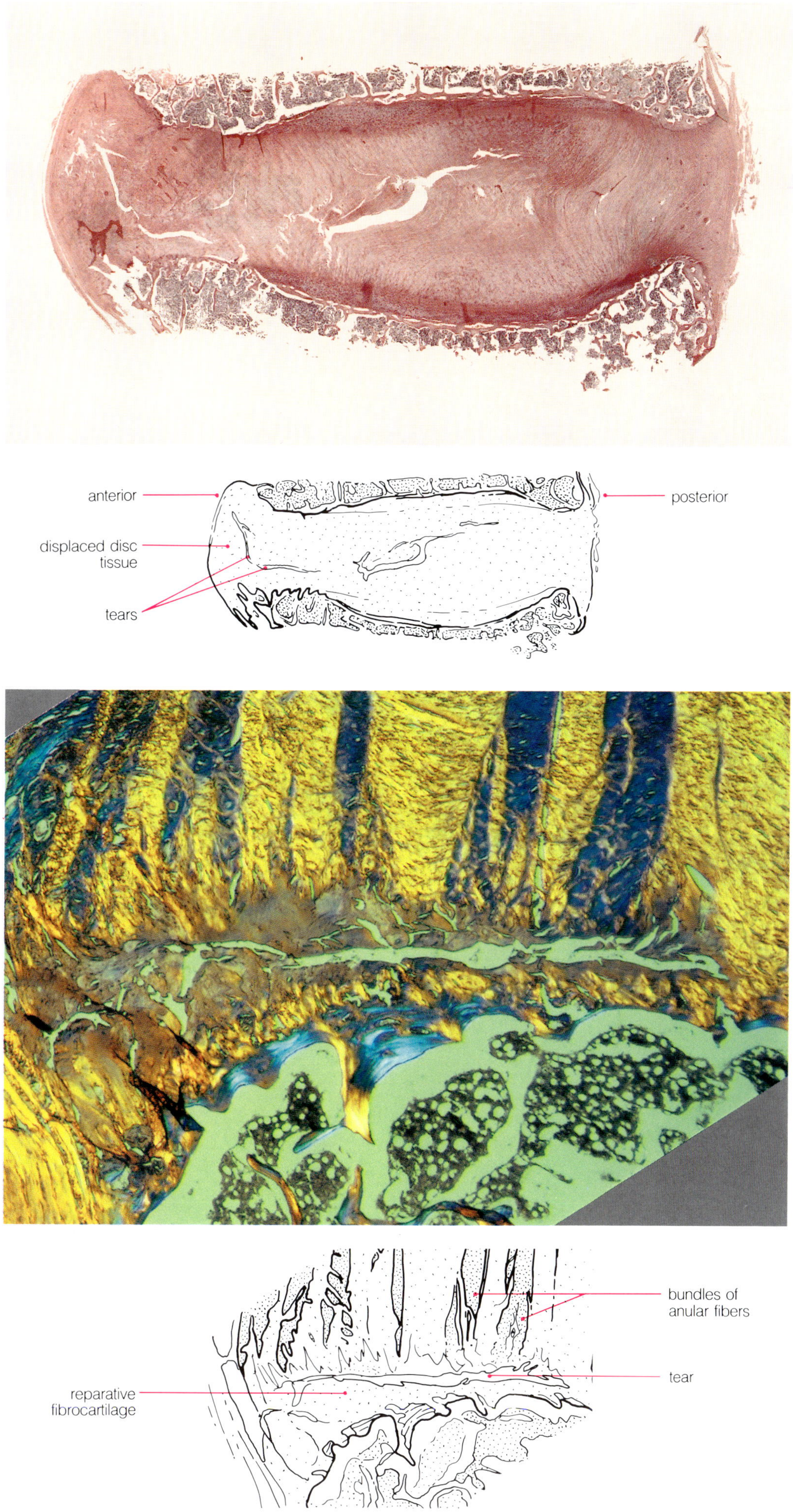

Figure 5.6 Photomicrograph (*top*) to show the early development (stage I) of spondylosis deformans. Note the peripheral tears in the anular fibers anteriorly, in addition to the anterior intervertebral disc displacement. (H & E stain, approximately 2 magnifications) Polarized photomicrograph (*bottom*) of the same, taken at the junction of the anulus fibrosus, subchondral bone, and anterior longitudinal ligament. At the insertion of the anulus into the bone, there is a linear tear through Sharpey's fibers. The defect is partially filled with reparative fibrocartilage. (Polarized light, × 1.5 objective, approximately 12 magnifications)

column (Fig. 5.7). These bony outgrowths extend first in a horizontal direction and then in a vertical direction, following the attachments of the ligament. Beaklike spurs are formed, which eventually may grow to bridge the intervertebral disc space (Figs. 5.8 and 5.9). The four stages of spondylosis deformans are summarized schematically in Figure 5.10.

The form and severity of the clinical manifestations related to vertebral osteophytes, while difficult to assess, will depend upon the size and location of the outgrowths and on their relationship to adjacent soft tissues and neurologic structures. Symptoms may include dysphagia, stiffness, and pain.

Osteophyte formation was noted by Schmorl to be less pronounced at sites of significant disc degeneration than it is in spondylosis deformans, an observation that has been emphasized by a number of investigators since Schmorl's time. It should be noted, however, that the characteristic changes of intervertebral disc degeneration (osteochondrosis) will in time become superimposed on those of spondylosis deformans (see Fig. 5.8). Osteophyte formation in spondylosis deformans should be differentiated not only from that seen in association with osteochondrosis, but also from the thin, vertically oriented syndesmophytes seen in ankylosing spondylitis and DISH (see Chapter 9).

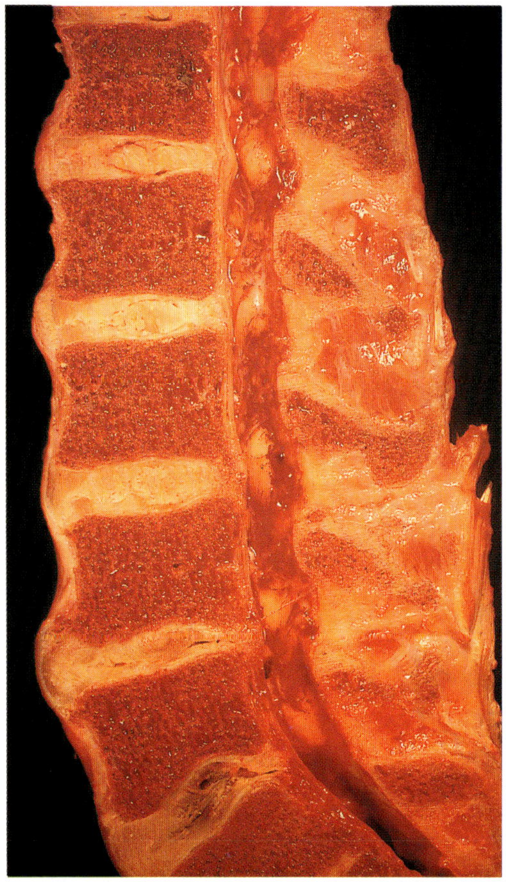

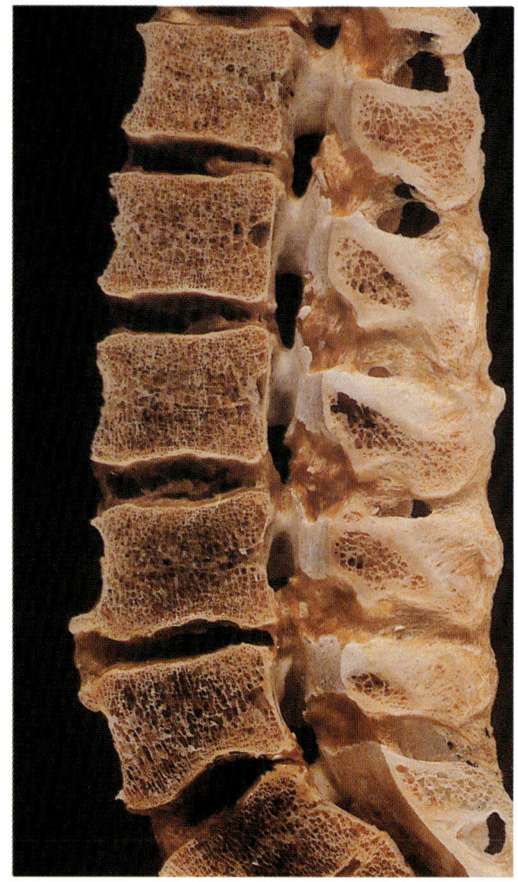

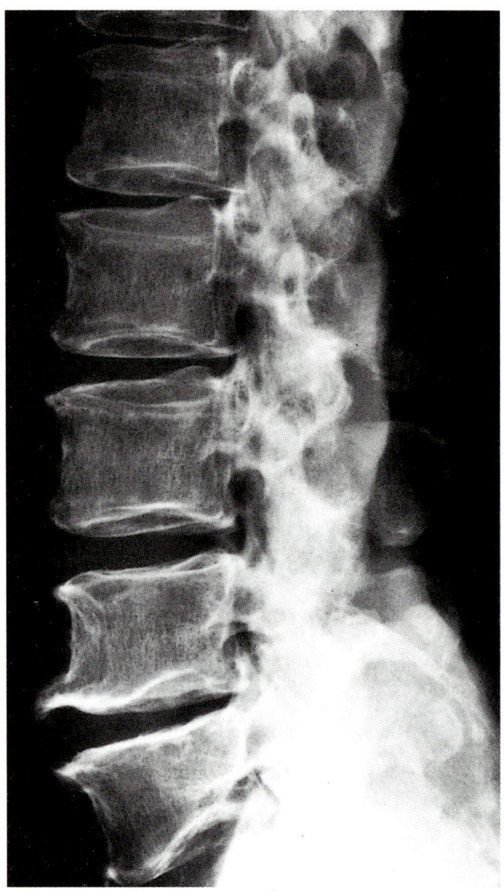

Figure 5.7 Photograph (*top left*) of a sagittal section of the lumbar spine in stage II spondylosis deformans. Note the anterior disc displacement of L4-5, with associated narrowing at the L4-5 disc space, compared to the levels above, and an anterior traction osteophyte. A macerated specimen (*top right*) of the same. A specimen radiograph (*bottom*) of this section shows the anterior osteophyte directed in a horizontal manner at the L4-5 disc space.

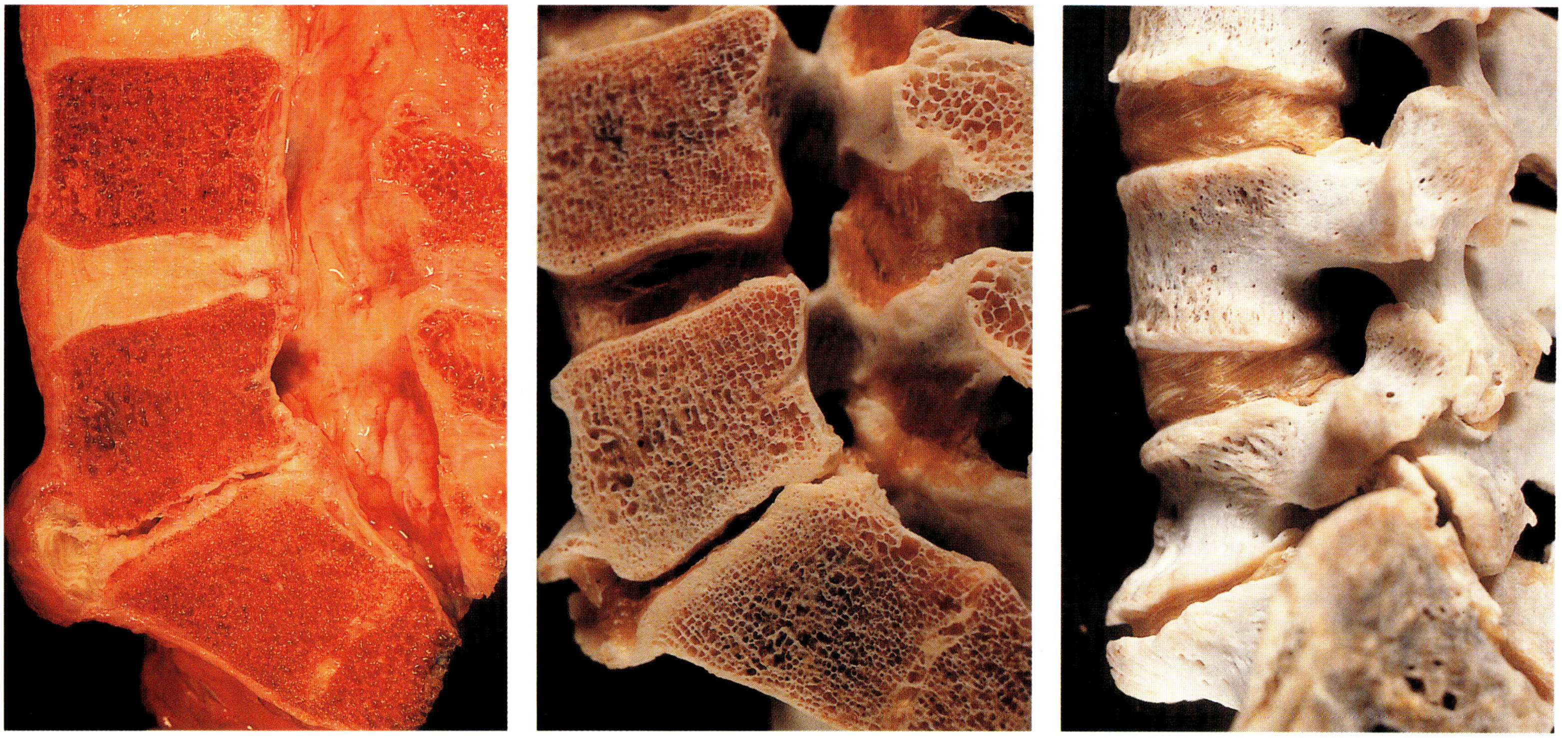

Figure 5.8 Photograph (*left*) of a sagittal section of the lumbosacral spine in stage III spondylosis deformans. Note the anterior herniation of the L-5 to S-1 disc, with narrowing of the intervertebral disc space. Note also the changes of intervertebral disc degeneration, i.e., osteochondrosis, superimposed upon those of spondylosis deformans. In the macerated preparation (*center*) of the same spine, the anterior beaklike spurs are well illustrated. The same specimen (*right*) viewed from the outside shows the anterolateral extension of the beaking osteophyte.

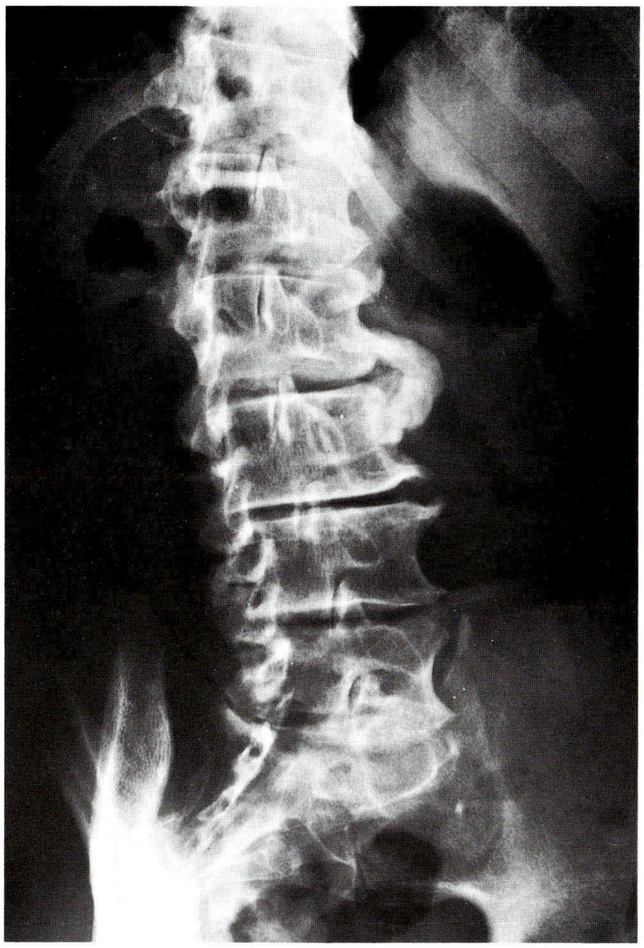

Figure 5.9 Oblique radiograph of a patient to illustrate the anterolateral osteophyte in stage IV spondylosis, which eventually has fused across the L2-3 disc space. Note also the horizontal osteophytes forming across L1-2 and L3-4, which are less involved by spondylosis deformans.

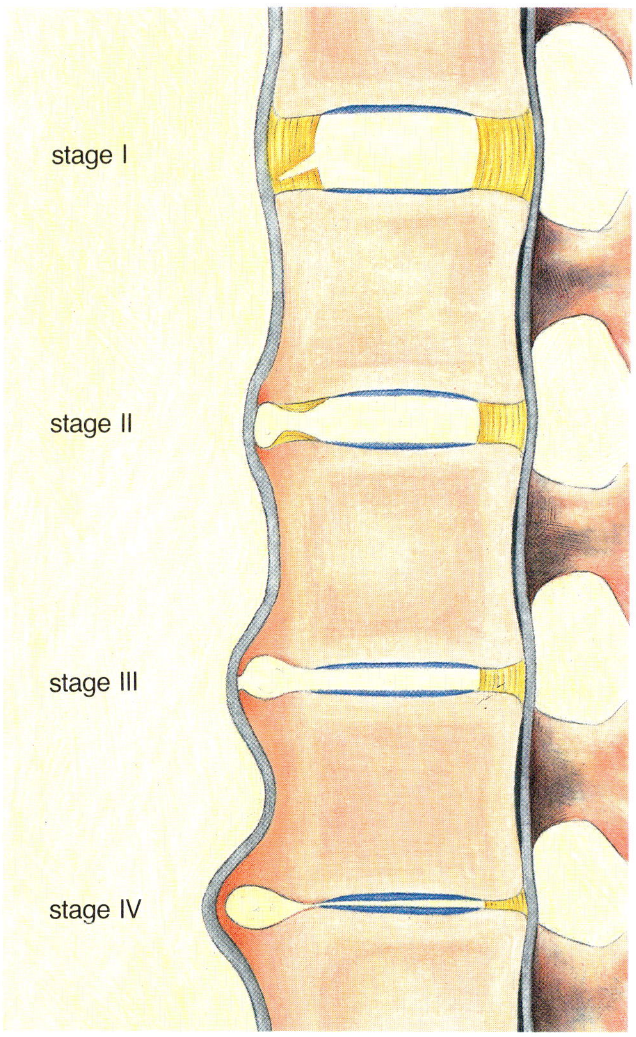

Figure 5.10 Schematic drawing to summarize the four stages of spondylosis deformans. In stage I, tears are seen in the anular fibers, anteriorly. In stage II, prolapse of the disc occurs, which elevates the anterior longitudinal ligament and the periosteum, resulting in bone production. In stage III, the horizontal osteophyte is beginning to extend in the direction of the ligament, thereby becoming more vertical to form beaklike spurs. In stage IV, eventual fusion of the osteophyte, anteriorly, is seen.

Posterior and Posterolateral Displacement

Intervertebral disc tissue also may displace posteriorly, to encroach on the spinal canal, or it may herniate posterolaterally into the intervertebral foramen, as first demonstrated by von Luschka and Schmorl (Fig. 5.11). Schmorl found that posterolateral herniations were present in 15.2% of all spines he examined at autopsy. The most common sites of involvement were in the lumbar and lower thoracic spines, with occasional involvement in the cervical spine. In our own autopsy material, over 50% of older individuals showed posterior disc bulging, mostly in the lumbar region of the spine (Fig. 5.12).

The basis of posterior disc displacement is found in the small tears that accumulate in the anulus of the disc as a result of the stress and strain of daily living. These clefts, especially the radial ones, prepare the way for displacement of the nucleus pulposus, either posteriorly or posterolaterally, following acute trauma.

Demonstration of posterior or posterolateral intervertebral disc protrusion, prolapse, or extrusion can be made radiographically or by employing CT, discography, or myelography (see Section 1; Figs. 1.12, 1.13, 1.16, and 1.17). Examination of autopsy material has shown that posterolateral disc displacement can occur unilaterally (Fig. 5.13) or bilaterally, with encroachment on the intervertebral foramina (Figs. 5.14 through 5.16). Posterior herniation of the disc also is accompanied by a loss of intervertebral disc space. Disc material removed at the time of surgery usually will show evidence of degeneration, along with regenerative clones of chondrocytes.

The displacement of disc tissue posteriorly and posterolaterally usually results in clinical symptoms, depending on the amount of disc tissue displaced and its proximity to neural structures. In clinical practice, acute posterior herniations of the disc are encountered mostly in the third and fourth decades of life. The typical presentation is that of nerve root compression with radiating pain, resulting from an acute inflammatory response to the displaced tissue. With rest, there is regression of edema and inflammation, and the pain usually subsides. Later recurrence of pain may result from further displacement of disc tissue or from scarring, which is sometimes accompanied by calcification and ossification. The relative infre-

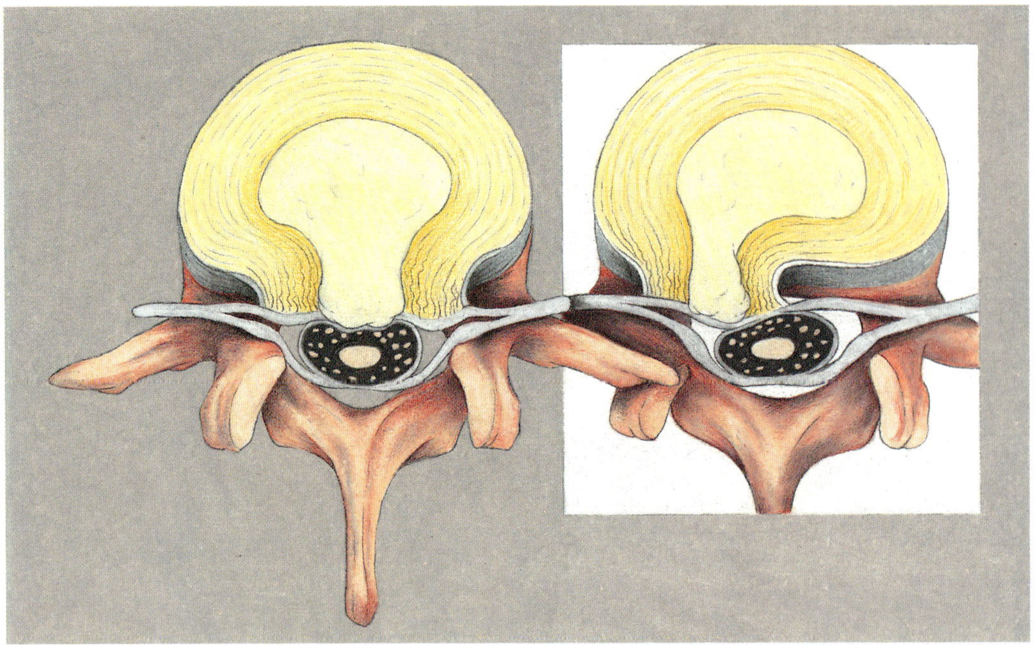

Figure 5.11 Schematic drawing to illustrate postero*central* disc herniation, with encroachment on the contents of the spinal canal. The right-hand figure illustrates postero*lateral* disc herniation, with encroachment on the nerve root as it goes through the intervertebral foramen.

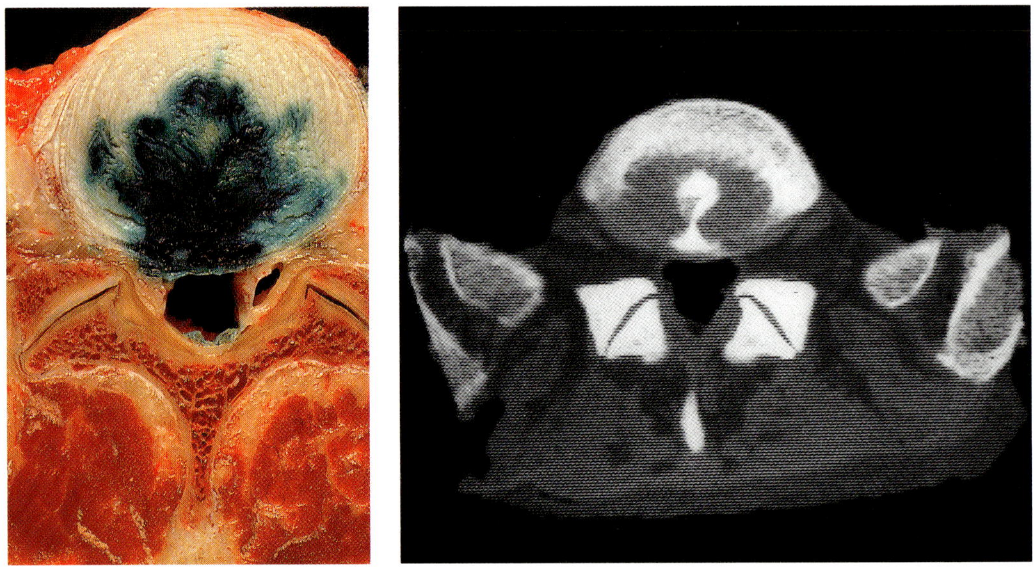

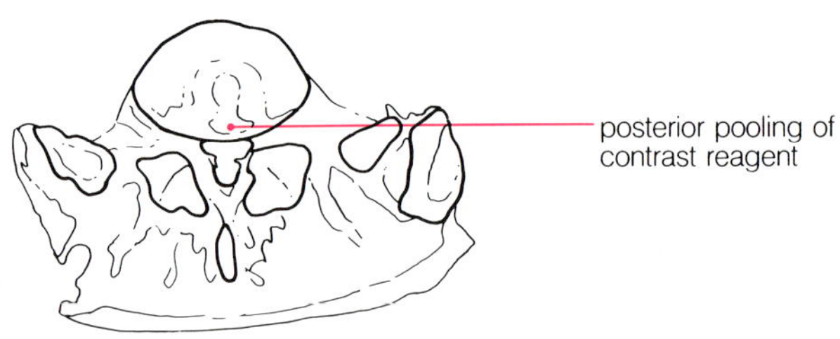

Figure 5.12 Photograph (*left*) showing the L3-4 disc of a young adult, in cross section. Note the posterior bulging of the disc, with loss of the normal posterior concavity and extension of contrast reagent posterocentrally. A CT discogram (*right*) of this specimen shows the pooling of contrast reagent posterocentrally, and posterior bulging of the intervertebral disc.

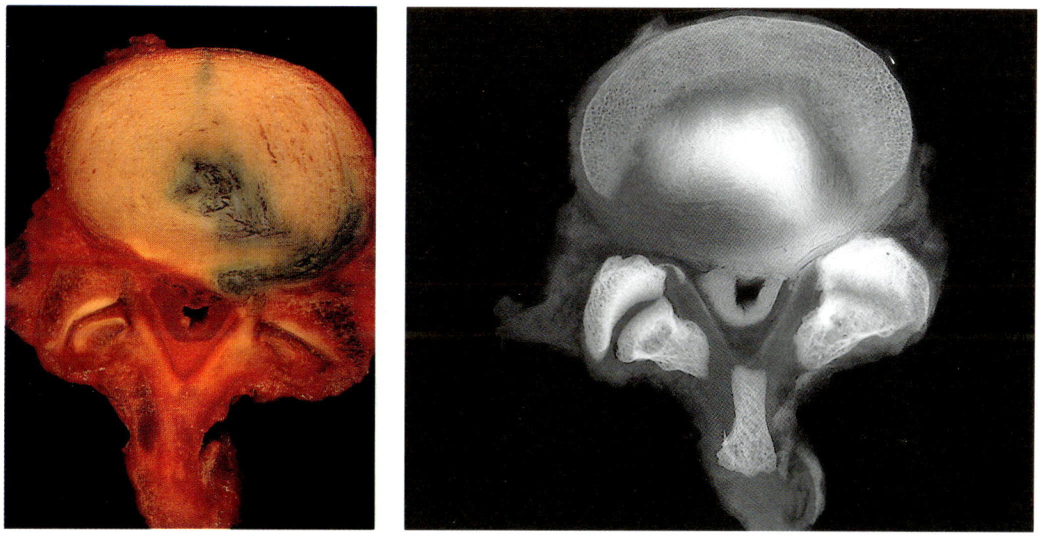

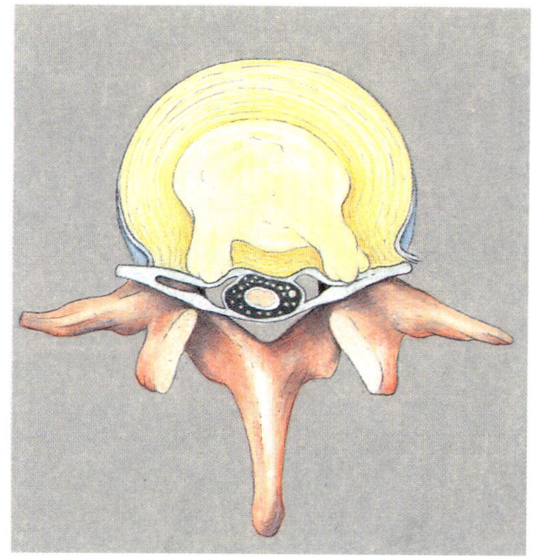

Figure 5.13 Photograph (*left*) of the L4-5 disc in cross section, following injection of contrast medium into the nucleus pulposus. Note the extension of the dye, posterolaterally. It is dissecting between the disc and the posterior longitudinal ligament, which appears to be intact. Note that there is a bulging that results in an impression upon the dura, with narrowing of the intervertebral foramen (lateral recess). In a CT scan (*right*) of the same specimen, the posterolateral bulging with encroachment on the lateral recess is well illustrated.

Figure 5.14 Schematic drawing showing bilateral posterolateral herniation. In this type of situation, bilateral symptoms may occur clinically.

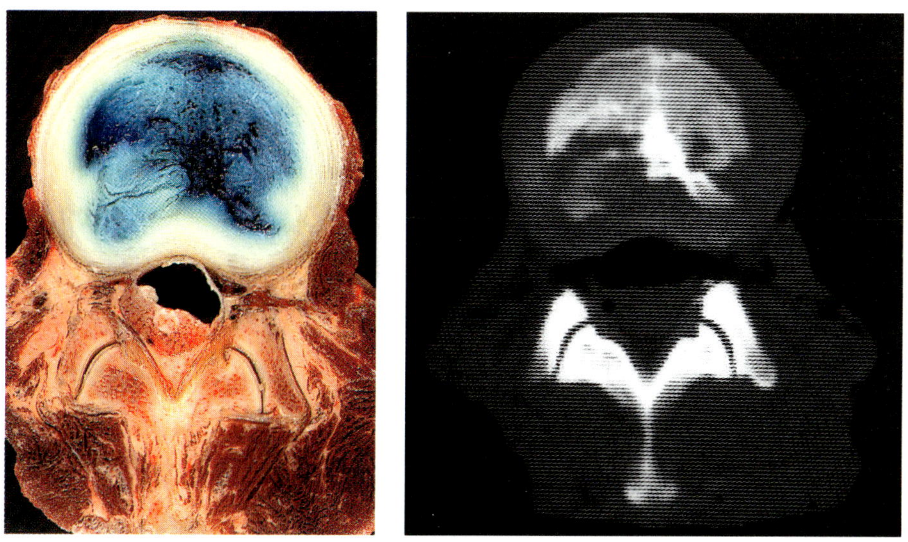

Figure 5.15 Photograph (*left*) of a cross section of the L1-2 disc space in a 30-year-old male. In this specimen, there is bilateral posterolateral protrusion, without prolapse of the nucleus through the anulus. No obvious bulging into the intervertebral foramina is seen at this time, and the posterior concavity of the disc is maintained. A CT scan (*right*) of the same specimen.

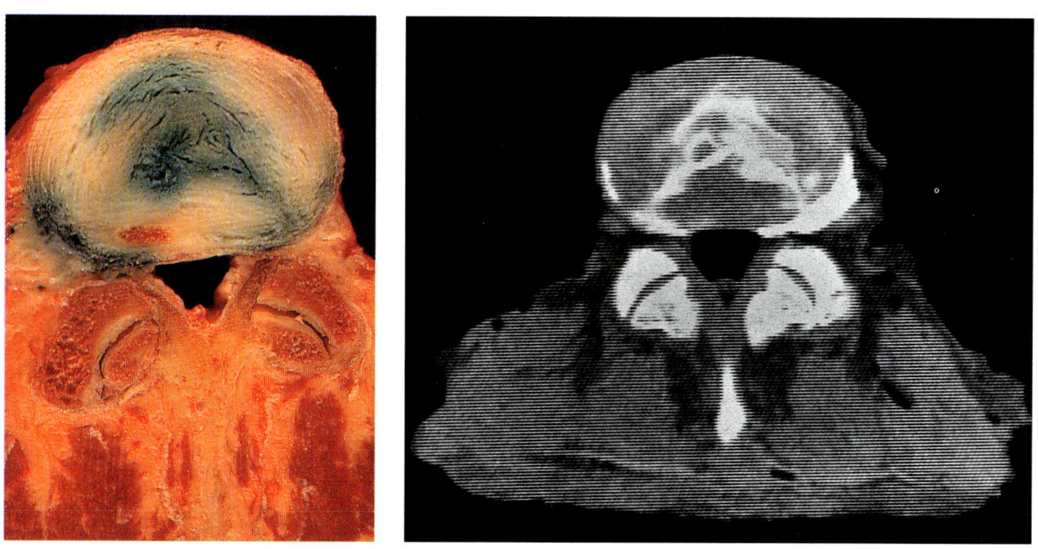

Figure 5.16 Photograph (*left*) of a cross section of the L4-5 disc space in a 50-year-old female. Following injection of contrast medium, bilateral prolapse of the nucleus pulposus is seen. On the left-hand side, the dye appears to have extended through the posterior ligament into the intervertebral foramen. A CT scan (*right*) of the same specimen confirms the extension of the dye through the posterior ligament on the left side.

quency of osteophyte formation in the posterior aspect of the vertebral body is thought to be due to the firm attachment of the disc to the posterior longitudinal ligament. This also may explain the relative rarity of severe neurologic deficits in central posterior disc prolapse.

One modality of treatment that has been used in cases of disease resulting from disc herniation is the injection of chymopapain into the nucleus pulposus, with the rationale that this will digest the noncollagenous proteins and thus reduce the pressure on the nerve root by the nucleus. The physical effect of chymopapain on disc tissue is demonstrated in Figure 5.17.

Intraosseous Displacement—Schmorl's Nodes

The herniation of disc substance through the cartilaginous end plate, into the adjacent vertebral body, will result in what are known as *Schmorl's nodes* (Figs. 5.18 and 5.19). This phenomenon was described first by von Luschka in 1858 and again by Schmorl in 1927.

These herniations, which are probably traumatic in origin, extend for a varying distance into the cancellous bone of the adjacent vertebral body. In older individuals, Schmorl's nodes tend to occur singly. When Schmorl's nodes occur in the young patient, the defects in the cartilaginous end plates may be developmental in origin and multiple, as seen in Scheuermann's disease (see Section 3, Chapter 10).

The clinical significance of Schmorl's nodes is that, as disc tissue escapes into the vertebral bodies, the intervertebral disc becomes degenerated and thinned, thereby placing strain on the facet joints, leading to spondylosis. In younger individuals herniations may occur suddenly, because of the turgor of the nucleus pulposus. However, in older individuals, where there is a loss of fluid in the nucleus, herniation usually occurs gradually.

The various stages of development of Schmorl's nodes can be demonstrated in anatomical specimens, especially in sagittal sections, and by fine-grain radiography or contrast injection studies into the intervertebral disc. Macerated specimens show the defects and the surrounding shell of condensed bone (Fig. 5.20).

Schmorl reported the incidence of these nodes to be 38%, being slightly more common in men than in women (39.9% and 34.3% respectively). On clinical radiographic examination of an adult population, Schmorl reported an incidence of 13%. This low incidence is due to an inability to recognize the cartilaginous nodes radiographically, until a reactive osseous shell has formed (Figs. 5.21 and 5.22).

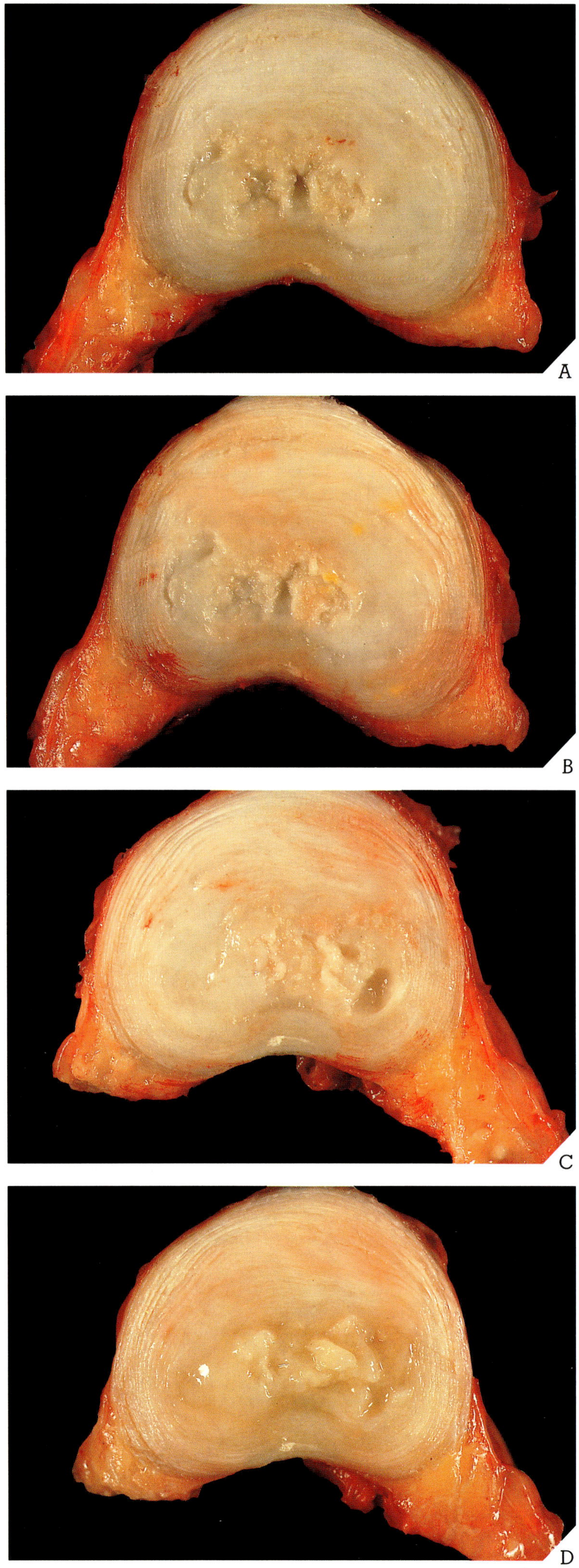
A B C D

Figure 5.17 Photographs of an intervertebral disc that has been transected through its central portion, with one-half being infiltrated with 3 cc of saline and the other half with 3 cc of chymopapain. Note the appearance of the disc before injection with saline (**A**) and after injection with saline (**B**). There is very little difference, if any, in the appearance of the tissue. However, when the disc before injection with chymopapain (**C**) is compared with that after injection of chymopapain (**D**), a marked swelling of the disc is seen, as it assumes a glassy and mucoid appearance.

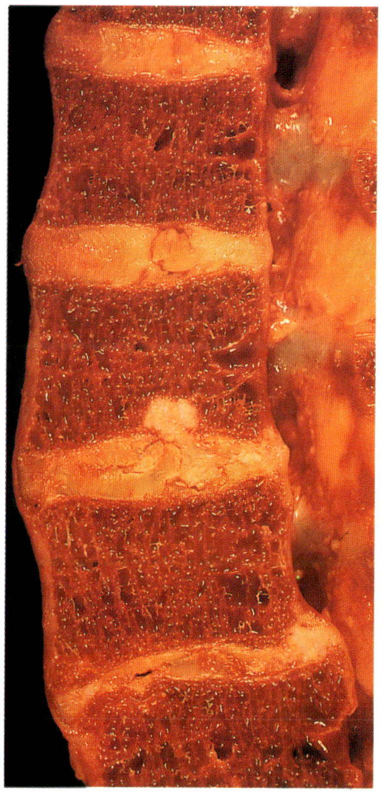

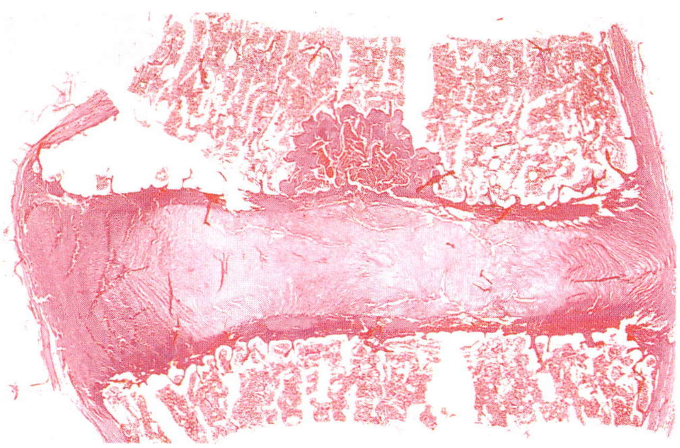

Figure 5.18 Photograph (*top*) of a sagittal section through the lumbar spine of an 83-year-old female. Herniation of the intervertebral disc into the lower surface of L-2 is clearly demonstrated. A photomicrograph (*bottom*) of the same specimen to show the extension of the intervertebral disc tissue through the cartilaginous and bony end plate of the vertebral body. At this time, there is no obvious reactive bony shell. (H & E stain)

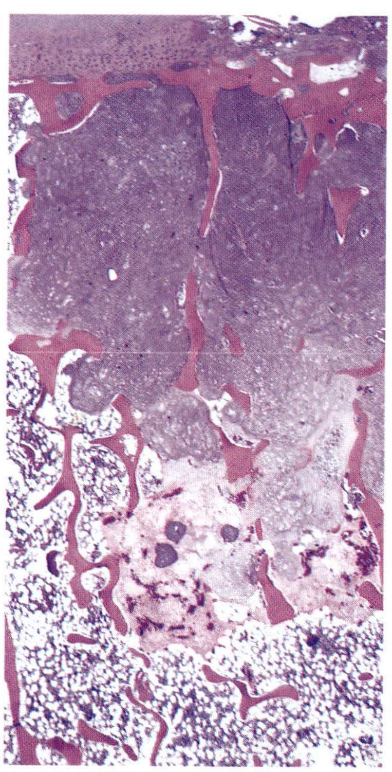

Figure 5.19 Photomicrograph to show a higher power view of another Schmorl's node. On microscopic examination alone, this could be confused with a cartilaginous tumor. (Courtesy of Dr. Howard Dorfman) (H & E stain, × 4 objective, approximately 30 magnifications)

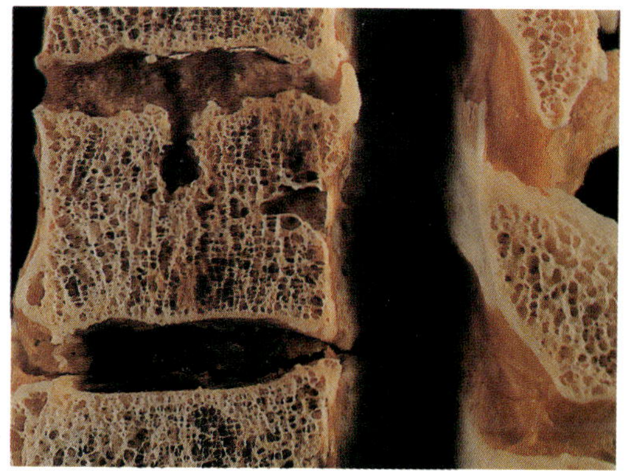

Figure 5.20 Photograph of a sagittal section through a macerated spine to show a defect in the central portion of the superior surface of the L-3 vertebral body. Note the lack of reactive bone around the defect, and, in addition, the irregularity of the bony end plate adjacent to the L2-3 disc.

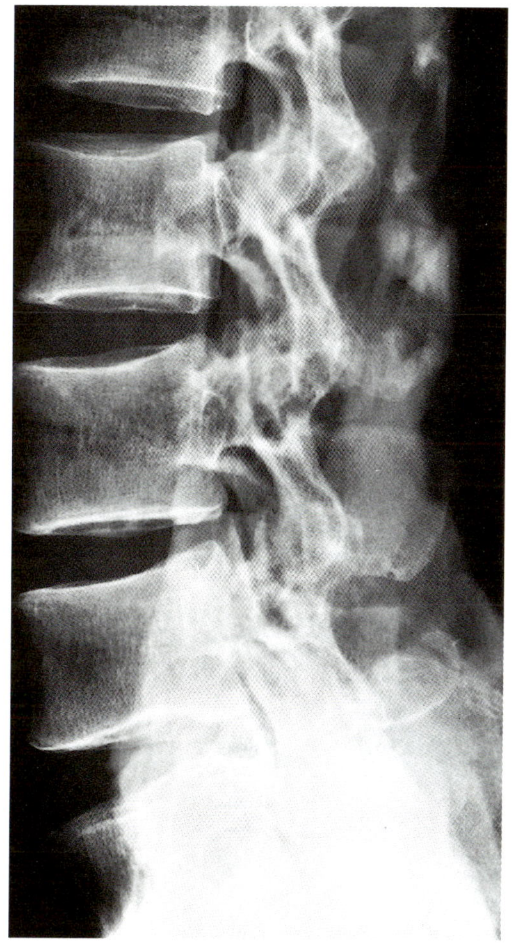

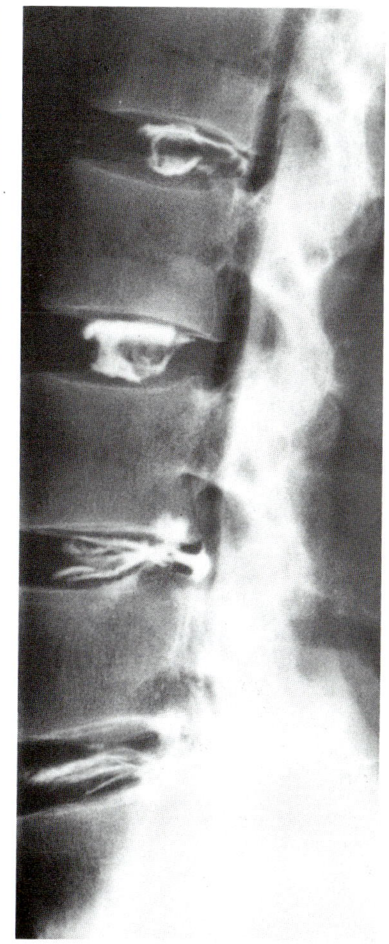

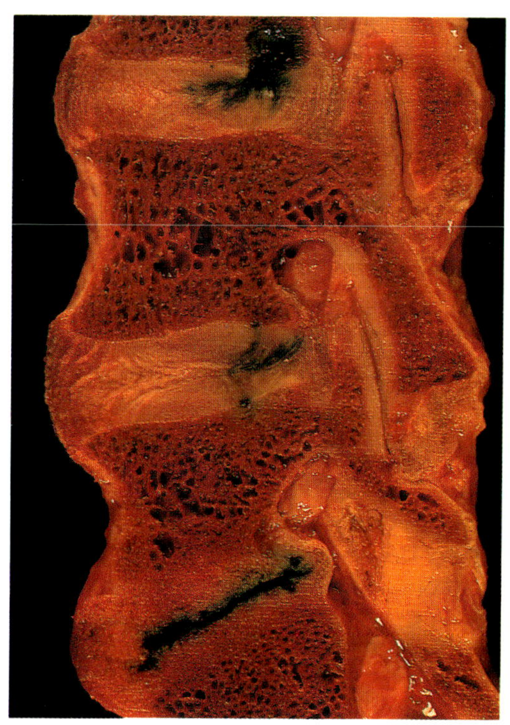

Figure 5.21 Specimen radiograph (*top left*) of the lumbar spine in a 67-year-old male. Schmorl's node cannot be demonstrated in this film. A lateral discogram of this specimen (*top right*) demonstrates clearly that not only is there a Schmorl's node on the posterior part of the inferior surface of L-3; there also is a central disc herniation. A sagittal section (*bottom*) through L3-4, after injection of contrast material, shows the herniation into the posterior part of the inferior surface of L-3.

In addition to developmental defects and traumatic or degenerative changes in the cartilaginous or bony end plates, Schmorl's nodes also are a common finding in conditions where weakening of the subchondral bone has occurred, such as in osteoporosis, hyperparathyroidism, or neoplastic disease (Fig. 5.23). In osteoporosis of the spine, the intervertebral discs frequently become ballooned because of the collapse of the cancellous bone of the vertebral bodies. These changes are seen most commonly in the thoracic and upper lumbar spine.

It has been reported that those Schmorl's nodes that form as a result of a congenital developmental defect of the end plate are generally regular and symmetrically located, whereas those that form as a result of bone loss or of degenerative changes in the end plate are irregular and often mushroom shaped.

A distinct variety of disc herniation of the Schmorl's type occurs in young people, resulting in a focal disturbance in the formation of the ring epiphysis (see Section 1, Chapter 4). This type of herniation, seen most commonly at the anterosuperior vertebral margin, generally is referred to as a *limbus* vertebra (Fig. 5.24). The defect often persists into adult life, where it usually is found incidentally, in lateral radiographs of the spine.

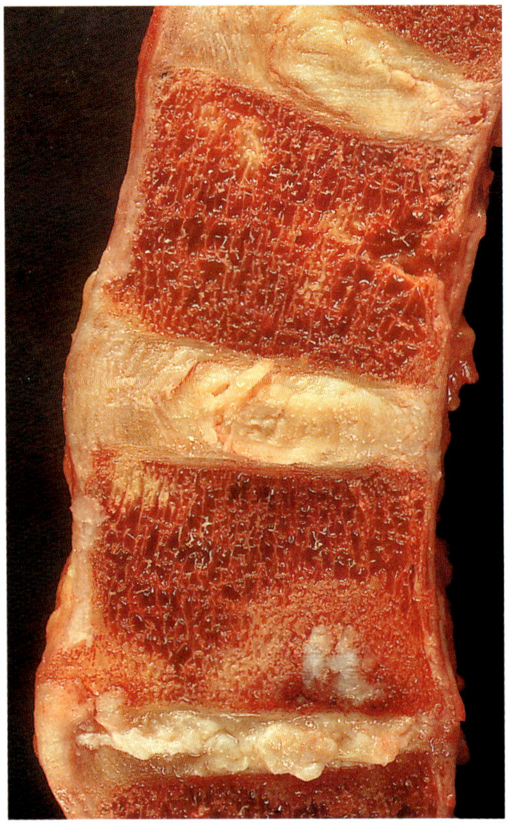

Figure 5.22 Photograph of a sagittal section through the lower lumbar spine of an 80-year-old male, demonstrating a posterior-inferior Schmorl's node, but in this instance, with considerable bony sclerosis around the herniated disc material.

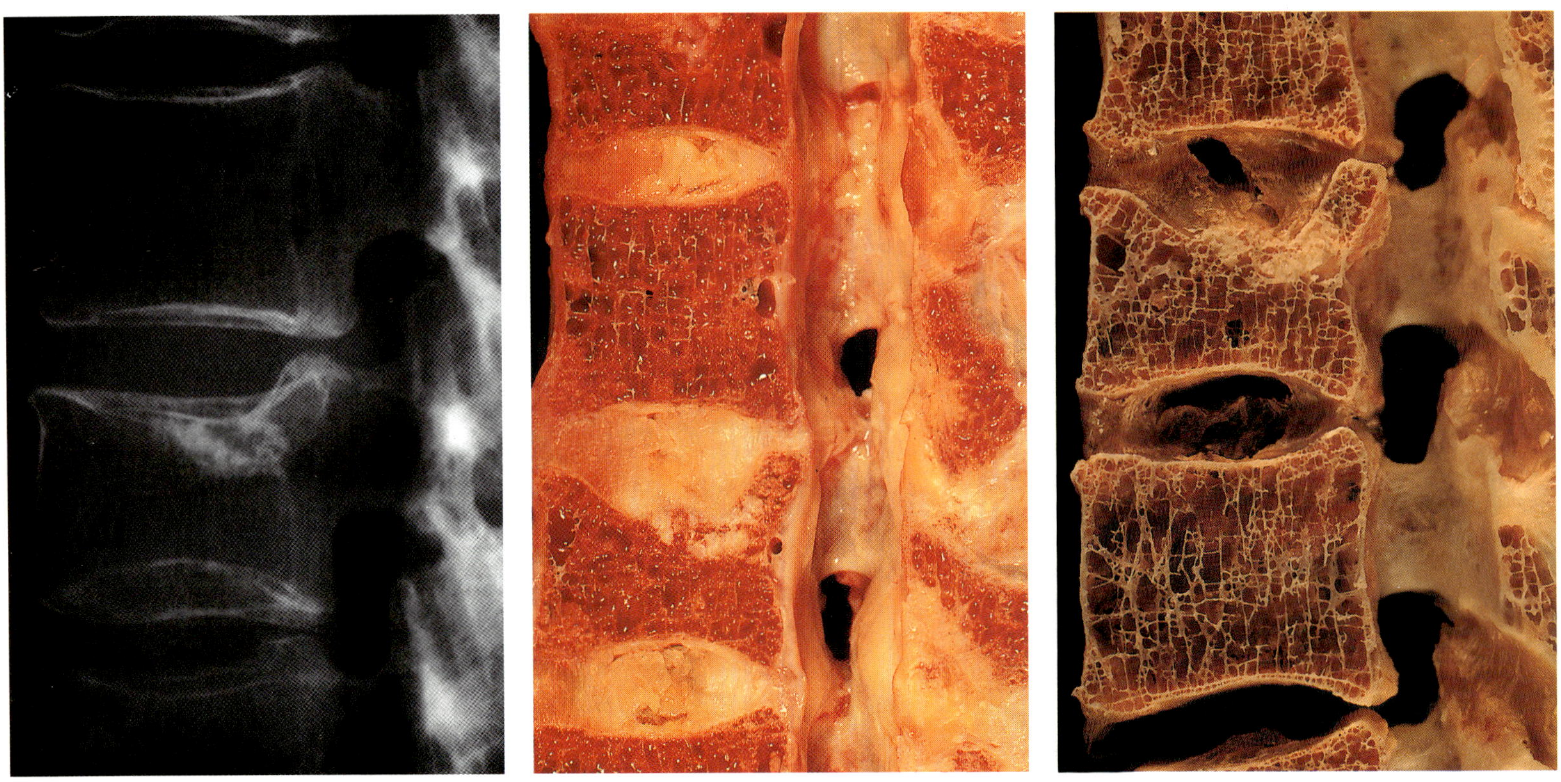

Figure 5.23 Specimen radiograph *(left)* of a portion of the thoracolumbar spine in a patient with severe osteopenia. Note that in T-11 collapse of the superior end plate is associated with an underlying osseous defect characteristic of a herniated disc. In a sagittal section *(center)* of the same segment, note also the widening of the disc below. In the macerated specimen *(right)*, note the reactive bone that has formed around the Schmorl's node.

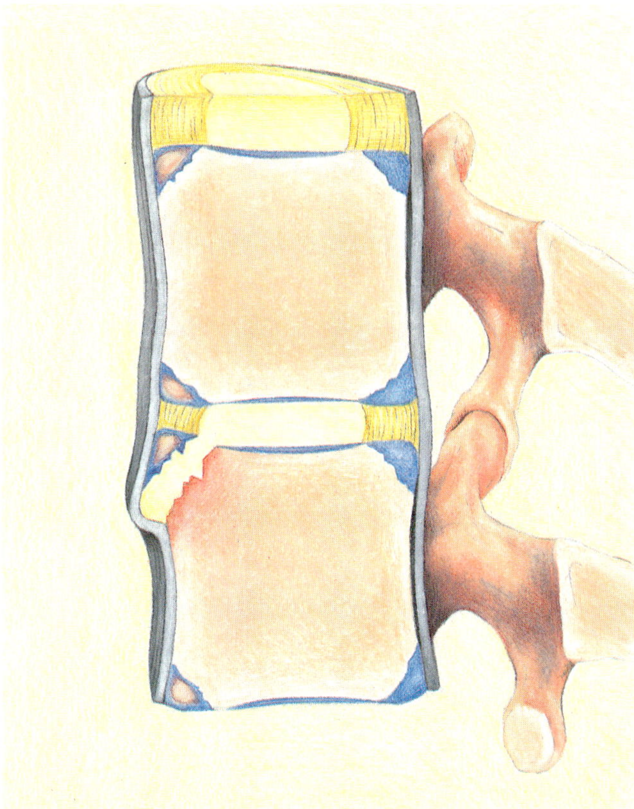

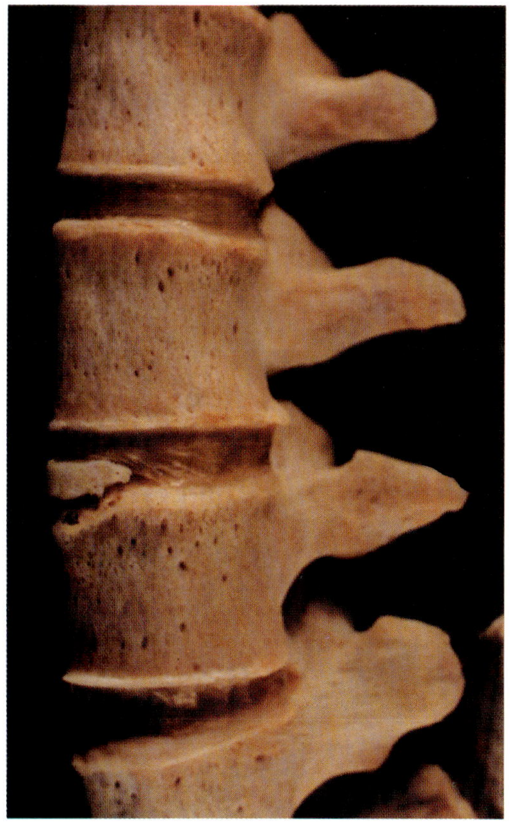

Figure 5.24 Schematic diagram (*top left*) to show the development of a limbus vertebra. The disc tissue extends between the vertebral body and the cartilaginous margin, separating the secondary center of ossification in the ring epiphysis from the rest of the vertebral body. Specimen photograph (*top right*) and radiographs (*bottom left* and *right*) to demonstrate a limbus vertebra in an adult. The secondary center at the anterior margin of the vertebral body has failed to fuse, because of the persistent intervening disc tissue. In the lower right radiograph, the bony defect is more obvious than in the left-hand view.

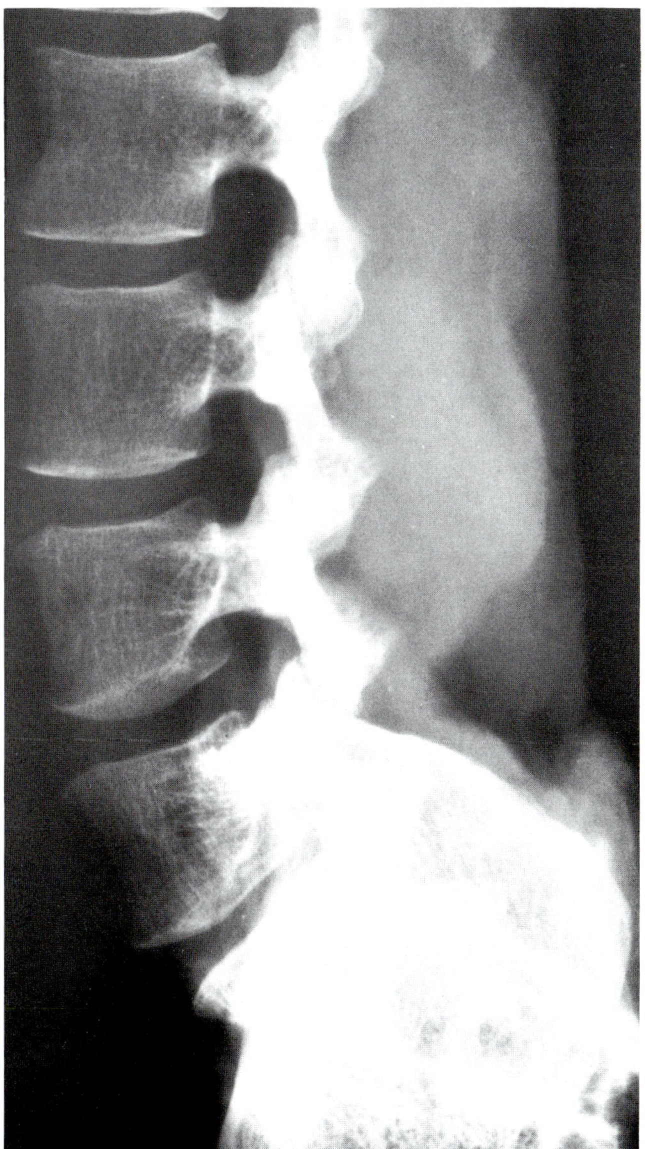

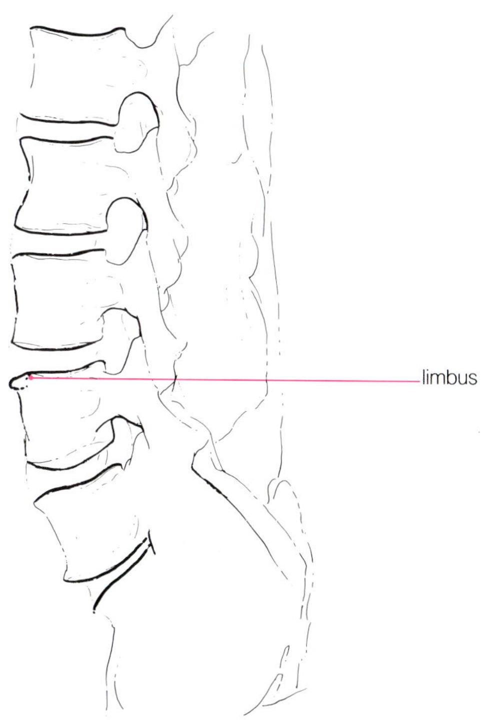

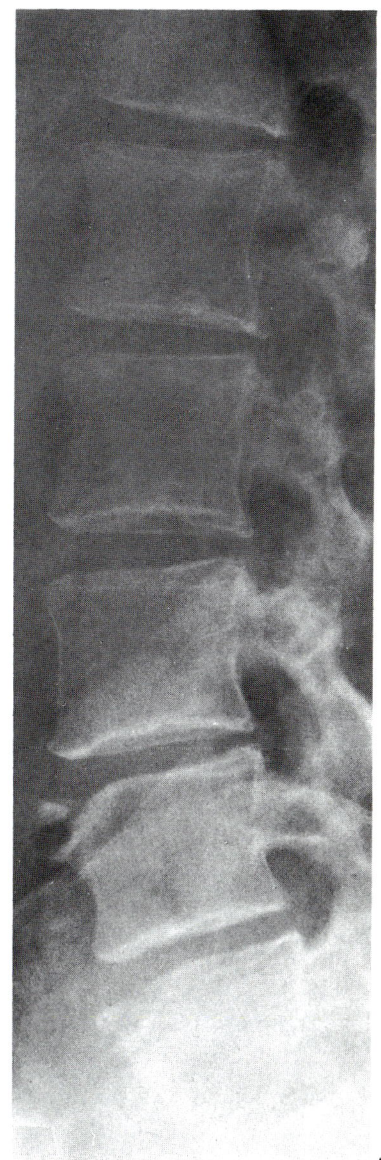

6 CHAPTER

DEPOSITION DISEASES AFFECTING THE SPINE

CALCIFIC DEPOSITS

The first description of intervertebral disc calcifications was given by von Luschka in 1858, who reported that at autopsy he had observed chalk-like deposits in intervertebral disc tissue, especially in the degenerative discs of elderly individuals. Such deposits were later demonstrated radiographically in cadavers, by Beneke in 1897, and later on clinical radiographs by Calvé and Galland in 1922.

The presence of intervertebral disc calcifications is now well documented in both children and adults. In children, intervertebral disc calcification mostly involves the cervical spine, and it is symptomatic in about 80% of affected children, with neck pain as the usual symptom (Fig. 6.1). About half of the cases of cervical disc calcification in children are preceded by a history of trauma (30%) or upper respiratory infection (15%). These childhood lesions generally go on to show resorption of calcium in the involved disc and resolution of symptoms. It has been shown by several investigators that the nucleus pulposus is the site usually affected by this condition, while the anulus fibrosus and the cartilaginous end plates are spared.

In the adult the story is quite different. The discs of the thoracolumbar spine are frequent sites of calcification (Fig. 6.2), while the lower

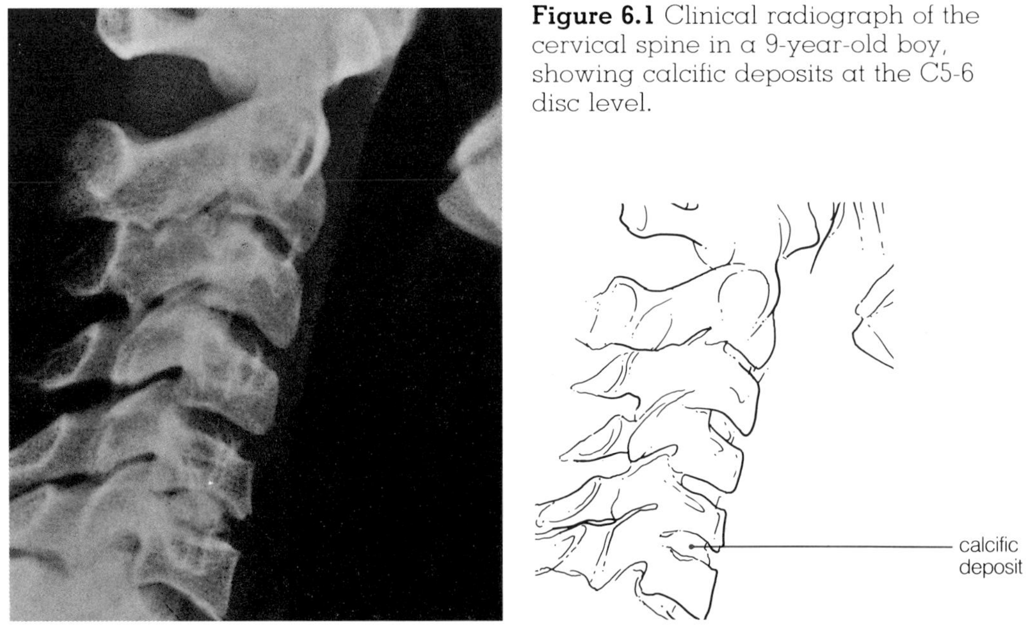

Figure 6.1 Clinical radiograph of the cervical spine in a 9-year-old boy, showing calcific deposits at the C5-6 disc level.

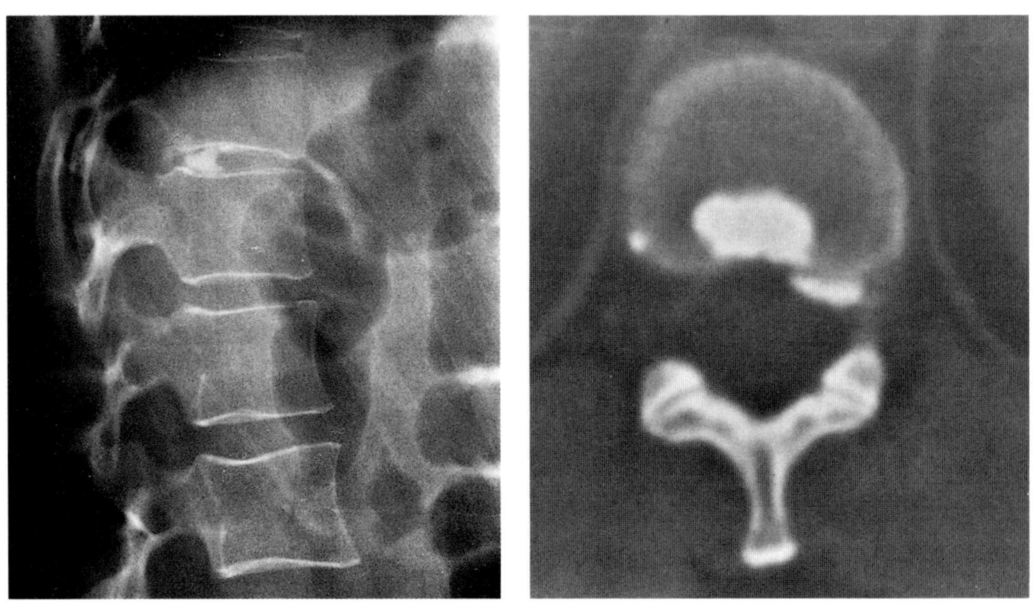

Figure 6.2 Clinical lateral radiograph (*left*) of a portion of thoracolumbar spine in a 41-year-old female, who complained of back pain. Disc calcification is seen in the T11-12 disc. In a CT scan (*right*) of this disc, the extent and location of calcification are clearly demonstrated. (Courtesy of Dr. Francis Denis)

lumbar and cervical regions of the spine are less commonly affected. Though generally asymptomatic, calcification of the intervertebral disc rarely may lead to clinical symptoms, with spinal cord or nerve root compression due to herniation of the calcified mass. Such deposits also may accelerate disc degeneration by interfering with disc nutrition and mechanical function.

In clinical practice, calcification is found incidentally in only 5 to 6% of individuals who have radiographs of the spine taken for one reason or another. On the other hand, at autopsy, Schmorl reported calcification in the anulus fibrosus in 71% of the spines he examined. However, calcification in the nucleus was in his experience relatively uncommon, occurring in only 6.5% of cases. He also reported that calcium deposits may occur at single or multiple levels. Our own autopsy studies generally are in agreement with those of Schmorl, with most deposits being found in the midthoracic and lower thoracic spine (Fig. 6.3). We also observed focal deposits of calcific material in the paraspinal ligaments, as well as in the facet joints.

In anatomical preparations, parasagittal and horizontal sections of the disc, followed by fine-grain radiographic examination (Figs. 6.4 through 6.6), are the best means of identifying calcific deposits. Microscopic, chemical, and x-ray diffraction studies of calcific material obtained from adult lumbar intervertebral discs have shown two main

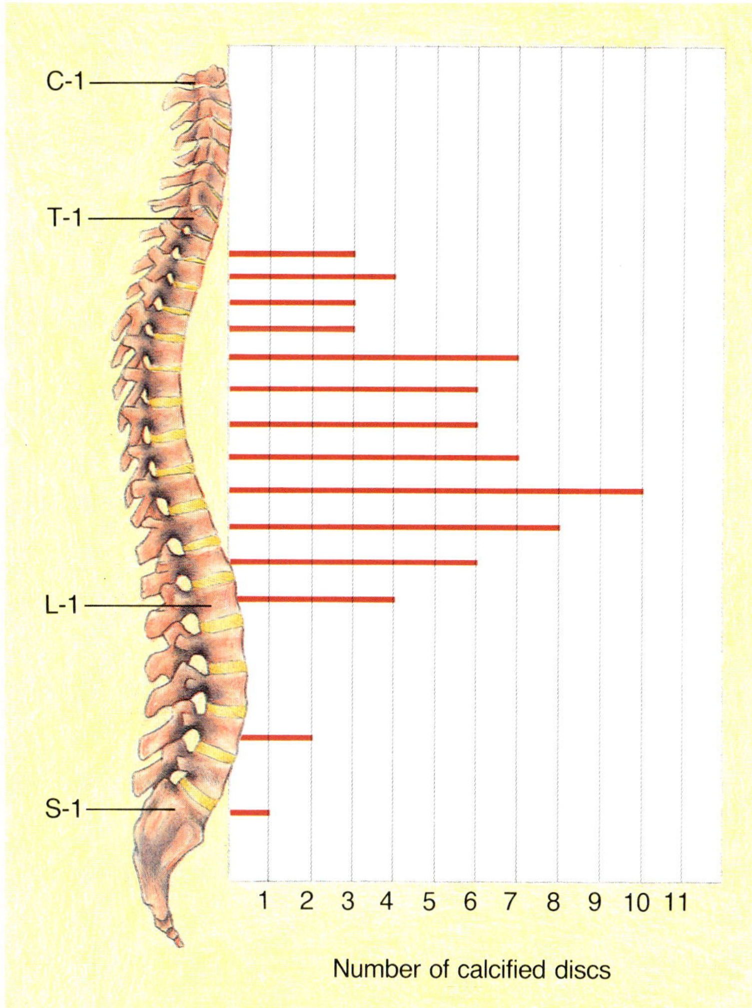

Figure 6.3 Histogram to illustrate the distribution of calcific deposits in the intervertebral discs of 17 out of 36 adult spines from patients over age 50, which showed calcific deposits. In these 17 spines, 70 discs were focally calcified, mostly in the lower thoracic spine. (Authors' own studies)

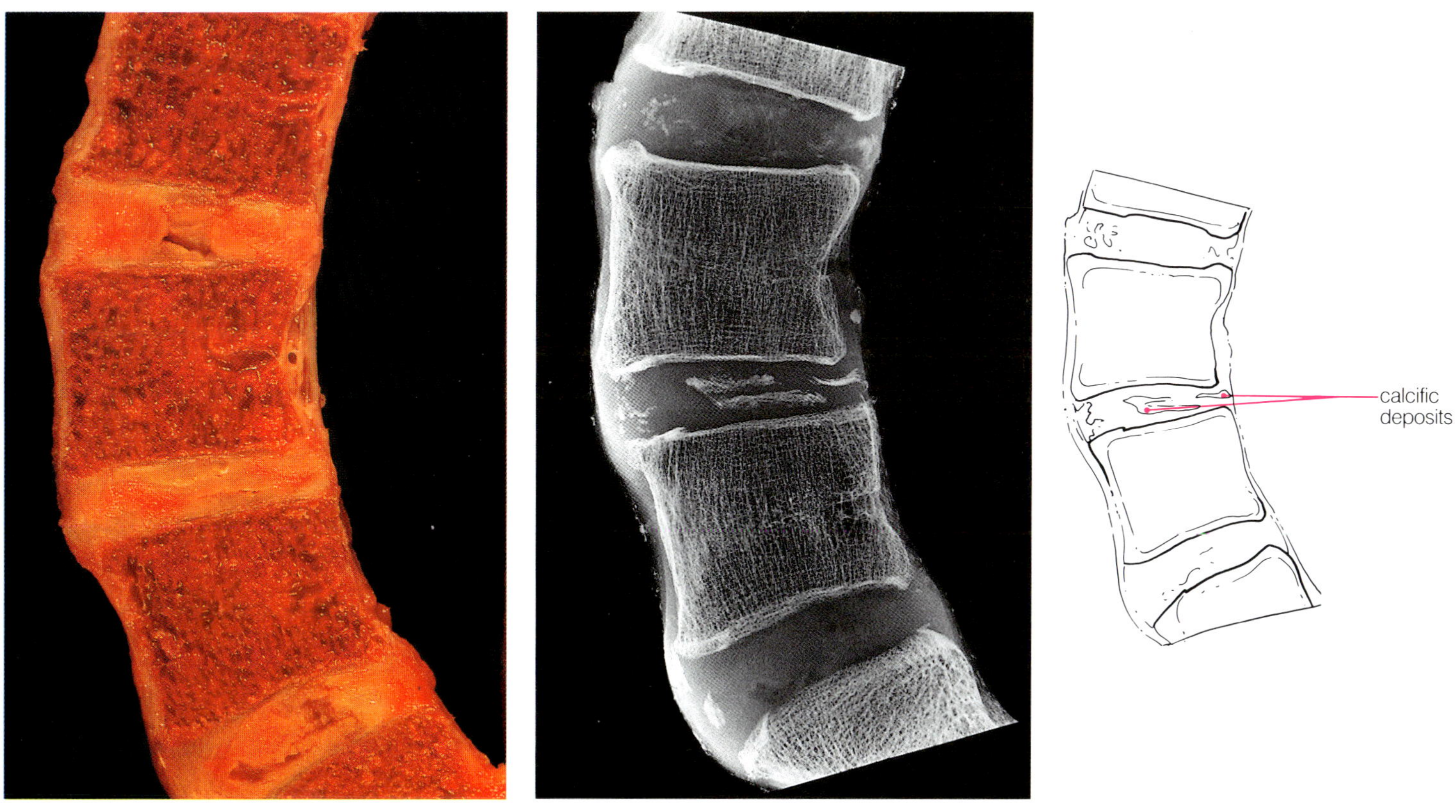

Figure 6.4 Photograph (*left*) of a parasagittal section through the lower lumbar spine. Flecks of chalky material may be seen at each disc level, though most obviously at L4-5. Radiograph (*right*) of the same specimen shows clearly that there is calcification within each of the discs. Since this is a thin slice, we can say that calcium deposits are located in both the central part of the disc as well as in the periphery.

types of calcific deposits: hydroxyapatite and calcium pyrophosphate dihydrate (CPPD) (Figs. 6.7 through 6.10).

Hydroxyapatite deposits are the most frequently encountered form of calcium deposit in disc tissue, and they are commonly associated with disc degeneration. However, apatite deposits occasionally may be seen in association with hyperparathyroidism, hypervitaminosis D, acromegaly, and ochronosis. It should be noted again that calcium deposits in children do not in general have any association other than that of trauma or infection.

At autopsy, CPPD deposits are found much less frequently, although when they do occur they are apt to be found at multiple levels. In surgically excised disc tissue, approximately 2 to 3% will show chondrocalcinosis when multiple sections are prepared.

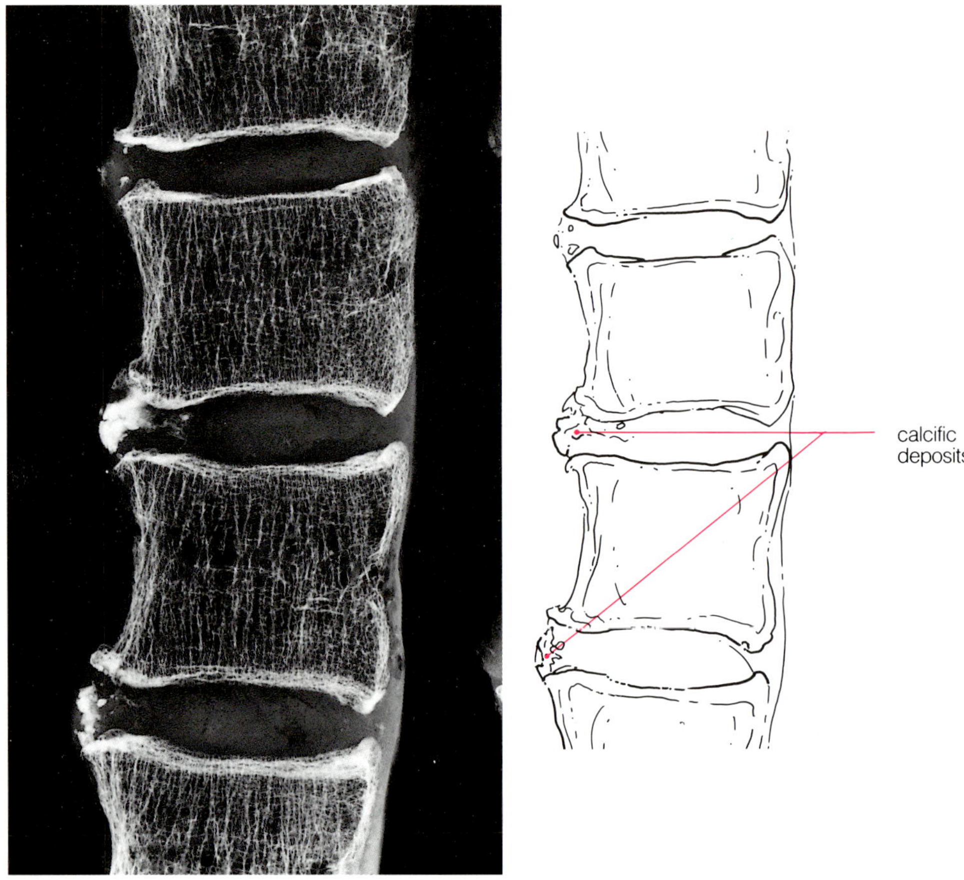

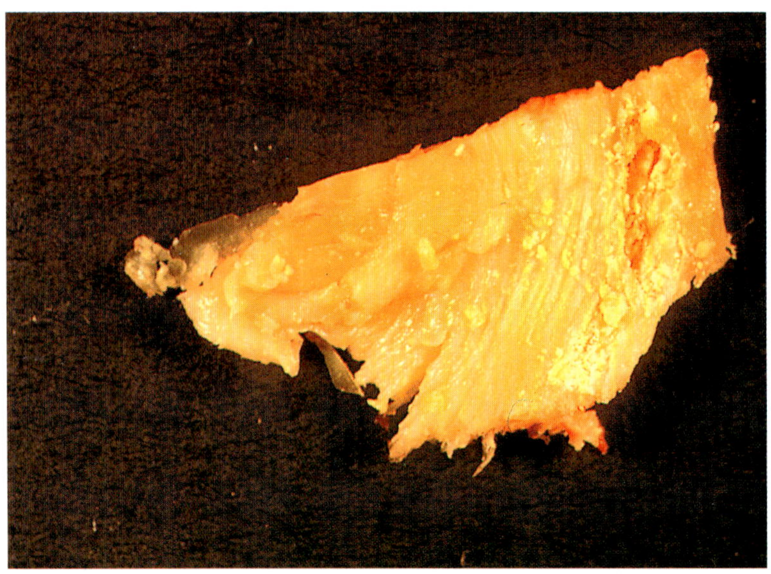

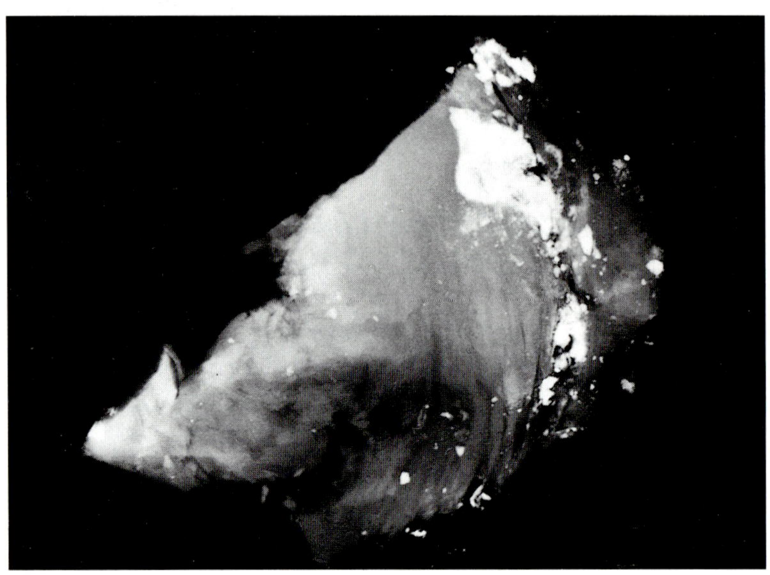

Figure 6.5 Radiograph (*top*) of a parasagittal section through the lower thoracic spine, with calcium deposits of different amounts present in the anulus. A photograph (*center*) of a transverse section through a portion of one of the calcified discs. A radiograph (*bottom*) of the transverse section of the same disc.

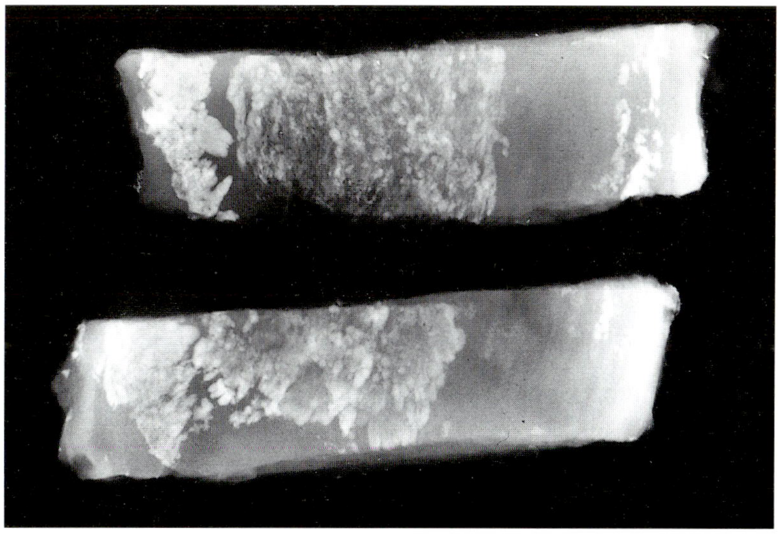

Figure 6.6 Fine-grain radiograph to demonstrate diffuse calcium deposits, which may not be obvious on macroscopic examination of disc tissue. These deposits were later shown to be due to calcium pyrophosphate dihydrate (CPPD) crystal deposition disease. Both the anulus and the nucleus are affected.

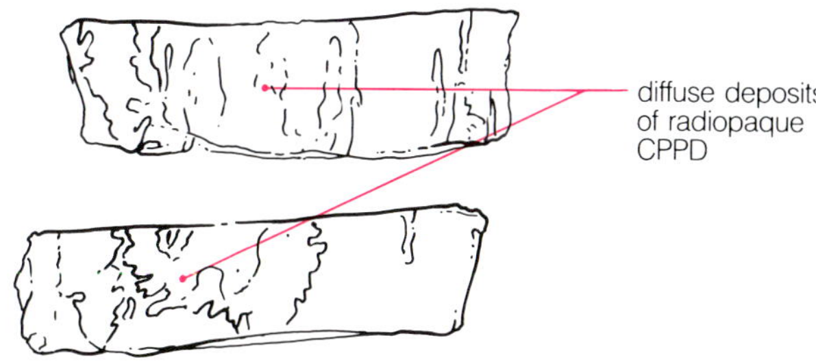

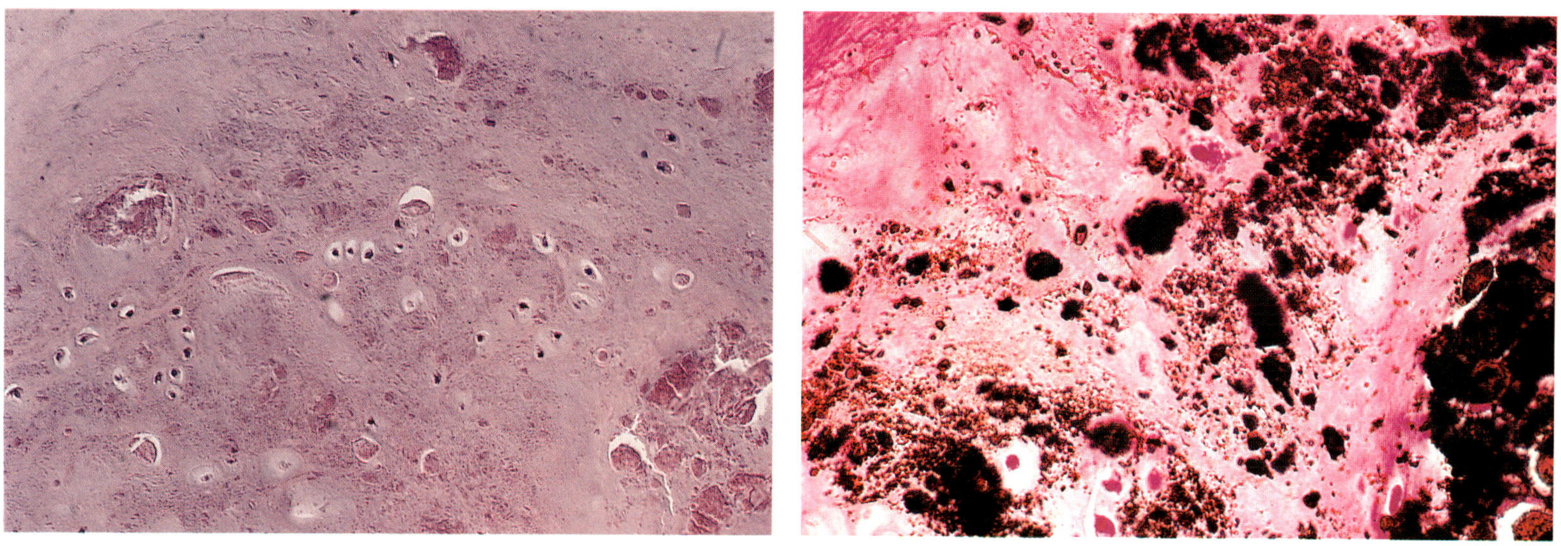

Figure 6.7 Photomicrograph (*left*) of an apatite deposit in the anulus fibrosus. The calcific tissue is granular and discrete, but no crystalline material can be recognized by light microscopy. (H & E, × 10 objective) A von Kossa stain (*right*) demonstrates the extent of the calcific deposits in this particular case.

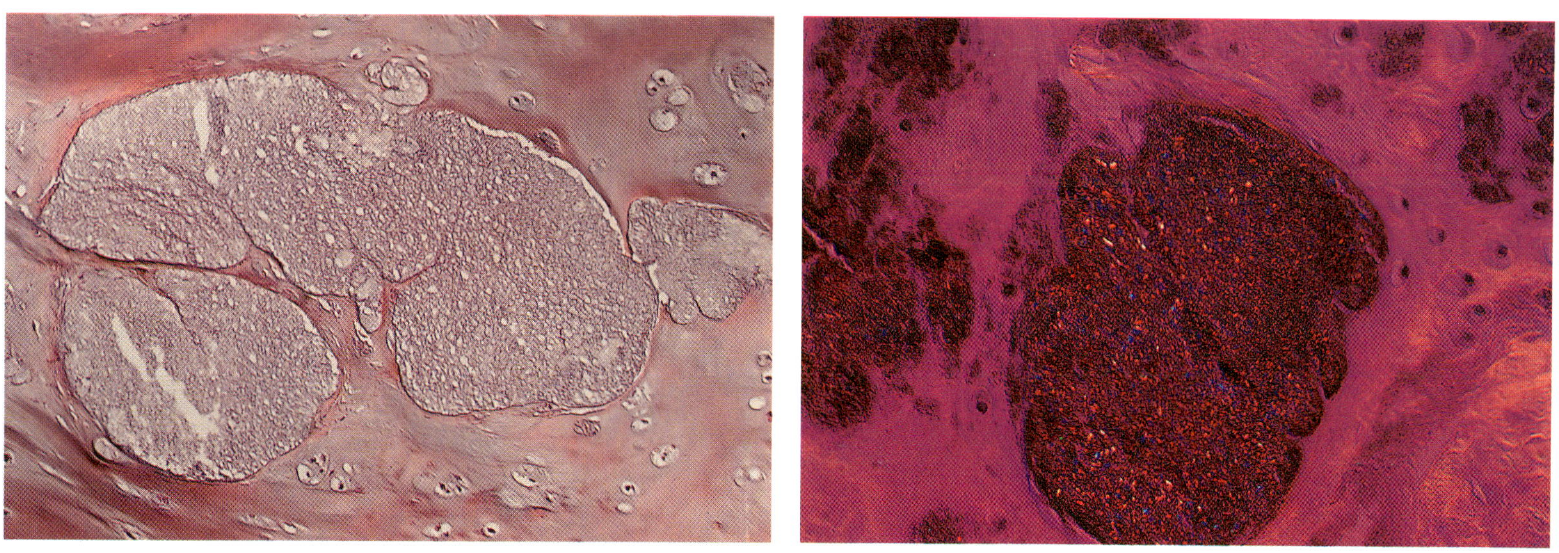

Figure 6.8 Photomicrograph (*left*) of a CPPD deposit in the nucleus pulposus. Note that the deposits are very well delineated, and display a fine granularity. (H & E, × 10 objective) When examined with polarized light (*right*), one of the CPPD deposits shows the weak positive birefringence characteristic of calcium pyrophosphate crystals. (Polarized light, × 10 objective)

In our experience, CPPD deposits tend to occur diffusely in the nucleus and anulus. Deposits may be associated with generalized familial chondrocalcinosis or with other metabolic disturbances such as hemochromatosis, hyperparathyroidism, and gout. CPPD may result in degenerative disc disease and even in degenerative spondylolisthesis (Fig. 6.11).

Gout

Spinal involvement by gout is very rare. However, in Schmorl's postmortem studies, as well as in those of others, the presence of urate deposits in the disc tissue, vertebral bodies, facet joints, and ligamenta flava of patients with a history of gout has been demonstrated, and in rare cases this has resulted in severe bony destruction and ver-

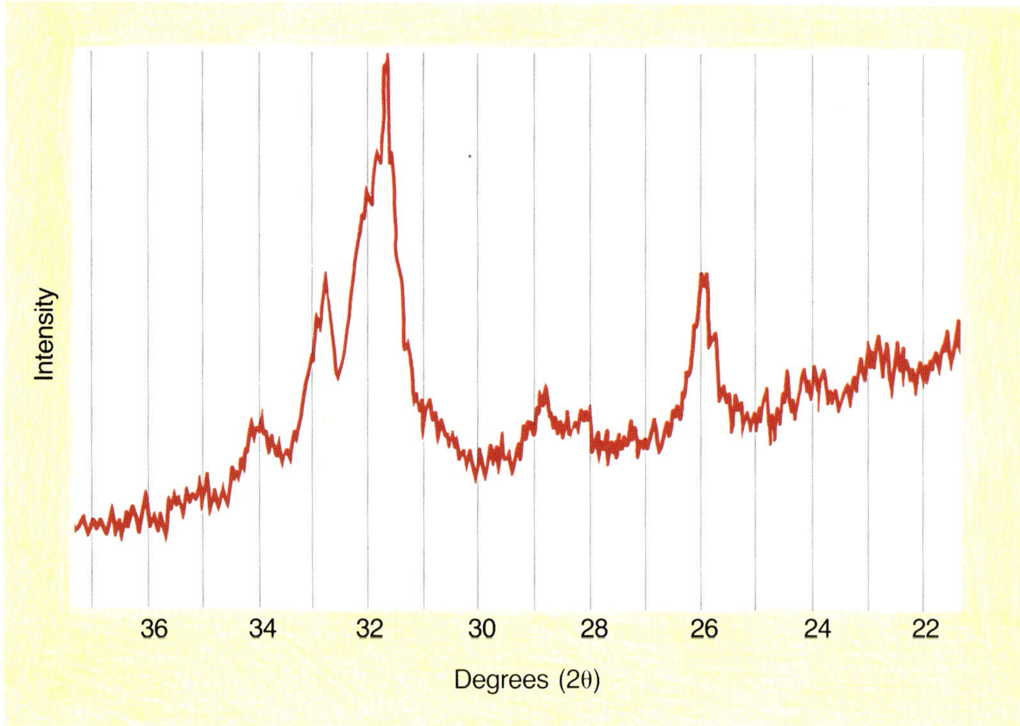

Figure 6.9 Tracing of the x-ray diffraction pattern of hydroxyapatite.

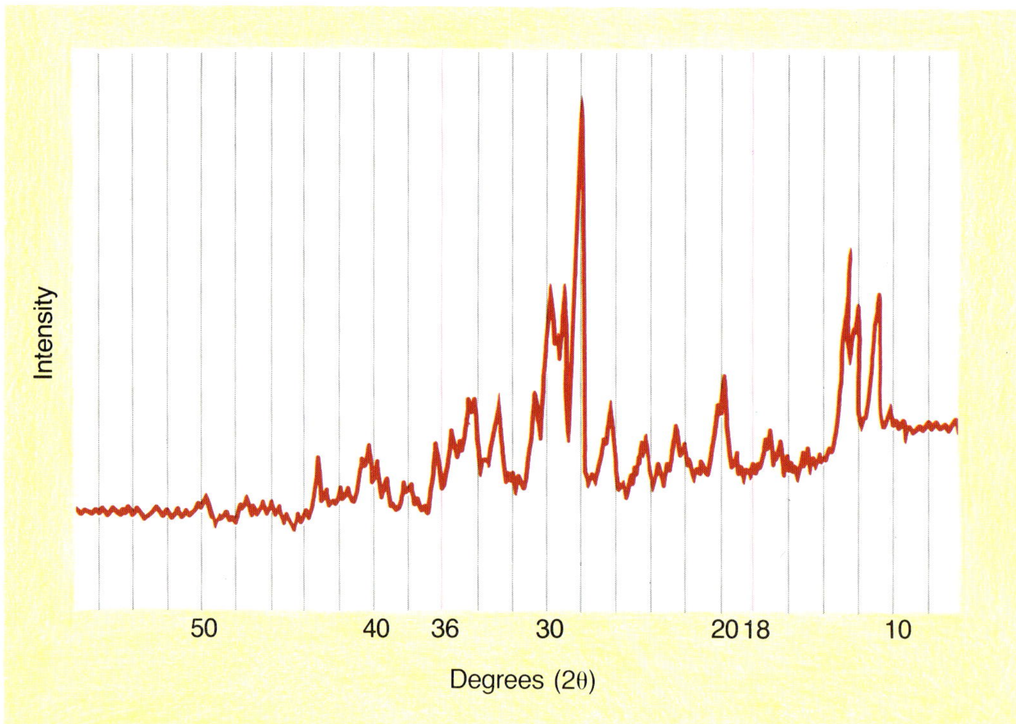

Figure 6.10 Tracing of the x-ray diffraction pattern of calcium pyrophosphate dihydrate (CPPD). The typical peaks for CPPD lie between 18 and 36. (Courtesy of Adele Boskey)

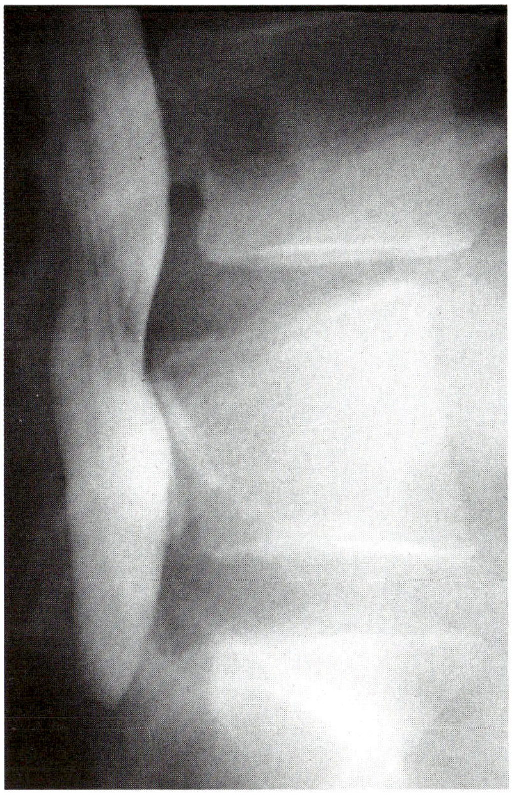

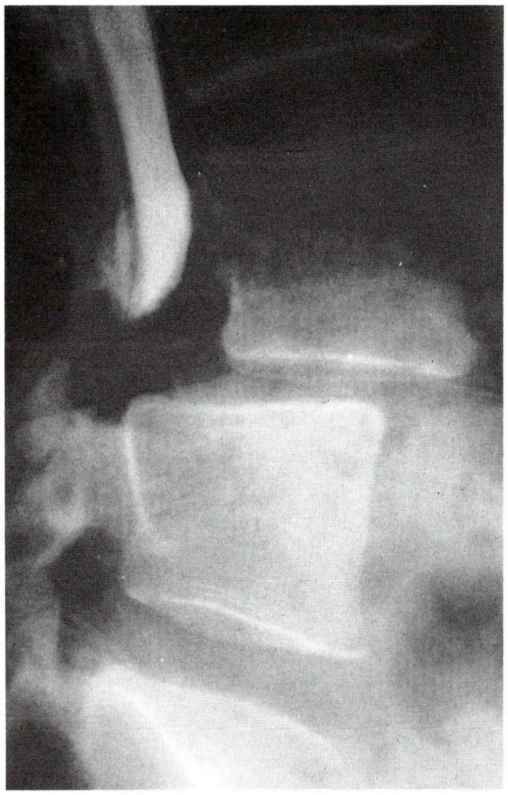

Figure 6.11 Lateral myelogram (*top left*) showing degenerative spondylolisthesis with marked instability in flexion. The same patient, seen two years later (*top right*), has developed a complete block from progression of the slippage. A photomicrograph (*bottom left*) of synovial tissue obtained from the facet joint demonstrates a calcific deposit (brown-black) in the surface of the synovium. (von Kossa stain, × 10 objective, approximately 160 magnifications) A photomicrograph (*bottom right*) of the deposits, taken with polarized light, demonstrates refractile crystals consistent with CPPD. CPPD deposits were also found in the disc tissue histologically and in the knees radiographically. (× 40 objective) (Courtesy of Dr. R. Lagier)

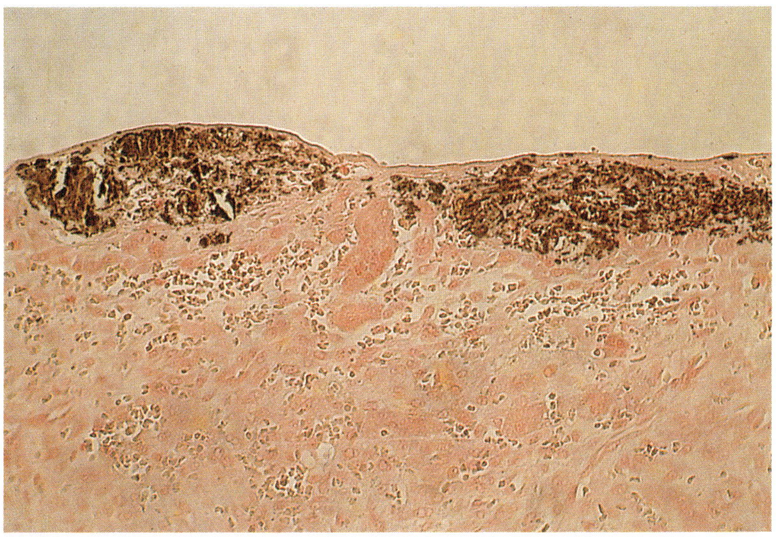

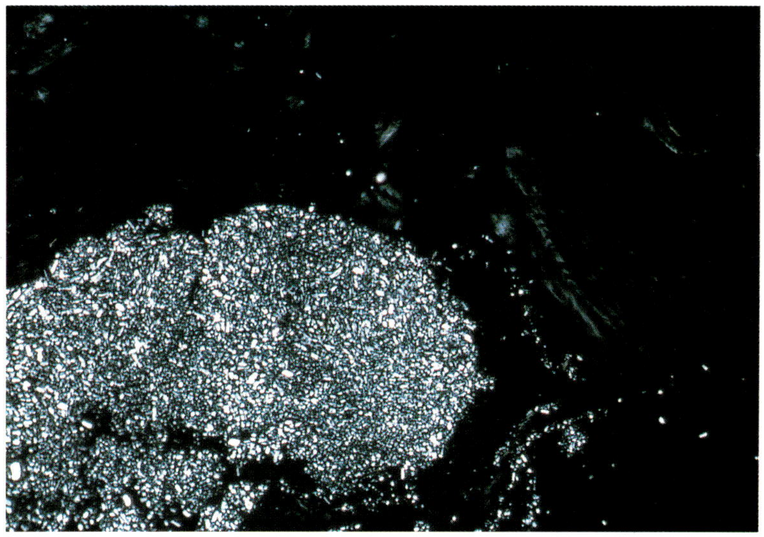

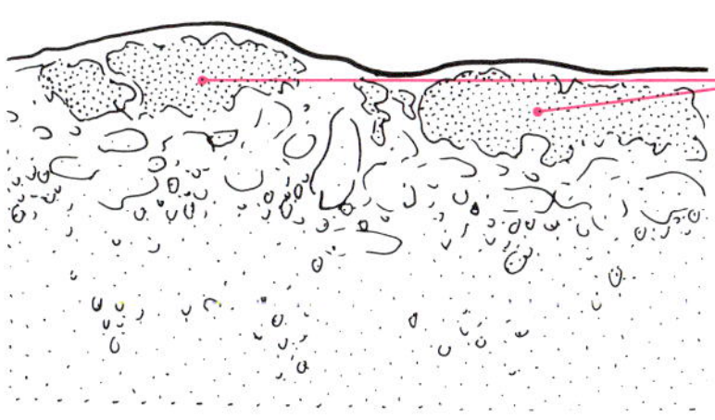

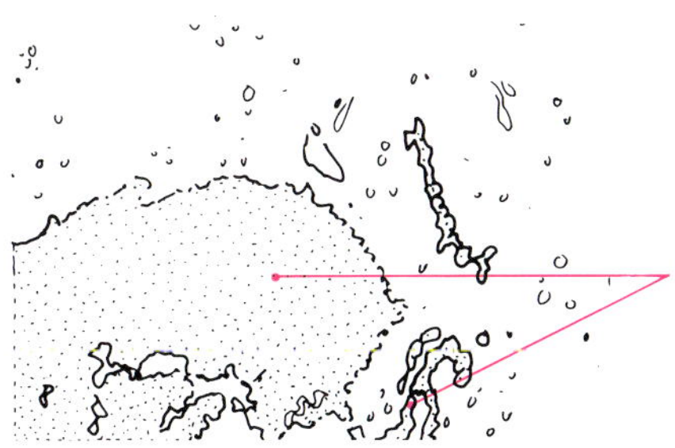

tebral body collapse (Fig. 6.12). In those patients with a history of the disease, gout should be included in the differential diagnosis of low back pain.

When gout affects the cervical spine, abnormalities may include erosions of the odontoid process or vertebral end plates, along with disc-space narrowing. Severe involvement and destruction of the odontoid process may result in atlantoaxial instability.

If gouty involvement of the spine is extensive, the tophaceous deposits may eventually surround the spinal cord and cauda equina, resulting in significant neurologic complications.

Ochronosis

The term ochronosis is used to describe an abnormal black-brown pigmentation of the cartilage and other connective tissues, which is the result of the failure to metabolize homogentisic acid due to an inherited deficiency of the enzyme homogentisic acid oxidase. The excess homogentisic acid is excreted in the urine (alkaptonuria) and on exposure to air becomes black (Fig. 6.13). It also accumulates in tissues, especially in connective tissue, where it alters the structure of the collagen, rendering it more brittle.

In general, the affected individual is asymptomatic until adult life, at which time ochronotic arthropathy may develop in the joints of the appendicular and axial skeleton. When the spine is involved, back pain and stiffness are the usual complaints, and usually there is a loss of the normal sagittal alignment, along with restriction of motion. Postural deformity eventually may simulate that of ankylosing spondylitis. In males especially, an initial presenting feature of the disease may be a herniated disc in the lumbar spine.

In anatomical preparations, the earliest findings of ochronosis are seen in the lumbar spine, as black-brown pigmentation of the intervertebral discs, which is more pronounced in the cartilaginous plate and anulus fibrosus (Figs. 6.14 and 6.15). Pigmentation also may be present in various vertebral ligaments.

In the spine, the natural history of the disease is one of a decrease in the disc-space height with subchondral sclerosis, bony proliferation around the vertebral bodies (in the form of osteophytes), and eventual bridging of the bodies. An association between intervertebral disc calcification and ochronosis is well recognized. Calcifications may occur at any segment of the spinal column but have a predilection for the intervertebral discs of the lumbar spine and involve both the anulus and the nucleus. X-ray crystallographic analysis of such deposits has shown them to be composed of hydroxyapatite.

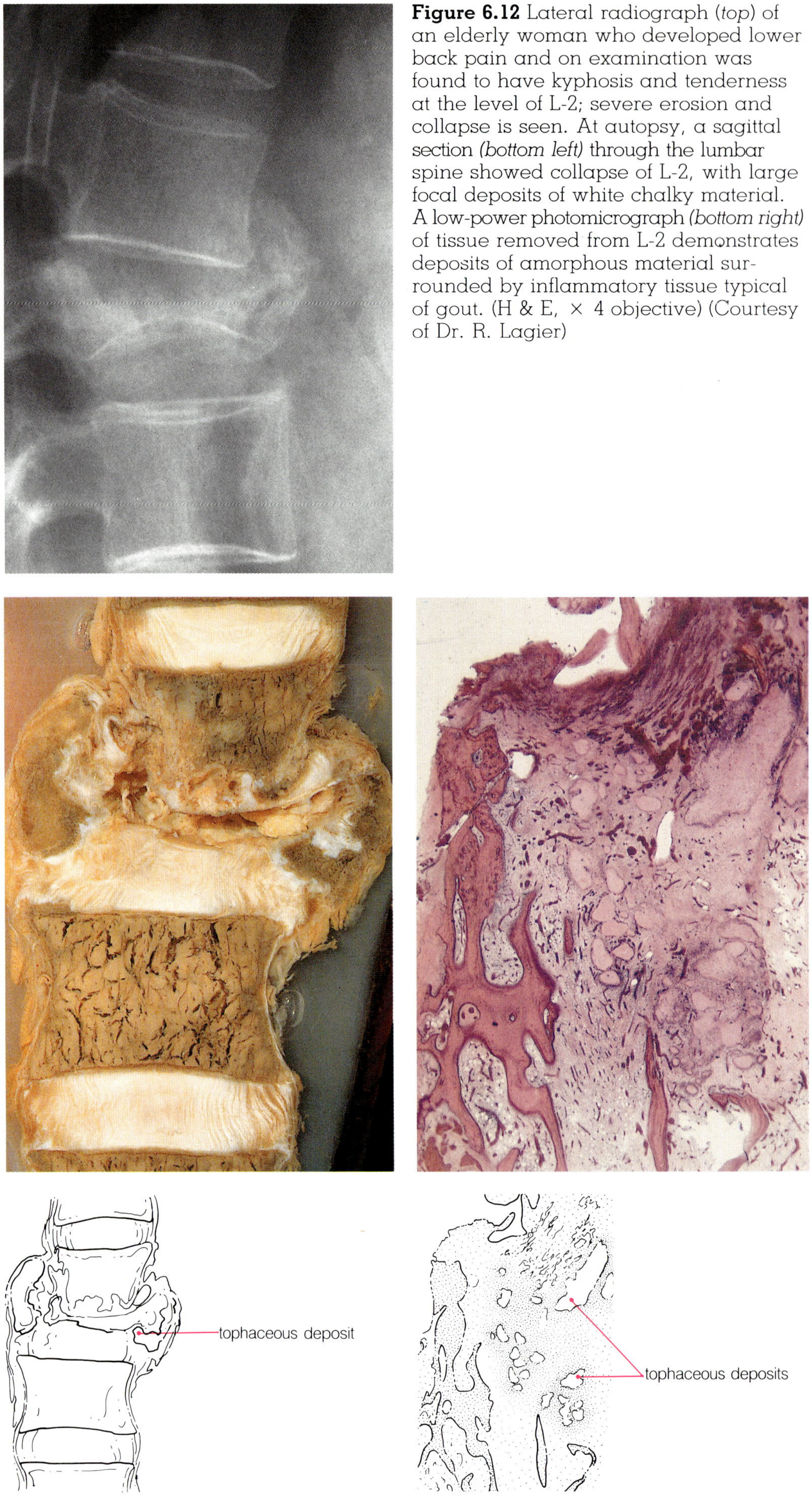

Figure 6.12 Lateral radiograph (*top*) of an elderly woman who developed lower back pain and on examination was found to have kyphosis and tenderness at the level of L-2; severe erosion and collapse is seen. At autopsy, a sagittal section *(bottom left)* through the lumbar spine showed collapse of L-2, with large focal deposits of white chalky material. A low-power photomicrograph *(bottom right)* of tissue removed from L-2 demonstrates deposits of amorphous material surrounded by inflammatory tissue typical of gout. (H & E, × 4 objective) (Courtesy of Dr. R. Lagier)

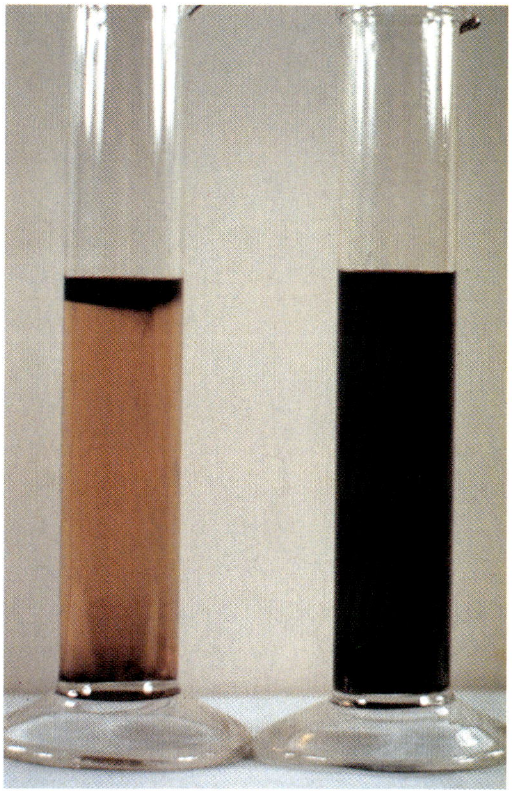

Figure 6.13 Photograph showing two flasks containing urine from a patient with ochronosis. In the flask on the left, the urine has been left to stand for 15 minutes. Some darkening is apparent at the surface, due to oxidation of homogentisic acid. In the flask on the right, after two hours, the urine has become entirely black.

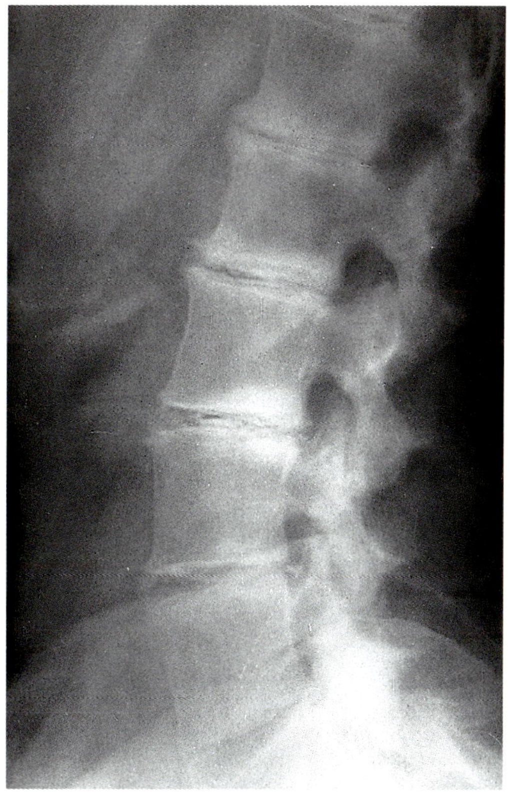

Figure 6.14 Radiograph of a patient with ochronosis shows narrowing of the disc spaces, many of which are seen to be calcified.

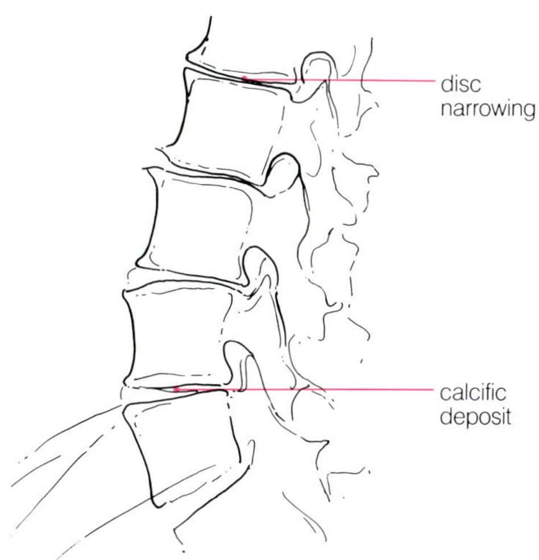

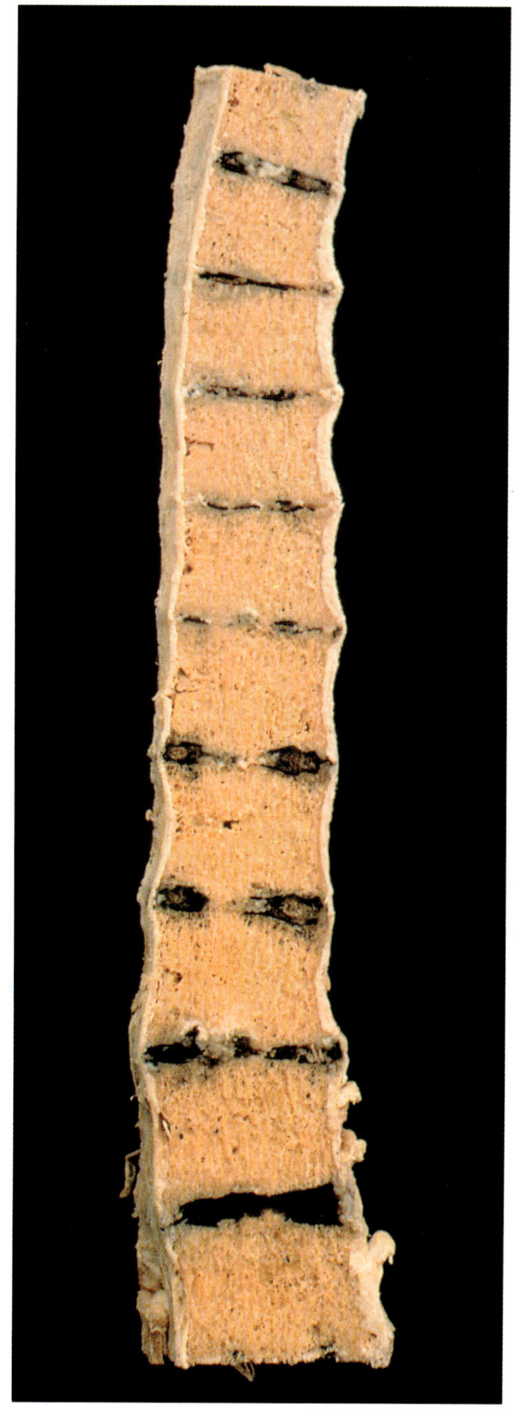

Figure 6.15 Photograph of a sagittally sectioned spine from a patient with ochronosis. Note the black pigmentation of the intervertebral discs, which also are seen to be narrowed.

7

CHAPTER

AGE-RELATED CHANGES AND DEGENERATIVE DISC DISEASE (OSTEOCHONDROSIS)

General Features

The form and function of the vertebral column are largely dependent on the integrity of the intervertebral disc. It was Schmorl in particular who first drew attention to the morbid changes in intervertebral disc tissue and to the relationship of these changes to vertebral body disease and to spinal disease as a whole. The age-associated structural changes that occur normally in the disc are to be distinguished from those that occur as a result of so-called morbid "degenerative" processes. While the changes that are observed in the nucleus and anulus with advancing age are associated with cartilaginous end plates that remain intact, there is good reason to believe that intervertebral disc degenerative disease, osteochondrosis, is closely related to damage occurring in the end plates (Fig. 7.1). In this chapter, age-associated changes will be discussed first, followed by a discussion of degenerative disc disorders.

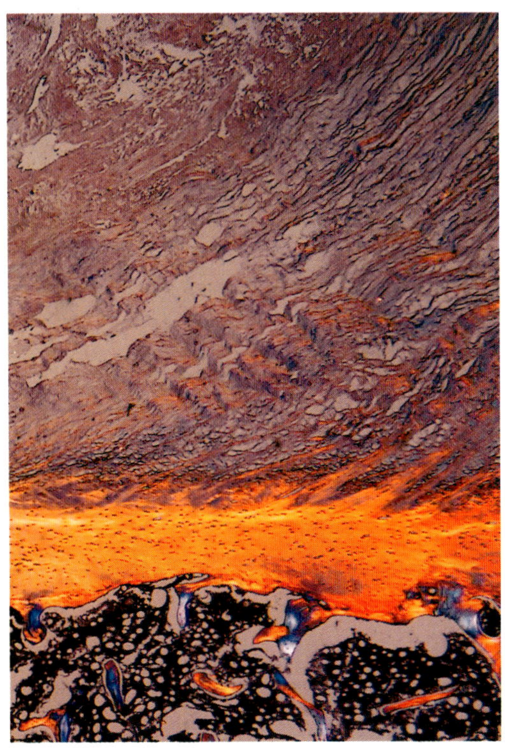

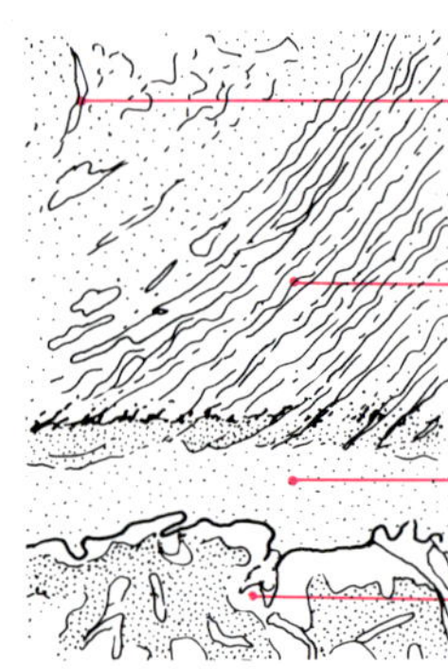

Figure 7.1 Photomicrograph to demonstrate the clear demarcation between the bone, the cartilaginous end plate, and the intervertebral disc tissue. A portion of the anulus is seen in the lower right, with a portion of the nucleus in the upper left. (Polarized light, × 1 objective, approximately 12.5 magnifications)

Age-Related Changes of the Intervertebral Disc

The disc of the young adult, with its bulging mucoid nucleus pulposus, dense collagenous anulus fibrosus, and well-defined cartilaginous end plates, can be differentiated clearly from that of the elderly person, with its shrunken, yellowed, dehydrated nucleus pulposus (Figs. 7.2 through 7.4). The transition between these states is not a sudden one, but, rather, occurs gradually, as a result of the normal aging process (see Section 1, Fig. 2.40).

To summarize this process briefly, during the first and second decades of life, the nucleus pulposus becomes increasingly well delineated, with its fluid content increasing in response to its increased functional role (Fig. 7.5). At this stage, microscopic sections of the disc tissue will stain strongly with Al-

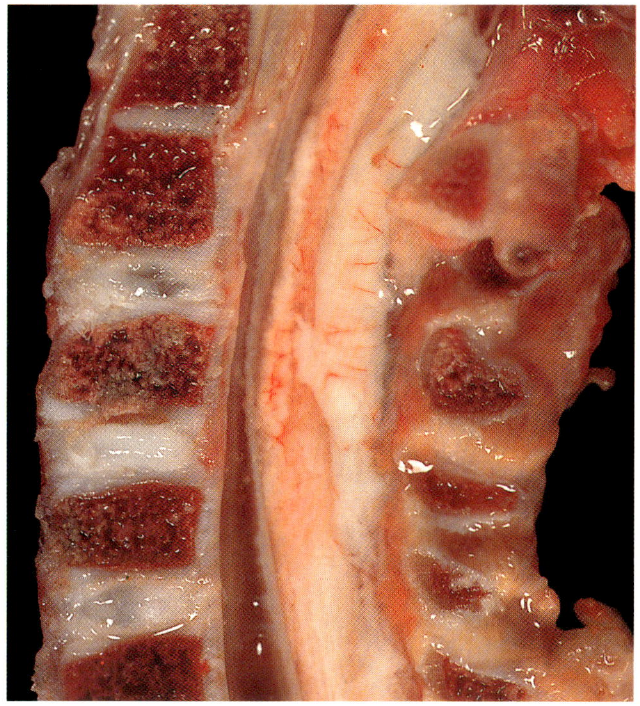

Figure 7.2 Photograph of a sagittal section through the cervical spine from a child. The bulging appearance of the cut surface of the disc, especially visible in C3-6, reflects the high water content of the tissue.

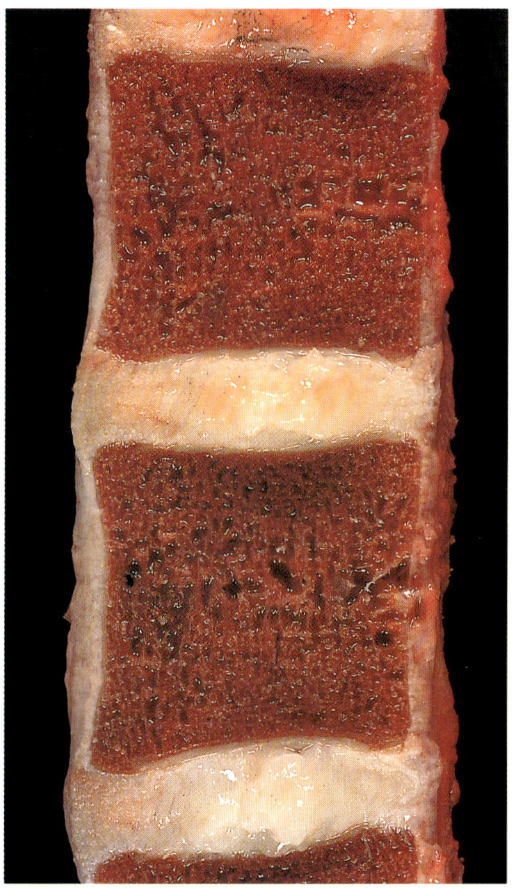

Figure 7.3 Photograph of a sagittal section through a portion of the upper thoracic spine of a 25-year-old male. Note the glistening, slightly bulging appearance of the normal disc in a young adult.

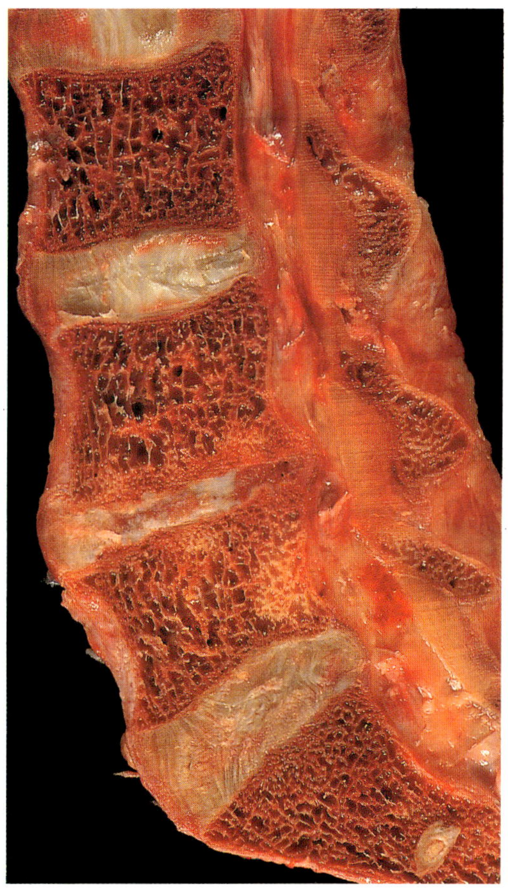

Figure 7.4 Photograph of a sagittal section through the lumbosacral spine in a 50-year-old male. The discs at the level of L3-4 and L-5 to S-1 show the discolored shrunken appearance normal to older discs. The L4-5 disc already shows the morbid changes of osteochondrosis.

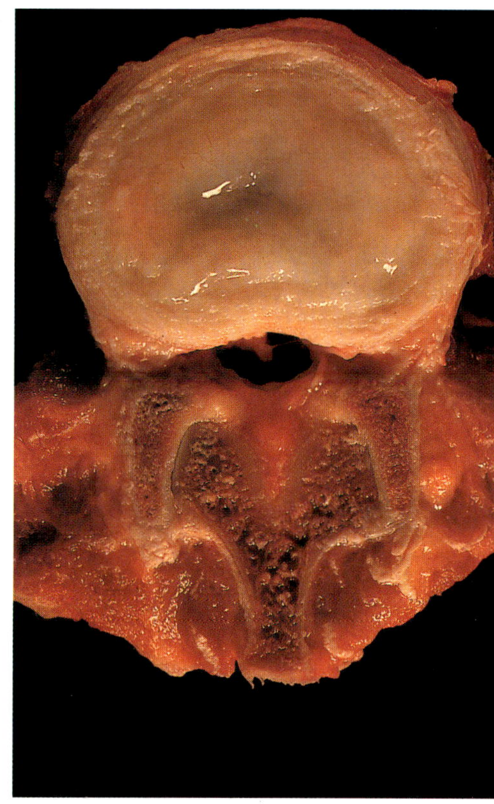

Figure 7.5 Photograph of a transverse section through the L1-2 disc from an adolescent. Note the clear demarcation between the mucoid nucleus pulposus and the laminated anulus fibrosus.

cian blue stain (Fig. 7.6). During the third decade, structural changes begin to appear in the anulus fibrosus such that concentric fissuring of the lamellae, loss of cellular detail, and swelling between the lamellae may be present. Similarly, the nucleus pulposus no longer shows its uniform mucoid appearance. Microscopic clefts and loose fibrillar changes become present as the nucleus begins to blend more with the anulus. By the end of the third decade the boundary may have become quite indistinct (Fig. 7.7). From the fourth decade on, there is a continuing, gradual loss of fluid from the nucleus pulposus. Microscopically, the homogeneous mucoid appearance of the youthful nucleus is lost, as it becomes a tangled mass of fibrous tissue and cartilage cells. Cut sections of the intervertebral disc at this time may show one solid fibrocartilaginous mass (Fig. 7.8).

With advanced age, a yellow-brown pigmentation, affecting both the anulus and the nucleus, is found. The Alcian blue stain, which is predominant in the healthy youthful disc, fades, and there is increased PAS staining of the disc tissue (Fig. 7.9). In older individuals, associated with the stiffening of the disc tissue, microscopic tears occur in the anulus fibrosus. Fibrocartilaginous metaplasia begins to appear around these tears, comparable to the cartilaginous metaplasia that is seen in the frayed knee menisci of older individuals (Fig. 7.10). These microscopic tears may herald the onset of spondylosis deformans (see Chapter 6).

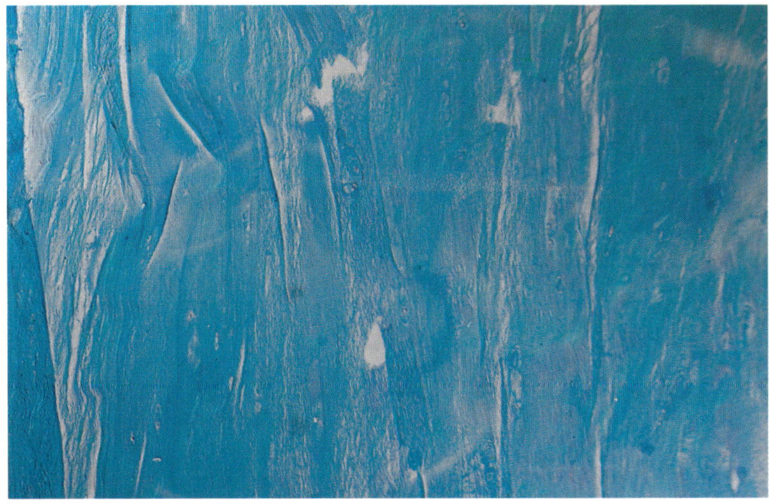

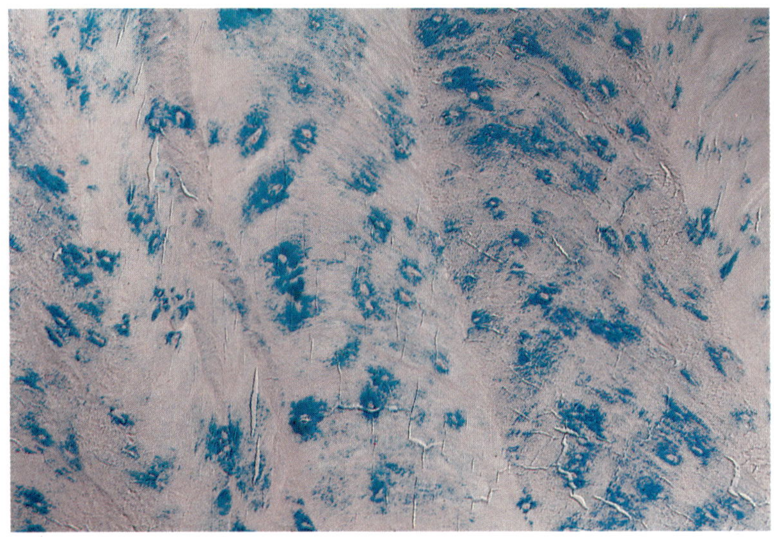

Figure 7.6 Photomicrograph (*top*) of a portion of the anulus fibrosus from an 18-year-old male. The disc is stained with Alcian blue, to demonstrate the sulfated mucopolysaccharide. (× 10 objective, approximately 250 magnifications) In a comparable section (*bottom*) from a 68-year-old male, diminished staining may be seen, with staining confined to the pericellular areas. This reflects a loss in the mucopolysaccharide content. (Alcian blue, × 10 objective, approximately 250 magnifications)

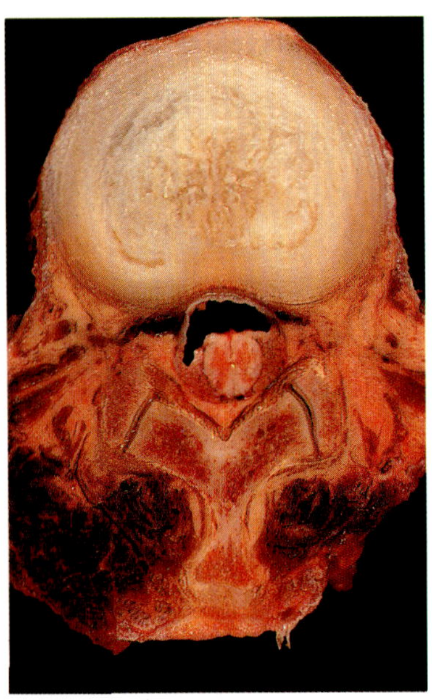

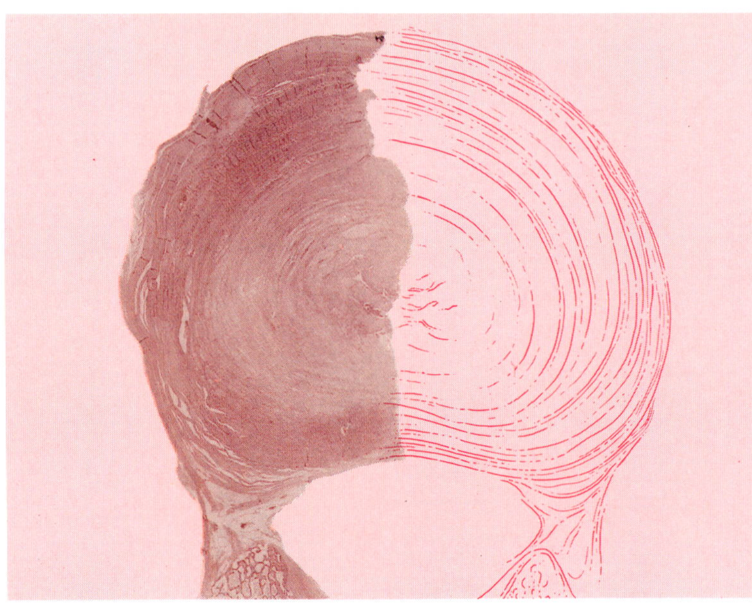

Figure 7.7 Photograph *(left)* of a transverse section through the L1-2 disc from a 28-year-old male. Note how the nucleus is denser and more shrunken in appearance, when compared to the nucleus seen in Figure 7.5. Note also that circumferential fissures have appeared. A photomicrograph *(right)* of a transverse section of half of the same disc shows the indistinct boundary between the anulus and the nucleus. (H & E, × 1 objective)

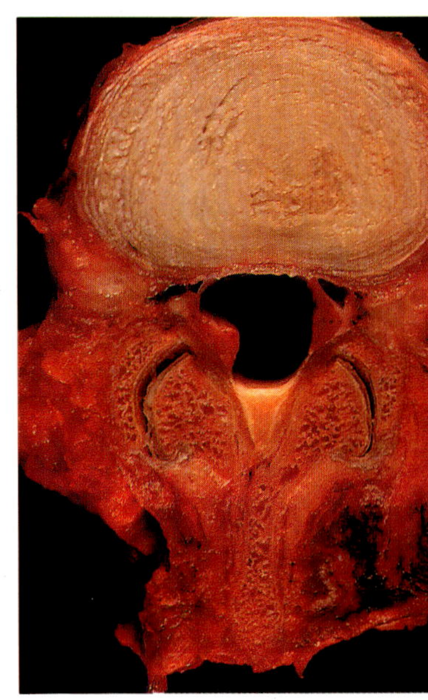

Figure 7.8 Photograph of a transverse section through the lumbar disc of a 70-year old. There is no clear distinction between the anulus and the nucleus.

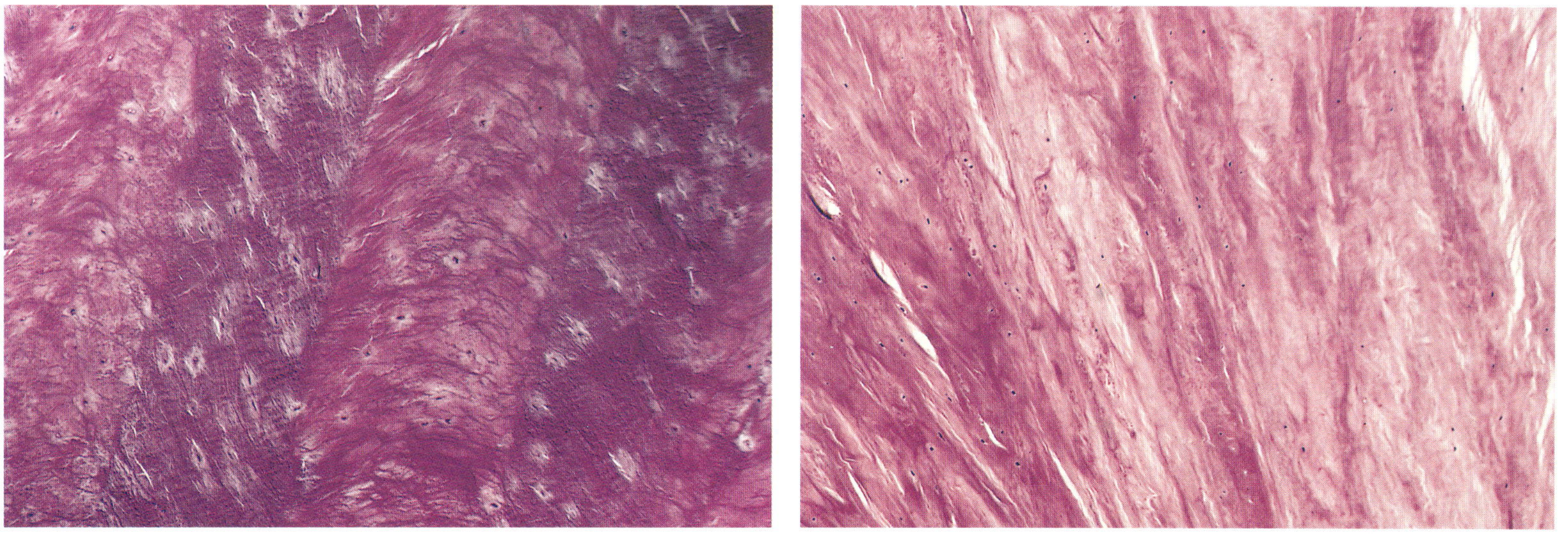

Figure 7.9 Photomicrograph (*left*) of a portion of the anulus fibrosus from a 68-year-old male. The tissue has been stained with PAS. (× 10 objective, approximately 250 magnifications) A photomicrograph (*right*) of a comparable section from an 18-year-old male shows less PAS staining. (These photographs should be compared with those in Figure 7.6.) (× 10 objective, approximately 250 magnifications)

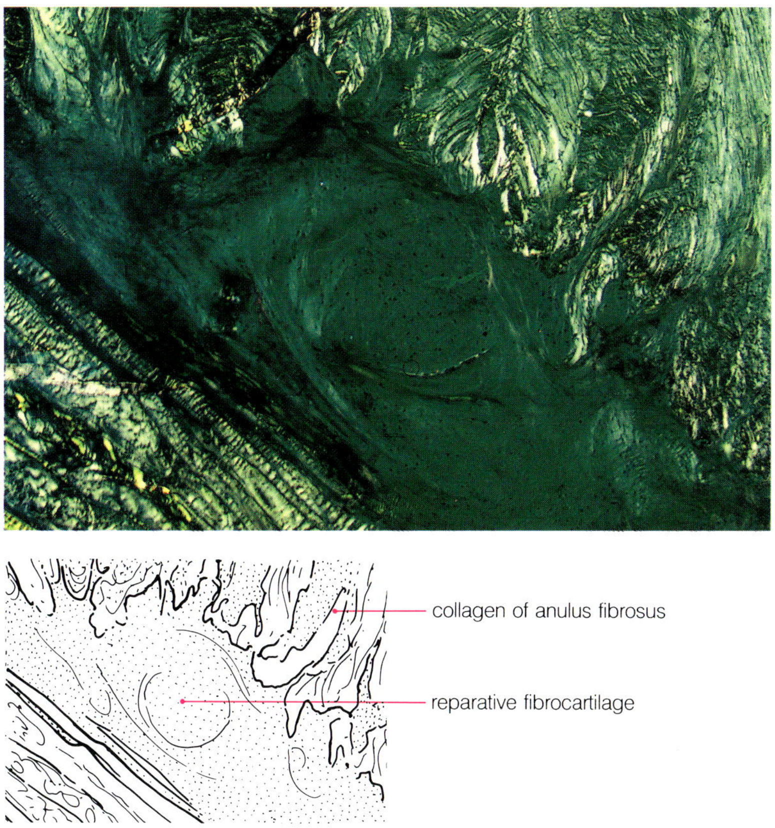

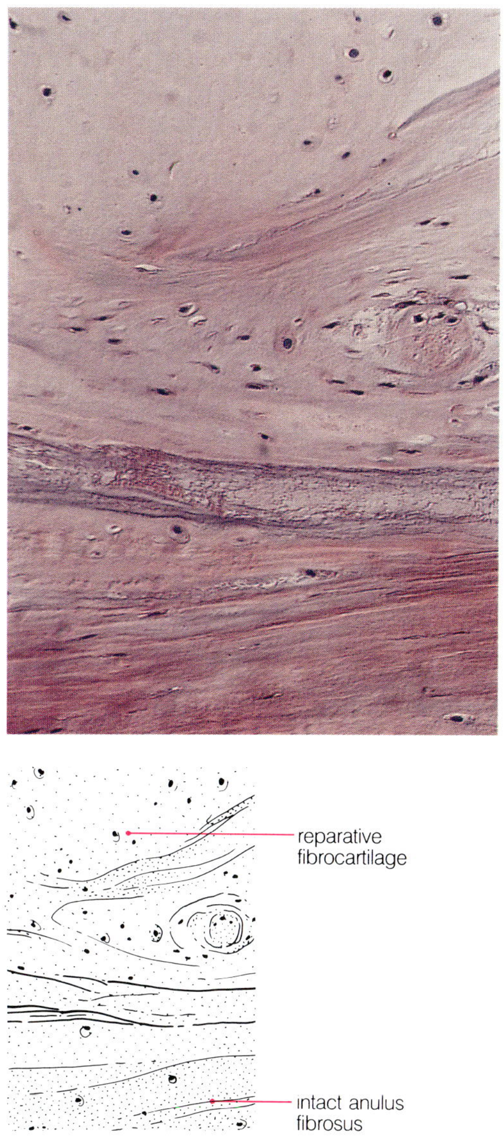

Figure 7.10 Photomicrograph (*left*) of a portion of the anulus fibrosus of an older individual. Note a disruption in the collagen structure, which has filled in with a less refractile material (reparative fibrocartilaginous tissue). (Polarized light, × 2.5 objective, approximately 50 magnifications) A higher power view (*right*) of this area shows the junction of the organized collagenous tissue and the disrupted area. Note the presence of chondrocytes in the area of repair. (H & E, × 10 objective, approximately 250 magnifications)

Osteochondrosis

Osteochondrosis is the term used to describe the pathologic changes that occur in the intervertebral disc as a result of disruption in the region of the end plate. Osteochondrosis is commonly found at autopsy in older individuals, and is not necessarily associated with clinical symptoms. In contrast to those changes observed in the disc as a result of advancing age, disruption of the end-plate region appears to be an essential prelude to progressive intervertebral disc degeneration.

As noted previously in the section on normal anatomy, the cartilaginous end plate is formed of hyaline cartilage and is attached to the underlying bony end plate of the vertebral body by a thin layer of calcified cartilage. Evidence of degeneration in the cartilaginous end plate is seen as microfractures in the bone-cartilage interface, an advancing of calcification into the cartilage from the bony surface, and an invasion of blood vessels from the subchondral bone into the cartilage, with subsequent endochondral ossification (Figs. 7.11 and 7.12). Note that all of these changes are also those seen in association with osteoarthritis in a diarthrodial joint. As a result of these changes, mechanical failure at the end plate compromises the mechanical function of the disc as a whole (see Section 1, Fig. 3.3) and may give rise to the herniation of disc material into the adjacent bone of the vertebral body (Schmorl's node).

With disruption of the cartilaginous end plate, the other disc components show a rapidly progressive degeneration, with focal necrosis, fissuring, calcification, radial or circumferential tearing in the anulus fibrosus (Figs. 7.13 and 7.14), and replacement of normal disc tissue by fibrous tissue. In the nucleus pulposus, replacement by fibrous tissue and amorphous material predominates. Large horizontal clefts develop in the central part of the disc tissue and may be seen on clinical radiographs, where often they are referred to by radiologists as the "vacuum phenomenon," though in fact they contain nitrogen gas (Fig. 7.15).

As already noted, extension of blood vessels through the subchondral bone and cartilaginous end plate also may occur. Injury to these vessels may result in hemorrhage into the intervertebral disc and in subsequent discoloration of disc material by blood pigments (Fig. 7.16). At autopsy these blood-pigment-stained discs, which might be quite prominent, are present in about 5% of individuals. Rarely several spinal levels may be involved (Fig. 7.17).

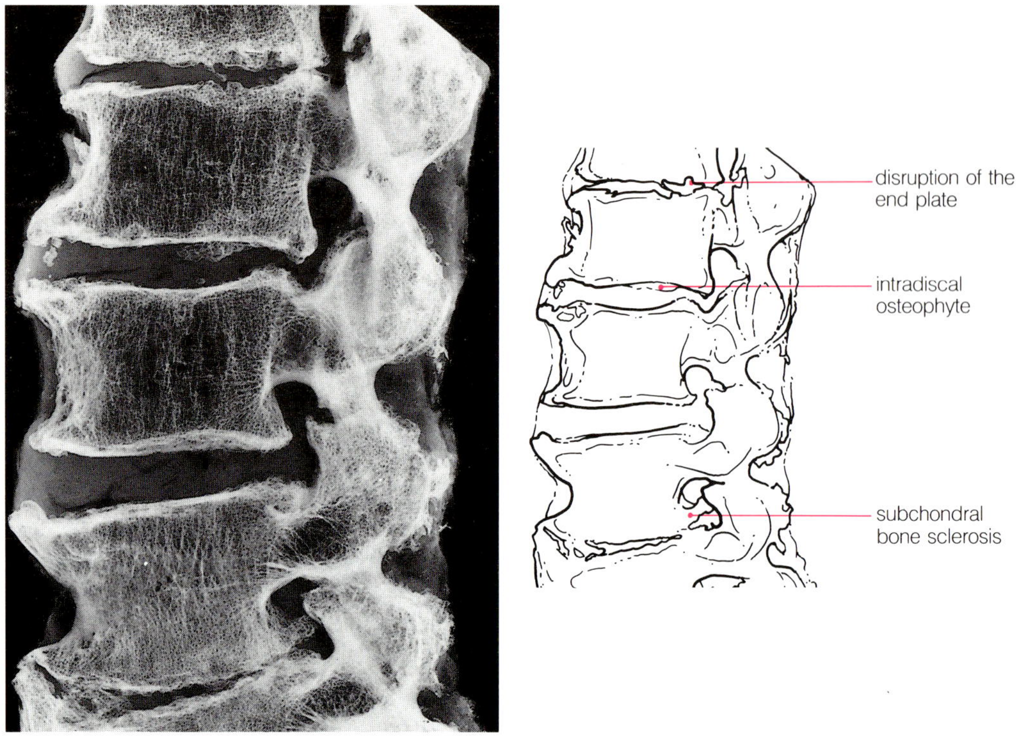

Figure 7.11 Specimen radiograph of a parasagittal section through a segment of lumbar spine (L1-4). In the L3-4 disc space, although there is obvious degeneration of the disc with cleft formation, the space is only slightly narrowed. The end plates are largely intact. In the L2-3 disc, there is partial ossification of the disc, adjacent to the superior end plate, and in L1-2, there is considerable disruption of the end plates, with ossification into the disc substance. In this specimen, there is also ossification of the anterior longitudinal ligament (ankylosing hyperostosis), which is probably an unrelated condition (see Chapter 9).

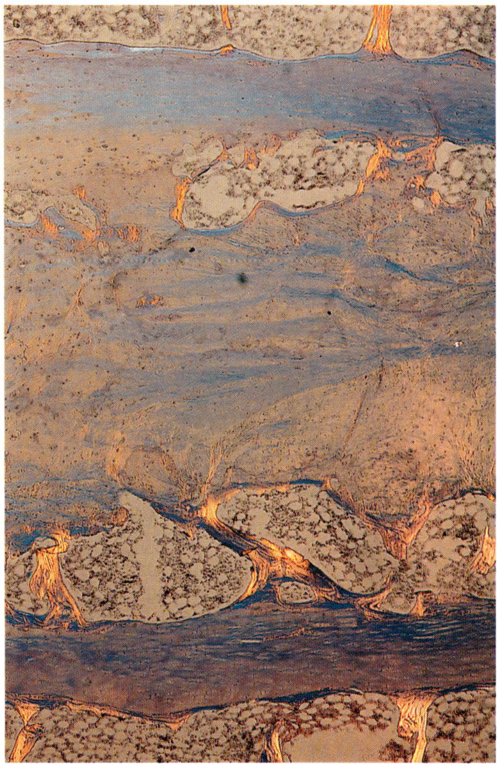

Figure 7.12 Polarized photomicrograph of a full-thickness section of the intervertebral disc. Bony osteophytes are seen extending into the nucleus pulposus on both sides of the disc. (Compare with Figure 7.11)

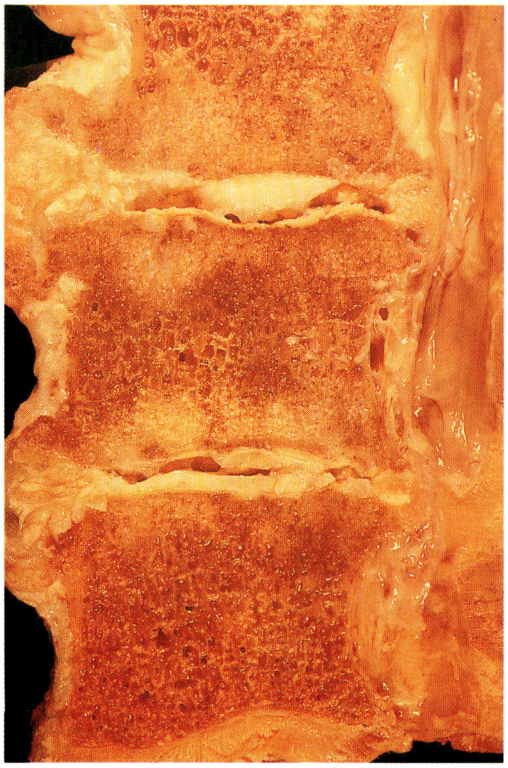

Figure 7.13 Photograph of a sagittal section through L3-5 of a 72-year-old male. Note the severe disc degeneration, along with irregularity of the end plates and adjacent sclerosis of the bone.

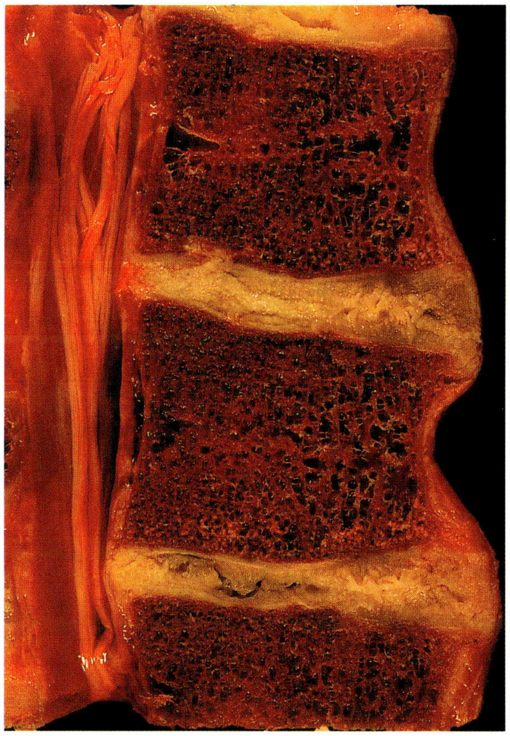

Figure 7.14 Photograph of a sagittal section through L-2 and adjacent discs, in a 43-year-old male. Note focal irregularities in the end plates and horizontal fissuring of the L2-3 disc.

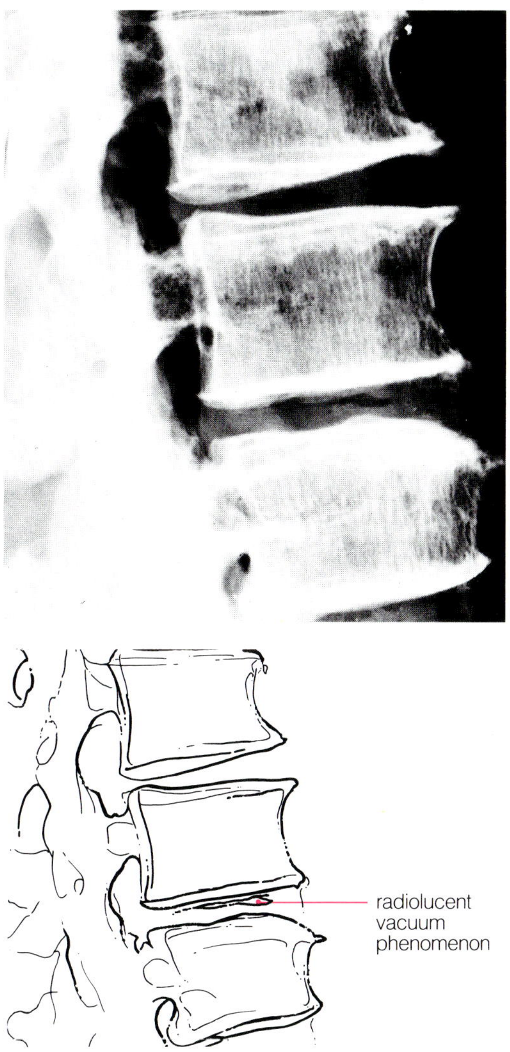

Figure 7.15 Specimen radiograph of the portion of spine illustrated in Figure 7.14. Note the radiolucent line, which corresponds to the cleft in the disc seen in the gross photograph. This line is generally referred to by radiologists as the "vacuum phenomenon."

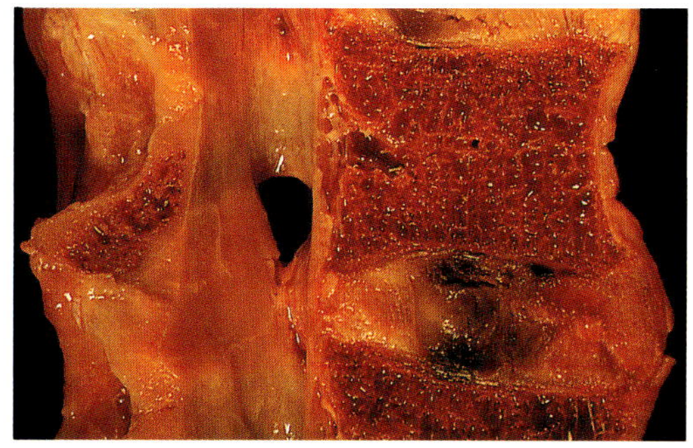

Figure 7.16 Photograph of a sagittal section through the L2-3 disc of a 78-year-old male. Note the brownish-black discoloration of the nucleus pulposus, resulting from intradiscal hemorrhage.

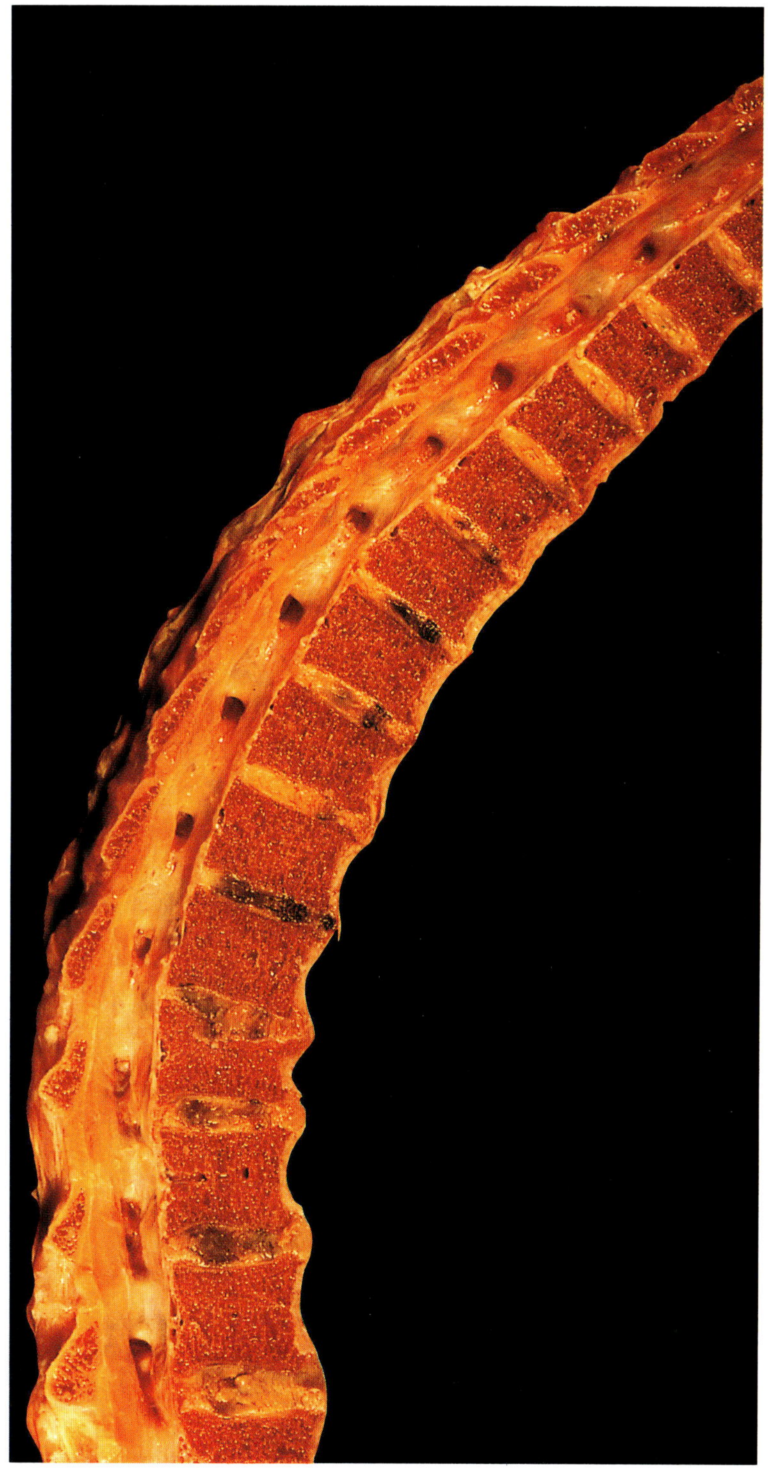

Figure 7.17 Photograph of a sagittal section of the spine of a 78-year-old male. Brown staining of several discs is obvious. These discs gave a positive heme test.

As disc tissue degeneration with subsequent narrowing of the disc space progresses, the formation of new bone is seen around the periphery of the disc, at the junction of the anulus and the vertebral body (Fig. 7.18). New bone formation also occurs as a result of endochondral ossification of the cartilaginous end plate, which contributes to the narrowing of the disc space (Fig. 7.19). It should be noted here that the bony outgrowths (osteophytes) seen in association with degenerative disc disease are not nearly as prominent as those seen in association with anterior disc herniation, which give rise to the condition referred to as spondylosis deformans (see Chapter 5).

Following vascular invasion, progressive breakdown of the disc-tissue contents will result in their resorption. At this stage the narrow space between the vertebral bodies will be occupied by a small amount of vascularized fibrous tissue, and the bone of the vertebral bodies on each side of the disc will become increasingly irregular and sclerotic (Fig. 7.20). Frequently, the final stage of the resorption process is the spontaneous fusion of adjacent vertebral bodies (Fig. 7.21).

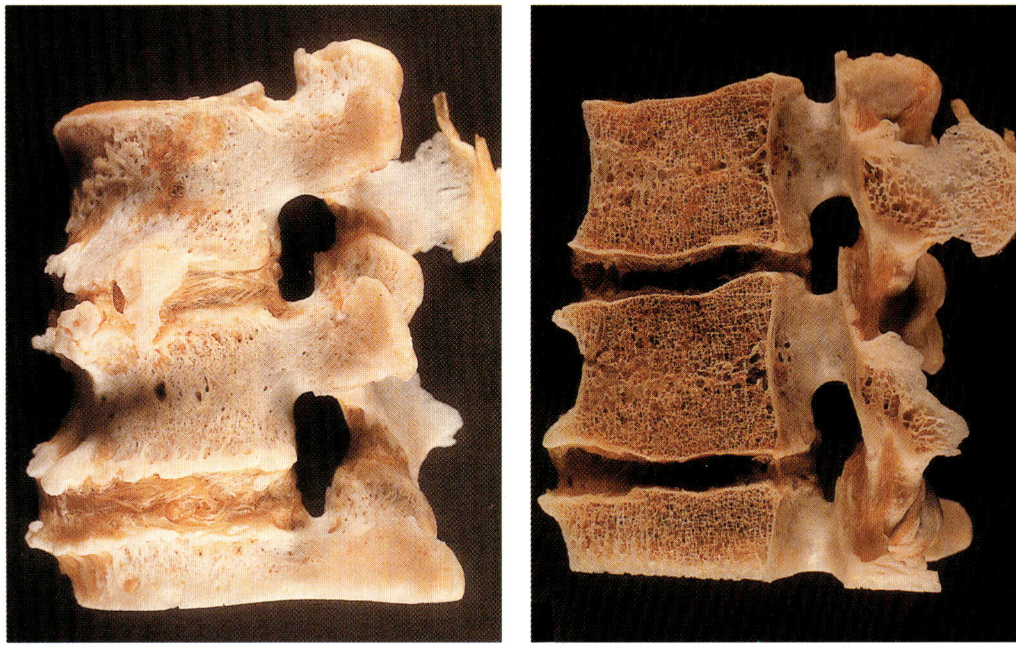

Figure 7.18 Photograph (*left*) of a portion of the macerated lumbar spine of a 43-year-old male. The development of peripheral osteophytes is demonstrated. A sagittal section (*right*) through this specimen shows marked irregularities of the end plates, with narrowed disc spaces and peripheral osteophytes.

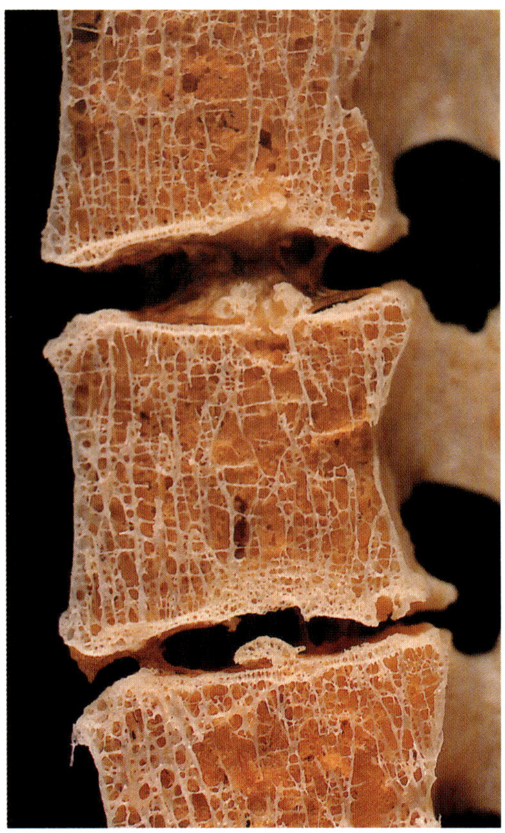

Figure 7.19 Photograph of a sagittal section through a portion of the macerated spine of an 83-year-old female. Ossification is seen extending into the disc space, which may eventually occlude the space entirely. In addition, note fractures through the end plate and associated bony sclerosis.

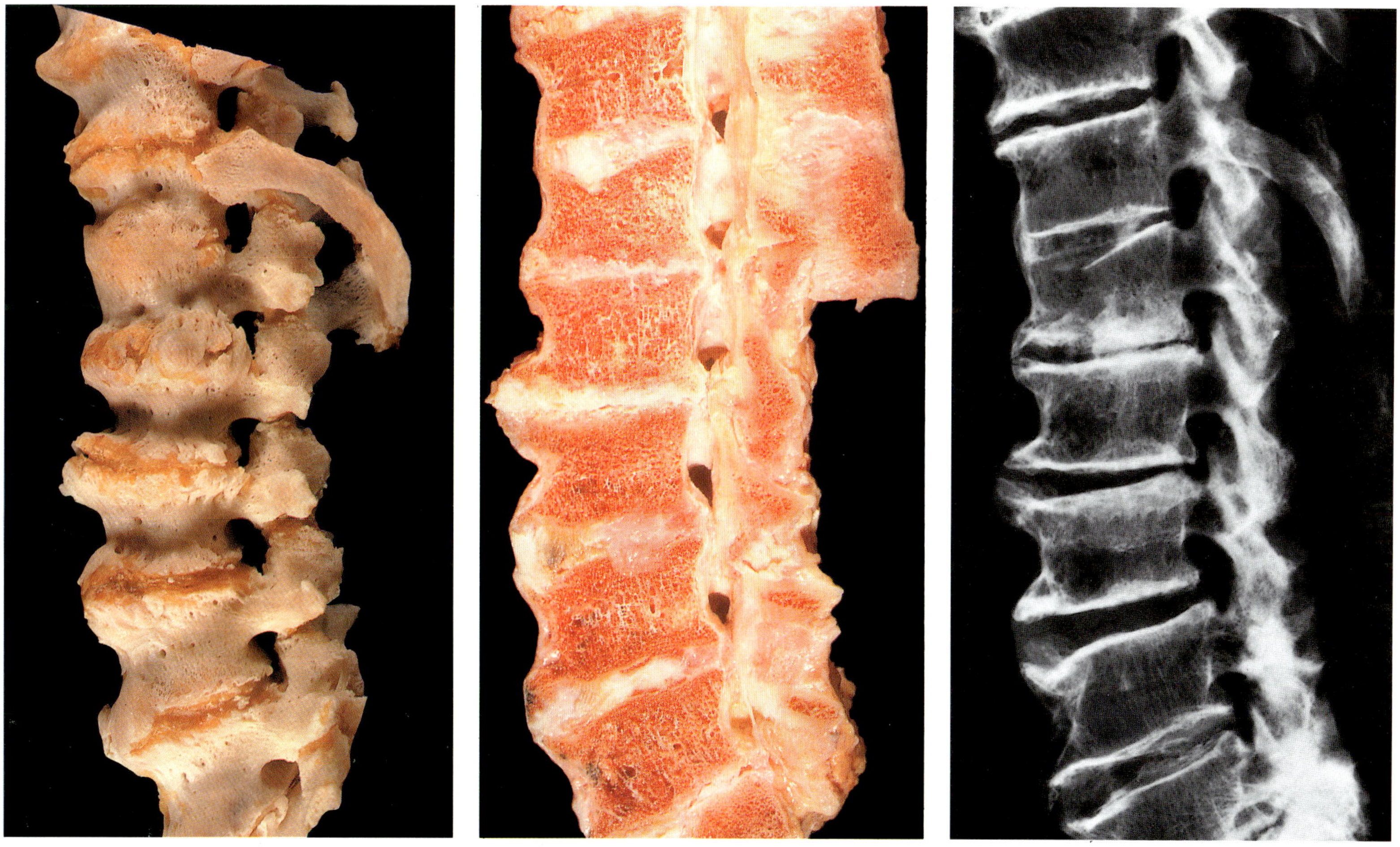

Figure 7.20 Photograph *(left)* of the macerated thoracolumbar spine of a 92-year-old male, to show severe osteophyte formation in a patient with osteochondrosis (degenerative disc disease). Note that in several areas the osteophytes have fused. Before maceration (*center*), a sagittal section of this case showed severe degenerative disc disease, although the severity is perhaps less obvious than in the macerated specimen. The specimen radiograph (*right*) shows the various features of osteochondrosis: disc degeneration involving end-plate fractures, narrowing of the disc space, osteophytosis (both peripheral and intervertebral), and end-plate sclerosis. Again, the severity of the disease seems less in the radiograph than in the macerated specimen.

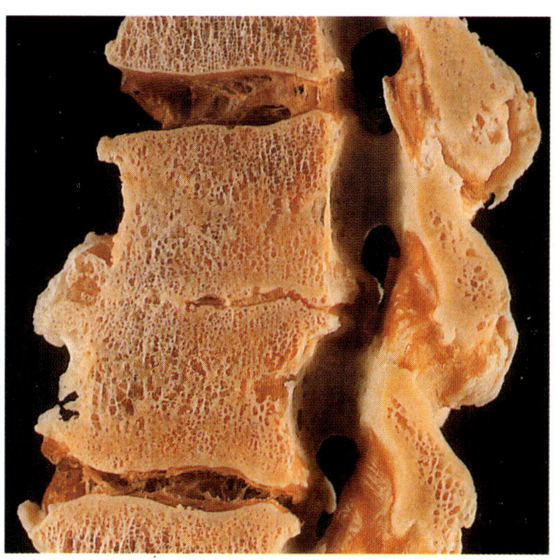

Figure 7.21 Photograph of a macerated sagittal section through L2-3 of a 79-year-old male, to show bony fusion across a severely degenerated disc. Note the mild to moderate changes in adjacent discs.

8 CHAPTER

DEGENERATIVE ARTHRITIS OF THE SPINE

Introduction

In the preceding chapter, age-related structural changes in the discs and intervertebral osteochondrosis were discussed as isolated phenomena. However, as should be apparent to the reader from the opening chapters of this book, alterations in the mechanics of one portion of the spine by a disease process, in general, will lead to more generalized alterations. In the case of osteochondrosis, subsequent changes will occur in the facet joints, intervertebral foramina, spinal canal, and ligaments. Spinal stability and function of the facet joints are likewise affected. The various aspects of this disease process, most commonly referred to as spondylosis, will be viewed in the present chapter. Osteoarthritis of the spinal articulations is rare before the age of 30. However, after the age of 45, osteoarthritis becomes more frequent, and is found in older individuals at autopsy in upward of 80% of spines examined.

Spondylosis

The clinical term "spondylosis" embraces degenerative disc disease, together with the associated vertebral osteophytosis, ligamentous disease, facet joint disease, and accompanying neurologic complications. In the older population, this condition is almost universally present and certainly it is one of the greatest single causes of loss of work, particularly among those who do heavy manual labor. Spondylosis occurs in all spinal segments, but is found most frequently in the more mobile segments of the spine (the cervical and lumbar segments). Moreover, each spinal level is affected to a different degree, as will be discussed in the sections that follow.

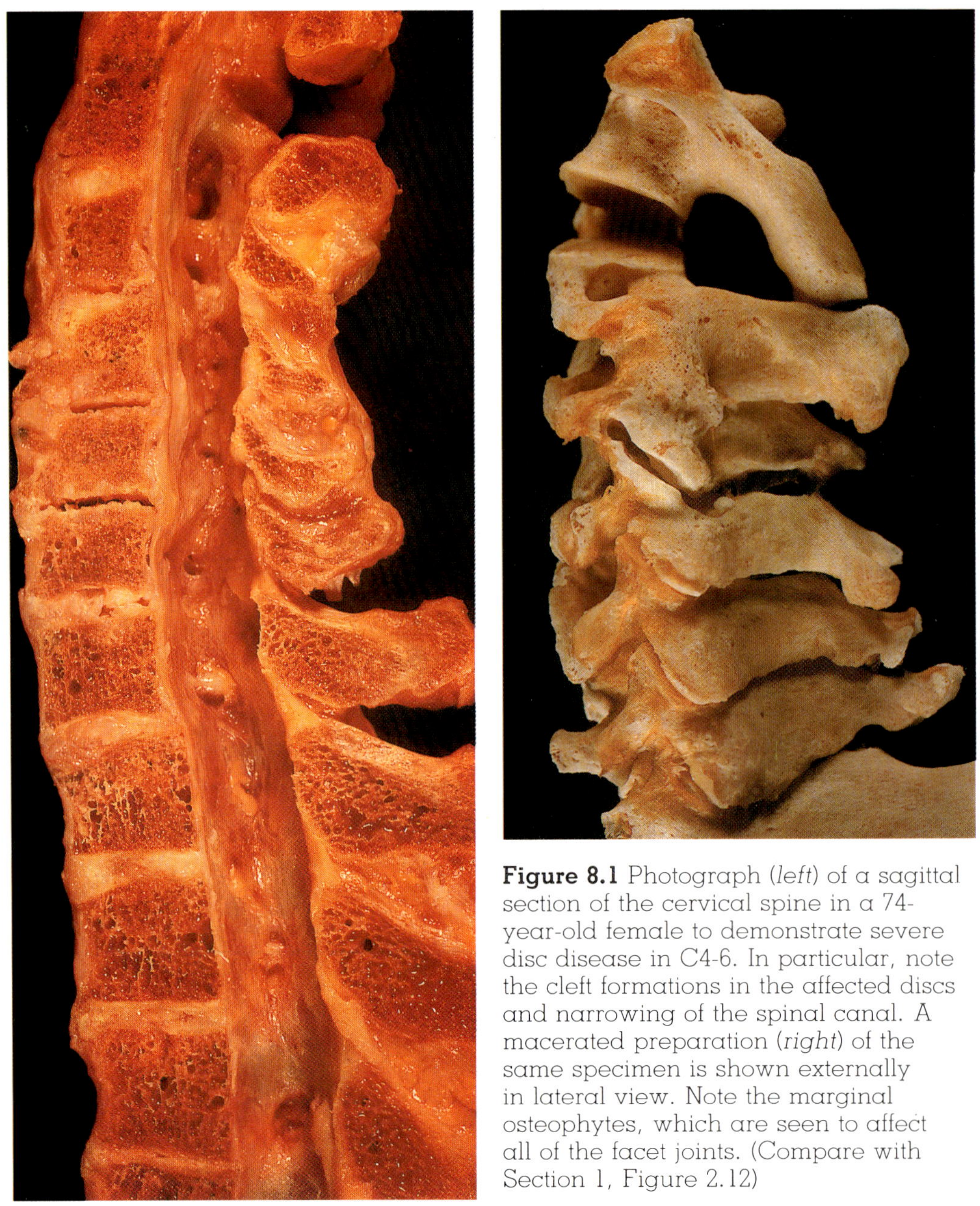

Figure 8.1 Photograph (*left*) of a sagittal section of the cervical spine in a 74-year-old female to demonstrate severe disc disease in C4-6. In particular, note the cleft formations in the affected discs and narrowing of the spinal canal. A macerated preparation (*right*) of the same specimen is shown externally in lateral view. Note the marginal osteophytes, which are seen to affect all of the facet joints. (Compare with Section 1, Figure 2.12)

CERVICAL SPONDYLOSIS

The cervical portion of the vertebral column possesses the greatest mobility and thus has the greatest susceptibility to functional stress and trauma. Therefore, clinical spondylosis of the cervical spine is very common and often is debilitating.

Degenerative arthritis of the zygapophysial (or facet) joints of the cervical spine generally is progressive, leading to the formation of osteophytes that may protrude into the intervertebral foramina, causing vascular congestion and subsequent irritation of the spinal nerve roots. With narrowing of the intervertebral disc space there is encroachment on the uncovertebral joints of Luschka, leading to degenerative changes. Uncovertebral osteophytes are particularly common at the lateral (especially at the posterolateral) lips of the superior surfaces of the mid to seventh cervical bodies (Figs. 8.1 through 8.4). Neck pain, either in the posterior or lateral portions, may be severe.

The clinical presentation of cervical spondylosis may include radicular symptoms,

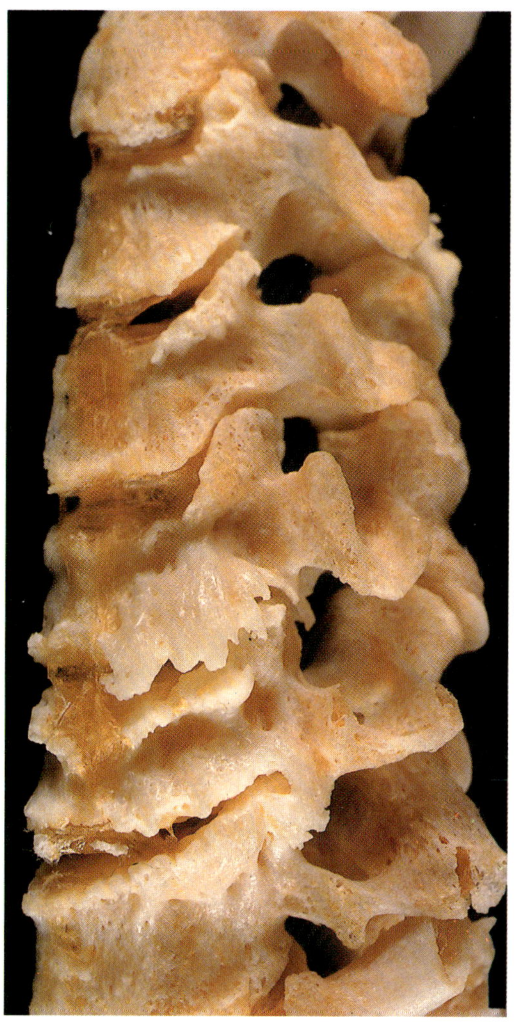

Figure 8.2 Photograph of the anterior oblique view of the macerated cervical spine of a 77-year-old female. There is marked osteophyte formation of the uncovertebral joints, particularly in the lower cervical region. Note the encroachment of the osteophytes on the intervertebral foramina, particularly at C5-7.

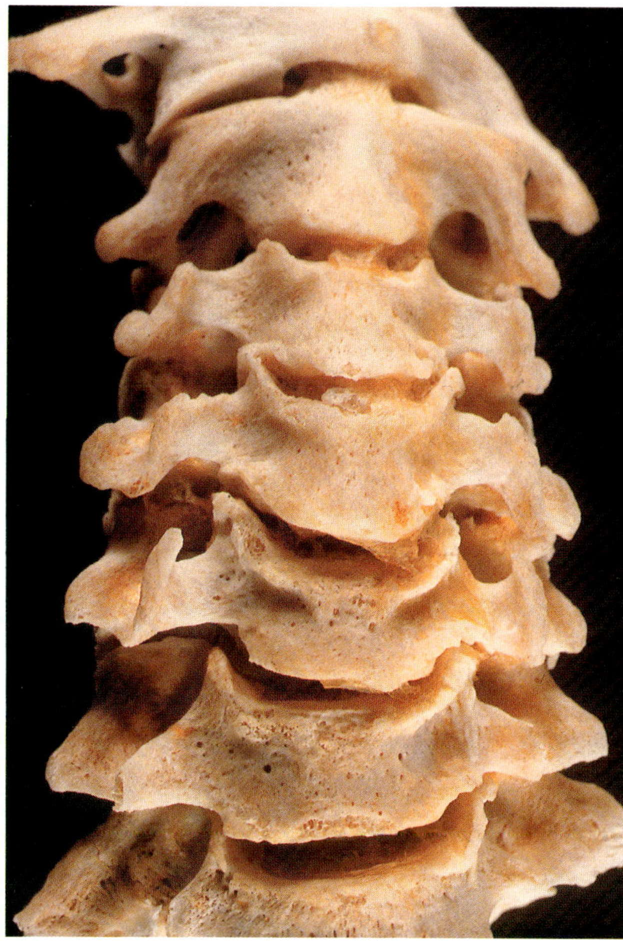

Figure 8.3 Photograph of a macerated preparation of the cervical spine in a 64-year-old woman in the frontal view. There are marginal osteophytes, particularly evident in the uncovertebral joints. (Compare with Section 1, Figure 2.21)

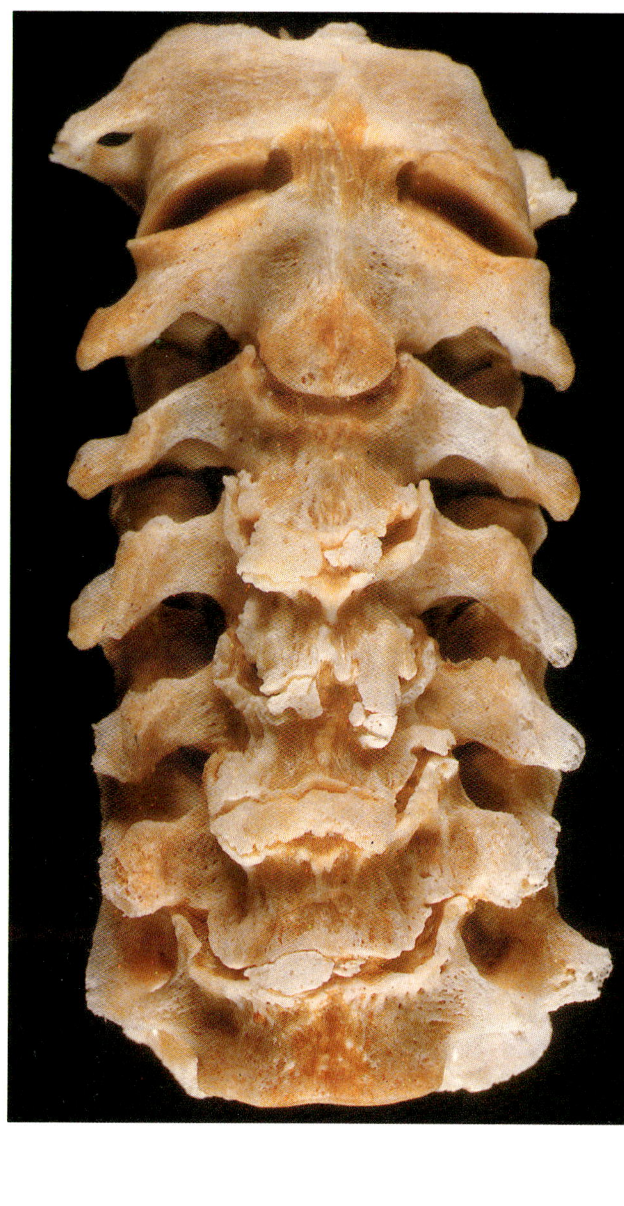

Figure 8.4 Photograph of a macerated specimen of the cervical spine in a 70-year-old female. Severe cervical spondylosis is seen.

due to herniation of disc material or to osteophyte encroachment on one of the nerve roots (most commonly the C-6 and C-7 roots). Symptoms of myelopathy, due to cord compression or ischemia, may result from acute midline disc herniation or from the multiple bony spurs that protrude posteriorly from the vertebral bodies into the spinal canal (Fig. 8.5). Vertebral artery insufficiency is yet another complication that may occur, as a result of osteophytes impinging on the vertebral artery within the transverse foramina of C2-6. This complication usually is compounded by the presence of arteriosclerosis in the vessels.

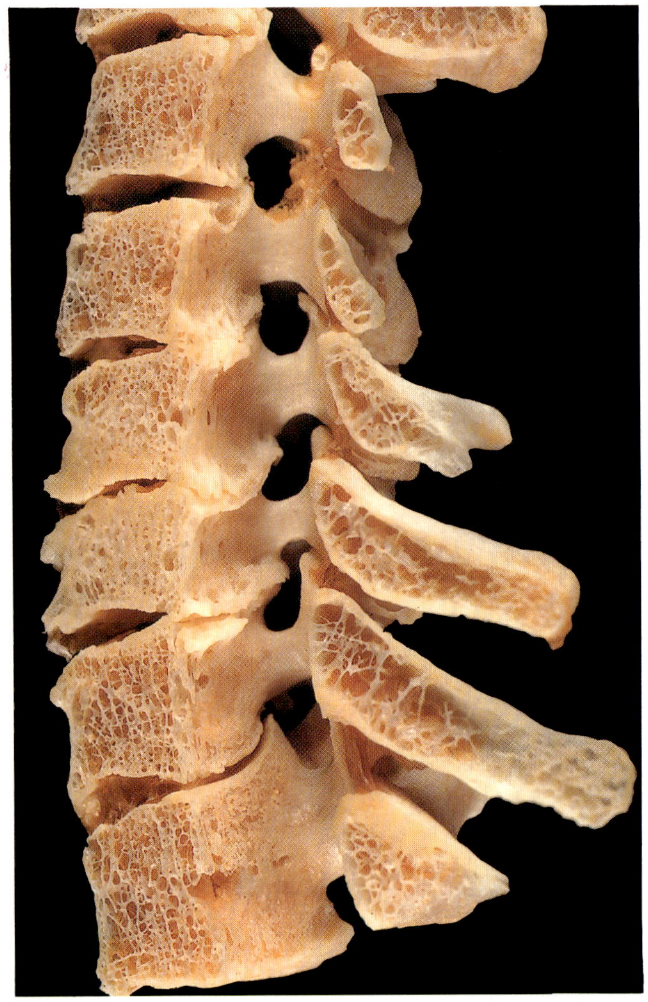

Figure 8.5 Photograph of a sagittal section of the macerated cervical spine of a 77-year-old female showing marked posterior osteophytosis, particularly in C4-6. Note the encroachment into the intervertebral foramen of C6-7.

THORACIC SPONDYLOSIS

In the thoracic region of the spine, which is less mobile in comparison to the cervical and lumbar regions, intervertebral disc disease is less marked. However, because of the thoracic kyphosis, the anterior edges of the bodies may compress the disc tissue to such an extent that the anterior portion of the disc is subject to increased degeneration. Concentric tears in the anterior parts of the disc, along the edge of the vertebral body rim, may

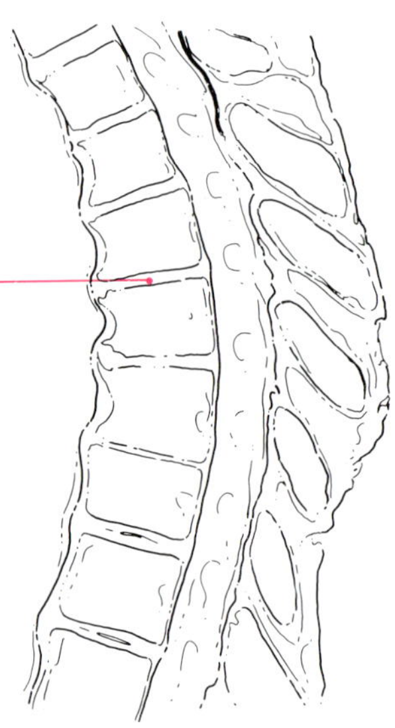

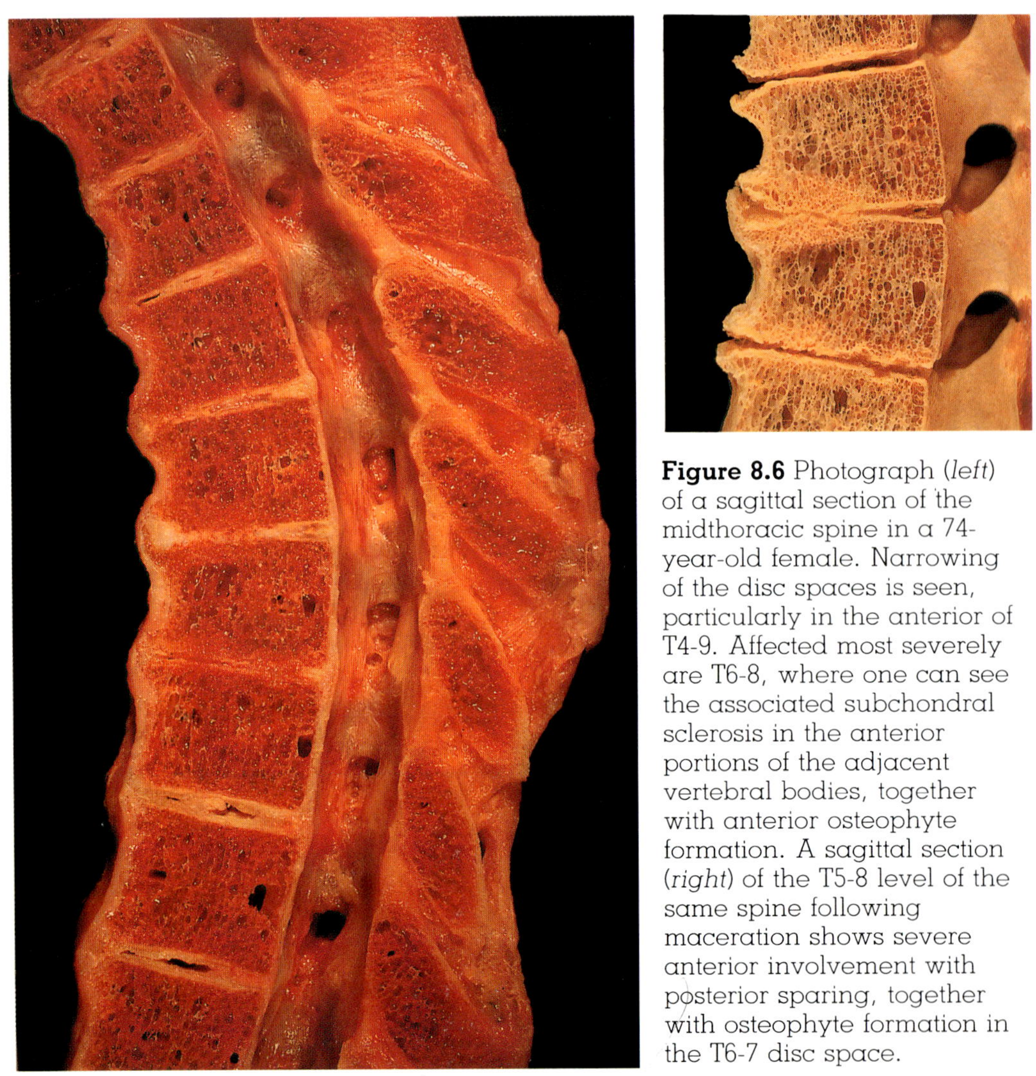

Figure 8.6 Photograph (*left*) of a sagittal section of the midthoracic spine in a 74-year-old female. Narrowing of the disc spaces is seen, particularly in the anterior of T4-9. Affected most severely are T6-8, where one can see the associated subchondral sclerosis in the anterior portions of the adjacent vertebral bodies, together with anterior osteophyte formation. A sagittal section (*right*) of the T5-8 level of the same spine following maceration shows severe anterior involvement with posterior sparing, together with osteophyte formation in the T6-7 disc space.

result in degenerative changes and in the proliferation of fibrous scar tissue and blood vessels at the disc margin (Fig. 8.6). Gradually, through the process of endochondral ossification, the anterior parts of the disc may be transformed into bone, resulting in a solid fusion between the vertebral bodies. When this occurs in the elderly, especially in association with osteoporosis, progressive kyphosis may develop in the midthoracic region (Fig. 8.7).

LUMBAR SPONDYLOSIS

Lumbar spondylosis, which occurs most frequently in males, is particularly prominent in the lower lumbar spine, where it represents one of the most common causes of low-back and leg pain. Lumbar disc degeneration follows a chronic course, with repeated injury playing a precipitating role. These degenerative changes result in alterations in the size and shape of the vertebral canal and its lateral recesses, with subsequent nerve root compression. The disease is found most often at the L4-5 level, which is the most mobile portion of the lumbar spine and also the narrowest portion of the vertebral canal in the lumbar spine.

In lumbar spondylosis a number of factors may contribute to nerve root and cauda equina impingement. These include:

Osteophyte formation around degenerate facet joints;

Disc narrowing, which results in narrowing of the vertical interpedicular distance, due to caudal migration of the pedicles with

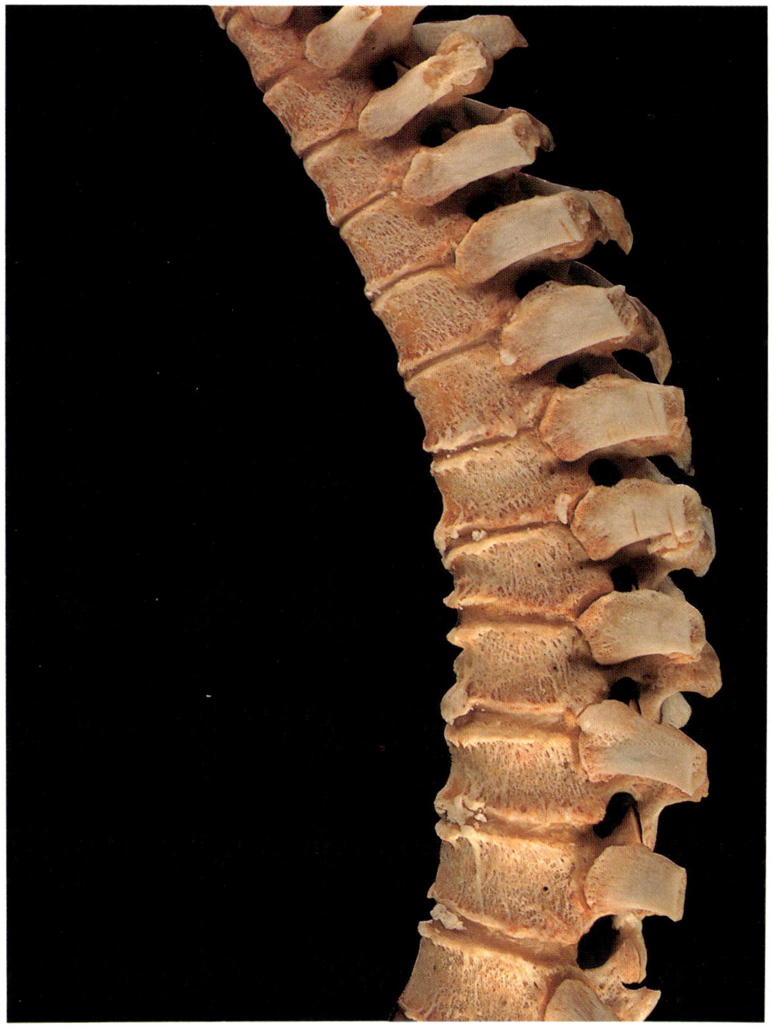

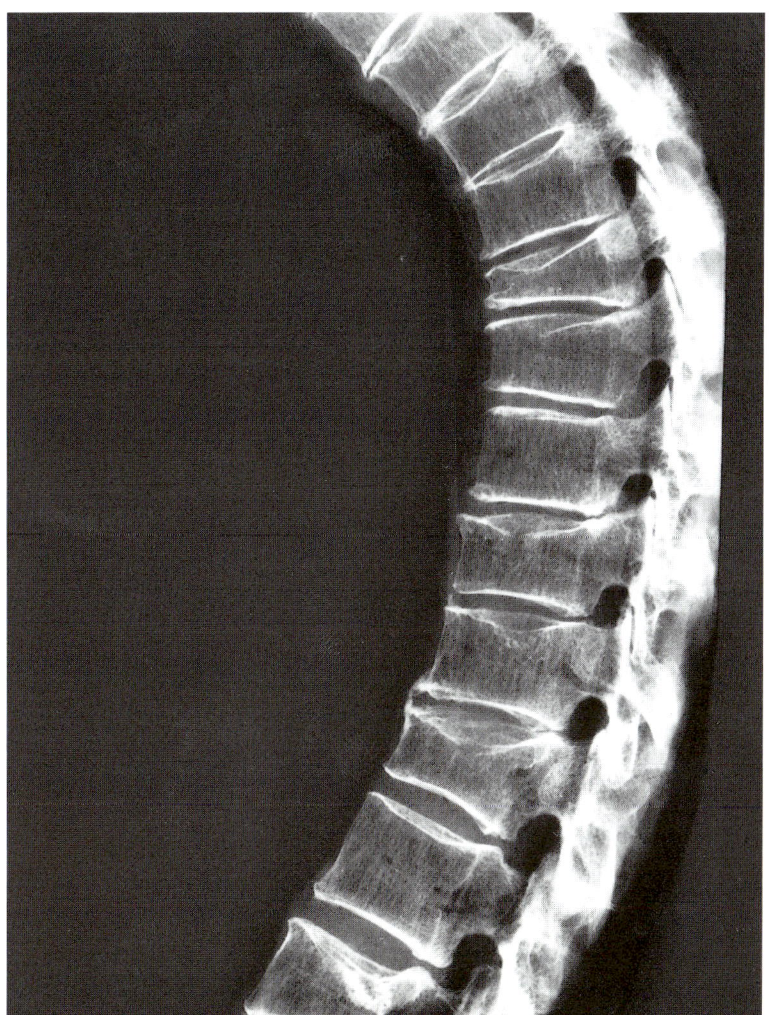

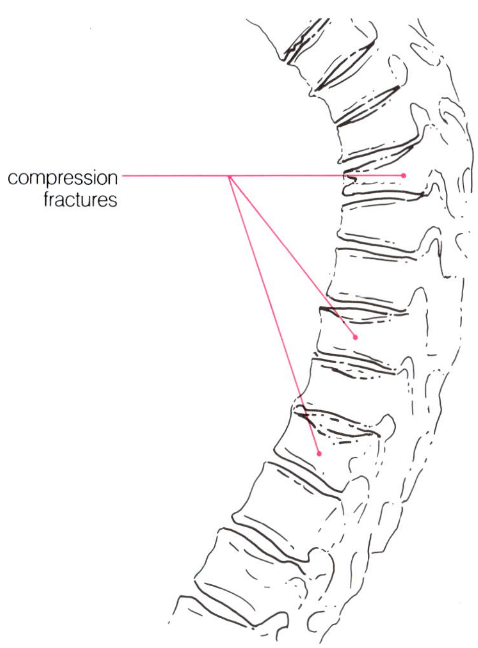

Figure 8.7 Photograph *(top)* of a macerated spine showing thoracic kyphosis. Note the marked disc narrowing and marginal disc calcification, anteriorly. A radiograph (*bottom*) of the same specimen demonstrates that the kyphosis is secondary to osteoporosis and compression fracturing of the spine.

subsequent "tethering" of the nerve roots (Fig. 8.8);

Progressive disc degeneration, resulting in subluxation of the vertebral bodies and posterior elements (degenerative spondylolisthesis).

The clinical manifestations produced by these structural abnormalities include sciatica and/or ischemia of the cauda equina, with pseudo- (neurogenic) claudication.

Facet Joint Arthrosis

Biomechanical studies have shown that in response to the combined compressive and torsional loads applied, the facet joints carry between 12 and 25% of the combined load. However, in the presence of disc narrowing from osteochondrosis, the load on the facet joints may increase to nearly 70% of the total load. These excessive loads result in the initiation of degenerative joint disease in the facet joints. The morphologic features of osteoarthritis seen in other diarthrodial joints—namely, capsular laxity, synovitis, cartilage fibrillation, cartilage loss with eburnation of

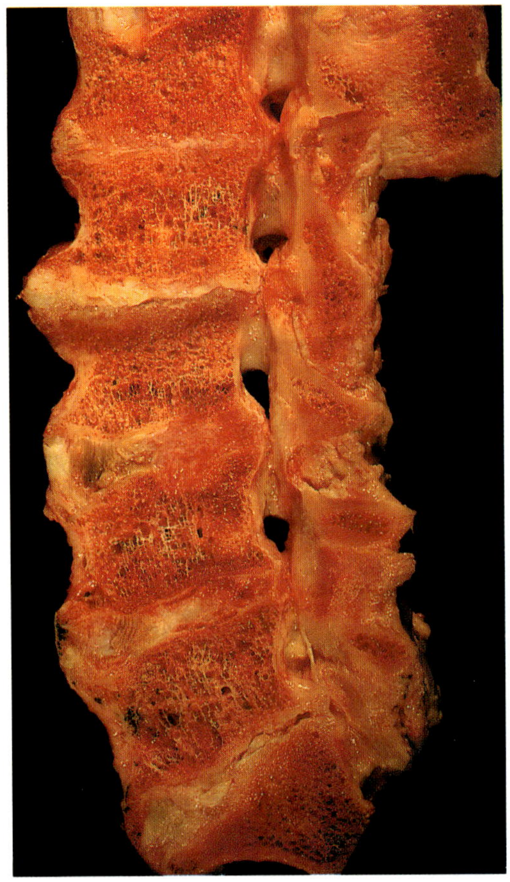

Figure 8.8 Photograph (*top*) of a sagittal section through the lumbar spine of a 92-year-old male to demonstrate varying degrees of disc degeneration. Disc narrowing, end-plate irregularities, subchondral sclerosis, and disc discoloration are seen, along with cleft formation with peripheral osteophytes and encroachment on the spinal canal and lateral recesses. The specimen radiograph (*bottom left*) shows encroachment on the intervertebral foramina by both posterior vertebral osteophytes and facet joint osteophytes, in association with varying degrees of intervertebral disc degeneration. In addition, note that the interpedicular distance is reduced, especially in the L4-5 and L-5 to S-1 region. An exterior view (*bottom right*) of this specimen following maceration shows extensive circumferential osteophytes, which posterolaterally can be seen to encroach on the intervertebral foramen, and focally to have resulted in bony fusion between adjacent vertebral bodies.

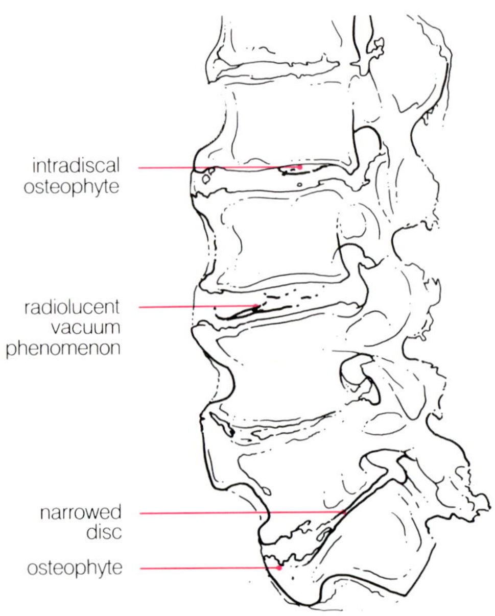

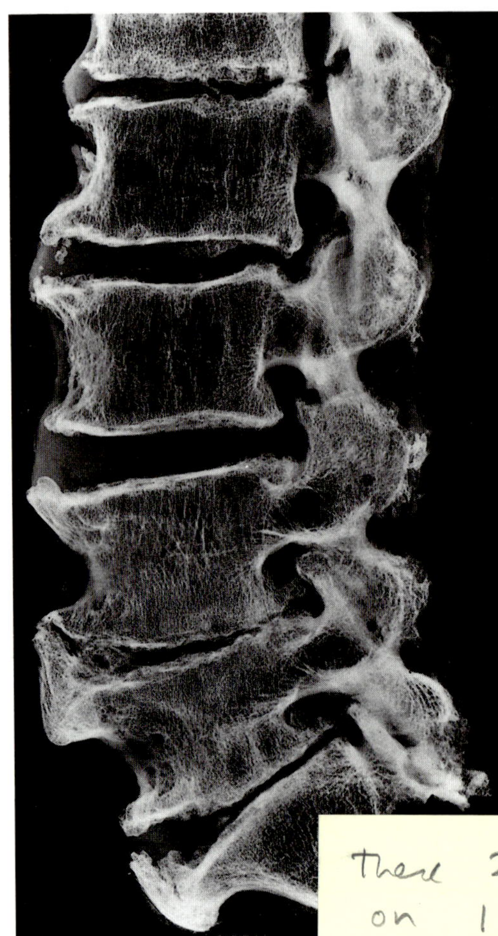

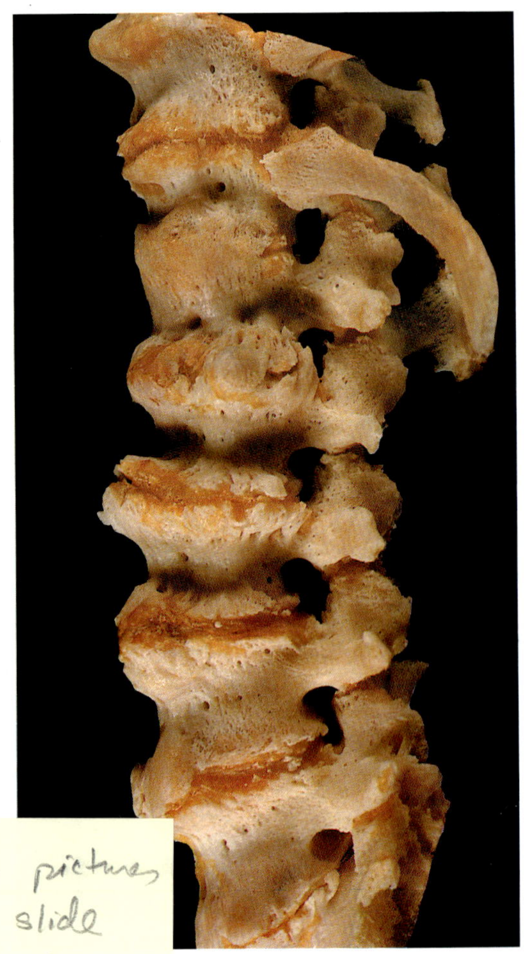

These 2 pictures on 1 slide (side by side as above)

the exposed bone, and marginal osteophyte formation—all are seen in association with facet joint disease (Figs. 8.9 through 8.11). It is possible that facet joint disease is a significant cause of low-back pain.

Degenerative Spondylolisthesis

Listhesis is a general term used to describe the displacement of a vertebral body on the one directly below it. In severe degenerative disc disease, the displacement of one vertebral body on another may occur in any direction, though anterior displacement, i.e., spondylolisthesis, is most common. Degenerative spondylolisthesis was first described by Junghanns in 1930, based on his examination of anatomical specimens from Schmorl's Institute. Junghanns called the degenerative disorder *pseudo*spondylolisthesis, to differentiate it from true spondylolisthesis, which occurs as a result of a defect in the pars interarticularis (see Section 3, Chapter 10). In 1963 Newman and Stone introduced the term "degenerative spondylolisthesis," as being more descriptive of the etiology than the term "pseudospondylolisthesis." Degenerative spondylolisthesis, unlike true spondylolisthesis, involves the whole of the neural arch. It is more prevalent in females than in males, and involves L4-5 mainly, though not exclusively. (True spondylolisthesis primarily involves L-5, with men and women equally affected.) The L4-5 segment is probably that segment affected most commonly by degenerative spondylolisthesis because it is at the apex of the lumbar curve and because it is the most mobile segment of the lumbar spine.

Degenerative spondylolisthesis results from degeneration of the facet joints, which in turn results from narrowing of the intervertebral disc space. Bony erosions of the articular surfaces of the facet joint result in a more horizontal disposition of the facets and in an increasing tendency toward forward slippage, potentiated by the narrowing of the disc space. Forward slippage is halted only when the inferior surface of the pars interarticularis (the isthmus) of the slipped ver-

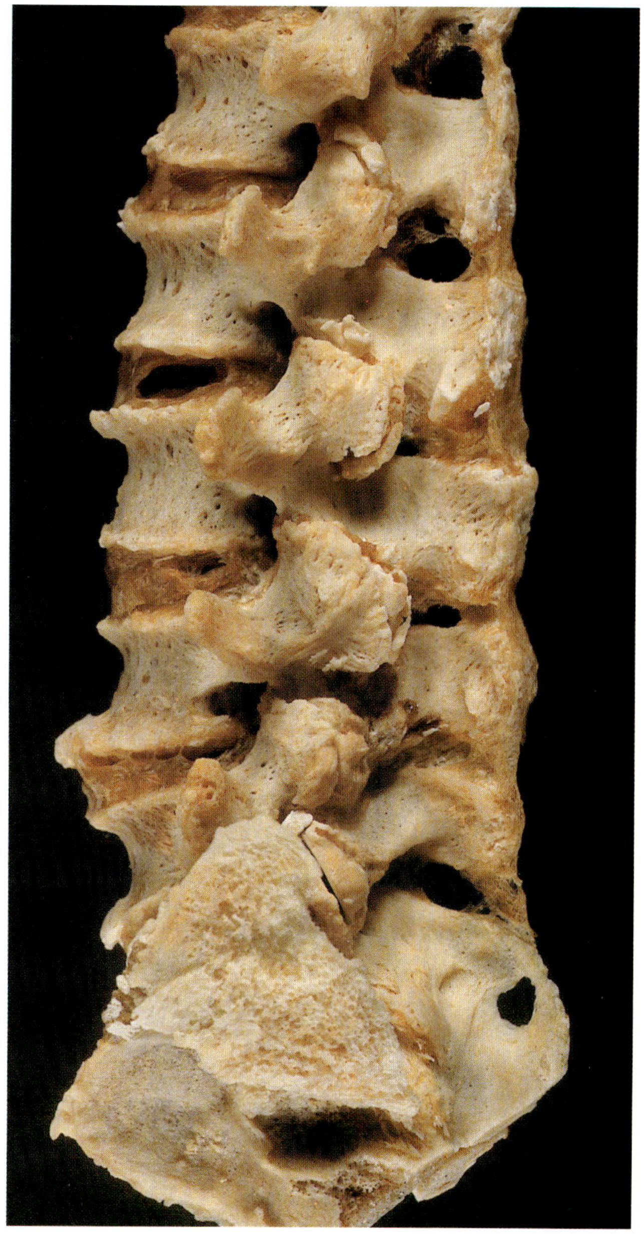

Figure 8.9 Photograph of a posterior oblique view of the lumbar spine of an elderly male, to demonstrate severe facet joint arthritis. Note the exuberant marginal osteophytes with their irregular serrated margins. (Compare with Section 1, Figure 2.15, showing normal facet joints)

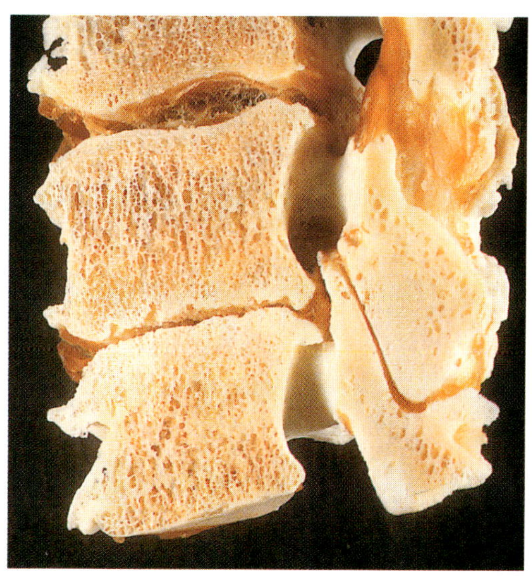

Figure 8.10 Photograph of a macerated sagittal section through L4-5 of a 79-year-old male to show severe narrowing of the facet joint, with associated subchondral sclerosis and osteophyte formation. Note the associated disc narrowing, posterior osteophytes, and lateral recess stenosis.

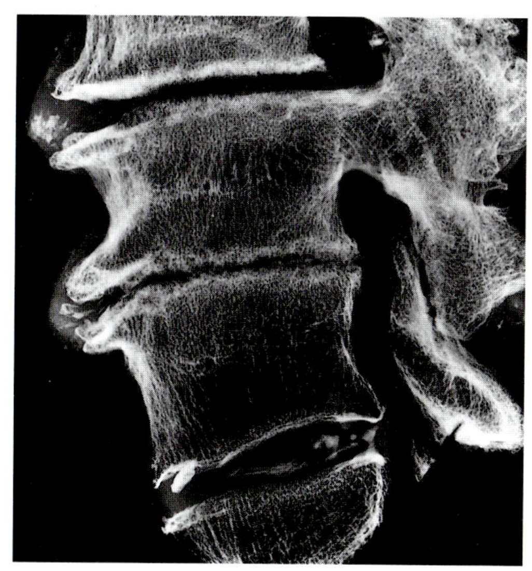

Figure 8.11 Specimen lateral radiograph of the lower lumbar spine of a 74-year-old female to show narrowing of the lower facet joint, with osteophyte formation. There is associated disc degeneration and stenosis of the lateral recess. The upper facet joint cannot be properly visualized because of its obliquity.

tebra abuts on the upper margin of the superior articular process of the vertebra below. Occasionally spontaneous fusion of the involved facet joints prevents further slippage. The effect of degenerative spondylolisthesis is spinal stenosis (Fig. 8.12). The extent of the process will determine its clinical symptoms; however, it should be noted that the majority of people affected by degenerative spondylolisthesis are symptom-free.

Degenerative Retrolisthesis and Lateral Listhesis

Retrolisthesis is the posterior displacement of one vertebra on the subjacent one. Degenerative retrolisthesis, like spondylolisthesis, affects the most mobile segments of the spine, i.e., the cervical and lumbar segments. Also like spondylolisthesis, this form of vertebral slippage was initially described by Junghanns. Junghanns observed this abnormality to be most common in the upper lumbar spine, with L2-3 involved most often (Figs. 8.13 and 8.14). With rotation or angular deformities, one also may see a lateral slippage associated with retrolisthesis (Fig. 8.15).

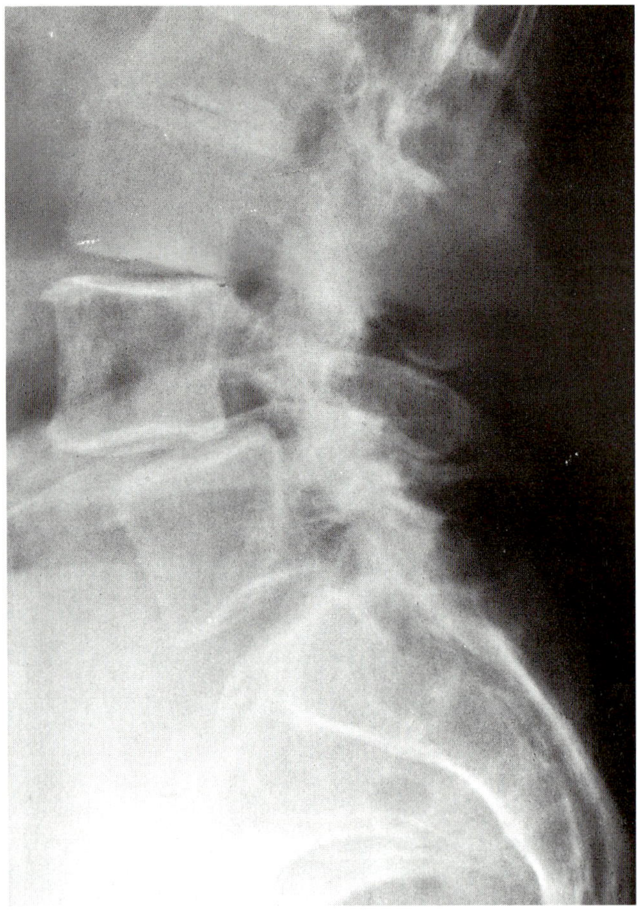

Figure 8.12 Lateral radiograph (*top*) of the lumbar spine of a 58-year-old woman with back pain and pseudoclaudication. At L4-5, degenerative spondylolisthesis is seen. Photograph (*bottom left*) of a sagittal section of a lumbar spine obtained at autopsy, to demonstrate degenerative spondylolisthesis (anterior slip) of L-3 and L-4 subsequent to degenerative disc disease. Note the r
a
S
C
r
tl

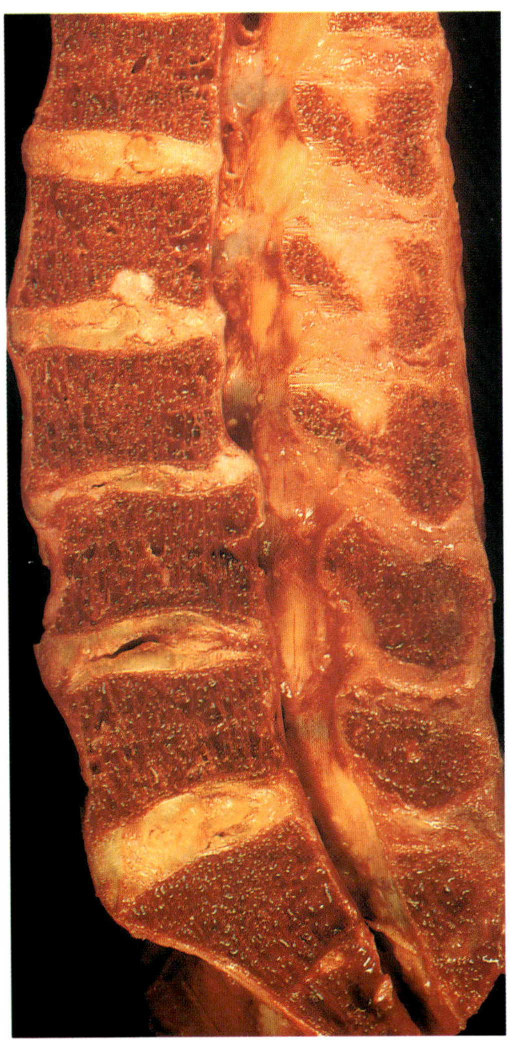

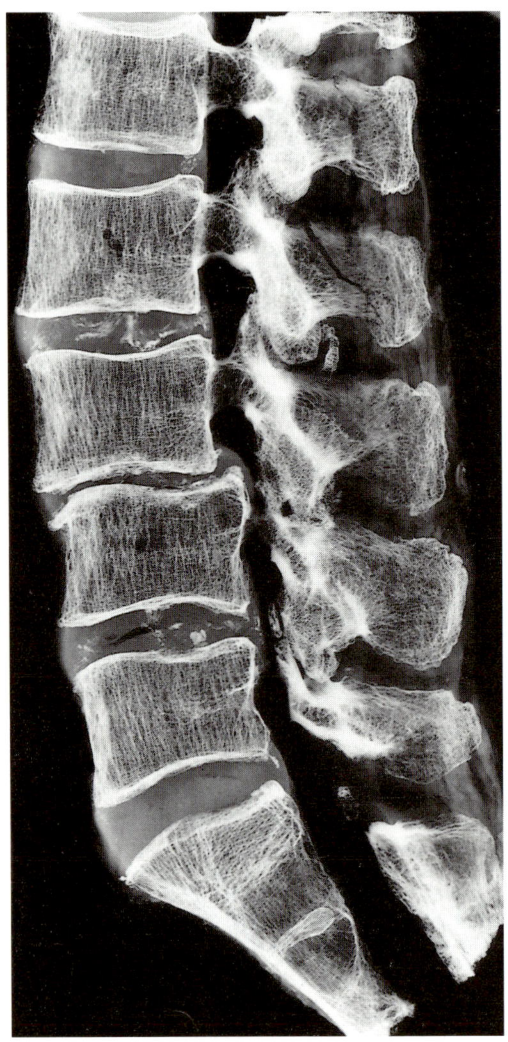

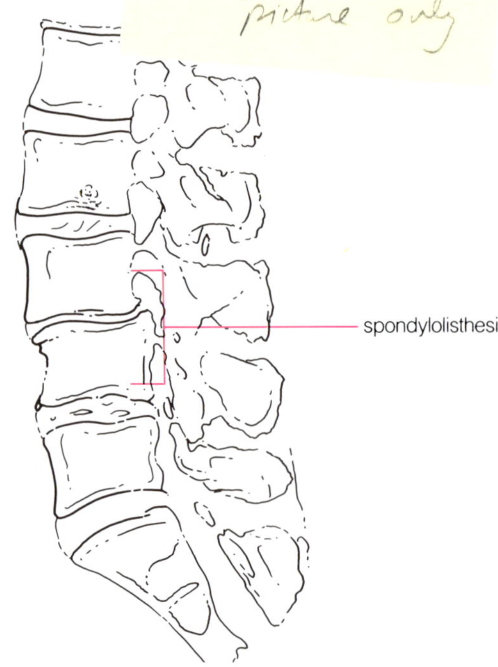

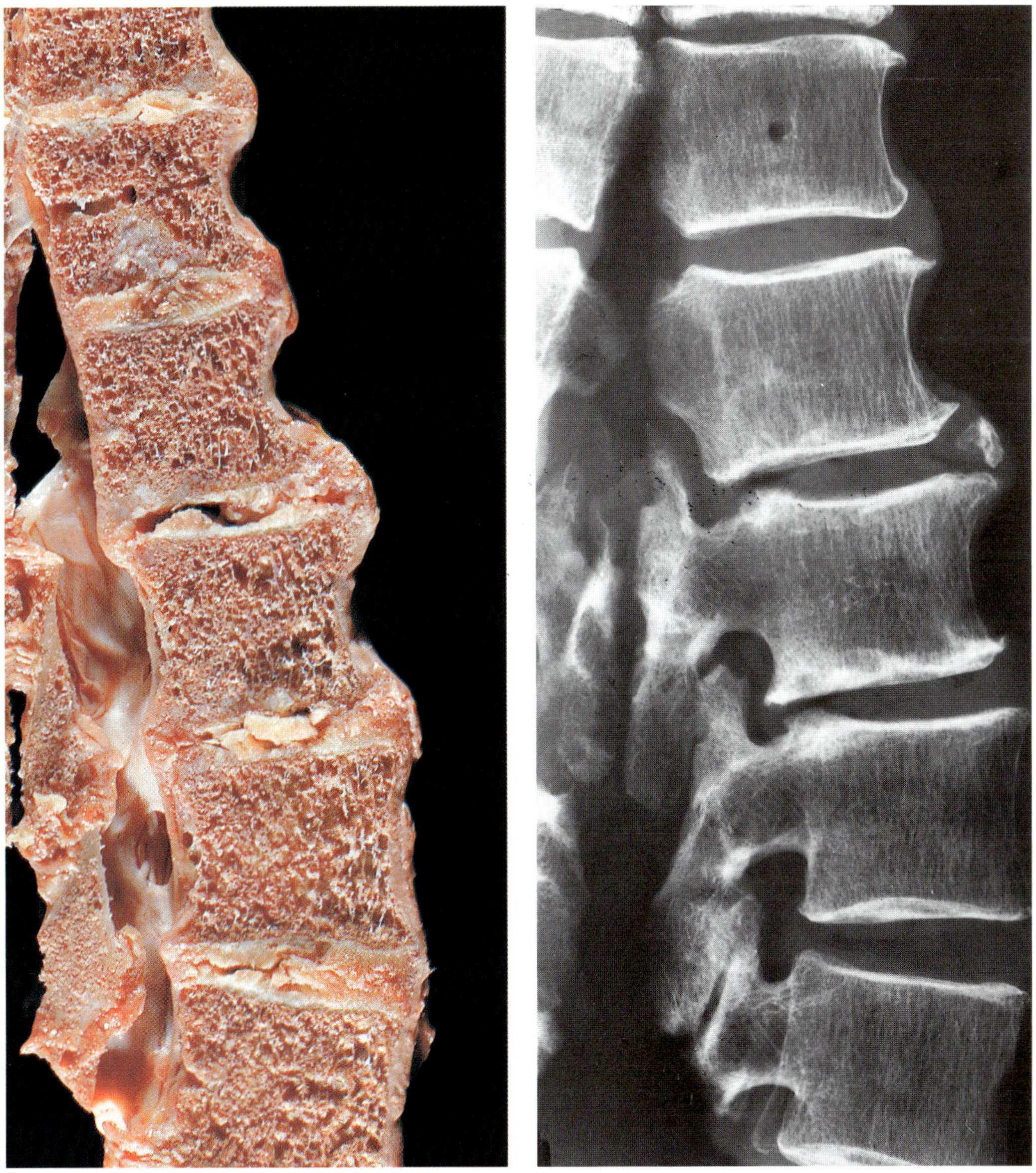

Figure 8.13 Photograph (*left*) of a sagittal section through the lumbar spine of an elderly patient to illustrate retrolisthesis at L2-3. Note the severe degenerative disc disease, which is associated with segmental stenosis. A radiograph (*right*) of the same specimen shows that in addition to the slip noted at L2-3, there is also a mild slip at L3-4.

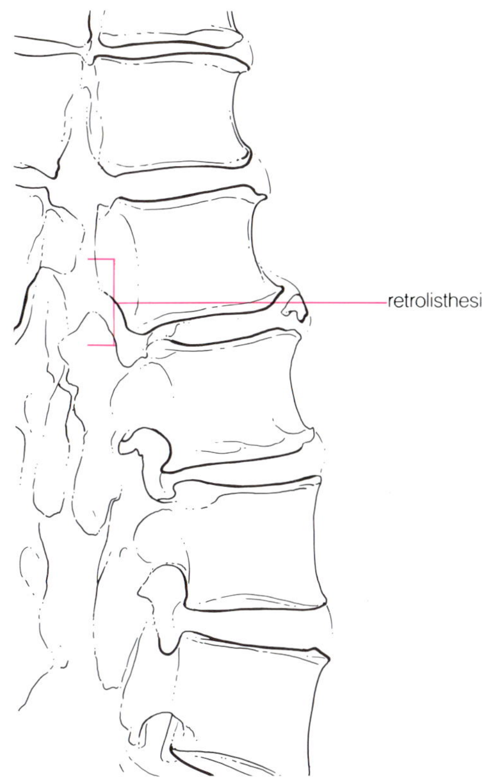

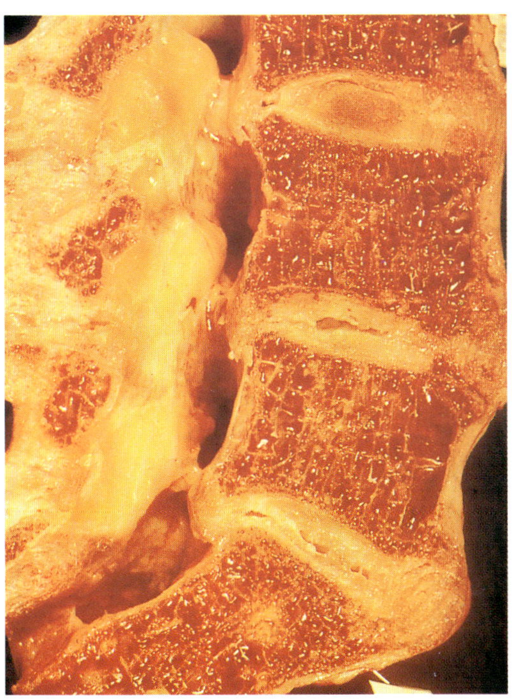

Figure 8.14 Photograph of a sagittal section through the lumbosacral spine in an 87-year-old female. There is posterior subluxation (retrolisthesis) to a slight degree, of L-5 on S-1, with associated narrowing of the spinal canal.

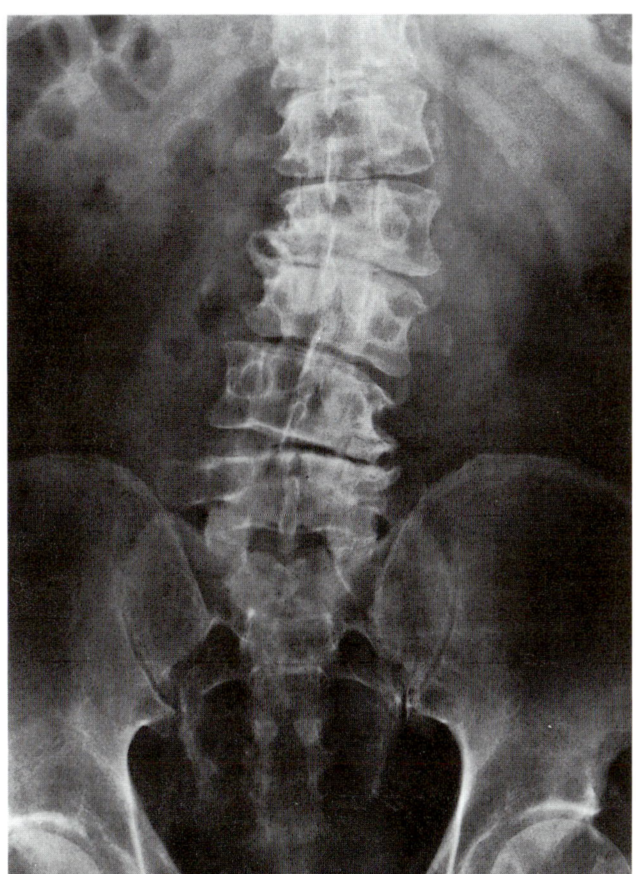

Figure 8.15 AP radiograph of a 72-year-old male, who presented with back pain and pseudoclaudication. This film demonstrates spondylosis at several levels. Lateral displacement also is present at several levels, but is most pronounced at L3-4. Note the associated scoliotic deformity.

Spinal Stenosis

GENERAL FEATURES

Spinal stenosis may result from developmental or acquired lesions or a combination of both, and it may affect the cervical, thoracic, or lumbar regions of the spine in both adults and children (Fig. 8.16). It may be symmetrical or asymmetrical, and central or confined to the lateral recesses. The narrowing seen in spinal stenosis may be produced by soft-tissue changes such as disc herniation (see Chapter 5), fibrous scar or tumor, or it may be the result of bony changes. The reduced volume and altered shape of the canal can lead to a spectrum of clinical syndromes arising from compression of neural elements within the spinal canal and intervertebral foramina.

CERVICAL STENOSIS

In general, an AP diameter of the spinal canal less than 11 mm, seen radiographically, is indicative of cervical stenosis (Fig. 8.17). Cervical stenosis may be related to congenital dysplasia, or it may be acquired in traumatic, infectious, metabolic, or neoplastic conditions. Degenerative cervical stenosis may develop from cervical disc degeneration, articular bony outgrowths of the facet joints, osteoarthritis of Luschka's joints, or osteophyte formation with encroachment on the spinal canal and neural foramina. Degenerative cervical stenosis is most common in the mobile mid- and lower cervical regions (Figs. 8.18 and 8.19). As noted previously, spinal stenosis is accentuated by the presence of degenerative spondylolisthesis or retrolisthesis.

THORACIC STENOSIS

Stenosis in the thoracic spine as a result of degenerative disease is much less frequent than in the cervical and lumbar regions. However, in rare circumstances, facet joint arthritis or congenitally short thickened laminae may lead to thoracic spinal canal stenosis with neurologic sequelae.

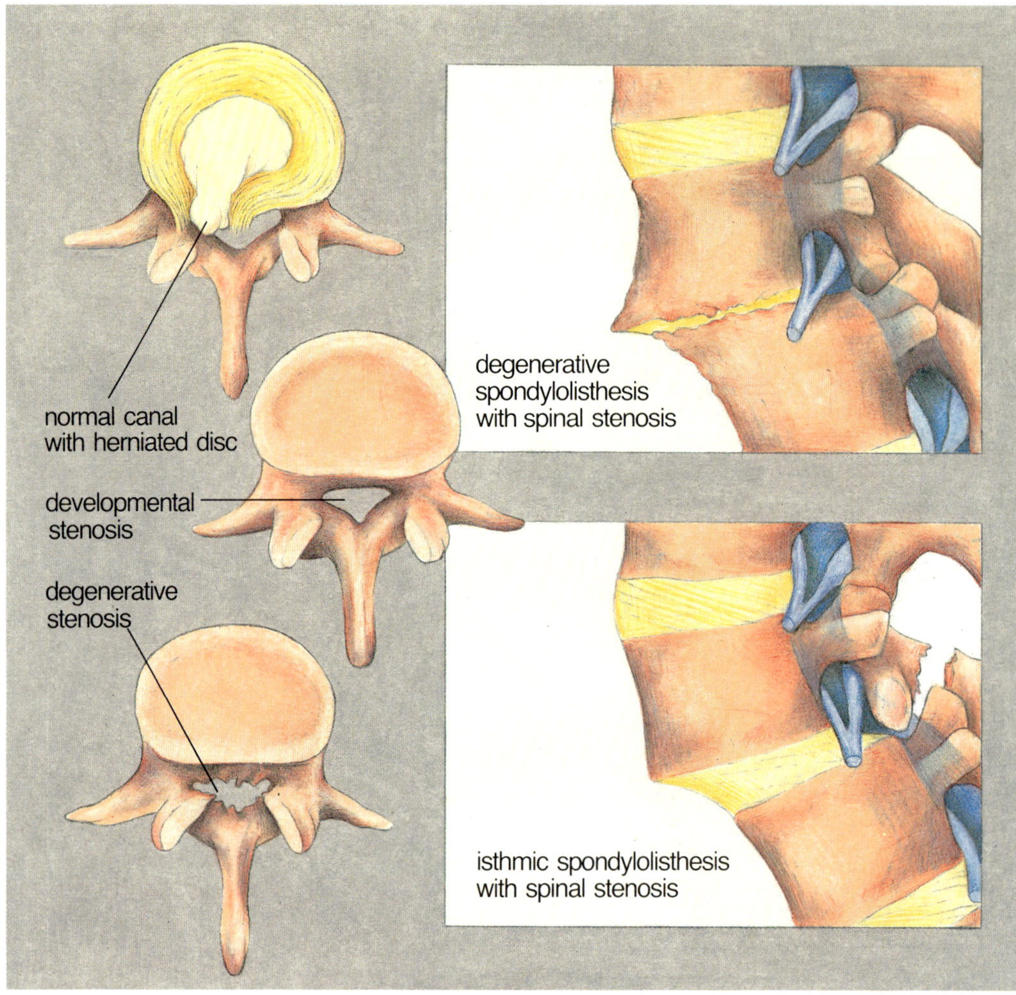

Figure 8.16 Schematic diagram to show the various forms of spinal stenosis. Illustrated are a normal canal with a herniated disc, developmental stenosis, degenerative stenosis, degenerative spondylolisthesis with lateral recess stenosis, and isthmic spondylolisthesis with lateral recess stenosis. Any of these different varieties of stenosis may occur with another, giving a picture of combined stenosis.

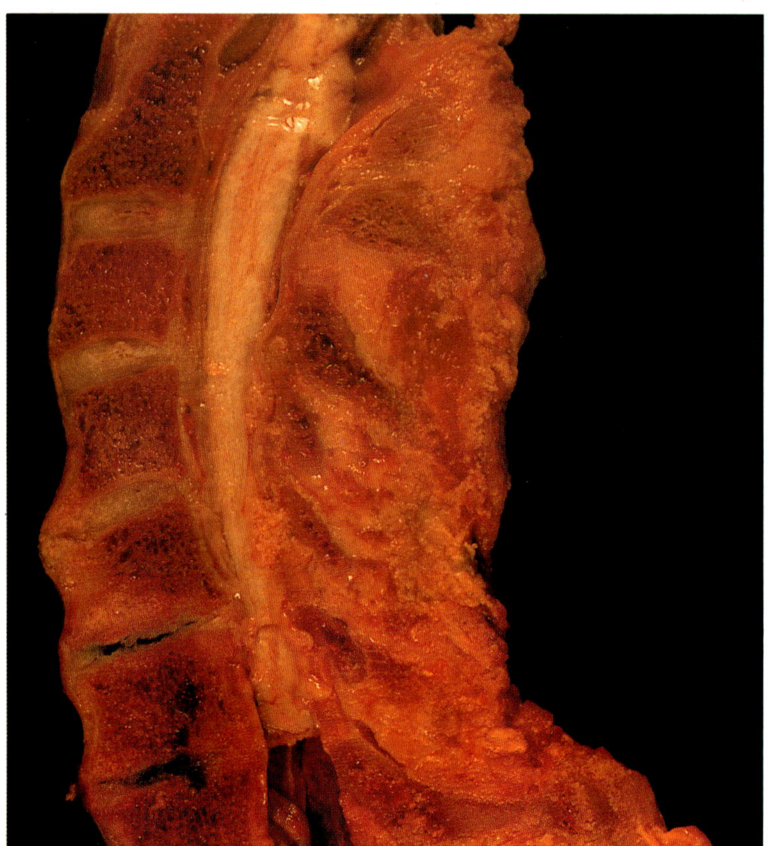

Figure 8.17 Photograph of a sagittal section through the cervical and upper thoracic spine of a 67-year-old male. There is a central stenosis [illegible]

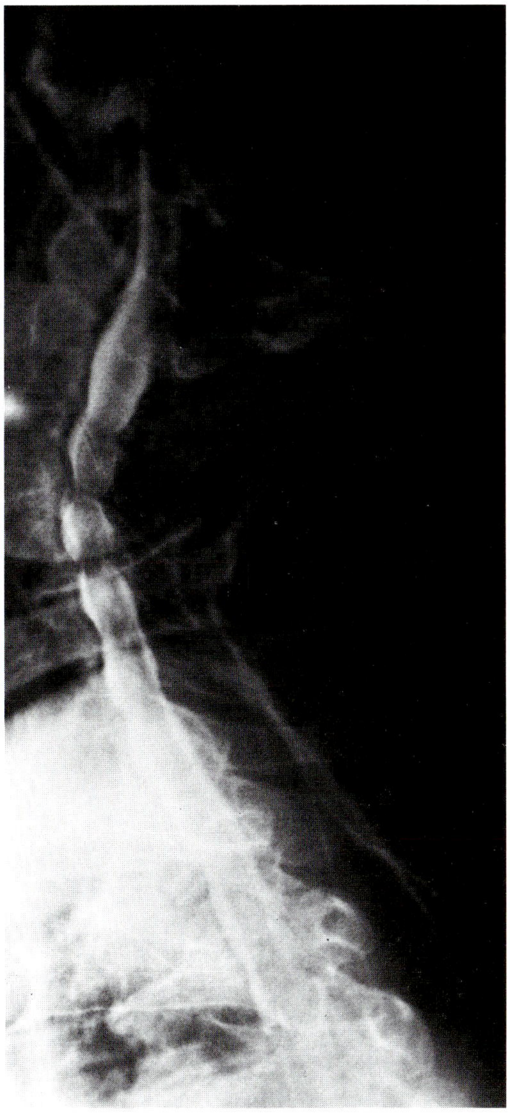

Figure 8.18 Lateral cervical myelogram (*top*) of a 69-year-old male who complained of symptoms referable to radiculopathy and myelopathy. In this myelogram, segmental narrowing can be seen from C-4 through C-7. A CT myelogram (*center*) at the level of C-2 shows a widened AP canal and a normally shaped cord. Another CT myelogram (*bottom*) of this same case, at the level of C5-6, shows marked narrowing of the AP diameter of the canal, with compression of the spinal cord, which is flattened in the AP diameter. The two crosses marked on the film indicate an 11-mm diameter.

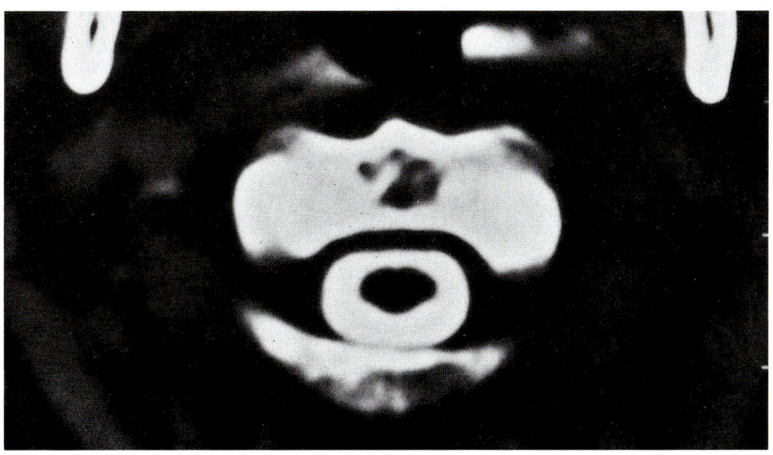

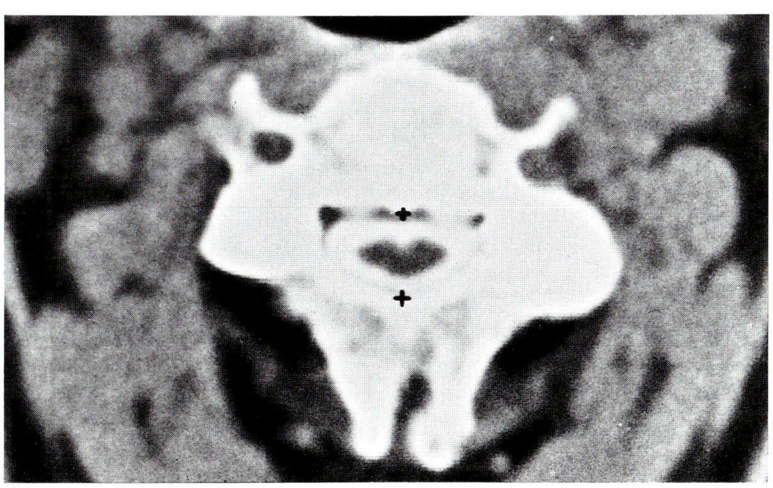

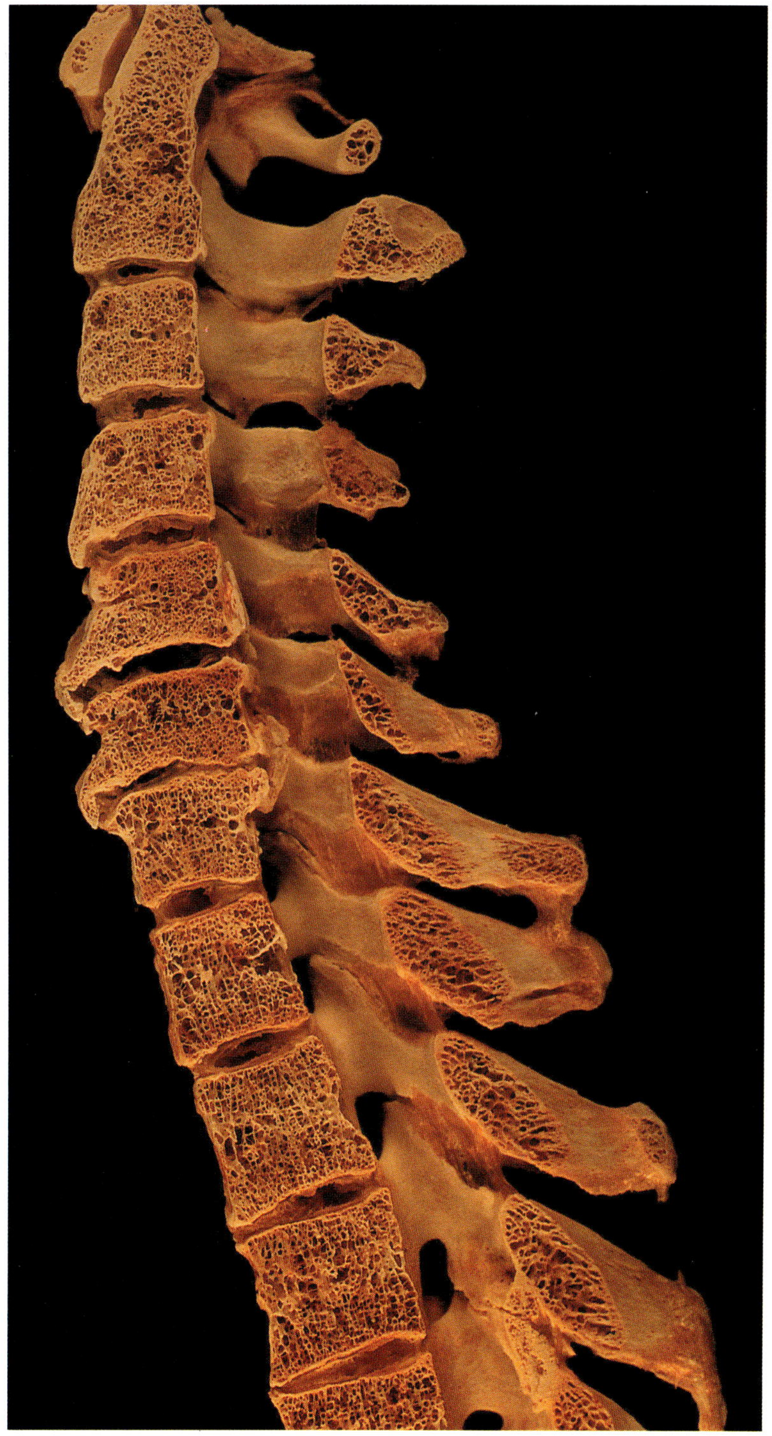

Figure 8.19 Photograph of a macerated specimen of the cervical spine in a 67 year old male. This photograph shows segmental narrowing of the spinal canal at the levels of C-5, C-6, and C-7.

LUMBAR STENOSIS

In the lumbar spine as in the cervical spine, developmental, acquired, or combined disease may lead to lumbar spinal stenosis with significant neurologic sequelae (Fig. 8.20). Developmental stenosis in the lumbar region may involve an isolated segment, causing a ringlike constriction of the region, or it may involve multiple levels or the entire lumbar segment. However, developmental stenosis in and of itself rarely causes symptoms. Combined stenosis is the most common form of lumbar spinal stenosis giving rise to clinical disease, and it is more common in the lumbar spine than in the thoracic or cervical spine (Figs. 8.21 and 8.22).

Lumbar spinal stenosis in the adult is indicated by an AP diameter of less than 13 mm or a transverse diameter of 20 mm or less, as measured radiographically, especially using CT. While the transverse diameter can be determined readily by conventional radiography, measurement of the sagittal diameter usually requires the use of myelography (Fig. 8.23) and/or CT scanning.

Most instances of lumbar spinal stenosis seen at autopsy are degenerative (Fig. 8.24). Such stenosis may involve the lateral recesses or central neural canal, with nerve root or cauda equina compression; as already noted, the L4-5 and L-5 to S-1 segments are the ones most commonly affected. However, it should be recognized that the abnormal and decreased mobility resulting from degenerative changes at these levels may predispose to progressive stenosis of the remaining portion of the lumbar spine.

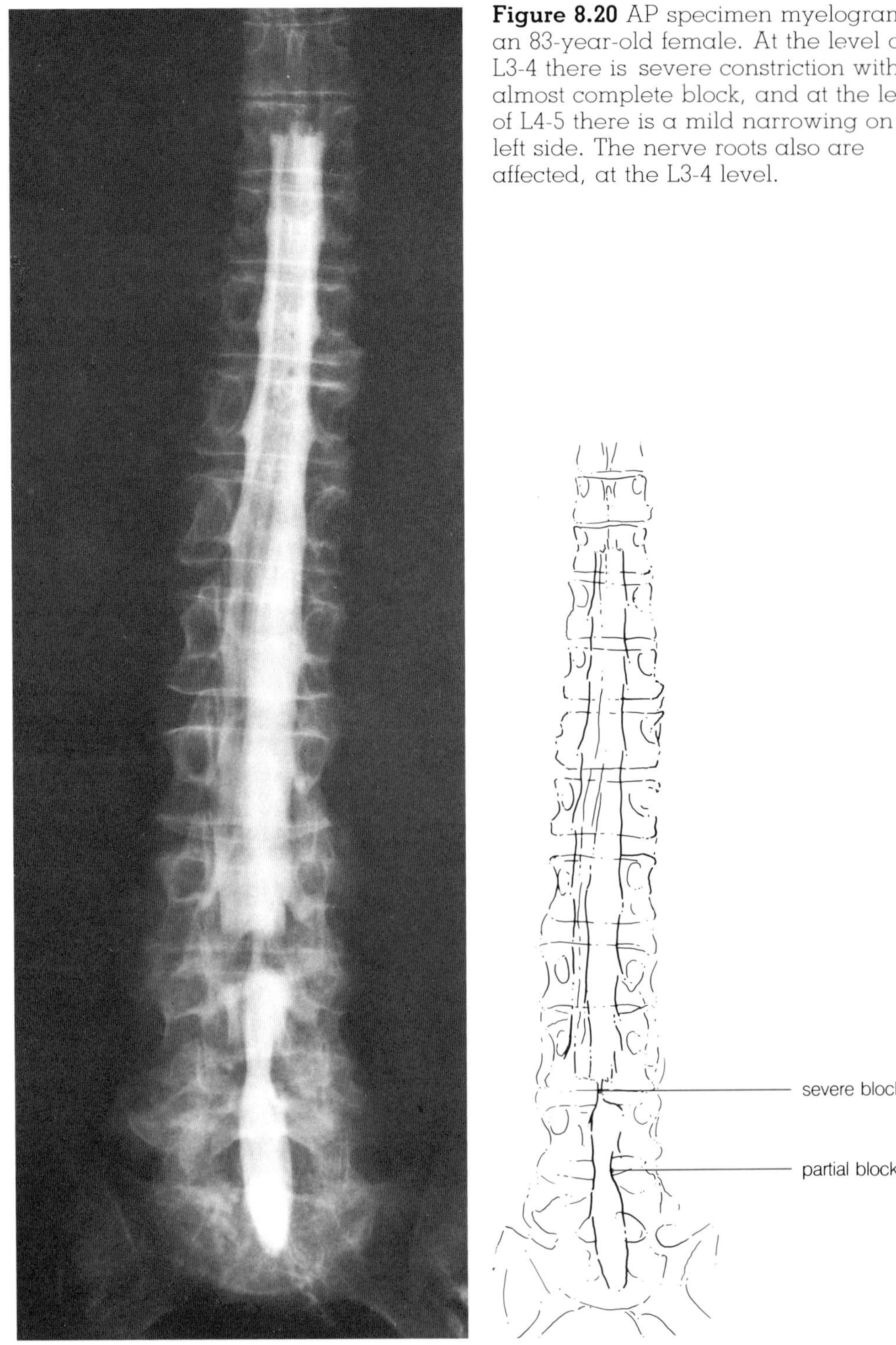

Figure 8.20 AP specimen myelogram of an 83-year-old female. At the level of L3-4 there is severe constriction with almost complete block, and at the level of L4-5 there is a mild narrowing on the left side. The nerve roots also are affected, at the L3-4 level.

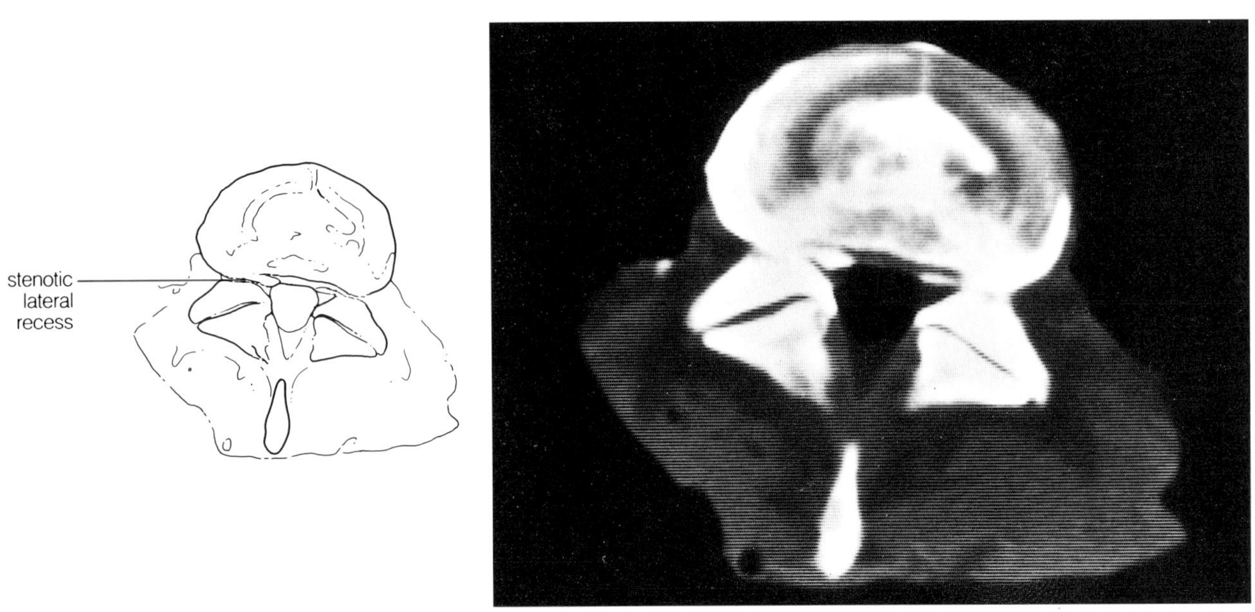

Figure 8.21 CT discogram at the level of L3-4, of a specimen obtained from an elderly male at autopsy, showing a combined stenosis with facet joint arthrosis and osteophytosis. There is also bilateral posterolateral disc herniation, with dye extending to the recesses behind the posterior ligaments.

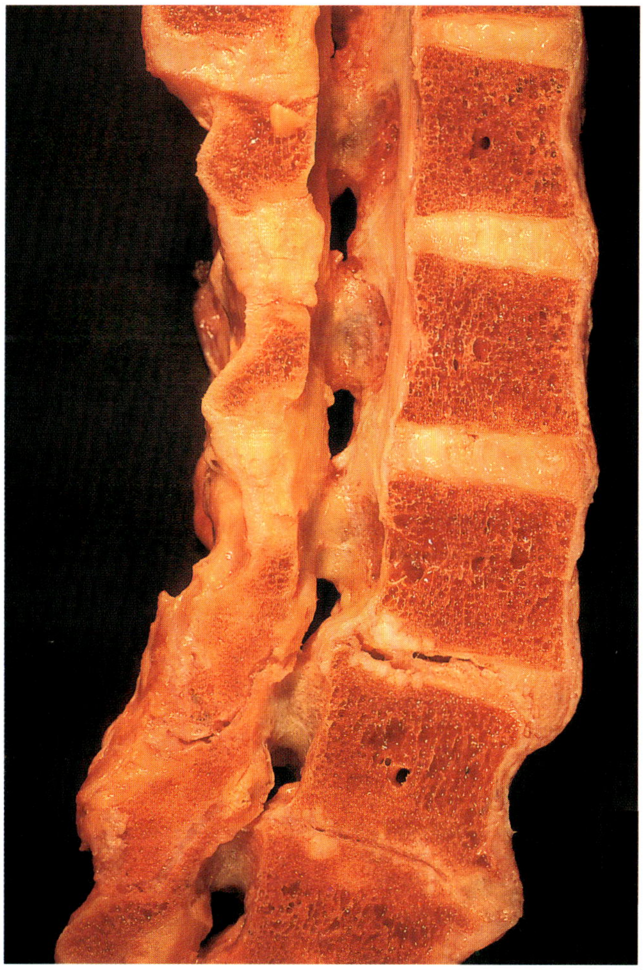

Figure 8.22 Photograph of a sagittal section through the lumbar spine of a 74-year-old female, showing degenerative disc disease in the lower three intervertebral disc spaces. In addition, there is spondylolisthesis with segmental spinal stenosis at the levels of L3-4, L4-5, and L-5 to S-1. Note also that in the upper lumbar spine, the canal is quite adequate. The intervertebral foramina also are narrowed at the affected levels.

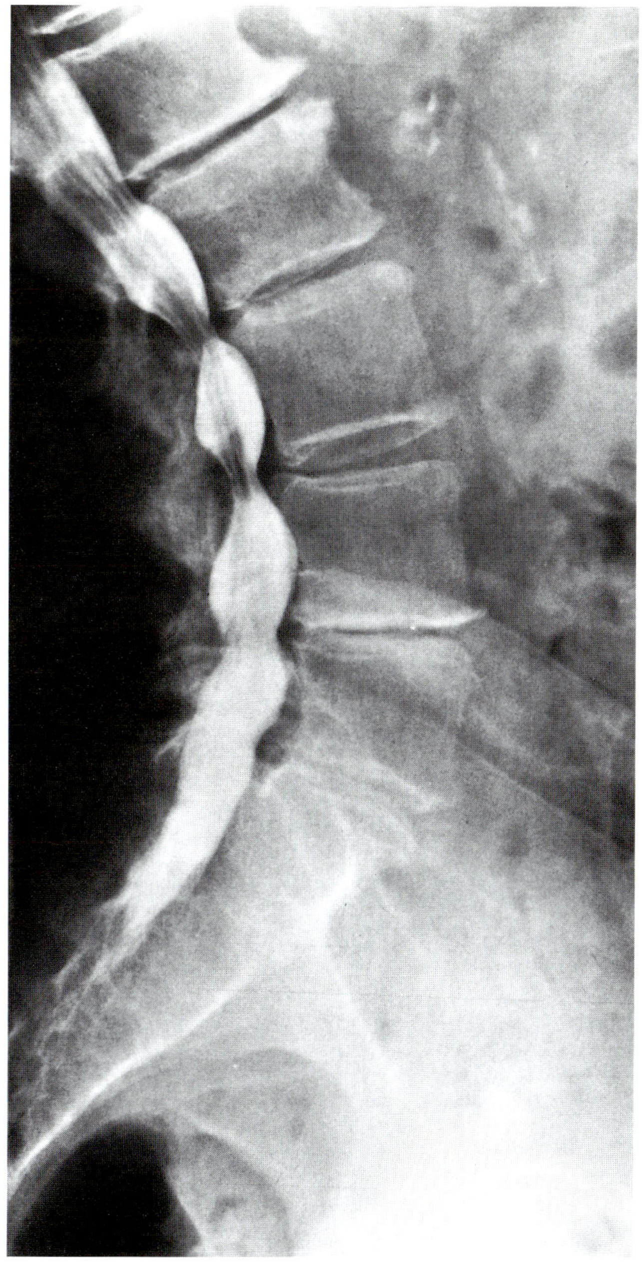

Figure 8.23 Lateral myelogram of a 60-year-old woman with complaints of both lower back and radiating leg pain, associated with activity. Note the segmental stenosis of severe degree, from L-2 through L-5, with associated disc degeneration and posterior osteophyte formation.

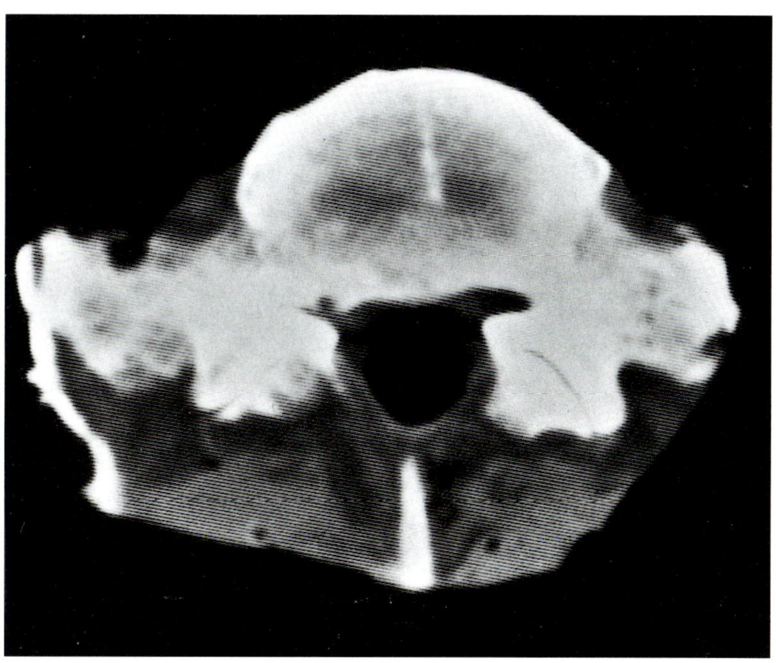

Figure 8.24 Specimen CT scan obtained from an elderly male, at the level of L4-5, to show severe degenerative changes in the facet joints, with osteophyte formation and lateral recess stenosis.

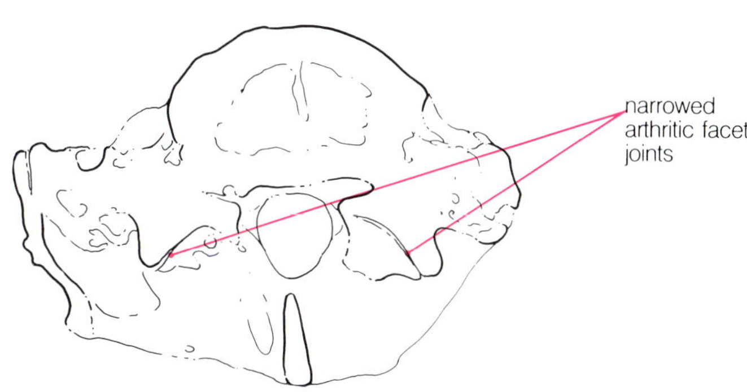

Neuropathic (Charcot) Spine

Trauma to the articulations, with their ultimate destruction, may occur due to impairment of pain or proprioceptive sensation, and is generally referred to as neuropathic arthropathy. Tabes dorsalis (neurosyphilis), diabetes, syringomyelia, paraplegia, peripheral neuropathy and congenital indifference to pain, as well as intraarticular steroid injections, are considered etiologic factors in the development of neuropathic arthropathy. Ten to 15% of patients with tabetic arthropathy of the peripheral joints also have involvement of the lumbar spine.

When the cervical spine is involved, syringomyelia is most frequently the underlying disease. Pain is the usual initial presentation, but it occurs not as a result of vertebral destruction, but rather as a consequence of the concomitant instability and stress placed on ligaments and neural structures. From the radiographic viewpoint, the progression usually is one of disc-space narrowing, sclerosis of the vertebral end plates, and osteophytosis (Fig. 8.25).

In advanced cases, the spine is characterized by extensive destruction of the discs, with sclerosis and fragmentation of the vertebral bodies and massive osteophytosis (Fig. 8.26). Subluxation and dislocation also may be present in the advanced disease state. However, the osteophytes that form are usually so huge and exuberant that they may help to stabilize the spinal segment affected.

Radiographic features, in conjunction with neurologic findings and spinal fluid and blood serology, will help to differentiate this disorder from those of intervertebral osteochondrosis (spondylosis), disc-space infection and rarely, neoplasm.

Histologic features include marked joint destruction with bone debris in the synovial tissue, and numerous loose bodies (Fig. 8.27). Occasionally, a severe form of chondrocalcinosis—pseudoneuropathic arthritis—may be difficult to distinguish from a Charcot joint. However, the finding of extensive CPPD disease elsewhere helps one to make the correct diagnosis.

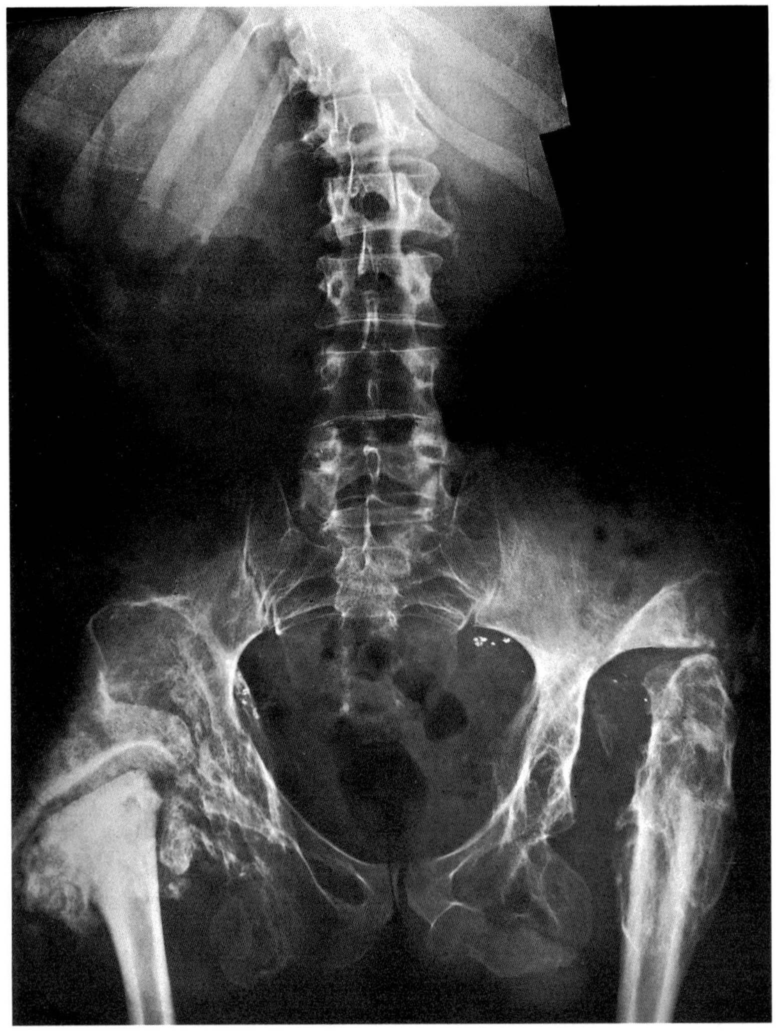

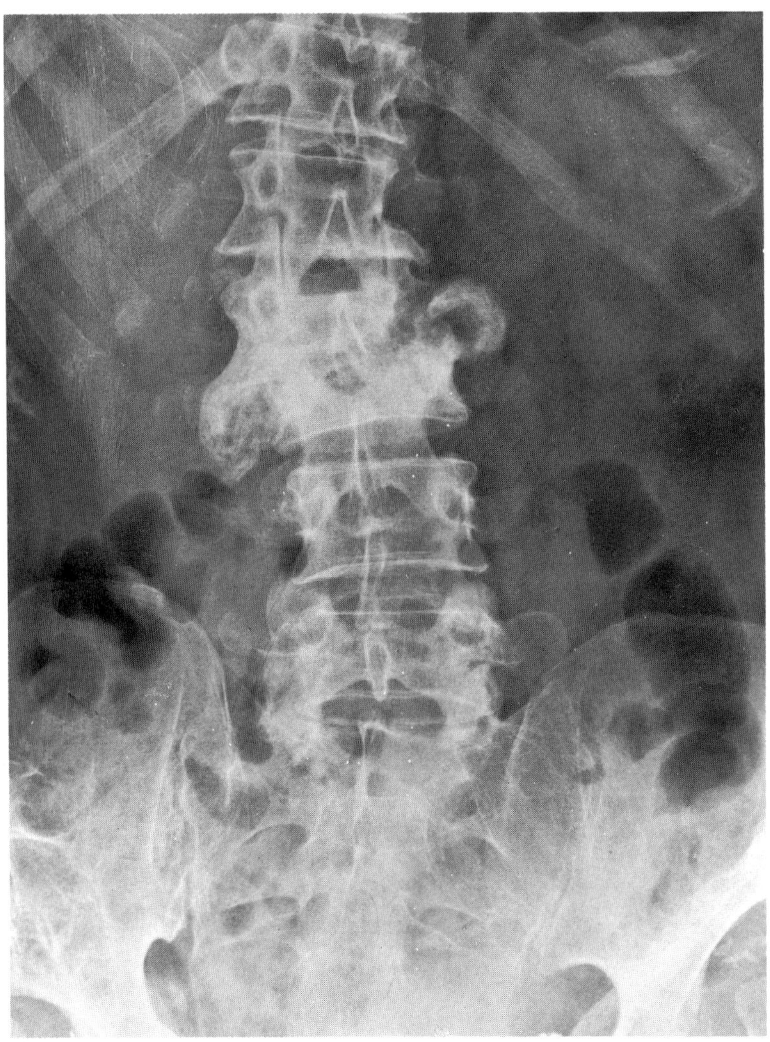

Figure 8.25 Radiograph (*top*) of the pelvis and thoracolumbar spine in a 30-year-old male with congenital syphilis and severe bilateral hip disease. Note that in the lumbar spine, at the level of L2-3, there is mild lateral subluxation. Radiograph (*bottom*) of the lumbar spine and pelvis in the same patient, 11 years later. Note that at L2-3, there is severe destruction and collapse of the bony elements, with large productive osteophytes characteristic of a Charcot joint.

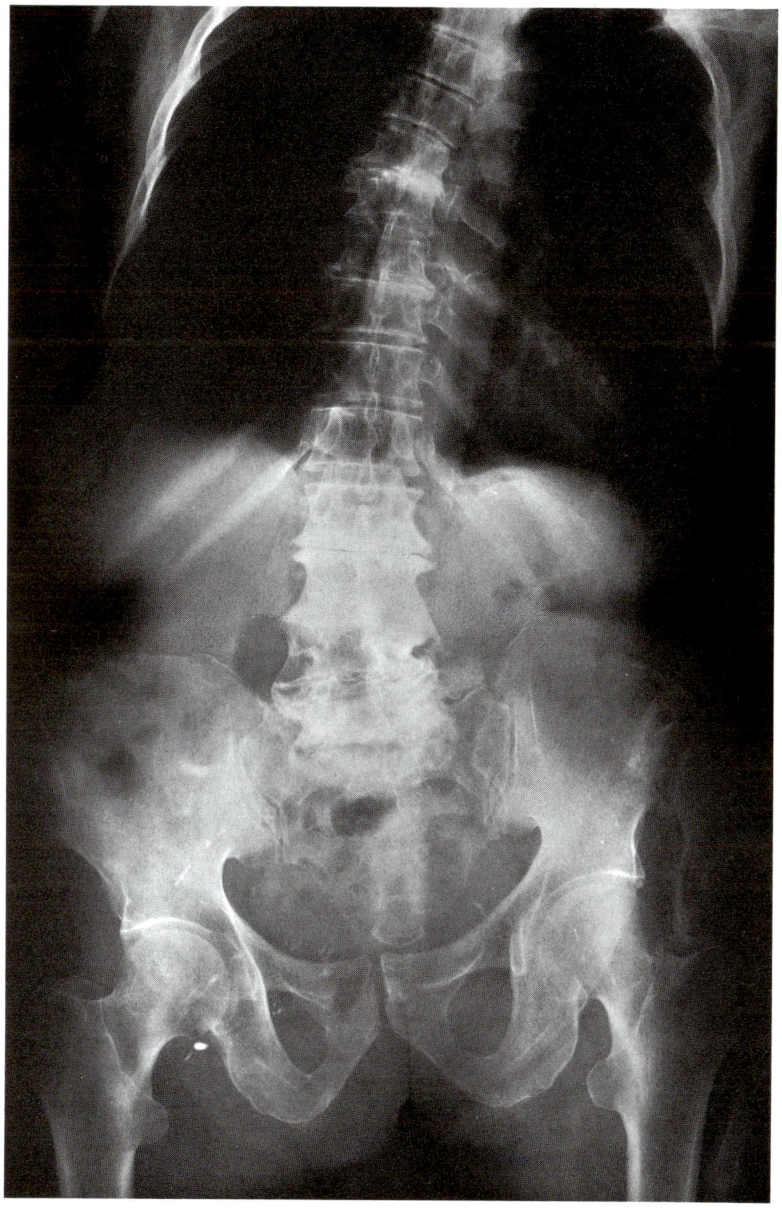

Figure 8.26 Radiograph of the thoracolumbar spine of a 55-year-old male with tabes dorsalis. In the lumbar spine, there is loss of the disc spaces, with bony collapse and sclerosis. Note that the hips are spared.

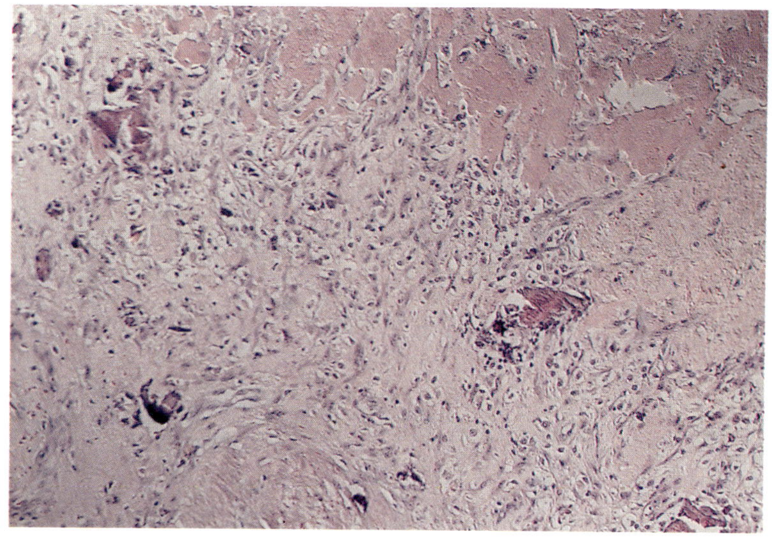

Figure 8.27 Photomicrograph of tissue obtained from around a Charcot joint. It is scarred and chronically inflamed with fibrinous exudation, and is filled by multiple irregular fragments of bone and cartilage. Such rapid breakdown of the joint is characteristic in patients with a Charcot joint.

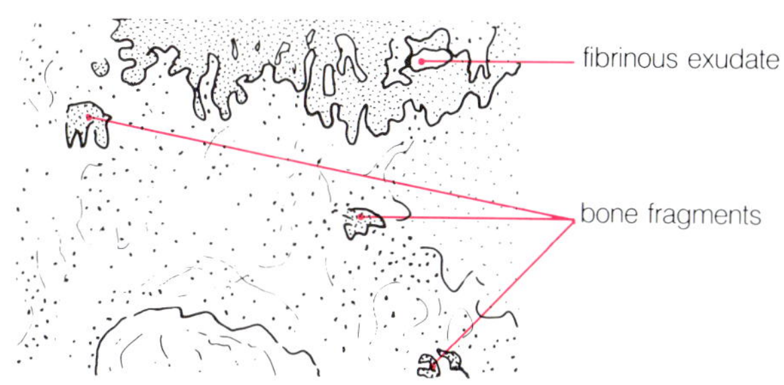

9
CHAPTER

INFLAMMATORY AND ANKYLOSING SPONDYLOARTHROPATHIES

General Features

In the spine, there are more than 130 articulations, including both the amphiarthroses as well as the synovial-lined diarthrodial joints. Consequently, many diseases affecting the spine will affect one or more of these joints, resulting in symptoms of joint dysfunction, i.e., arthritis.

In the earlier chapters of this section, we explained the process by which intervertebral disc disease leads to osteoarthritis of the spine, which in turn may result in neurologic complications. In the present chapter, we will discuss features of the most common inflammatory and ankylosing diseases of the spinal articulations, and emphasize how different segments of the spine are affected by the different disease entities.

Inflammatory Spondylitis

RHEUMATOID ARTHRITIS

Rheumatoid arthritis is a systemic chronic inflammatory disease that is more common in women than in men (approximately 4:1) and which usually presents between the ages of 25 and 55 years. Its principal targets are the lymphoid system, the synovial joints, and the small blood vessels (Figs. 9.1 and 9.2). In rheumatoid disease, the arthritis of the peripheral articulations tends to be bilateral and symmetrical, with a predilection for the hands, wrists, and feet. In the spine, the cervical articulations usually are the ones affected most significantly clinically, although changes in the thoracolumbar spine and in the sacroiliac joint, though uncommon, also may occur.

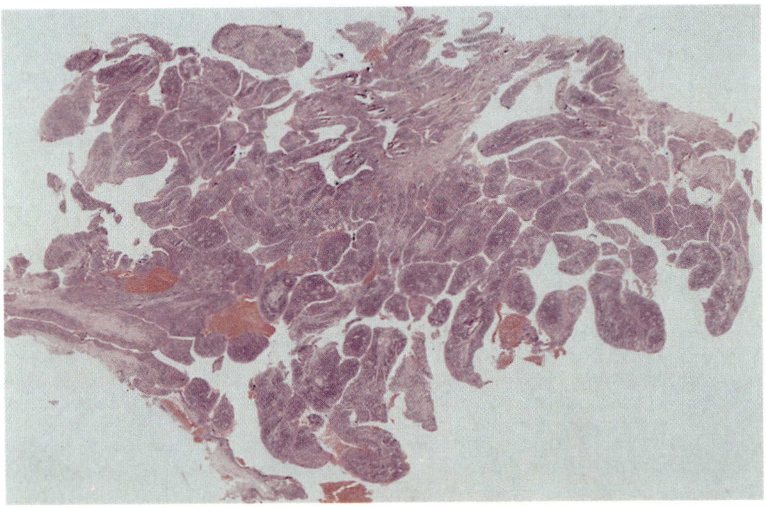

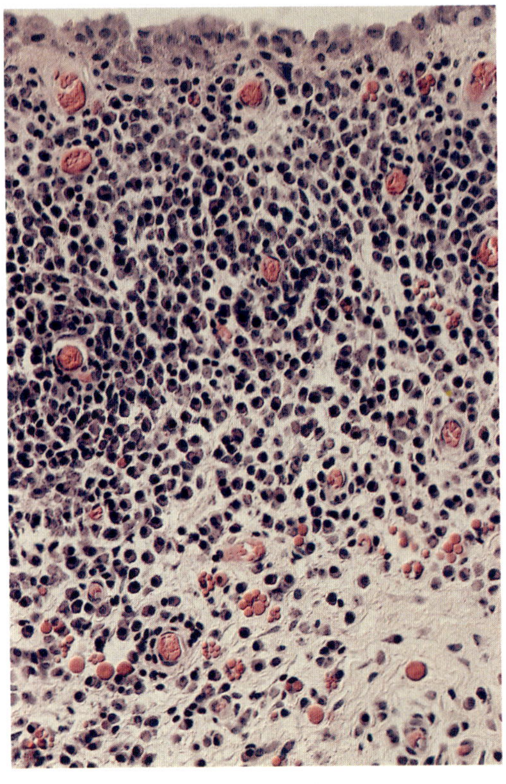

Figure 9.1 Photomicrograph (*top*) at low power of synovial tissue obtained from a patient with rheumatoid arthritis shows the typical papillary appearance, hypervascularity, and cellular infiltration. (H & E, × 1.25 objective) A photomicrograph (*bottom*) of a rheumatoid synovium at higher power shows the hypoplastic synovial lining and the infiltration by chronic inflammatory cells, mostly plasma cells, many of which contain eosinophilic cytoplasmic inclusions (Russell bodies). (H & E, × 10 objective)

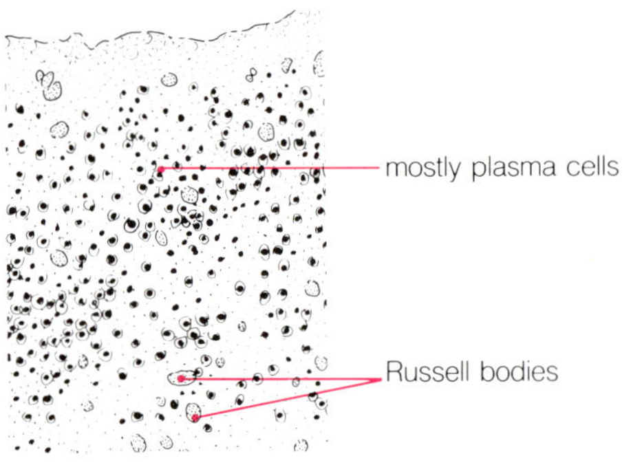

The clinical course of rheumatoid arthritis may be complicated by several other entities, including osteoporosis and infection. Osteoporosis may be aggravated by the administration of steroids used in the treatment of rheumatoid arthritis. In some cases, the use of corticosteroids may result in osteonecrosis, which in time may lead to a Charcot joint or be predisposed to infection (Fig. 9.3). Infections are frequent in the rheumatoid patient, especially with the use of steroids and other immunosuppressive agents; quite commonly these infections are clinically silent.

The Cervical Spine

Approximately 60 to 70% of all rheumatoid arthritis patients at some time during their illness develop symptoms and signs relating to the cervical spine. Pain is the most common symptom, and in association with atlantoaxial subluxation it may be referred to the temporal, auricular, or orbital regions. Also in the cervical region, neurologic signs may occur as a result of nerve root involvement and/or cord compression. Vertebrobasilar artery insufficiency too may occur, leading to transient blindness, vertigo, loss of consciousness and, occasionally, sudden death (see Section 1, Fig. 2.55).

From the radiographic point of view, the entire cervical spine often is involved. Lesions may be evident not only in the synovial articulations but also in the joints of Luschka, in the disc space, and at the tendon and ligamentous attachments. Bony erosion and apophysial joint-space narrowing are common, and may be followed by fibrous ankylosis and occasionally by bony ankylosis (Fig. 9.4). Erosions of the odontoid process

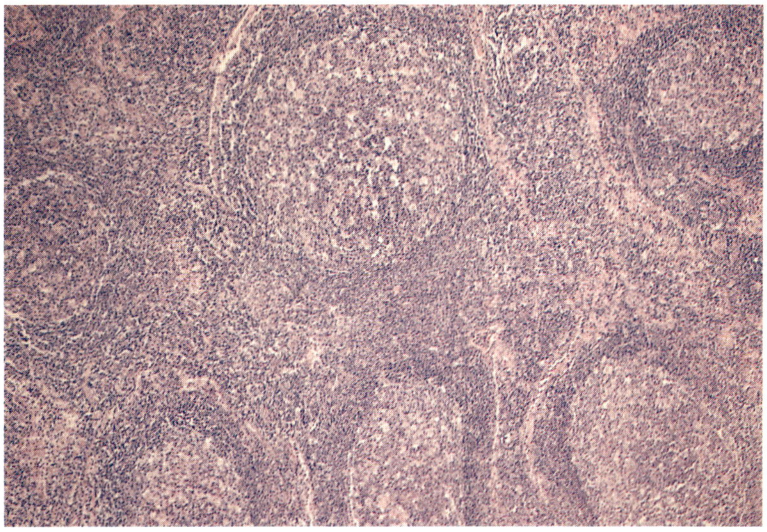

Figure 9.2 Photomicrograph of an enlarged lymph node from a patient with rheumatoid arthritis demonstrates nodular hyperplasia. (H & E, × 4 objective)

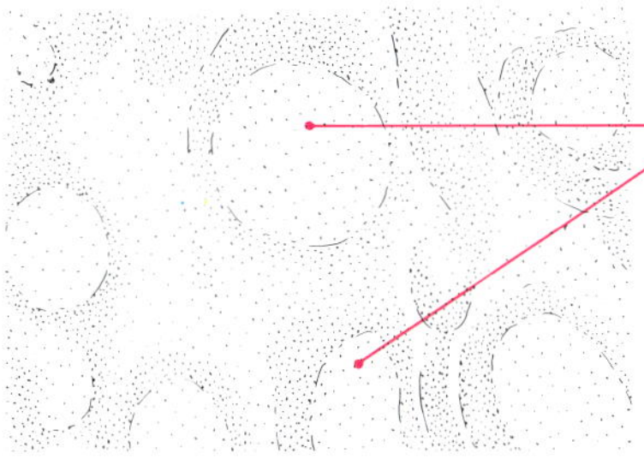

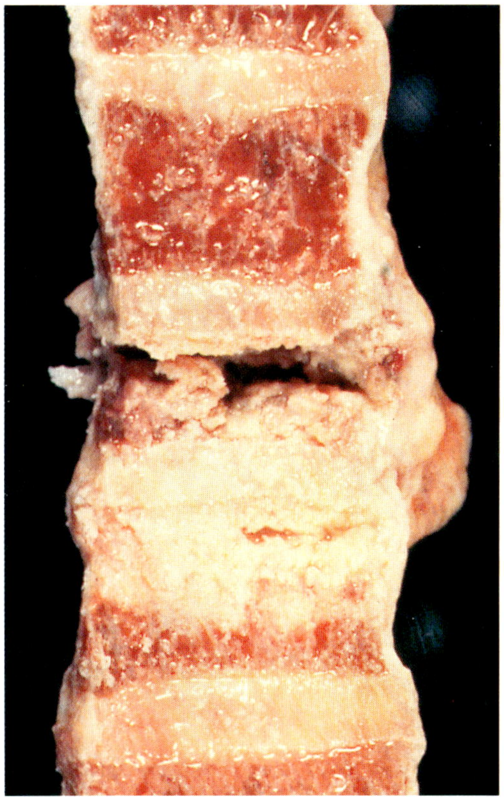

Figure 9.3 Photograph of a segment of lower thoracic spine from a patient with rheumatoid arthritis treated with cortisone. There is a generalized osteopenia, but, in addition, osteonecrosis of two adjacent vertebrae has resulted in collapse of one of the vertebrae. (Courtesy of Dr. Vorachai Sirikulchayanonta)

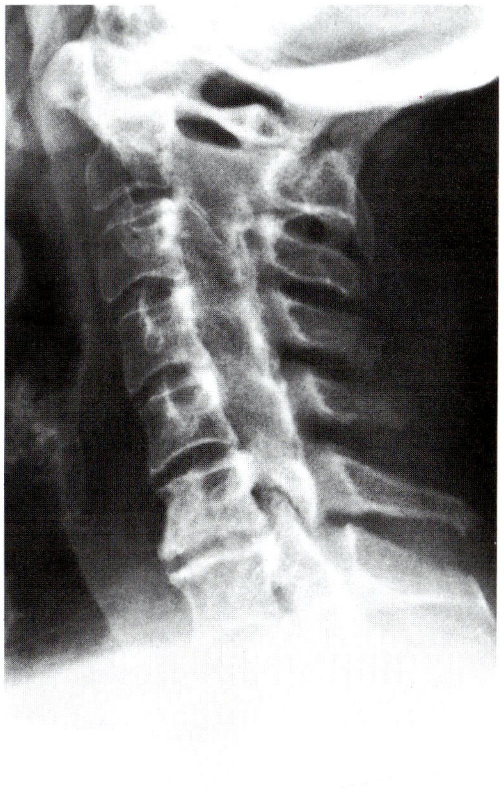

Figure 9.4 Lateral radiograph of the cervical spine of a 50-year-old woman with rheumatoid arthritis. In C-2 through C-6, note the fusion of the facet joints. There is narrowing of the spinal canal at the level of C1-2, due to anterior displacement of the atlas. The spine as a whole is osteopenic.

occur in one-third of patients with rheumatoid arthritis in those areas that are in intimate contact with inflamed synovial membrane, i.e., between the anterior arch of the atlas and the odontoid process, between the odontoid process and transverse ligament of the atlas, and at the tip of the odontoid process where the apical ligament is attached (Fig. 9.5). As a result of such erosions, three major complications may occur:

1. Fracture of the odontoid following minimal trauma
2. Disappearance of the odontoid if the erosion is severe enough
3. Atlantoaxial subluxation and/or basilar invagination

Basilar invagination is due to the vertical displacement of the odontoid process of C-2 (Fig. 9.6). Such a displacement results from destruction and collapse of the bony and articular structures between the occiput and the atlas (Fig. 9.7), and between the atlas and the axis (Fig. 9.8). On occasion, such dis-

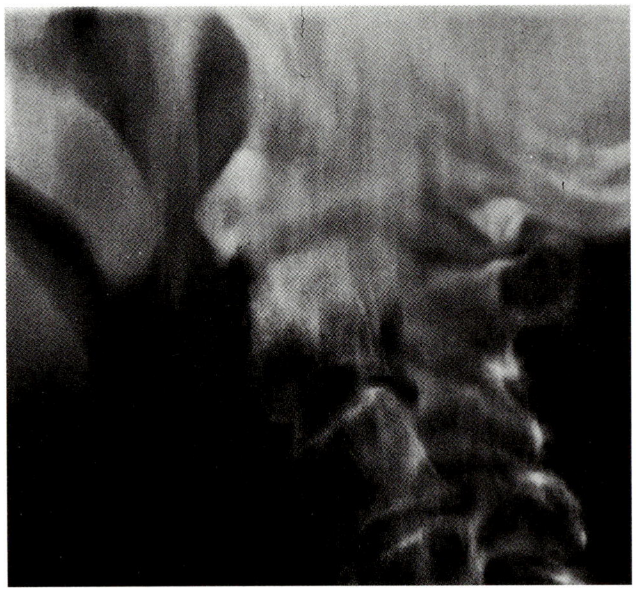

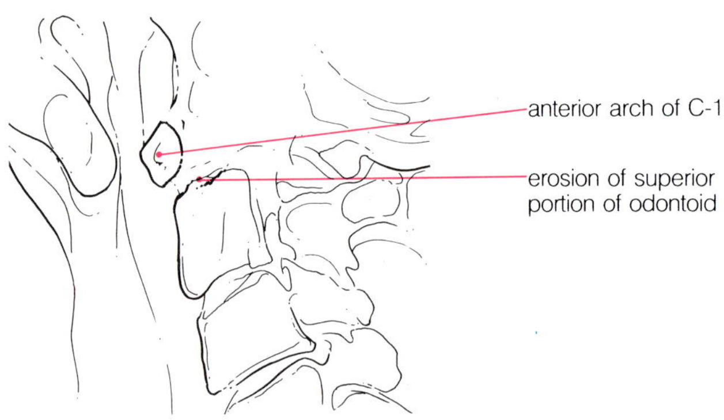

Figure 9.5 Lateral tomogram of the upper cervical spine of a man with rheumatoid arthritis to show erosion of the odontoid. The upper half of the residual body of C-2 is irregularly sclerotic.

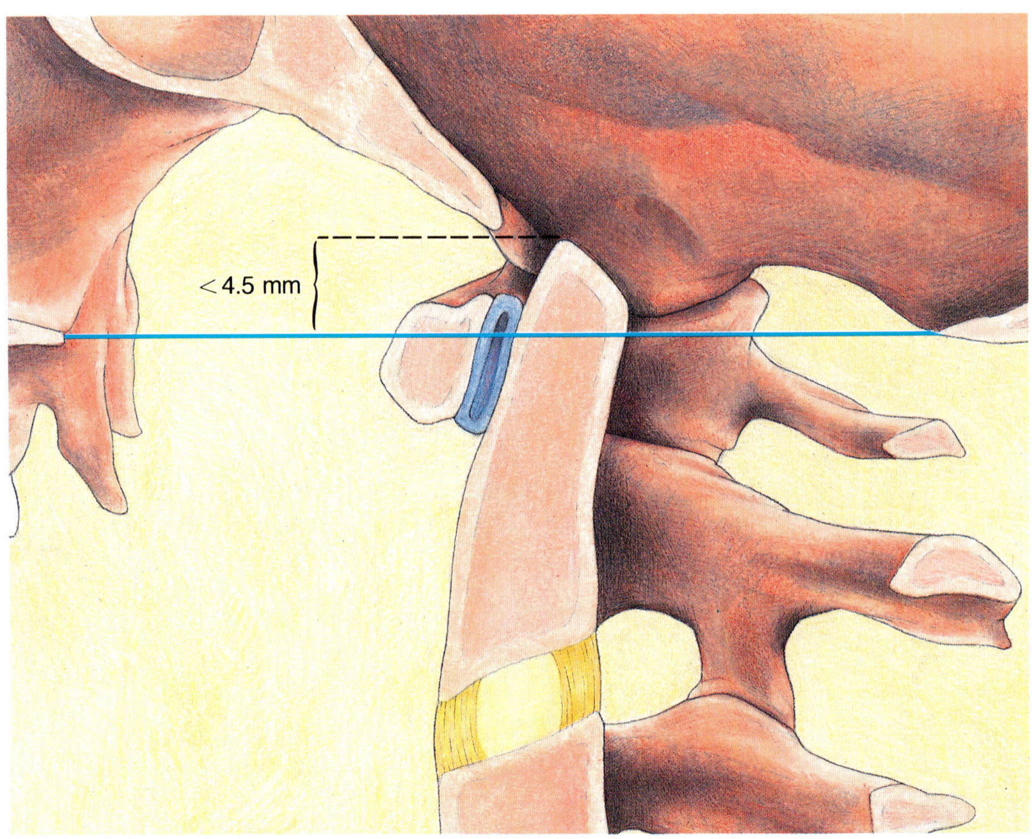

Figure 9.6 Schematic drawing of a midsagittal section through the upper cervical spine and the base of the skull, to show the normal relationships between the anterior arch of C-1, the odontoid, and the foramen magnum. The reference line shown, McGregor's line, is useful in the interpretation of clinical radiographs. The line is drawn from the upper surface of the posterior edge of the hard palate to the most caudal point of the occipital curve of the skull. The tip of the odontoid should not extend more than 4.5 mm above this line.

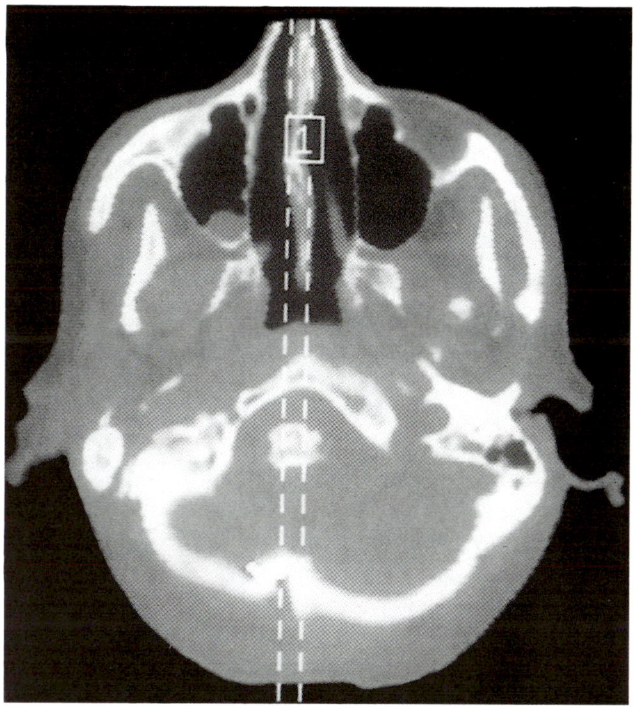

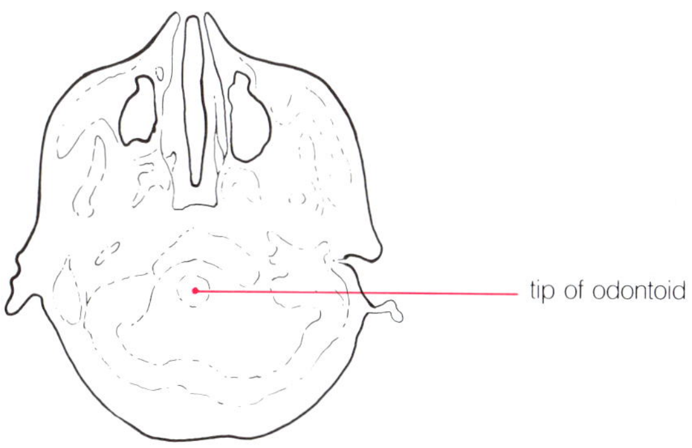

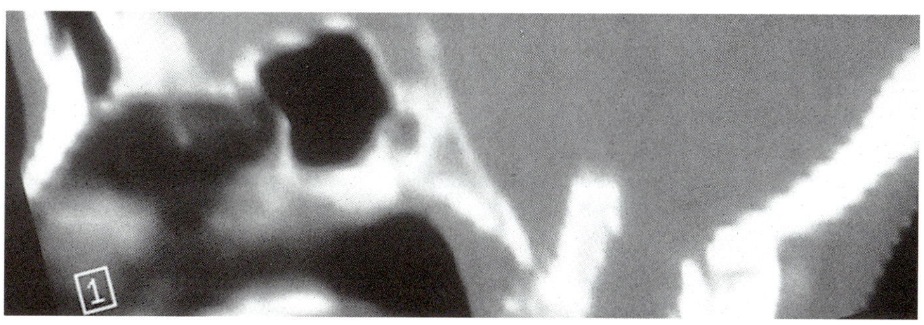

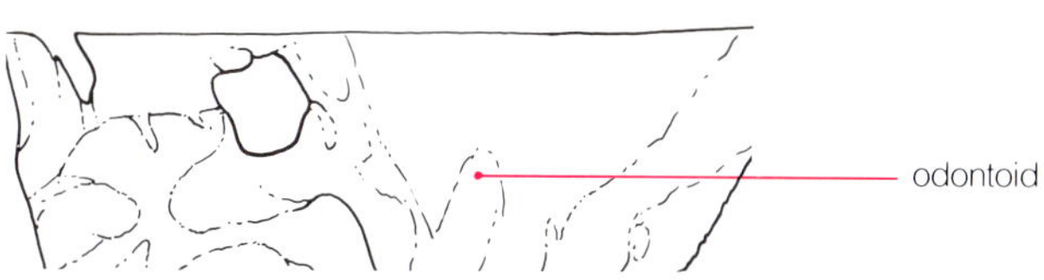

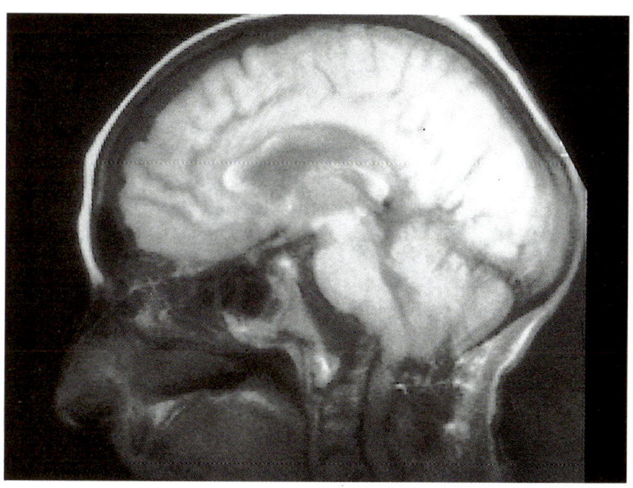

Figure 9.7 CT scans (*top* and *center*) of the base of the skull in a woman with rheumatoid arthritis and complaints of transient episodes of loss of consciousness. In both the sagittal reconstruction and the transverse section, displacement of the odontoid into the base of the skull is obvious. An MRI (*bottom*) of the same patient shows encroachment of the odontoid on the medulla oblongata.

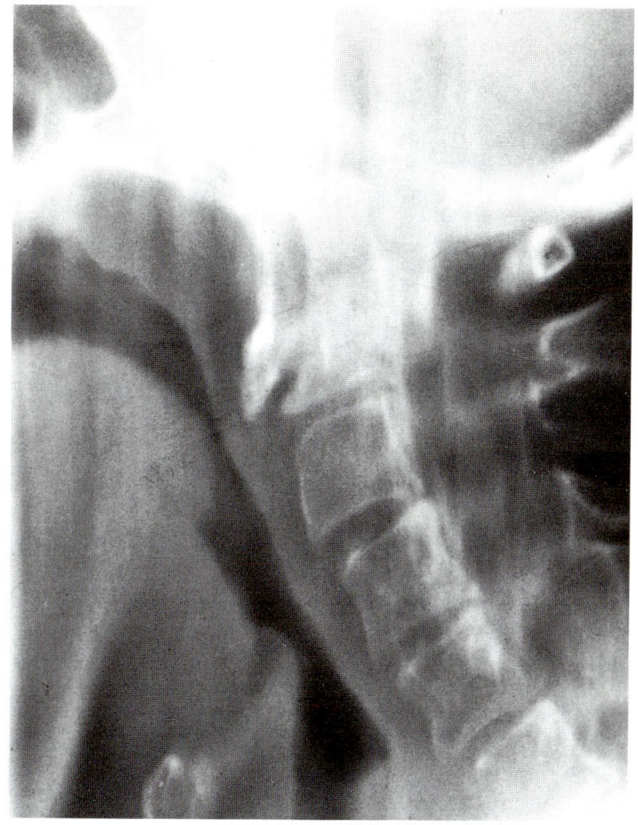

Figure 9.8 Lateral tomogram of the upper cervical spine in extension, in a patient with rheumatoid arthritis. Note that the lower border of the anterior arch of C-1 is at the level of the upper margin of the C2-3 disc space, indicating atlantoaxial instability.

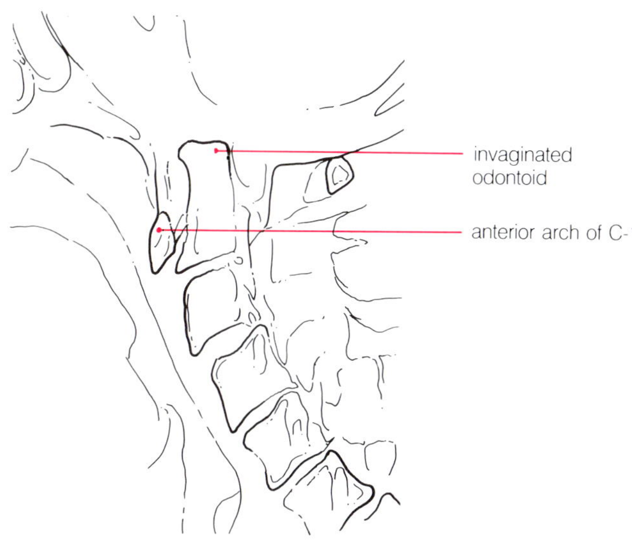

placement may be fatal (Fig. 9.9).

A characteristic radiographic finding in rheumatoid arthritis (which also may be one of the earliest findings) is an increased distance between the anterior arch of the atlas and the odontoid process of the axis, occurring in about 25% of patients. Normally, this distance, as measured radiographically in the adult, should not exceed 3.5 mm (Figs. 9.10 and 9.11).

Atlantoaxial subluxation may result from inflammation of the synovial lining of the transverse ligament, with subsequent erosion of the odontoid posteriorly, or it may result from stretching and rupture of the ligament by the inflammatory process. With subluxation at the C1-2 junction as a critically important complication of cervical spine involvement, lateral radiographs of the neck in flexion and extension, as well as tomographic studies, should always be obtained in the rheumatoid patient with suspected cervical spine involvement. On occasion, a lateral subluxation of the atlantoaxial joint also may be observed and in such cases, an asymmetry between the odontoid and the atlas will be seen on AP open-mouth view (Fig. 9.12). Subaxial subluxations also may occur and are particularly common at the C3-4 and C4-5 levels (Fig. 9.13).

Bywaters (1981) has described the presence of bursal spaces located between the cervical interspinous processes in approximately 50% of all individuals. These spaces occur most frequently at the level of C6-7 but also may be found in other spinal levels, especially in the lumbar region. Their presence in the cervical spine appears to be related to the closeness of the spinous processes to one another. These bursae may be involved in the rheumatoid process, and erosions of the spinous processes may be seen in the lower cervical and upper thoracic spine in about 10% of patients.

The Thoracolumbar Spine

Clinical evidence of involvement of the thoracic and lumbar segments of the spine is relatively infrequent. Radiographs sometimes will show intervertebral disc-space narrowing, irregularities of the subchondral end plate, and erosions and sclerosis in these sites. Such discovertebral changes may result from a number of factors. These include:

1. Apophysial joint synovitis with instability
2. Costovertebral joint synovitis in the thoracic spine, with extension to the vertebral body and to the intervertebral disc (discitis)
3. Enthesitis resulting from inflammation of ligamentous insertions and extension into the vertebral body and the intervertebral disc
4. Neuropathic alterations secondary to steroid therapy

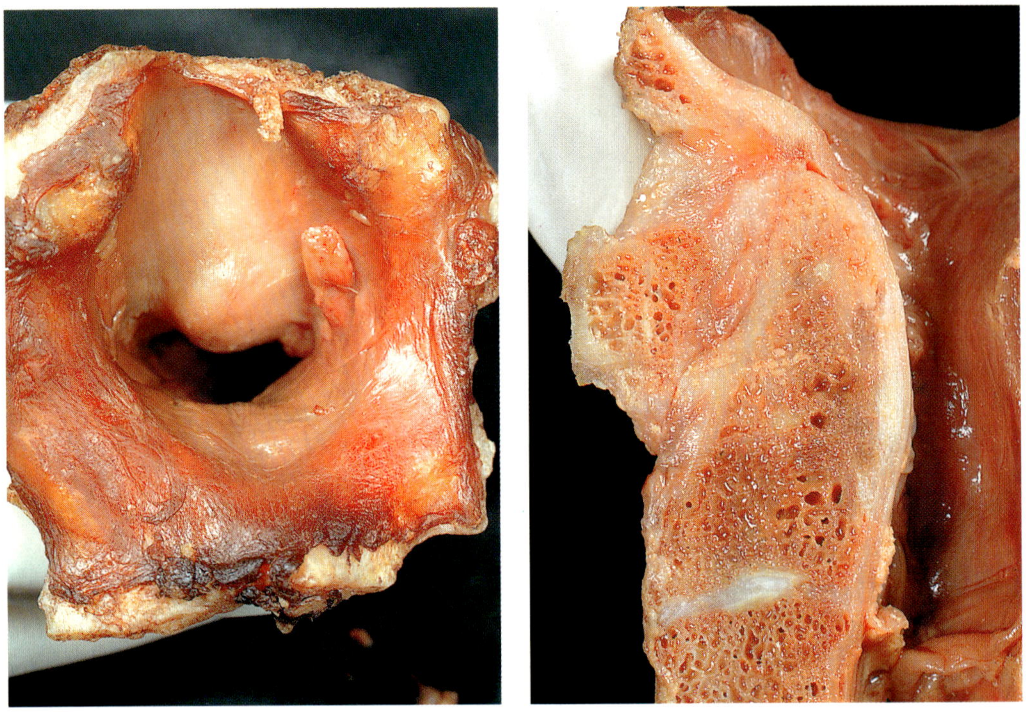

Figure 9.9 Photograph (*left*) of the base of the skull seen from above, in a patient with rheumatoid arthritis who died suddenly in a minor automobile accident. The odontoid process is protruding through and narrowing the exit of the foramen magnum. Photograph (*right*) of a sagittal section of the same specimen. The vertical displacement has been reduced. Note the increased space between the anterior arch of the atlas and the odontoid, as well as the decreased diameter of the spinal canal. The transverse ligament and the posterior longitudinal ligament were not found. The reddish-brown color of the dura is due to chronic hemorrhage.

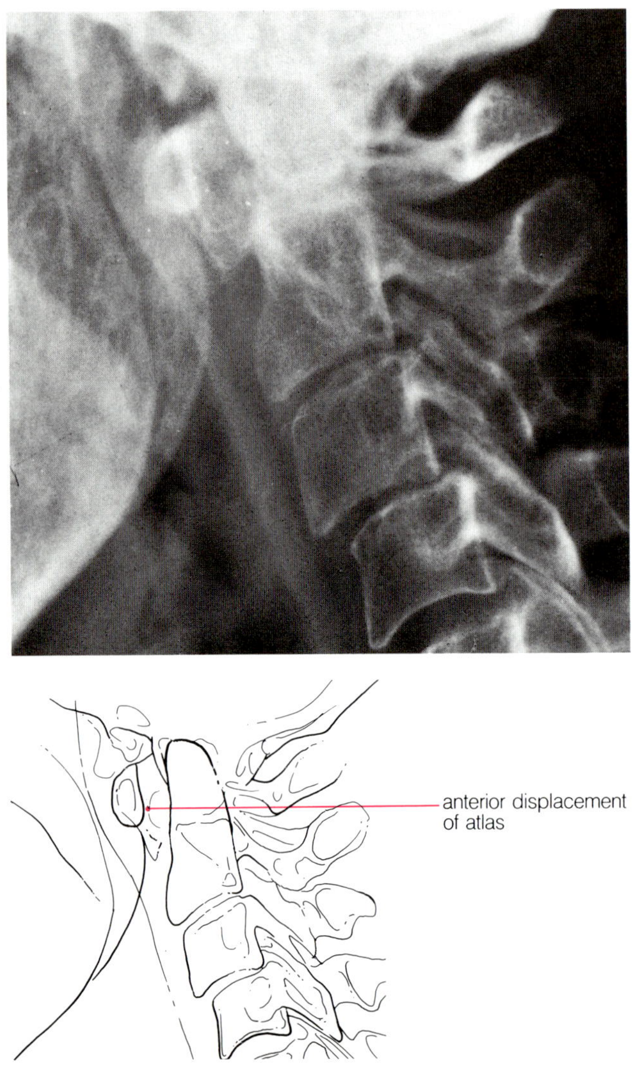

Figure 9.10 Lateral radiograph of the upper cervical spine in flexion, in a 45-year-old woman with a clinical diagnosis of rheumatoid arthritis and complaints of occipital pain. The space between the atlas and the anterior border of the odontoid measures 10 mm, reflecting anterior displacement of the atlas on the axis. Note also the anterior displacement of C-3 on C-4.

Any of these conditions may be aggravated by trauma. Rheumatoid nodules in the extradural space also have been described, giving rise to compression of the spinal cord.

The Sacroiliac Joint

In rheumatoid arthritis, lesions of the sacroiliac joint are clinically infrequent and generally are mild. However, asymptomatic radiographic abnormalities may be present in one-third of patients with long-standing disease. Erosions tend to be seen on the iliac side of the joint and are well marginated and superficial. They may be unilateral or bilateral. Joint-space narrowing occasionally may result in complete obliteration of the articulation and in osseous fusion. Ossification of the sacroiliac ligament is common in rheumatoid arthritis.

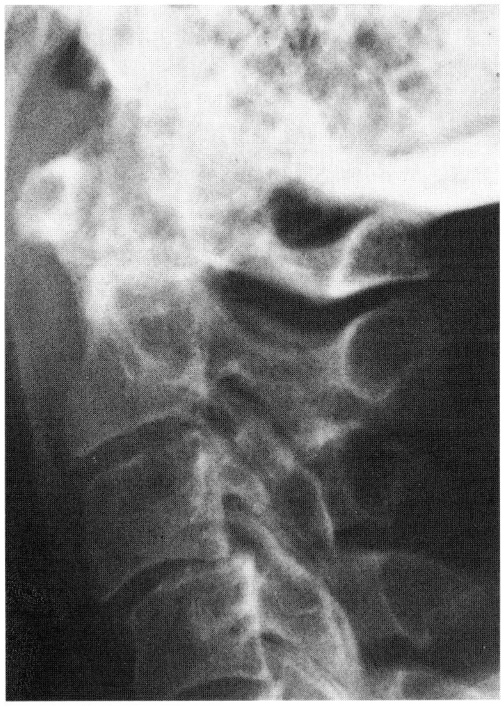

Figure 9.11 Lateral radiograph of the upper cervical spine in extension, of the patient seen in Figure 9.10. In extension the displacement of the atlas on the axis is reduced, and the space between the atlas and the odontoid measures 4 mm.

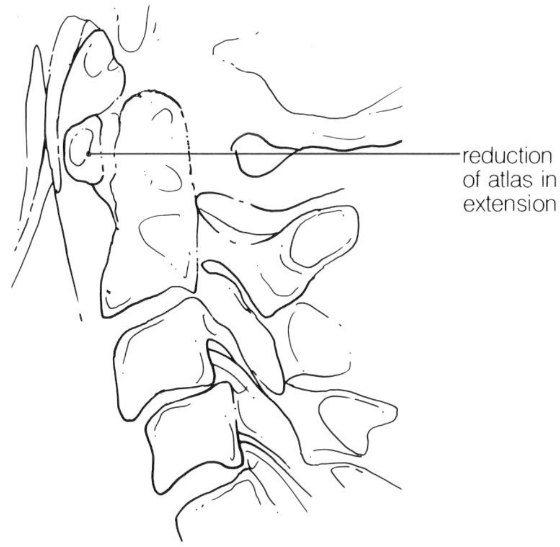

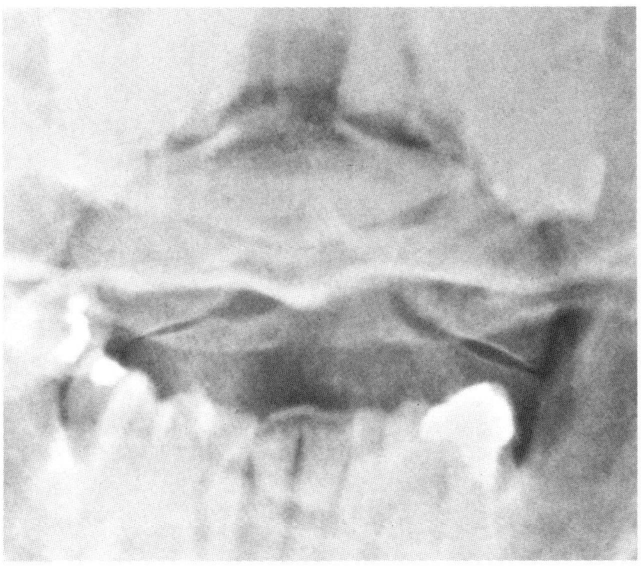

Figure 9.12 Radiograph taken through the open mouth of a man with rheumatoid arthritis demonstrates lateral displacement of the odontoid, with reference to the lateral masses of C-1.

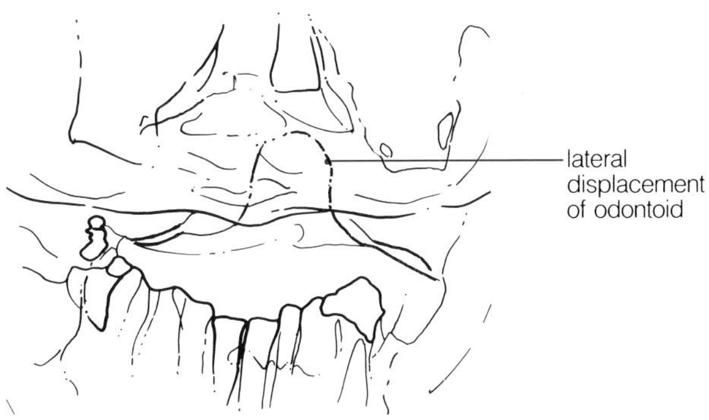

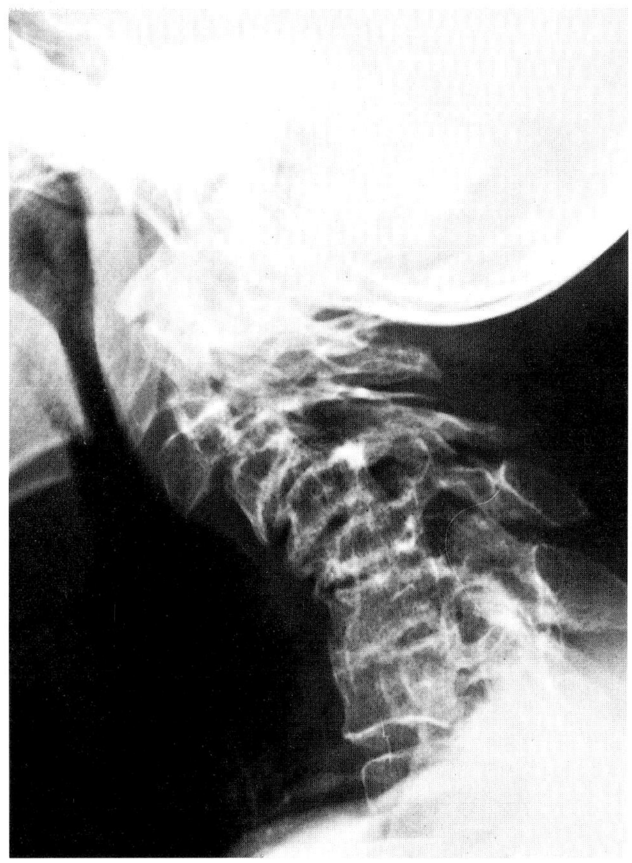

Figure 9.13 Lateral radiograph of the cervical spine of a female with rheumatoid arthritis demonstrates subaxial subluxation at multiple levels. Note the deformities of the vertebral bodies.

SERO-NEGATIVE INFLAMMATORY SPONDYLITIS

Inflammatory spondylitis commonly is seen in patients who have a negative test for rheumatoid factor. Many, but not all, of these patients are likely to be suffering from systemic disorders such as psoriasis or inflammatory bowel disease.

Characteristically, the distribution and morphology of articular lesions observed in the spine in these conditions are different from those of rheumatoid arthritis. Whereas in rheumatoid disease the lesions are most obvious in the cervical region, in the sero-negative spondylitidies, sacroiliitis and involvement of the lumbar and lower thoracic spine are more common (Fig. 9.14). Osteoporosis is not usually seen, and in marked contrast to rheumatoid disease, there is bony proliferation and on occasion intraarticular osseous fusion. Paravertebral ossification, a characteristic finding in ankylosing hyperostosis (see below), is also a radiographic feature of sero-negative spondylitis. These paravertebral calcifications or ossifications are vertical in disposition in comparison to traction osteophytes, which are mainly horizontal. They occur in the anterior longitudinal ligament, as well as in the peripheral fibers of the anulus fibrosus. They are referred to radiographically as *syndesmophytes*, and depending upon the involvement or lack of involvement of the peripheral portion of the anulus fibrosus, they are described as being either marginal or nonmarginal (Fig. 9.15). These syndesmophytes usually occur in the thoracic and upper lumbar areas of the spine, and may produce prominent outgrowths that merge with the underlying bone and disc tissue (Fig. 9.16), giving rise to the appearance described as a "bamboo spine."

Psoriatic Spondylitis and Reiter's Syndrome

Peripheral arthritis associated with psoriasis is well recognized, usually affecting young men and women in approximately equal numbers. Although the etiology and pathogenesis of psoriasis and psoriatic arthropathy are unknown, a genetic predisposition has been described. Specifically, in patients with psoriatic spondylitis, there is a 90% incidence of the HLA B27 antigen (the antigen associated with ankylosing spondylitis). Radiographic manifestations of sacroiliitis or of thoracolumbar spondylitis are seen in approximately 20% of psoriatic patients and may precede the appearance of psoriasis of the skin by weeks or months.

In Reiter's syndrome, spinal involvement occurs less frequently than in psoriasis, although a higher percentage of patients may show radiographic evidence of sacroiliitis. The radiographic changes in Reiter's syndrome rarely may resemble those of ankylosing spondylitis, although the involvement in Reiter's usually is patchy and nonpro-

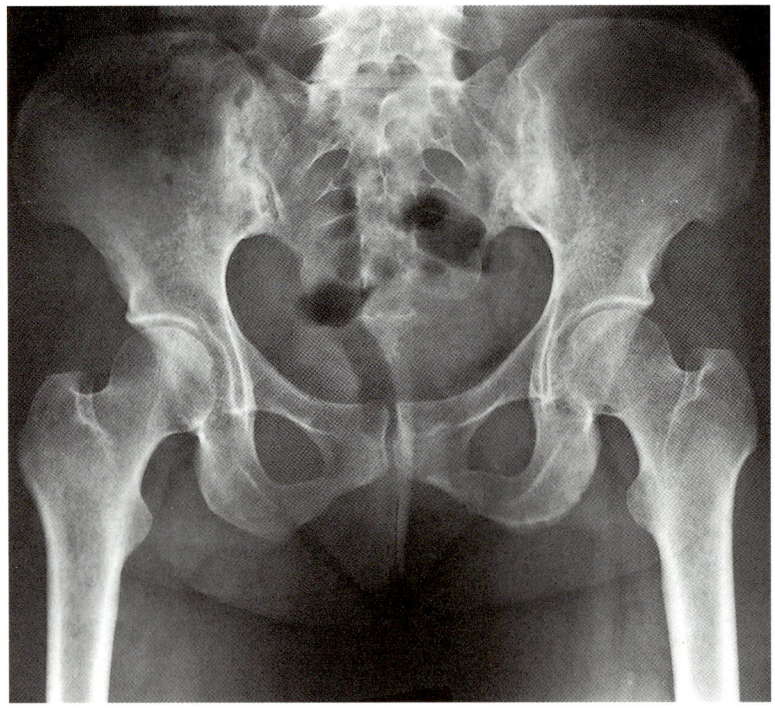

Figure 9.14 AP radiograph of the pelvis of a young woman with a clinical diagnosis of Reiter's syndrome to demonstrate bilateral sacroiliitis. Note the lack of clear margination of the sacroiliac joint, together with the irregular marginal bony sclerosis.

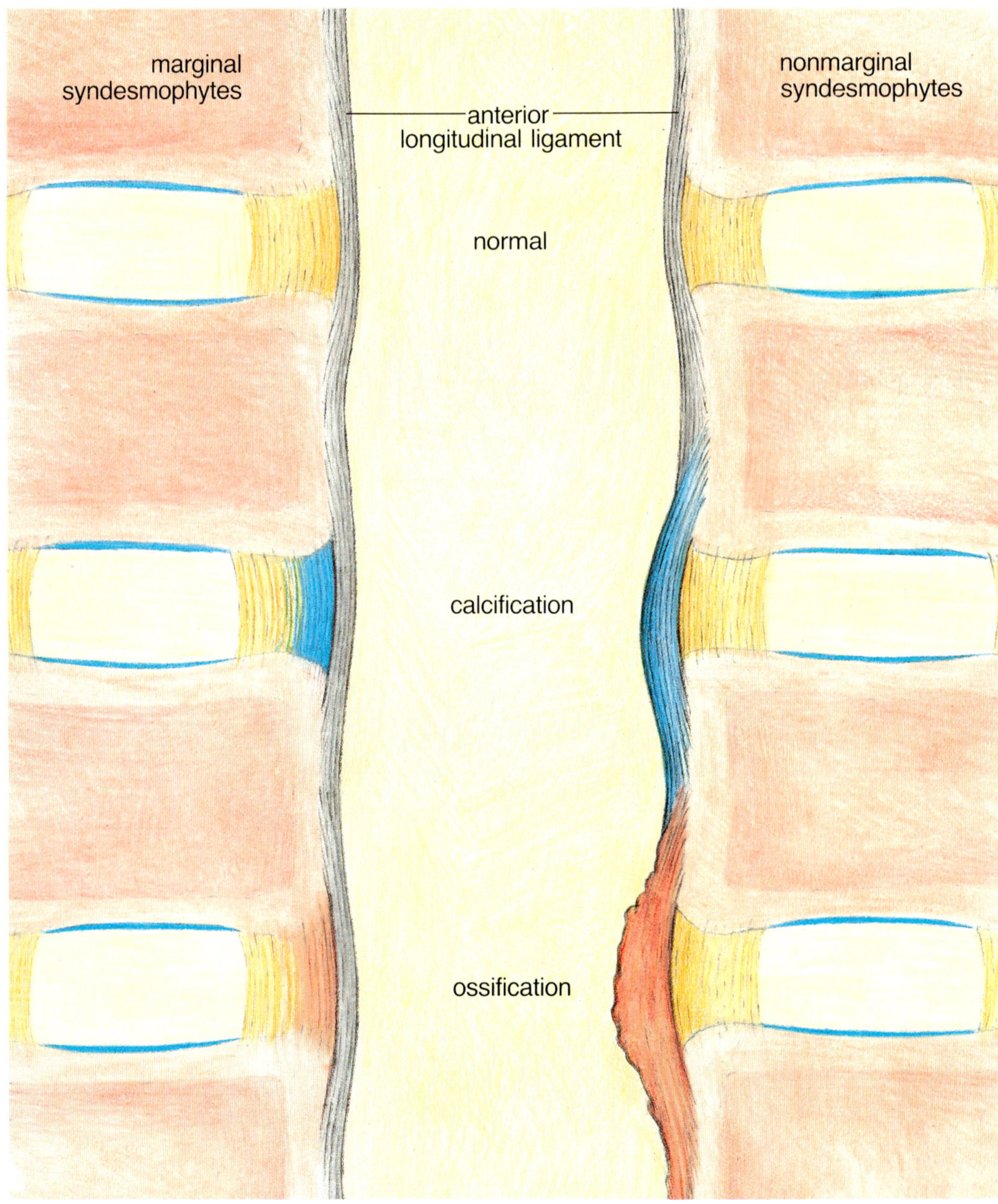

Figure 9.15 Schematic drawing of the development of syndesmophytes. Calcification of the anterior longitudinal ligament may become secondarily ossified.

gressive, while in ankylosing spondylitis it is ascending and progressive. In addition, the distinguishing features of Reiter's syndrome—namely, urethritis, conjunctivitis, oral lesions, and keratoderma—do not occur in ankylosing spondylitis.

ANKYLOSING SPONDYLO-ARTHROPATHIES

ANKYLOSING SPONDYLITIS

General Features

Ankylosing spondylitis—also known as Marie-Strumpell disease, spondylitis ankylopoietica, and pelvospondylitis ossificans—is a systemic ankylosing arthropathy that primarily affects Caucasian men in their late adolescent or young adult years. Recent epidemiologic studies suggest that the incidence of asymptomatic sacroiliac changes in young women may be more common than previously thought.

Although the onset of the disease is usually insidious, its manifestations may evolve clinically in one of three patterns:

1. In the axial skeleton, chiefly in the lumbar and sacroiliac joints
2. In the peripheral joints, predominantly in the hips, knees and heels, especially among adolescents
3. As recurrent iritis, aortic valvular disease, fatigue and other systemic features, without obvious arthritis

The spinal disease may progress in an ascending fashion to involve the thoracic and cervical vertebrae, along with other axial articulations, such as the pubic symphysis and ribs. Pain may be present on deep inspiration, along with a loss of chest expansion due to rib cage involvement. Sacroiliac joint tenderness is an early finding, followed by the later development of limited motion of the lumbar spine. Atrophy of the trunk muscles also occurs, and patients therefore may seek to ease back pain by assuming a bent posture; therefore, a tendency toward thoracic kyphosis is common (Fig. 9.17).

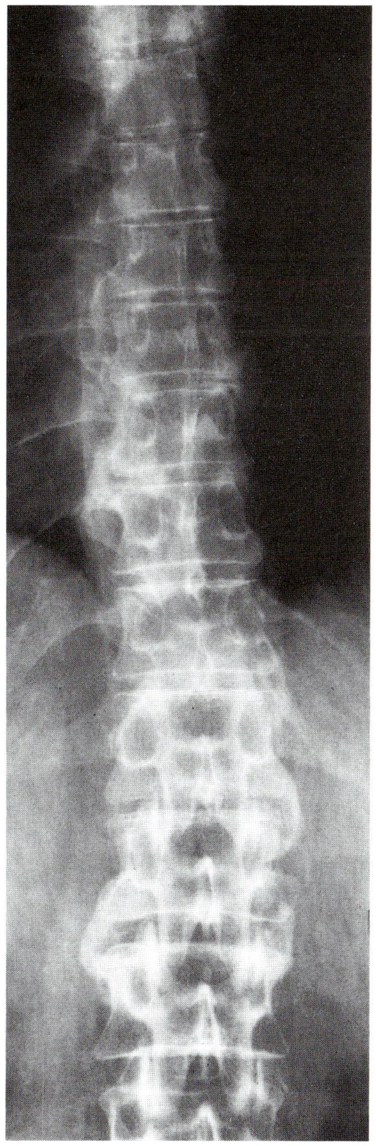

Figure 9.16 AP radiograph of the thoracolumbar spine of a man with a clinical diagnosis of psoriasis. Note the relatively intact disc spaces and the nonmarginated syndesmophytes bilaterally in the lower thoracic and upper lumbar spine. The facet joints do not appear to be involved.

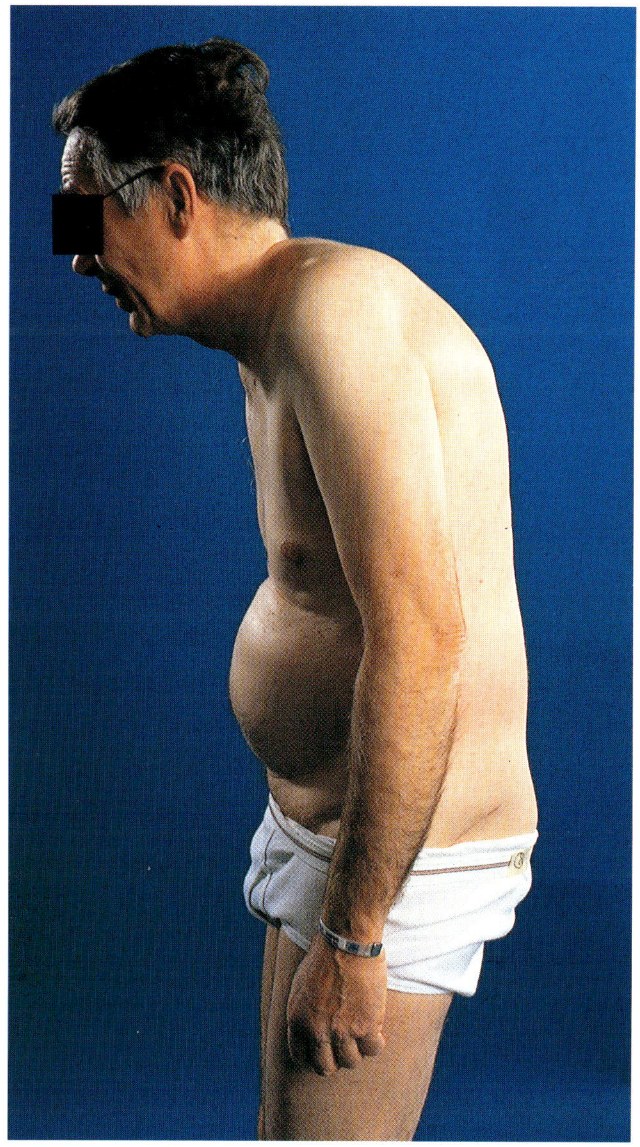

Figure 9.17 Clinical photograph of a patient with ankylosing spondylitis to demonstrate the typical attitude, with increased thoracic kyphosis, loss of lumbar lordosis, and a forward thrust of the head. (Courtesy of Dr. David S. Bradford)

Either transient or chronic involvement of the peripheral joints has been reported in 50% of cases, especially in the hips and knees, but it is not commonly found in the small joints of the hands and feet. The natural course of the disease generally is one of slow progression without remittance (Fig. 9.18).

HLA B27 occurs in 90 to 95% of patients with ankylosing spondylitis, compared to a 6 to 9% incidence in the normal population. Other laboratory findings may include elevation of the ESR, as well as mild hypochromic anemia (in less than one-third of cases). Elevated levels of serum creatinine phosphokinase (CPK) of muscle origin occur in about one-third of patients with ankylosing spondylitis.

Bachman, after reviewing a large series of spinal radiographs, reported a 2% incidence of ankylosing spondylitis in the general population. Involvement of family members is more common in subjects affected with ankylosing spondylitis than in control subjects; it is rare in blacks. Thus there is both a familial and a racial predisposition to this disease.

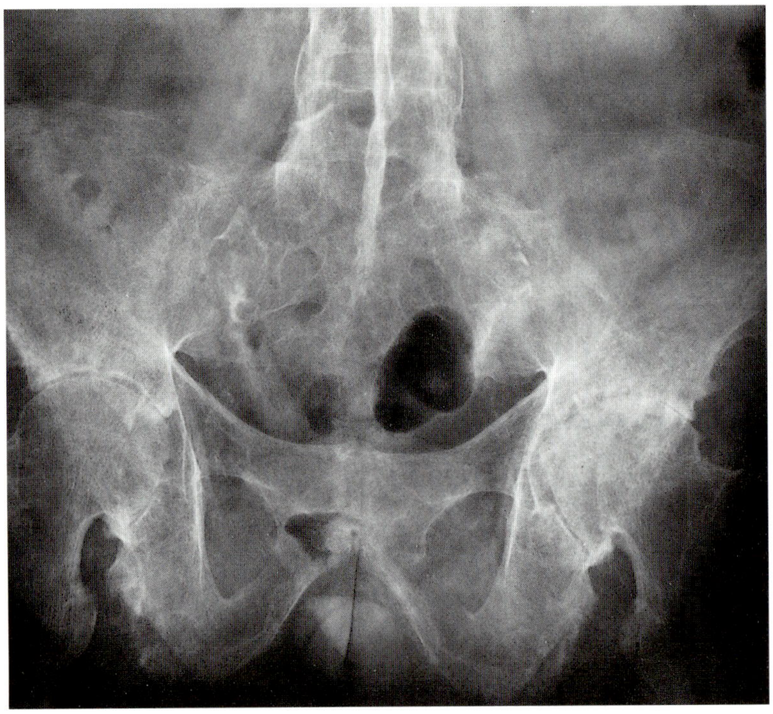

Figure 9.18 AP radiograph of the lower lumbar spine, pelvis, and hips of a man with advanced ankylosing spondylitis. Note the generalized osteoporosis with fusion of the spinous processes, intervertebral discs, sacroiliac joints, and symphysis pubis, and severe concentric degeneration with partial fusion in both hips. Thus, the entire skeletal unit has been transformed into one continuous osseous mass.

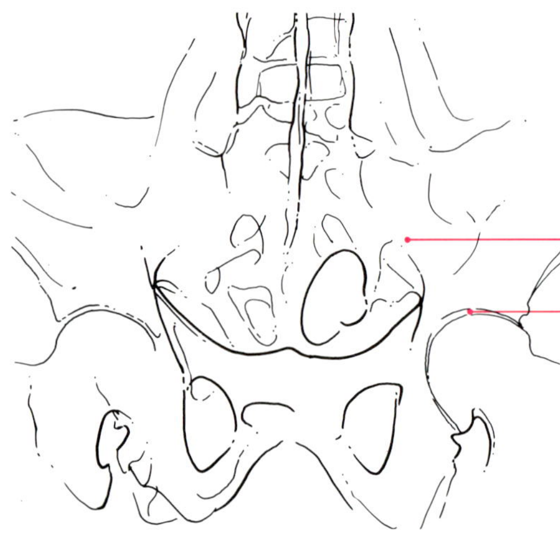

Radiographic Findings

An early and characteristic radiographic finding of ankylosing spondylitis is symmetrical sacroiliitis, in which the bony margins become indistinct and subsequently undergo condensation resulting in partial or complete fusion. Other early radiographic changes in the spine include apophysial irregularities, osteopenia of the vertebrae and squaring of the vertebral bodies on the lateral view, and marginal syndesmophytes.

In the early phase of the disease, the discs appear to be fairly well preserved but in the end stage they are clearly bridged centrally by bone tissue. As the disease progresses, the apophysial joints of the spine generally are completely ankylosed (Fig. 9.19). The intervertebral foramina also show narrowing, and the spine always shows an increase in the thoracic kyphosis, which frequently is markedly accentuated. Prominent ossification of paravertebral ligaments usually does not develop.

As the spine becomes fused, so the cancellous bone becomes increasingly porotic and the cortices of the vertebrae become more prominent. This, together with the ossifications along the peripheral parts of the disc, transforms the segmented column of the normal spine into a tube-like osseous rod referred to as a bamboo spine (Figs. 9.20 and 9.21).

Some of the radiographic findings in ankylosing spondylitis are similar to those of the sero-negative spondyloarthropathies previously discussed; however, the findings of osteitis and of vertebral body squaring are unusual in psoriatic spondylitis, as is facet joint involvement. However, in post-Reiter's spondylitis, the radiographic findings may become indistinguishable from ankylosing spondylitis, with the passage of time.

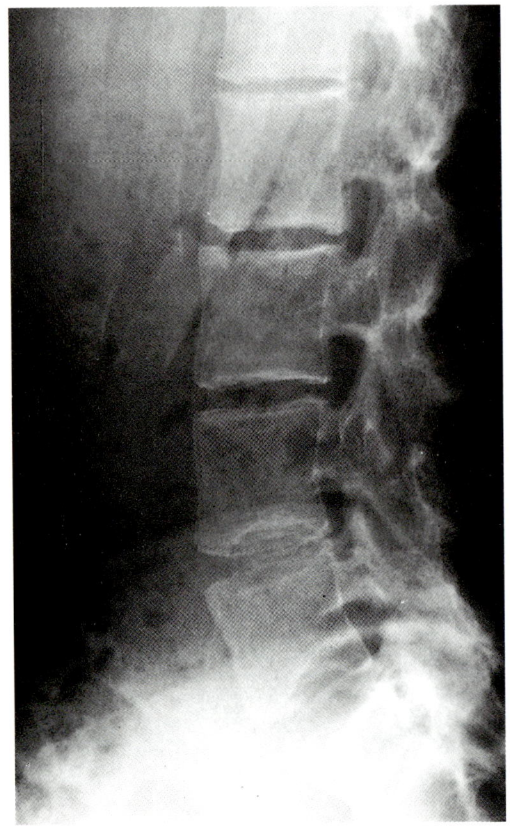

Figure 9.19 Lateral radiograph of the lumbosacral spine in a young man with ankylosing spondylitis. The apophysial joints are fused throughout this spinal segment, and the vertebral bodies have a square appearance and show some osteopenia. The disc spaces appear to be preserved, and there are no obvious syndesmophytes.

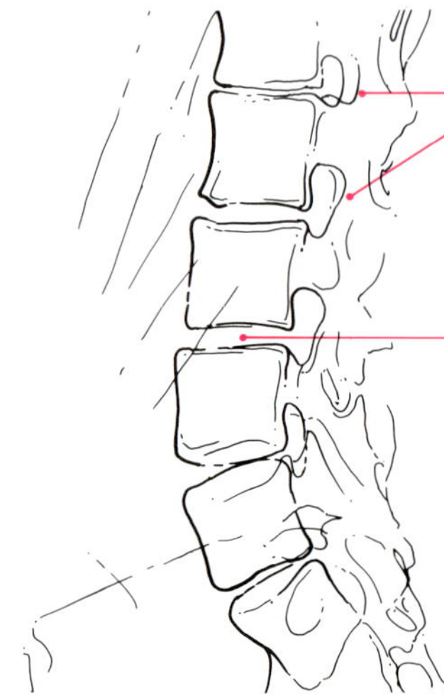

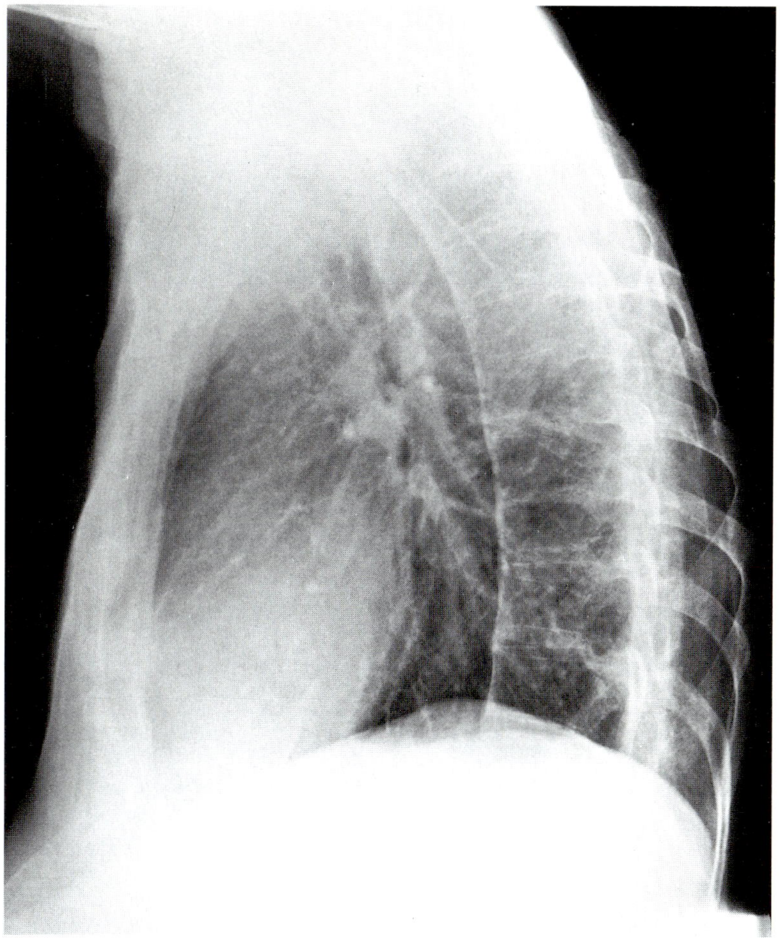

Figure 9.20 Lateral radiograph of the thoracic spine in a 40-year-old male with ankylosing spondylitis. The vertebral bodies are fused throughout via the disc spaces. Anteriorly, there is a continuous sclerotic cortex formed by the thickened anterior cortex of the vertebral bodies and the ossified peripheral fibers of the anulus fibrosus.

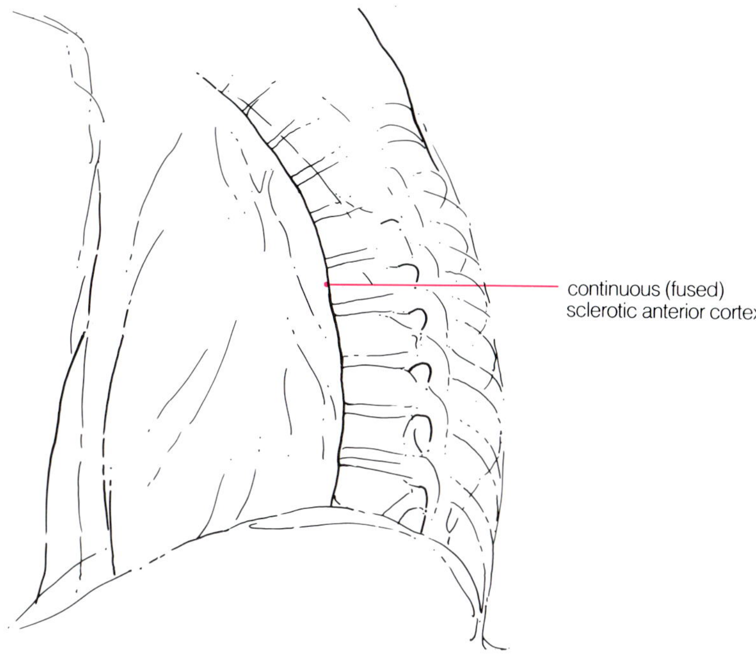

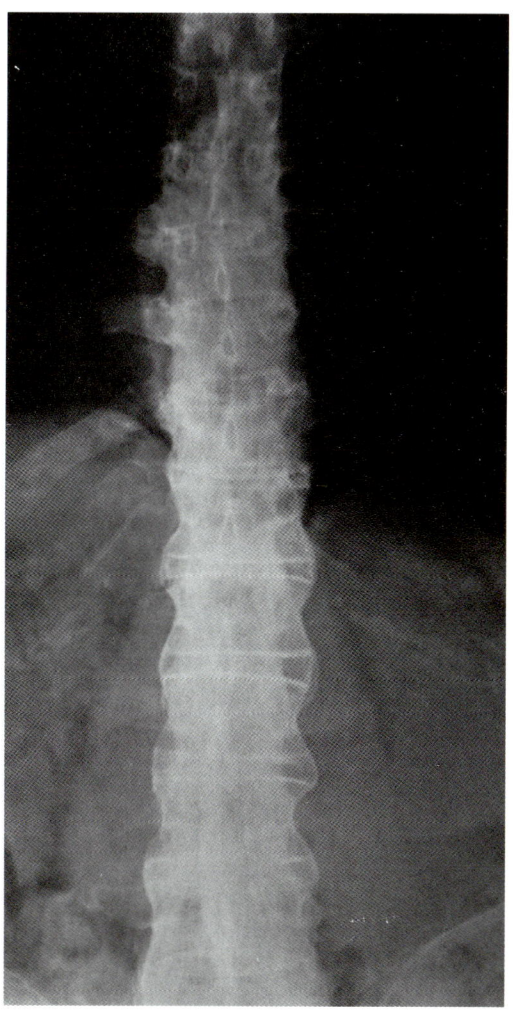

Figure 9.21 AP radiograph of the thoracolumbar spine in a 69-year-old male with ankylosing spondylitis to show a "bamboo spine." Note the ossification of the interspinous ligament.

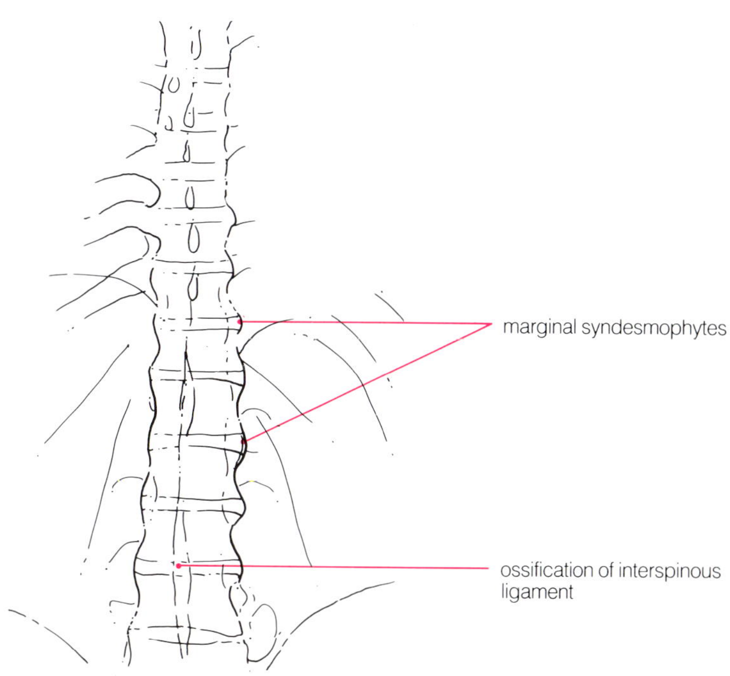

Pathologic Features

An understanding of the pathogenesis of ankylosing spondylitis has been limited by the lack of biopsy material and by the infrequency with which the spine is examined at autopsy. Cruickschank (1971) postulated that in affected joints, there initially was an osteitis localized in the subchondral bone, a stage that he associated with the radiologic finding of osteopenia. He further postulated that the cartilage and bone were then destroyed from beneath, and subsequently infiltrated by granulation tissue. Radiographically, this would appear as an erosion of the bony end plate and as a widening of the cartilage space. Eventually, ossification and bridging of the cartilage space would result, leading to ankylosis. In postmortem studies of the intervertebral disc, Cruickschank reported ossification to be the most significant change, which he described as occurring particularly in the anterior part of the disc although occasionally the posterior portion was involved.

In our own experience, examination of the spine at autopsy of a patient with end-stage ankylosing spondylitis will show fusion of the apophysial joints and intervertebral discs, resulting in a rigid immobile vertebral column with accentuated kyphosis (Fig. 9.22). However, unlike ankylosing hyperostosis or DISH (see below), ossification of the paravertebral ligaments is not a prominent feature (Fig. 9.23).

Biopsies of tender areas in the iliac crest, greater trochanter, and patella in patients with ankylosing spondylitis have been reported to show chronic inflammatory infiltrates at the bony ligamentous junctions, i.e., enthesitis. In addition, it also has been noted that there may be an accelerated endochondral ossification of the hyaline cartilage (Fig. 9.24). Symmetric or asymmetric pulmonary fibrosis also has been reported to occur in patients with ankylosing spondylitis. Amyloidosis of the secondary type has been reported in about 8% of cases coming to autopsy. At the present time, morphological information on ankylosing spondylitis is extremely scant and there is an urgent necessity for more anatomical studies of this condition.

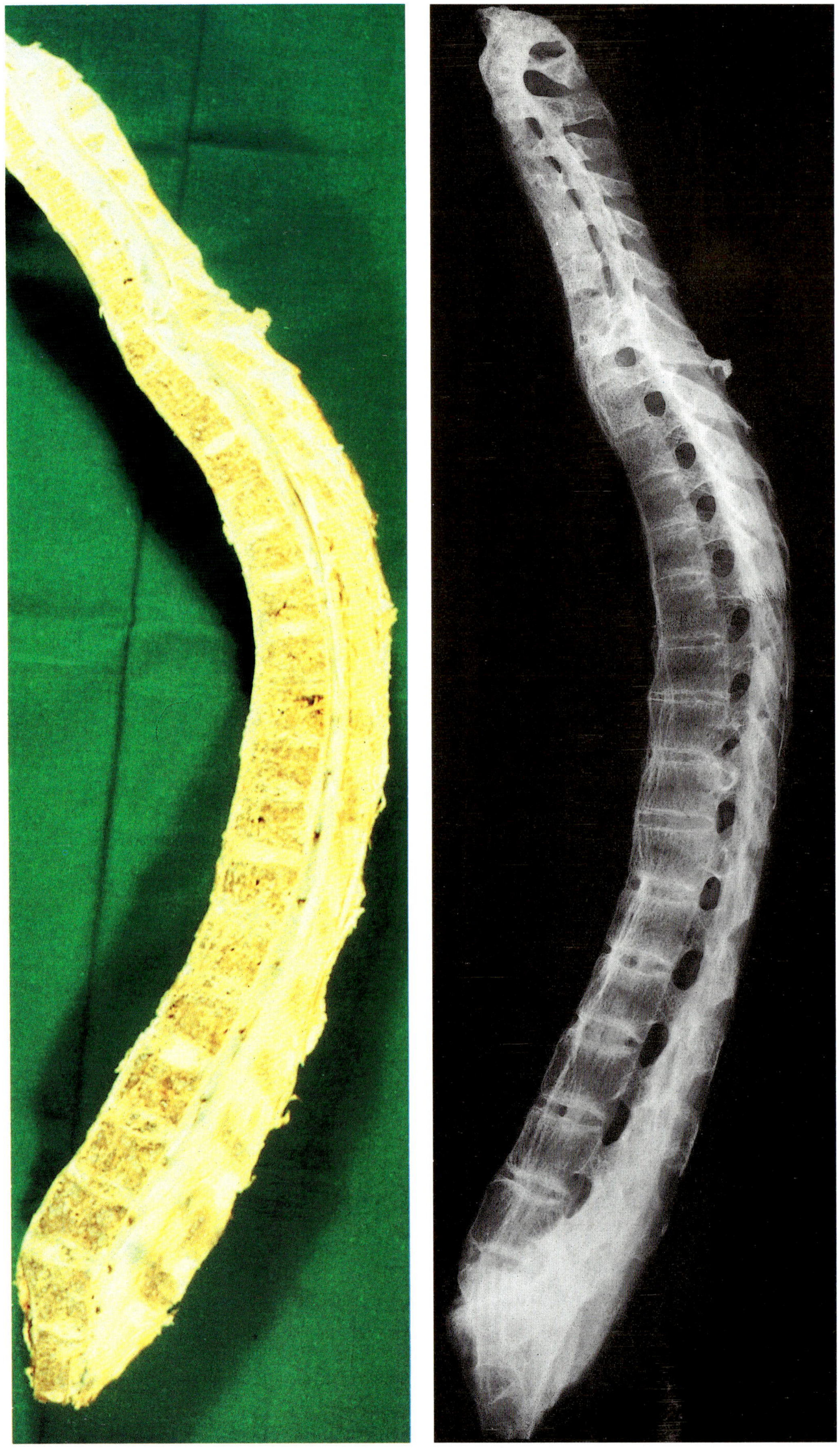

Figure 9.22 Photograph (*left*) of a sagittal section through the vertebral column of a patient with ankylosing spondylitis. There is complete fusion of the spine, and accentuated kyphosis and loss of lumbar and cervical lordosis. At the C-7 to T-1 level, there is an angular deformity of the spinal canal, resulting from a healed fracture at this site. A specimen radiograph (*right*) of the same patient shows complete fusion of the apophysial joints, as well as fusion across the intervertebral disc spaces.

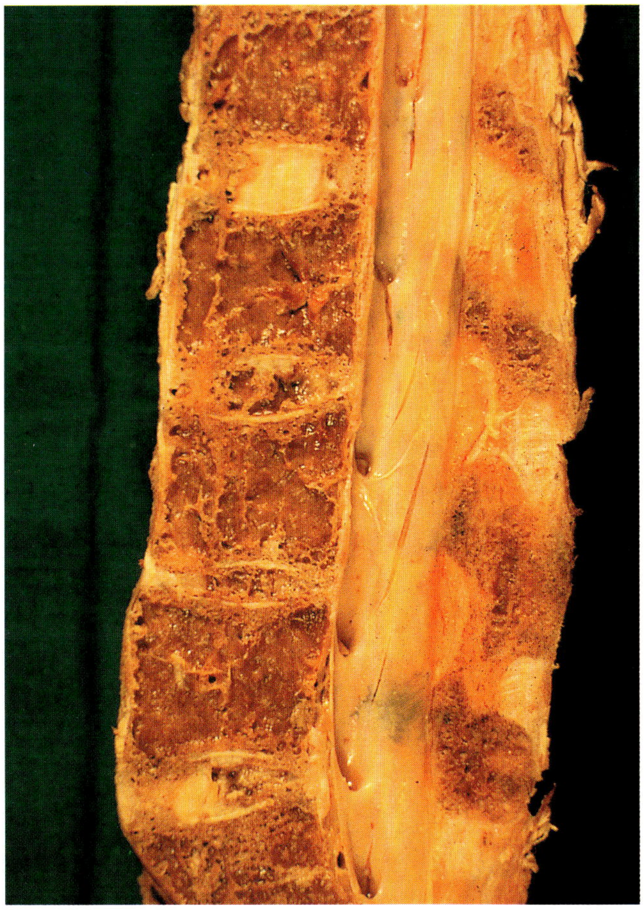

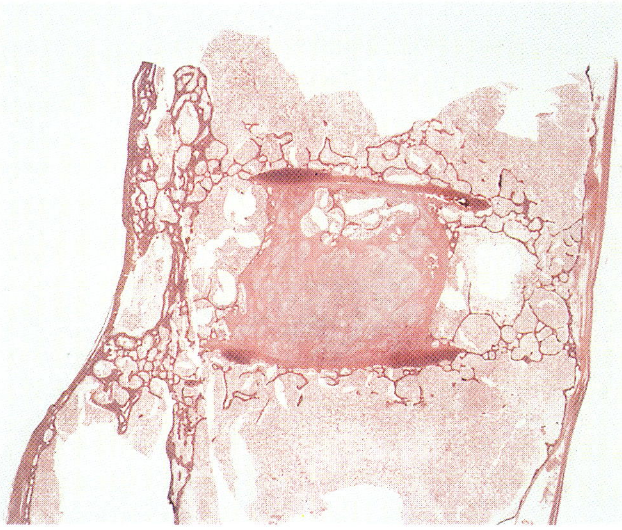

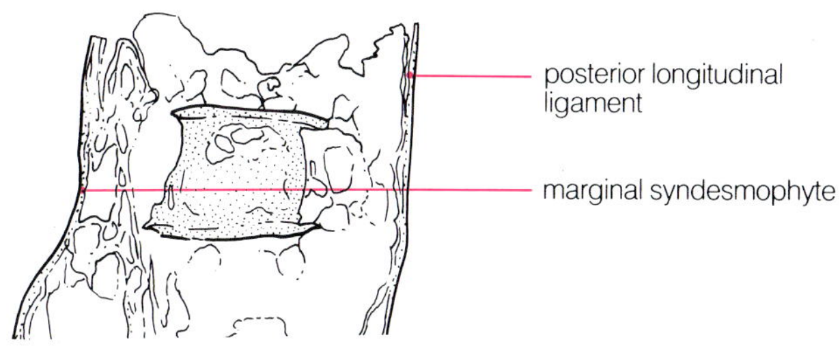

Figure 9.23 Photograph (*left*) of a sagittal section through the lumbar spine of the patient illustrated in Figure 9.22. Fusion of the intervertebral disc spaces, mainly peripherally, is apparent. The paravertebral ligaments, both anteriorly and posteriorly, are spared. A photomicrograph (*right*) of the lumbar disc and adjacent vertebral bodies in this case shows an absence of ossification in the anterior and posterior longitudinal ligaments, with severe osteoporosis of the vertebral bodies. The fusion is confined to the intervertebral disc.

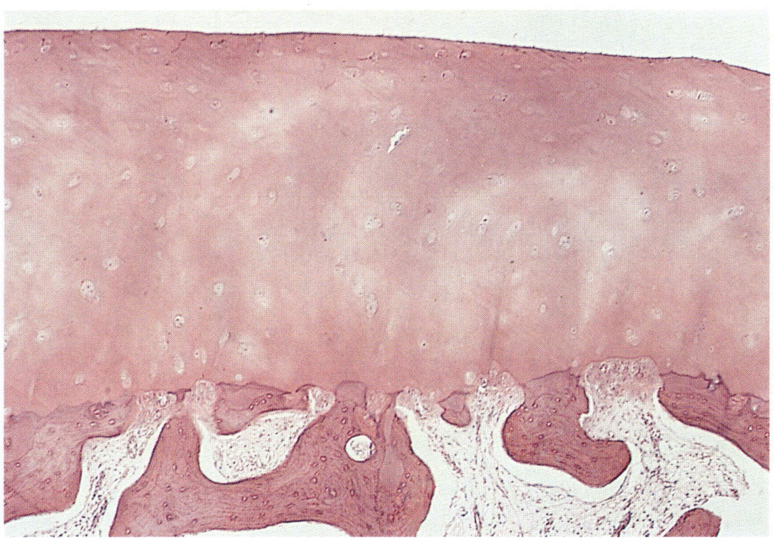

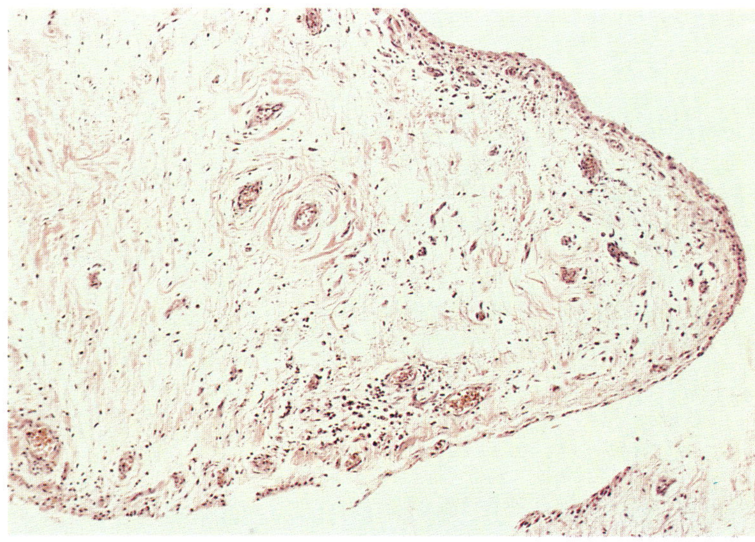

Figure 9.24 Photomicrograph (*left*) at low power of a representative portion of the articular cartilage and underlying bone of the femoral head in a patient with ankylosing spondylitis associated with bilateral hip disease. The articular cartilage is being invaded by blood vessels from the subchondral bone, and in the marrow spaces there is a diffuse, chronic inflammatory infiltrate. Similar changes might be seen in rheumatoid arthritis. (H & E, × 4 objective) However, unlike what one would expect to see in rheumatoid arthritis, a photomicrograph (*right*) of the synovium of the hip joint in the same case shows no significant inflammation or synovial proliferation. (H & E, × 10 objective)

ANKYLOSING HYPEROSTOSIS OF THE SPINE

General Features

Ankylosing hyperostosis of the spine, also known as Forestier's disease or diffuse idiopathic skeletal hyperostosis (DISH), is an ankylosis of the vertebral column that occurs as a result of ligamentous ossification without significant disc disease (Figs. 9.25 and 9.26). It usually is manifest in older men, with clinical symptoms that generally are mild. Since the first half of the 19th century, when it was first recognized, various names have been proposed for this ankylosing disease, including "spondylitis ossificans ligamentosa" and "physiologic vertebral ligamentous ossification" (so-named by Smith and his colleagues, who thought it was due to spinal immobility and degenerative changes in older patients). Bechterew (1844) also recognized this form of ankylosis, sometimes called by his own name, but he mistakenly considered it to be a form of ankylosing spondylitis (Figs. 9.27 and 9.28).

Forestier (1950) and his collaborators better delineated both the anatomical and clinical findings of this condition and proposed that it be called senile ankylosing hyperostosis of the spine, since most cases were found to occur in older individuals. Later, once the condition was identified in young adults, the term "senile" was eliminated. More recently however (1975), the term diffuse idiopathic skeletal hyperostosis (DISH) has been proposed by Resnick, in recognition of the frequency with which extraspinal ligamentous involvement occurs around the shoulder, elbow, knee, hip, and heel, and which may in fact be more extensive and more clinically significant than the spinal involvement. This term, broader in scope, generally has been accepted as perhaps the more appropriate one.

Radiographic Features

The diagnostic radiographic criteria originally proposed by Forestier included the presence of focal spinal ankylosis, intact vertebral end plates, normal intervertebral disc height, and most importantly, flowing ossification of the anterior longitudinal ligament, especially along the right side of the thoracolumbar region. He also noted the absence of sacroiliac or facet joint sclerosis or

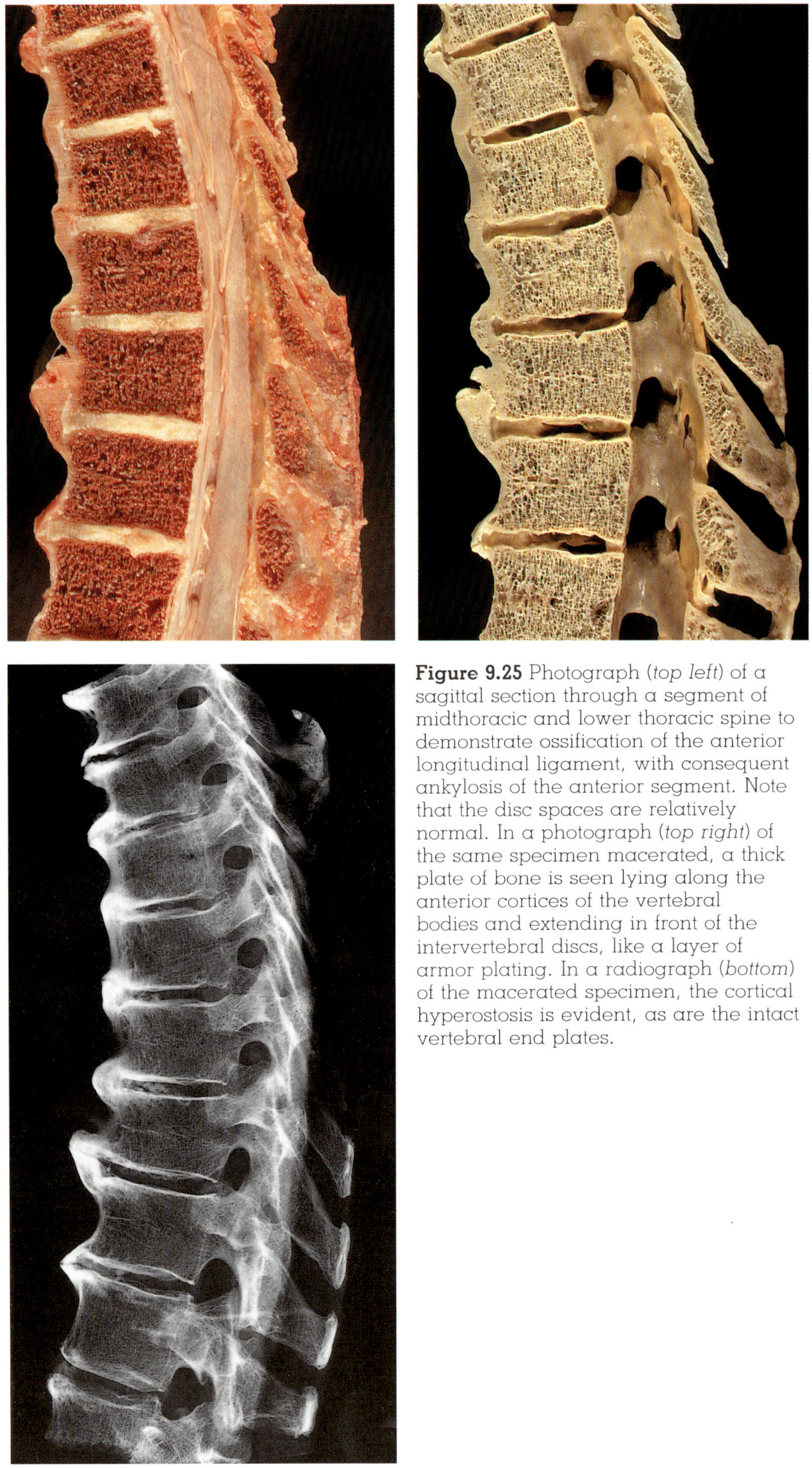

Figure 9.25 Photograph (*top left*) of a sagittal section through a segment of midthoracic and lower thoracic spine to demonstrate ossification of the anterior longitudinal ligament, with consequent ankylosis of the anterior segment. Note that the disc spaces are relatively normal. In a photograph (*top right*) of the same specimen macerated, a thick plate of bone is seen lying along the anterior cortices of the vertebral bodies and extending in front of the intervertebral discs, like a layer of armor plating. In a radiograph (*bottom*) of the macerated specimen, the cortical hyperostosis is evident, as are the intact vertebral end plates.

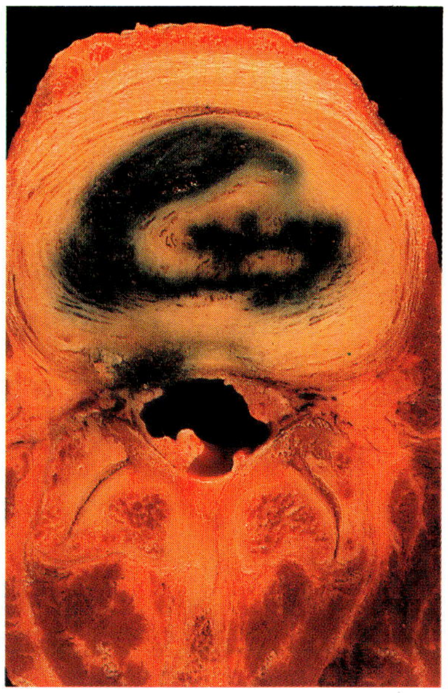

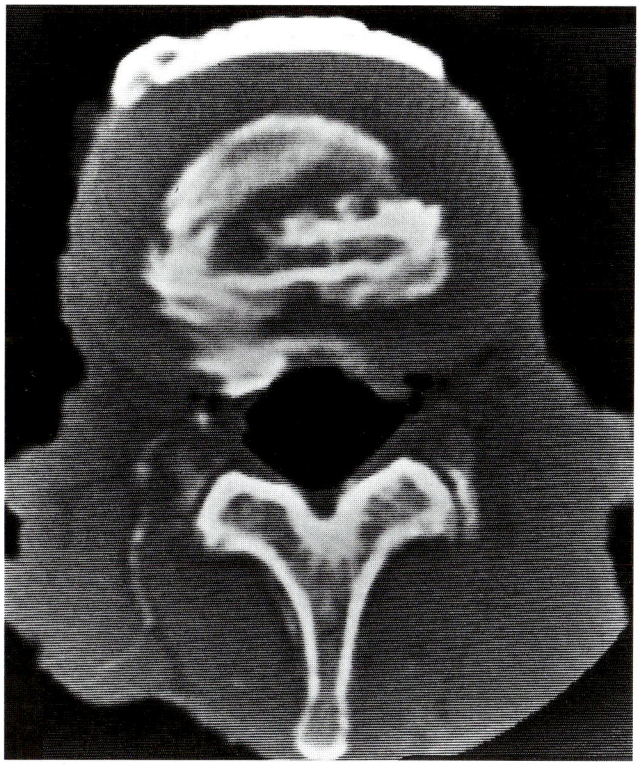

Figure 9.26 Photograph (*left*) of a section through the L2-3 disc, following injection of contrast agent into the disc. While the disc appears normal and the anulus fibrosus is intact, anterior to the anulus is a plate of osseous tissue, which represents a section through the ossified anterior longitudinal ligament. In a CT scan (*right*) through this same area (L2-3), the clear demarcation between the anulus and the ossified anterior longitudinal ligament is obvious. Note that the facet joints are normal.

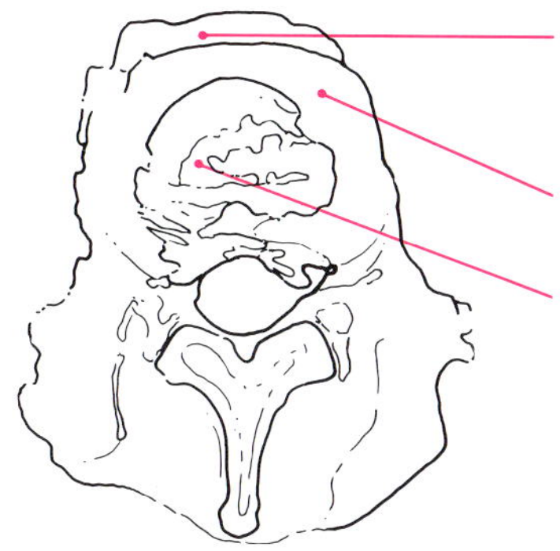

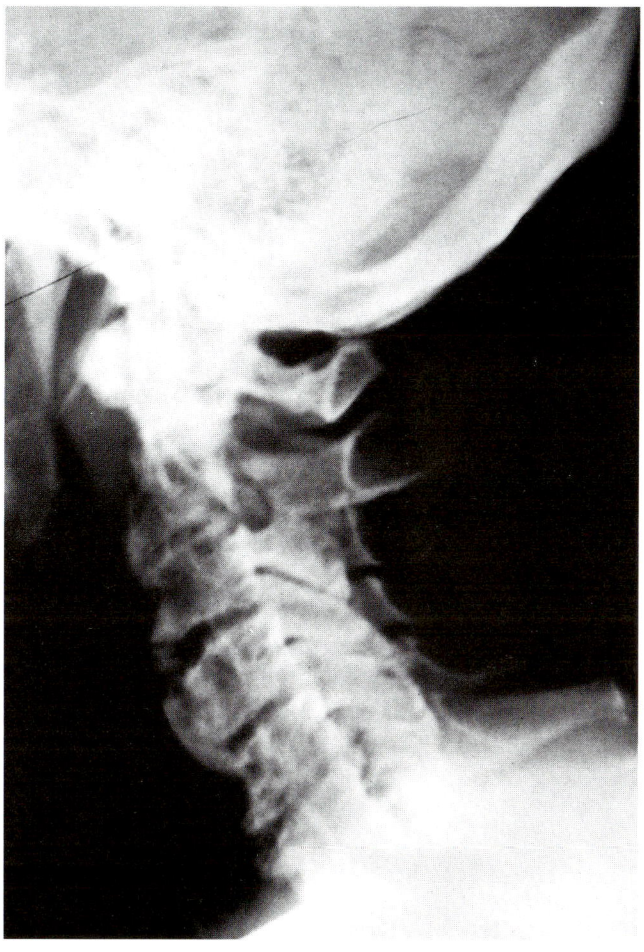

Figure 9.27 Lateral radiograph of the cervical spine of an elderly male who complained of difficulty in swallowing. There is an irregular severe anterior hyperostosis, which is largely the result of ossification of the anterior longitudinal ligament typical of DISH. Neither the disc spaces nor the facet joints appear fused and the bone is not osteopenic, thus ruling out a diagnosis of ankylosing spondylitis. This radiograph should be compared with Figure 9.28.

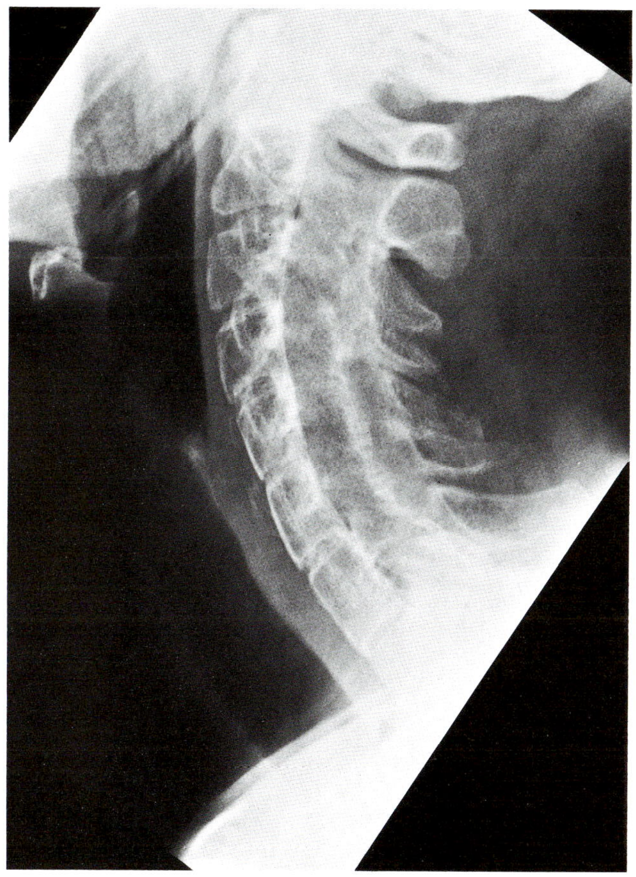

Figure 9.28 Lateral radiograph of the cervical spine of a 50-year-old male with ankylosing spondylitis. Note the complete fusion of the facet joints, and the osseous bridging of the intervertebral disc spaces. The bone is osteopenic and there is no obvious ligamentous calcification or ossification.

ankylosis (Fig. 9.29). According to Forestier, the evolution of the disease may cover as many as three to four decades, with end-stage disease becoming evident in the seventh decade.

Using Forestier's criteria (with the additional requirement that at least four contiguous vertebral bodies be involved), Resnick and co-workers have reported that in older individuals there is a radiographic incidence of 12%. Relative preservation of the disc height in the involved area and intact end plates distinguish patients with ankylosing hyperostosis from those with intervertebral osteochondrosis. Absence of facet joint and sacroiliac joint sclerosis and fusion differentiates the disorder from ankylosing spondylitis.

Pathologic Findings

On the basis of his own studies, including anatomical dissections, Forestier proposed three stages in the disease process. These stages are as follows:

I. Early spinal involvement, characterized by ligamentous calcification, with periosteal new bone present at the anterior vertebral body margins without ankylosis (Fig. 9.30)
II. Developed disease manifested typically by vertebral "flamelike" ossification of the anterior longitudinal ligament in front of the disc, nonmarginal syndesmophytes, clearly demonstrated in lateral oblique radiographs (Figs. 9.31 and 9.32)

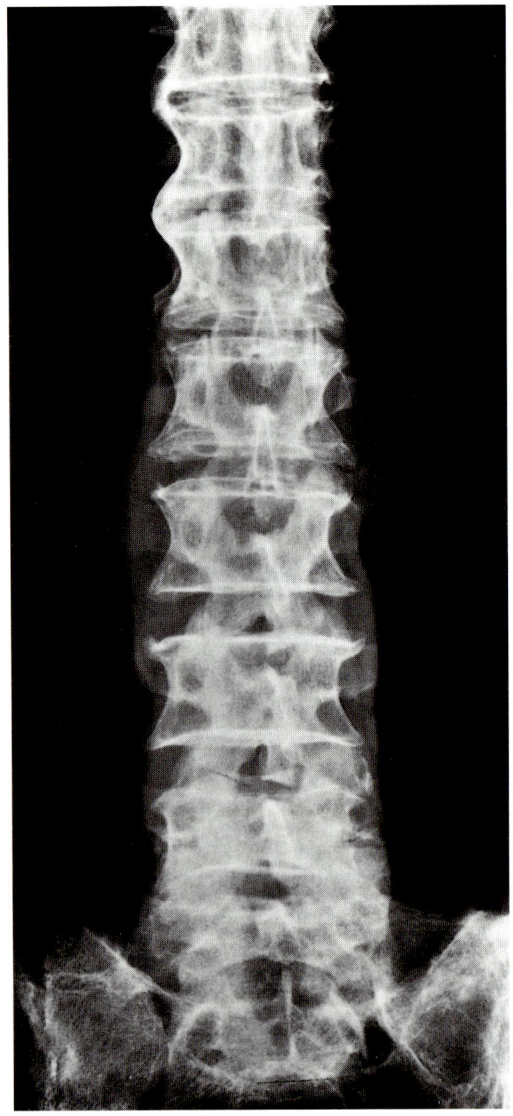

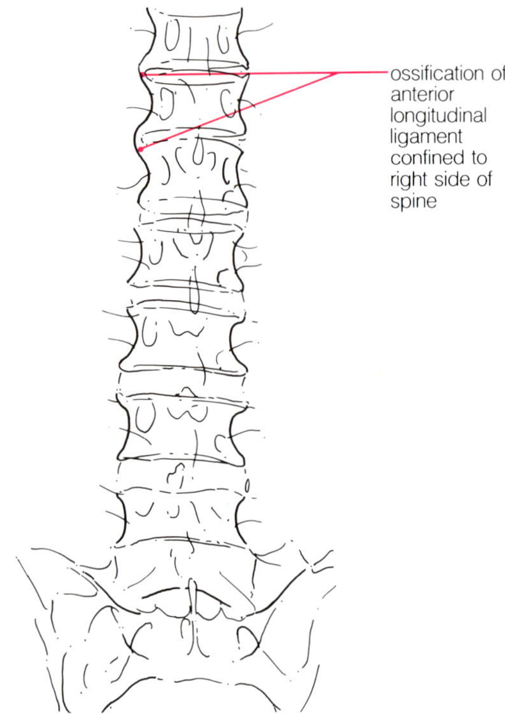

Figure 9.29 Specimen radiograph of the lower thoracic and lumbar spine and the sacroiliac joints removed from an elderly male. There is right-sided cortical hyperostosis and ligamentous ossification, with ankylosis of the lower thoracic spine. Early symmetrical changes are present in the lumbar spine. Note that the sacroiliac joints are not affected, differentiating this condition from ankylosing spondylitis.

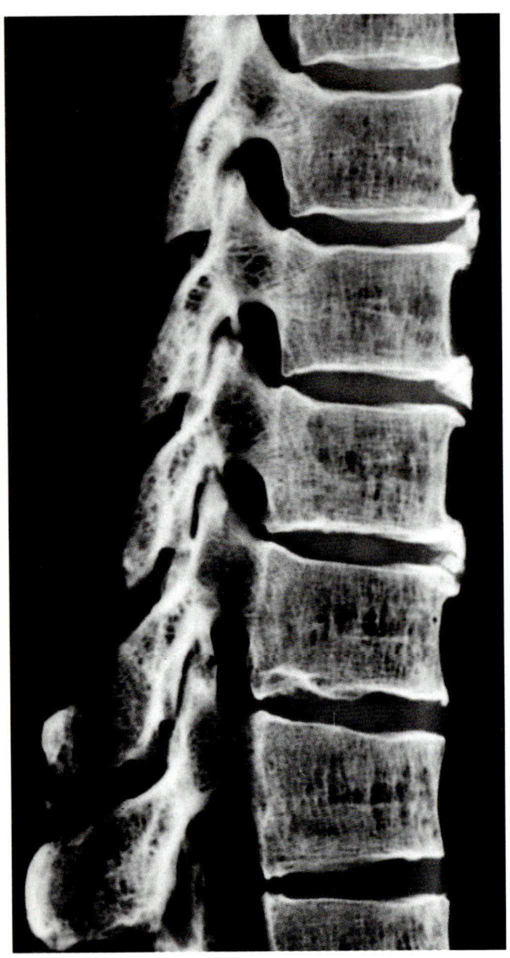

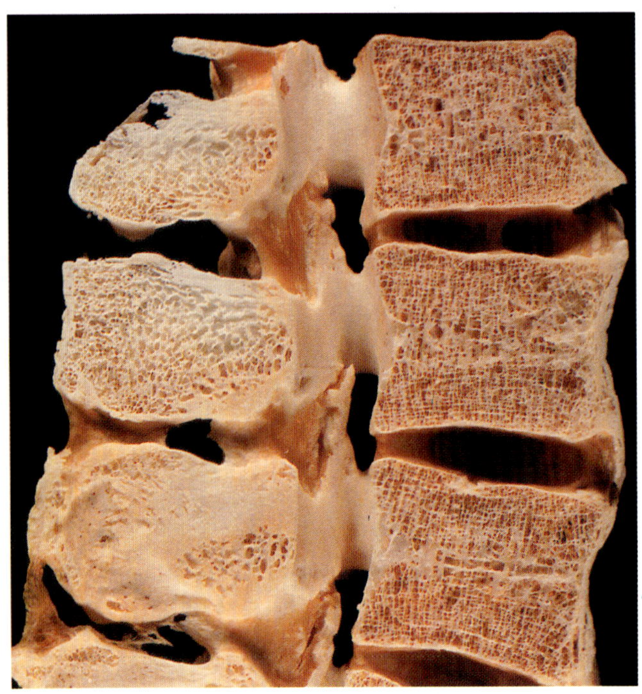

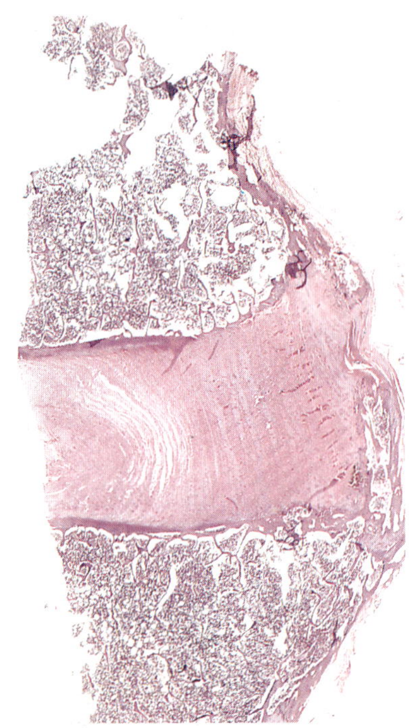

Figure 9.30 Fine-grain radiograph (*left*) of a sagittal section of the thoracic spine to illustrate early involvement by DISH. Note the prediscal isolated triangular ossicles. A sagittal section (*center*) through L-1 through L-3 of this specimen illustrates that the anterior cortices of both L-2 and L-3 are thickened. Note also the ossification in the supraspinous ligament overlying L-3. The disc spaces are well maintained, with intact bony end plates. A photomicrograph (*right*) of the L2-3 disc space illustrates ossification of the anterior longitudinal ligament extending in front of the disc. The disc itself is normal.

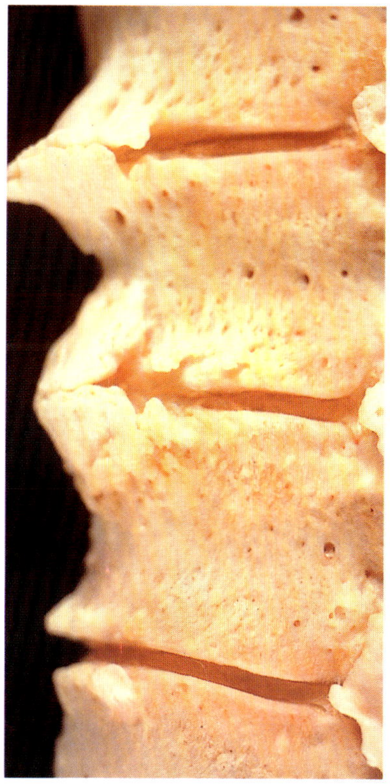

Figure 9.31 Photograph of a lateral view of a segment of thoracic spine to illustrate prediscal "flamelike" ossification. It is not as yet completely ankylosed.

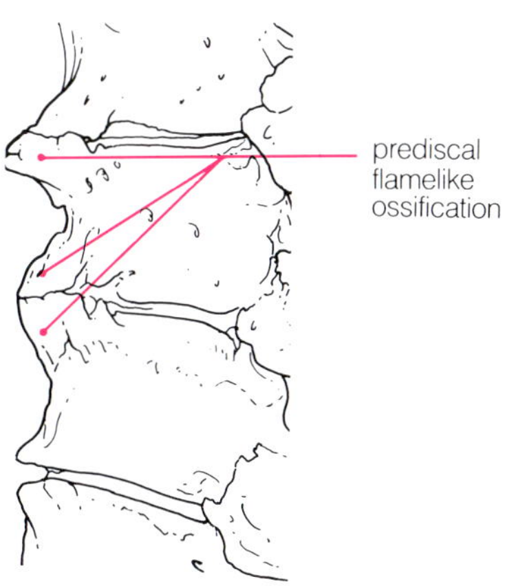

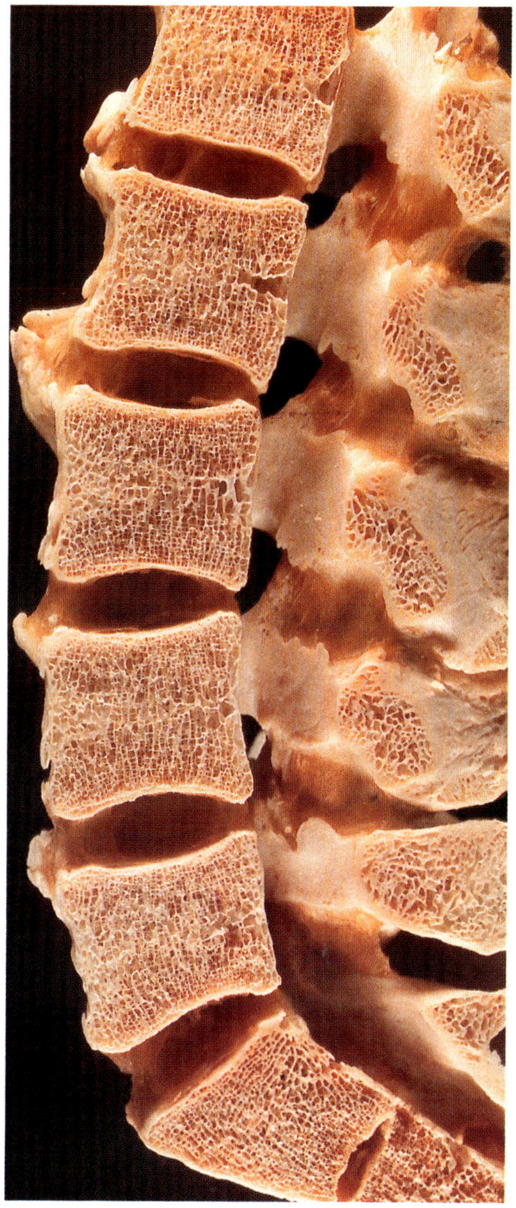

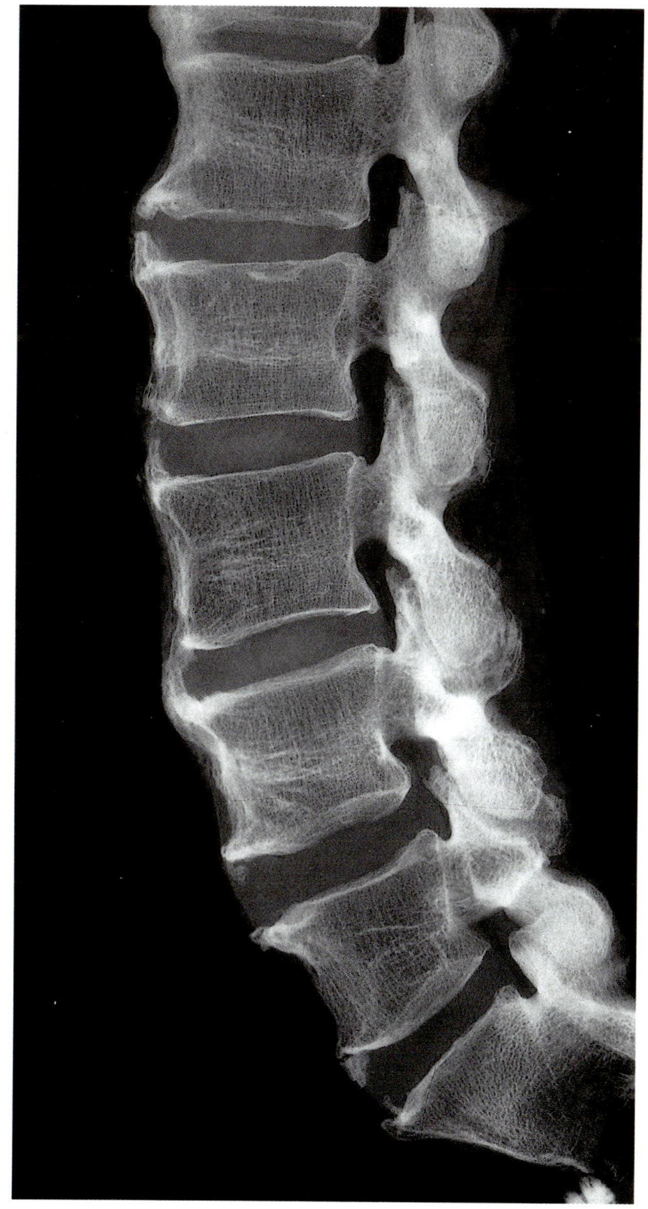

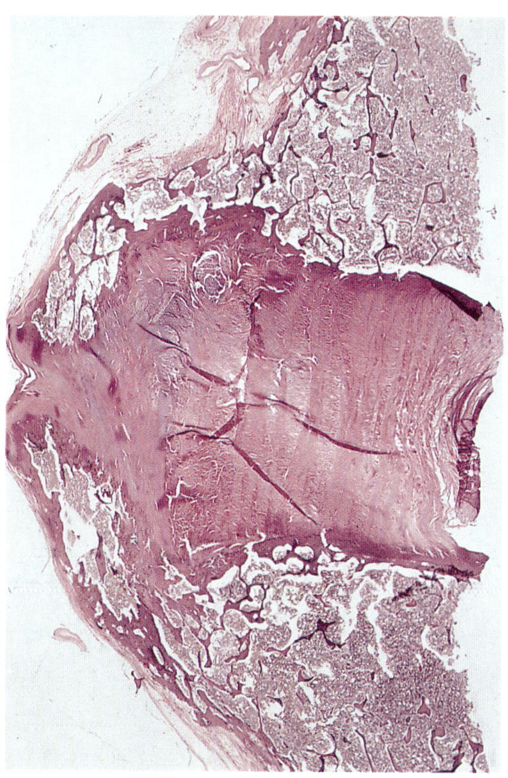

Figure 9.32 Photograph (*top left*) of a macerated sagittal section through a segment of the lumbosacral spine again illustrates "flamelike" prediscal ossification, with normal discs. A radiograph (*top right*) of the same specimen. In a photomicrograph (*bottom*) of the L2-3 disc space, cortical hyperostosis is well seen in L-2. The prediscal ossified tissue is not completely fused. (This figure should be compared with Figures 5.8 and 9.23.)

III. End-stage disease found usually in the thoracic segment and characterized by ankylosis resulting from ossification of the longitudinal ligament; this adds a thick layer of new bone to the vertebral body surface, likened to armor plating (Fig. 9.33) (This armor plating is characteristic of ankylosing hyperostosis and is not seen in ankylosing spondylitis)

All of these stages may be demonstrated in one specimen (Fig. 9.34).

In our experience, approximately one-third of the older adult population has ankylosing hyperostosis at necropsy, more than half of these showing end-stage disease. The thoracic spine is involved twice as often as is the lumbar spine, which in turn is involved twice as frequently as the cervical spine. Unlike the thoracic region where the right side of the spine is predominantly affected, symmetric right- and left-sided involvement is seen characteristically in the cervical and lumbar regions.

Although ankylosing hyperostosis occurs independently of disc disease, the disc spaces nevertheless may be mildly narrowed. Disc calcification also may be present, on occasion. Osteoporosis in general is not a common association.

Clinical and Laboratory Findings

In ankylosing hyperostosis, clinical symptoms are rare in association with spinal involvement; however, patients with severe involvement of the cervical spine may develop dysphagia. A peculiar variant of cervical ankylosing hyperostosis has been described particularly in the Japanese literature, in which ossification of the posterior longitudinal ligament (OPL) occurs, sometimes leading to cord compression (Figs. 9.35 through 9.37). In patients who have undergone total hip replacement, a higher incidence of heterotopic bone formation following surgery has been found in patients with

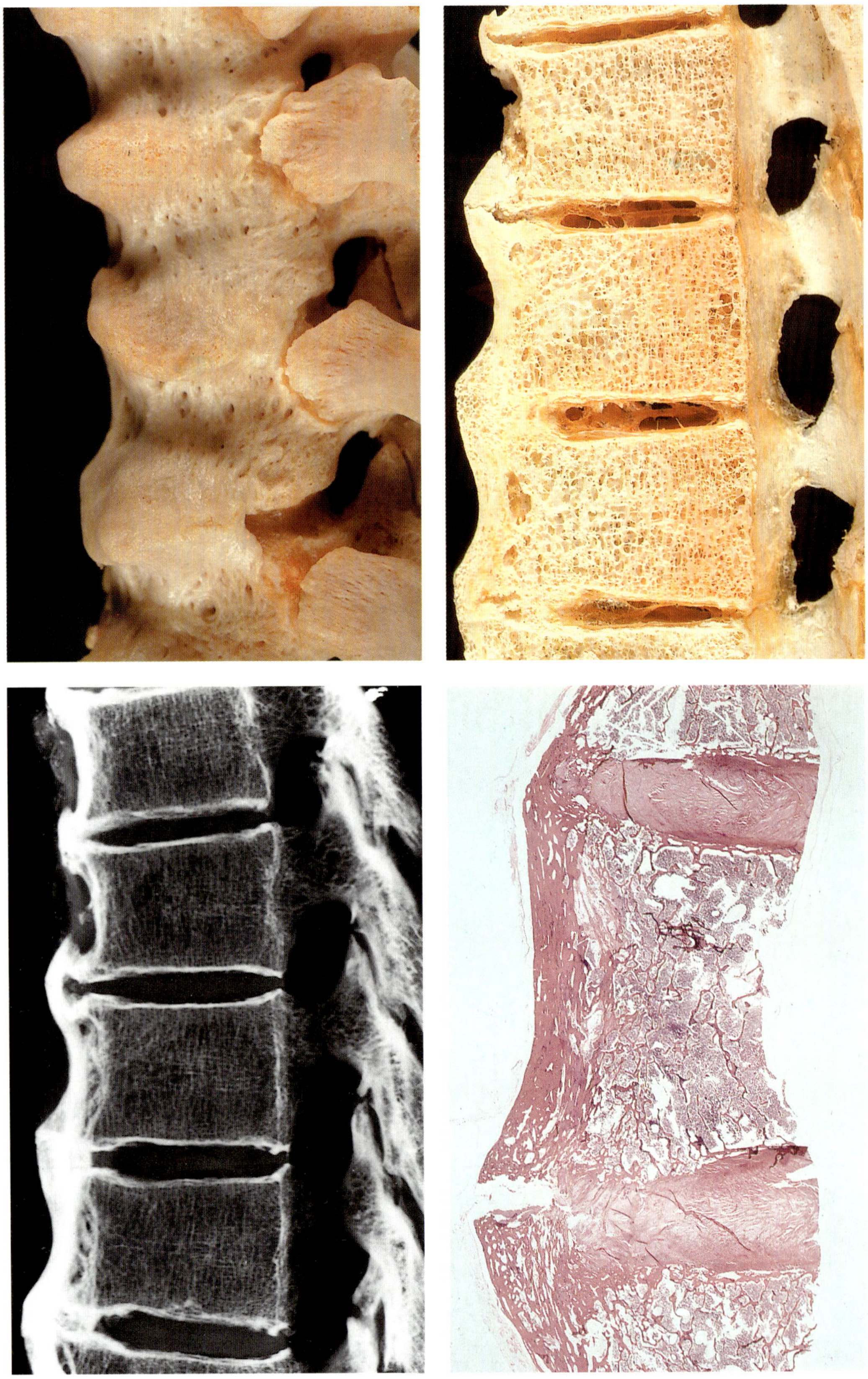

Figure 9.33 Photograph (*top left*) of a lateral view of a segment of thoracic spine to show bony ankylosis and "armor plate" thickening of the anterior surface. The lower two facet joints can be seen, and are uninvolved by the disease. A sagittal section (*top right*) of the same specimen. In a radiograph (*bottom left*) of the same specimen, note that the ossification appears to be confined to the anterior longitudinal ligament, and the facet joints are uninvolved. A photomicrograph (*bottom right*) of a section of the same specimen.

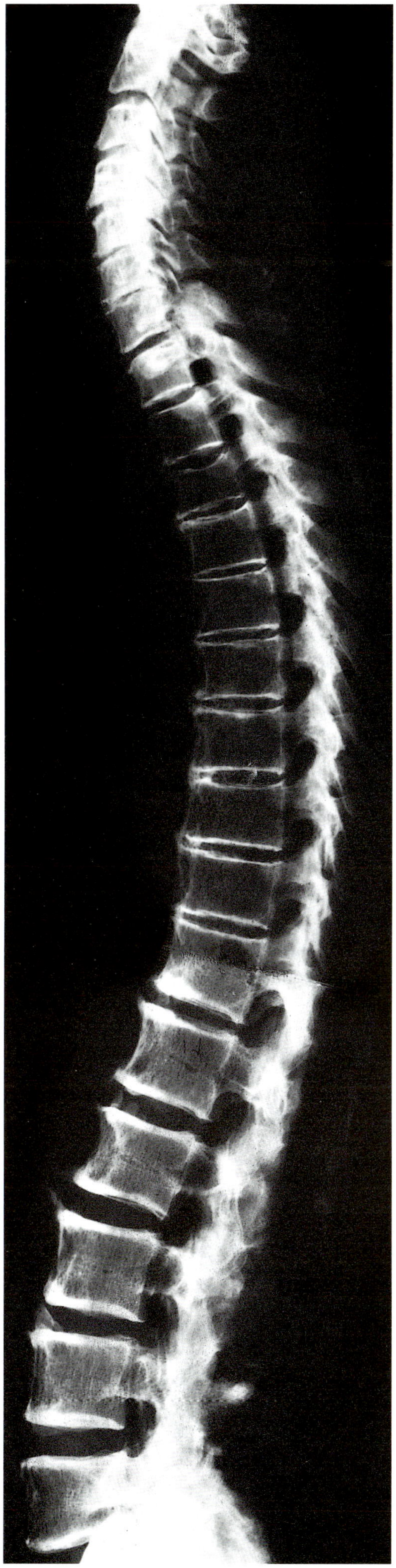

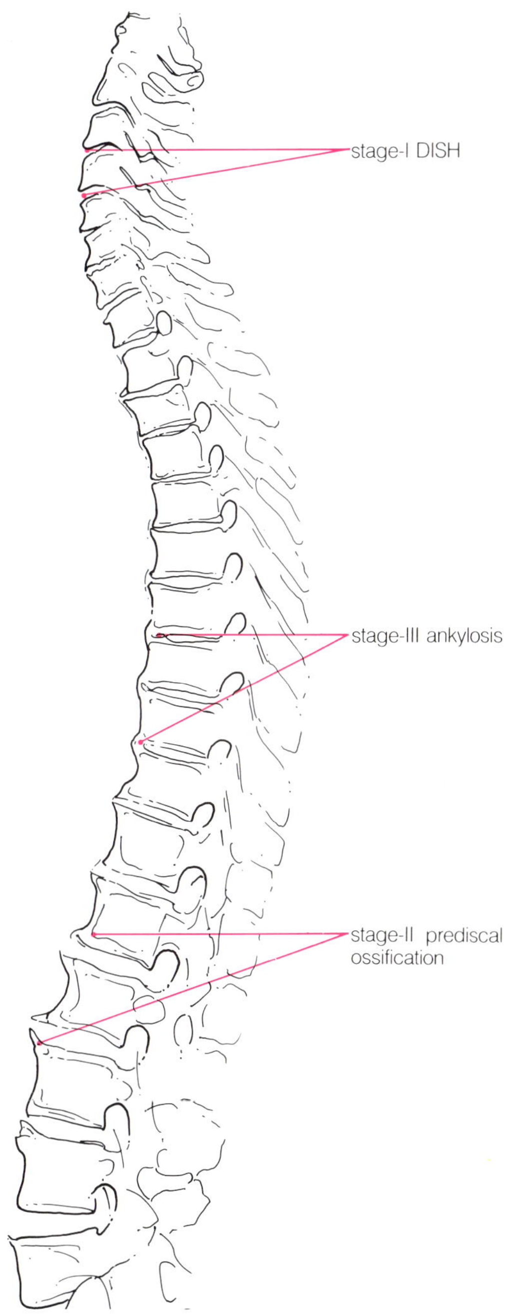

Figure 9.34 Lateral radiograph of the spine from a 65-year-old male to illustrate different degrees of spinal involvement in ankylosing hyperostosis. In the cervical spine, there is minimal stage-I involvement of C-3 and C-4, while in the upper thoracic spine, there are early changes of cortical hyperostosis. In the mid- and lower thoracic spine, stage-III changes are seen, with flowing ossification of the anterior longitudinal ligament and resultant ankylosis of that segment of the spine. The underlying cortex can be clearly distinguished. In the lumbar spine, there are stage-II changes, with prediscal flamelike ossifications.

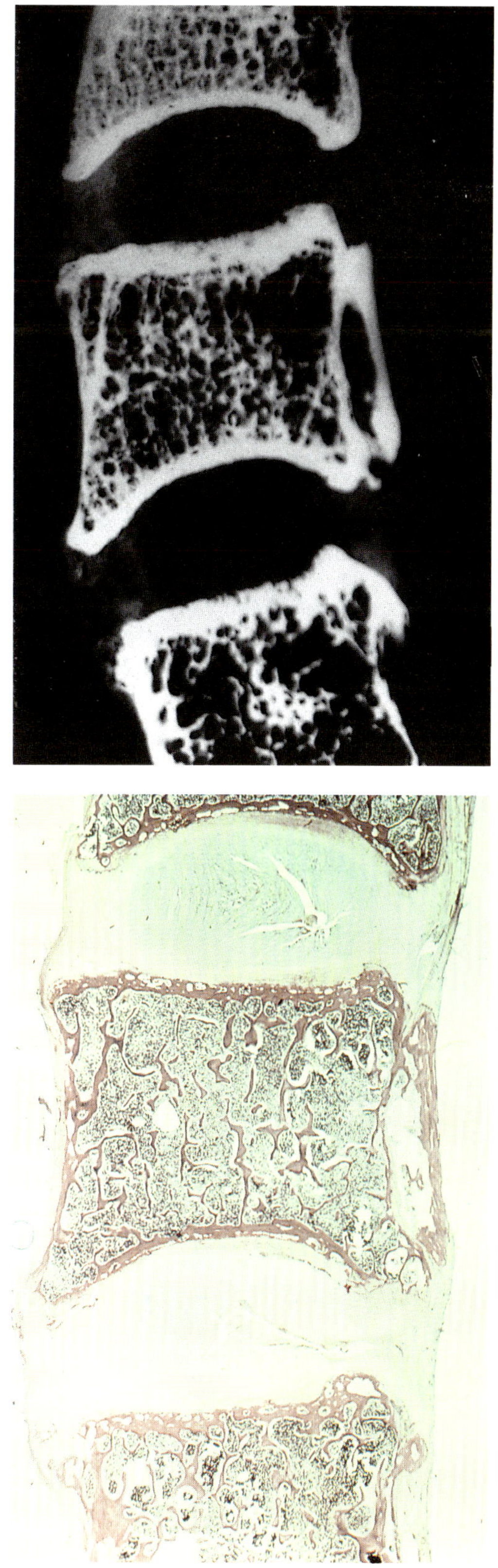

Figure 9.35 Radiograph (*top*) of a sagittal section through a portion of the cervical spine from a Japanese patient with OPL. Note the ossification of the posterior longitudinal ligament (seen to the right), which is clearly demarcated from the posterior cortex. The disc spaces are normal, and there is no anterior hyperostosis. A photomicrograph (*bottom*) from the same case to show the ossification of the posterior ligament. (Courtesy of Professor Terayama)

preexisting ankylosing hyperostosis (Fig. 9.38).

Although the etiology of ankylosing hyperostosis remains unknown, advancing age is considered to be a common factor. We consider that the disease is a spinal manifestation of a more diffuse ossifying diathesis of the ligamentous and tendonous insertions. Bony outgrowths, especially along the spine, also may accompany certain endocrine disorders such as acromegaly, hypoparathyroidism, and diabetes mellitus. However, patients with ankylosing hyperostosis do not show any specific laboratory findings, although the ESR may be minimally elevated and a significant number will have an abnormal glucose tolerance test. An increased incidence of HLA B8 in patients with ankylosing hyperostosis has been reported, occurring in approximately 42% of cases. (Of interest is the relationship between HLA B8 and many endocrine disorders.) Hyperostosis has been produced experimentally in cats by the use of high doses of vitamin A; fluoride intoxication also may produce ligamentous ossification and ankylosis.

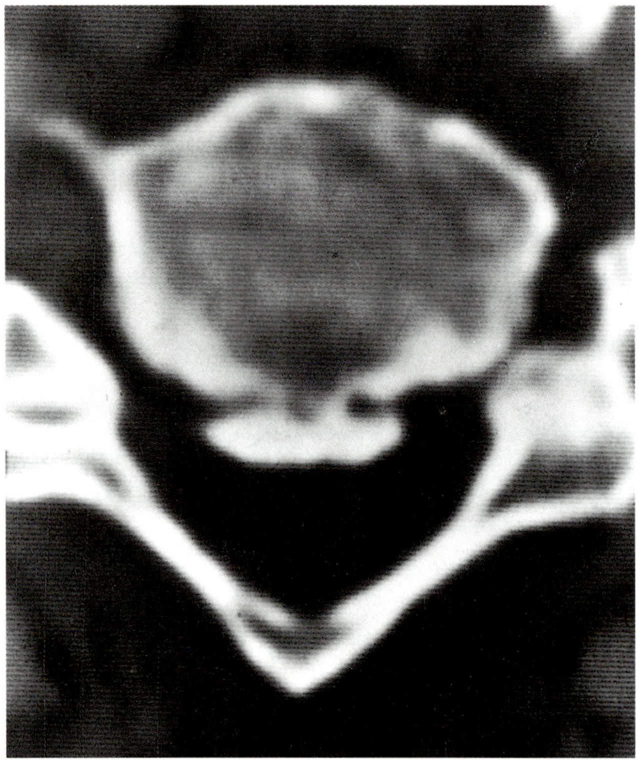

Figure 9.36 CT scan of the upper cervical spine of a patient with OPL and encroachment on the cervical canal. Following minor trauma, this patient presented with myelopathy.

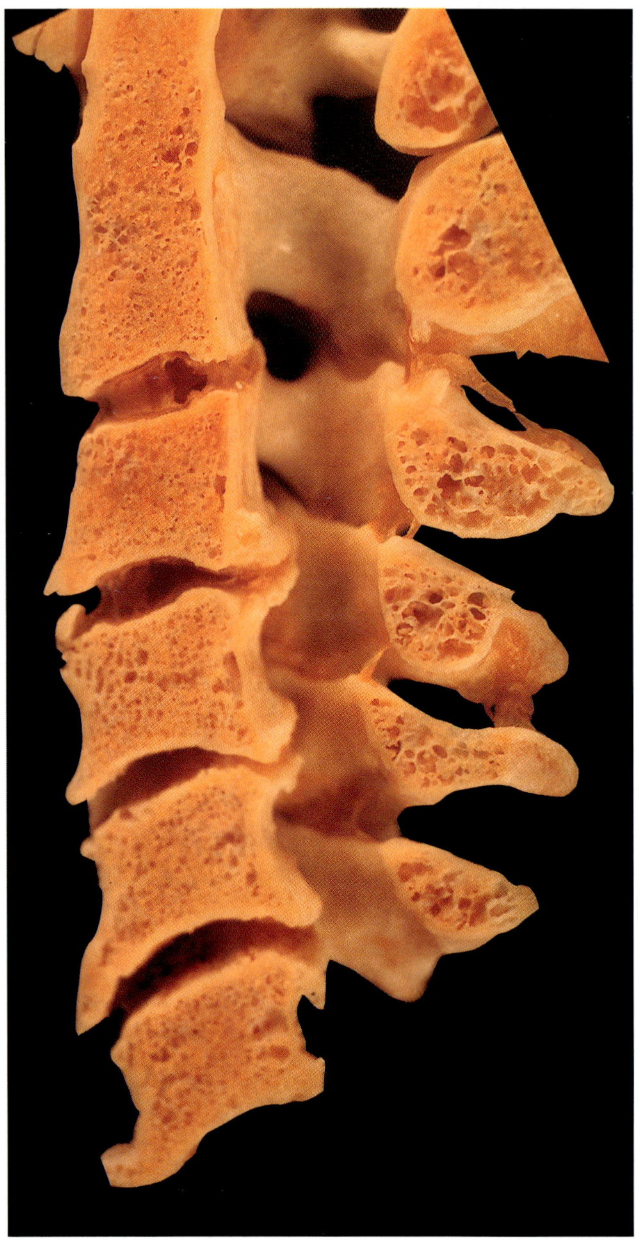

Figure 9.37 Photograph of a sagittal section through the cervical spine, which demonstrates both ossification of the anterior longitudinal ligament (DISH), as well as severe ossification of the posterior longitudinal ligament (OPL).

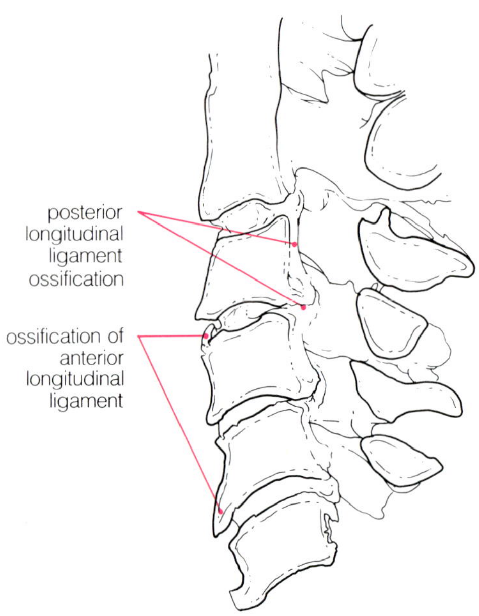

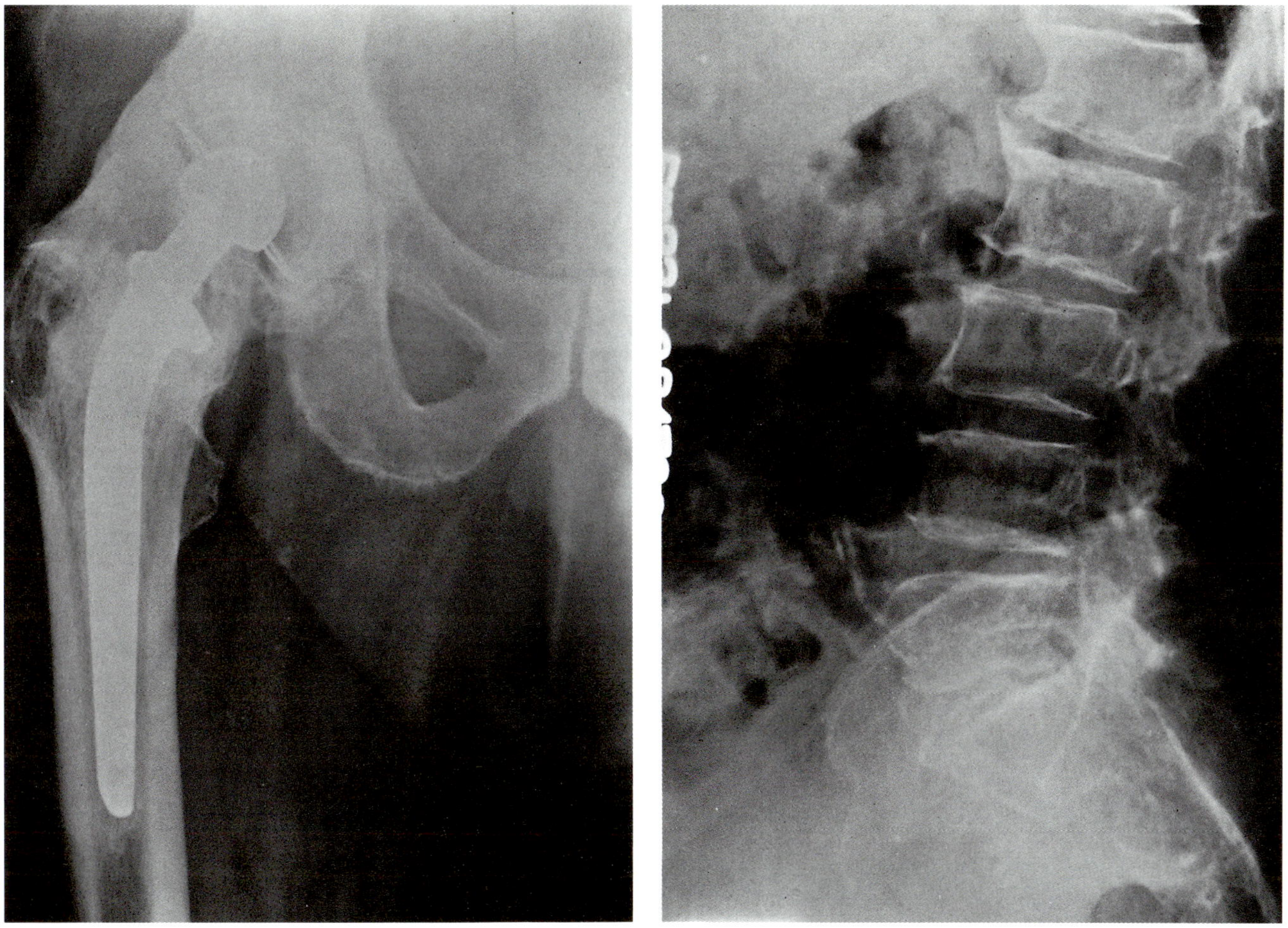

Figure 9.38 Postoperative radiograph (*left*) of a 65-year-old male with total hip replacement three years previously. Total bony ankylosis of the joint from ectopic ossification is seen. A lateral radiograph (*right*) of the lumbar spine of this patient shows the anterior cortical hyperostosis and nonmarginal syndesmophyte formation typical of ankylosing hyperostosis (DISH).

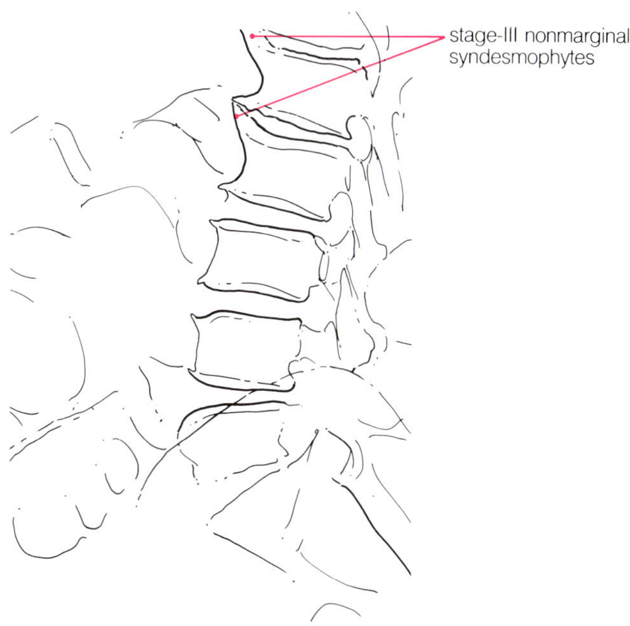

3 SECTION

DISEASES OF THE BONY ELEMENTS

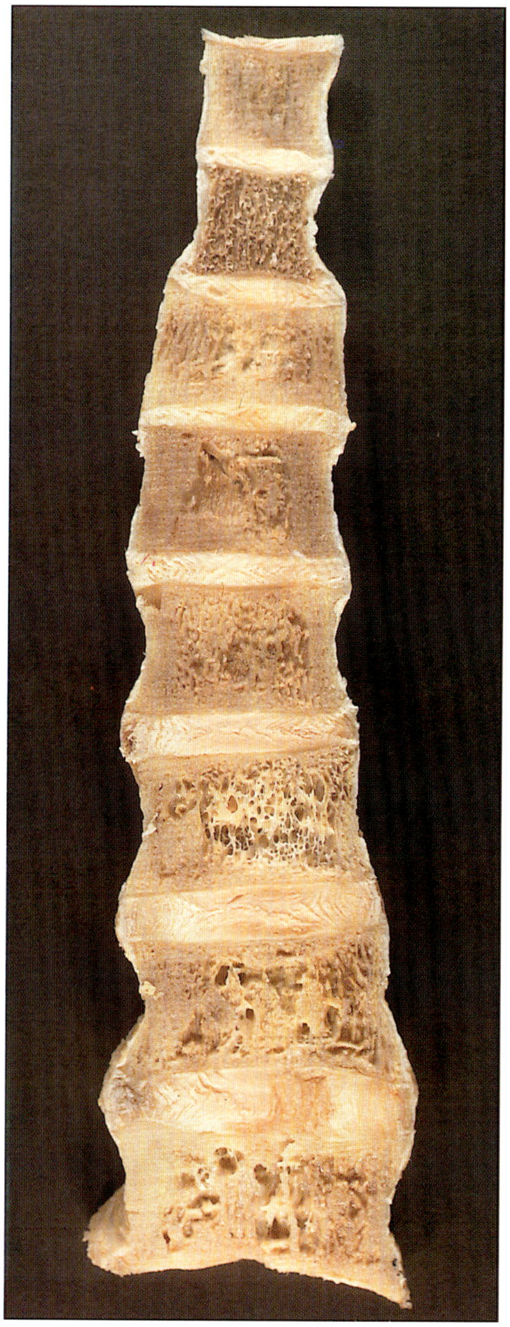

In this final section on diseases affecting the vertebral column, we will deal with those conditions that originate in the bony tissue rather than in the joints. We will concentrate on the more common conditions, recognizing that "While pigs might fly, they are very rare birds in most of our practice."

The first chapter in this section deals with the more common developmental abnormalities; the second with the effects of metabolic and hematologic diseases of the spine; the third with infection, and the fourth and fifth chapters deal with the benign and malignant tumors most likely to be met with in the spine.

10 CHAPTER

DEVELOPMENTAL AND ACQUIRED MALFORMATIONS

INTRODUCTION

An understanding of the normal development of the spine (as discussed in Section 1, Chapter 4) is prerequisite to any understanding of developmental malformations. A defect in formation and/or segmentation of the spine will result in a *primary* deformity, with the clinical implications of the defect depending on its location; such primary abnormalities are classified according to their location and the anatomical defect. When *secondary* deformity of the vertebral column is present, then the direction and magnitude of the deformity often are included in the classification. As will be seen throughout this chapter, many malformations of the vertebral column also are associated with malformations of the nervous system, the urogenital system, and the extremities.

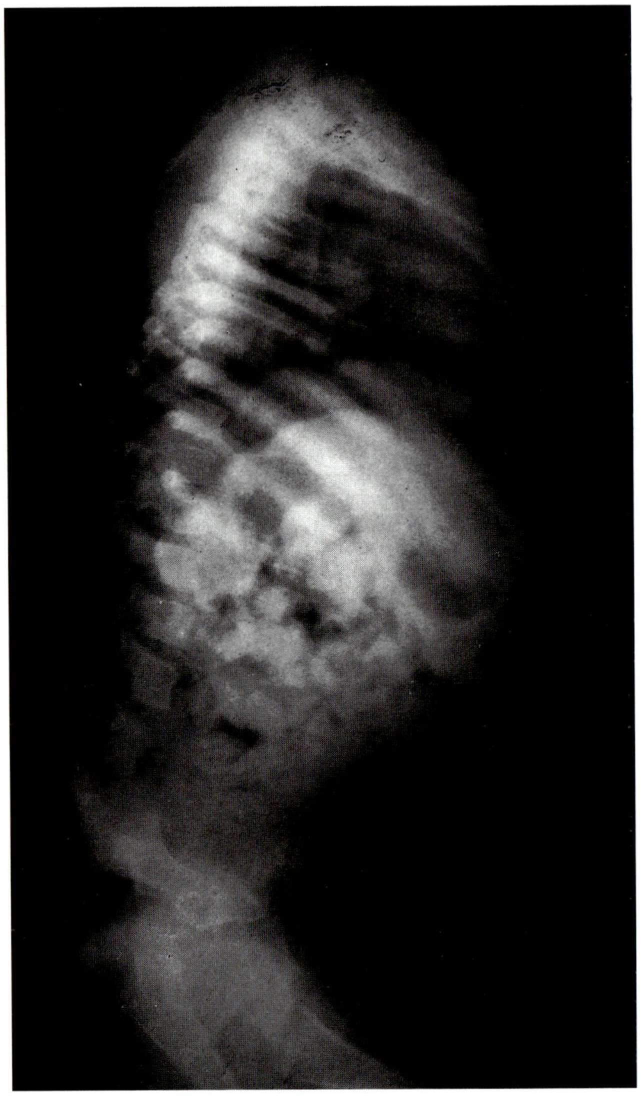

Figure 10.1 Lateral radiograph of a young child to demonstrate congenital absence of the lower lumbar spine and sacrum. The pelvis is hypoplastic.

SEGMENTAL MALFORMATIONS

AGENESIS

Agenesis of one or more vertebral bodies is rare, and when it occurs above the level of T-12 it usually is incompatible with life. Clinical cases therefore almost always involve the lower lumbar and lumbosacral regions of the spine. Both the vertebral bodies and the vertebral arches are affected.

Lumbosacral agenesis results in severe handicap with contractual deformities and functionless lower limbs. The thoracic cage usually is symmetrical, with T-12 being the most distal spinal segment. There is a narrow pelvis below it, and the femora may be well formed or atrophic (Fig. 10.1). Autopsy studies have shown the absence of the major motor nerves as well as an atrophy of muscle. However, even in the absence of the lumbosacral plexus, there may be sensory innervation from the thoracic level to the lower limbs.

A number of theories have been put forward to explain the pathogenesis and etiology of lumbosacral agenesis. Among these theories are that:

1. The defect results from a partial failure in development of the notochord and the neural ectoderm; this theory is supported by experiments in which agenesis was produced by partial resection of the distal segment of the developing neuroectoderm.
2. The failure in development may result from abnormal insulin levels; this theory is based on findings of cases of agenesis in diabetic mothers, particularly in those who suffered from diabetic coma during their first trimester.
3. The failure in development in some cases may be genetic.

CONGENITAL BLOCK VERTEBRAE

Failure of segmentation of the cartilaginous anlage of the vertebral column results in absence of the intervertebral disc and in the formation of "block vertebrae." Generally, both the vertebral bodies and the posterior arches are affected; less commonly only the bodies are fused. In most cases the block vertebrae have a height equivalent to the number of vertebrae fused (including their discs), without significant loss of height (Fig. 10.2). The block vertebrae change the mobility of the involved segment, leading to increased stresses on the intervertebral discs above and below the affected area, with the early development of degenerative disc disease. Although block vertebrae may appear anywhere in the vertebral column, they are more common in the cervical spine (Figs. 10.3 through 10.5).

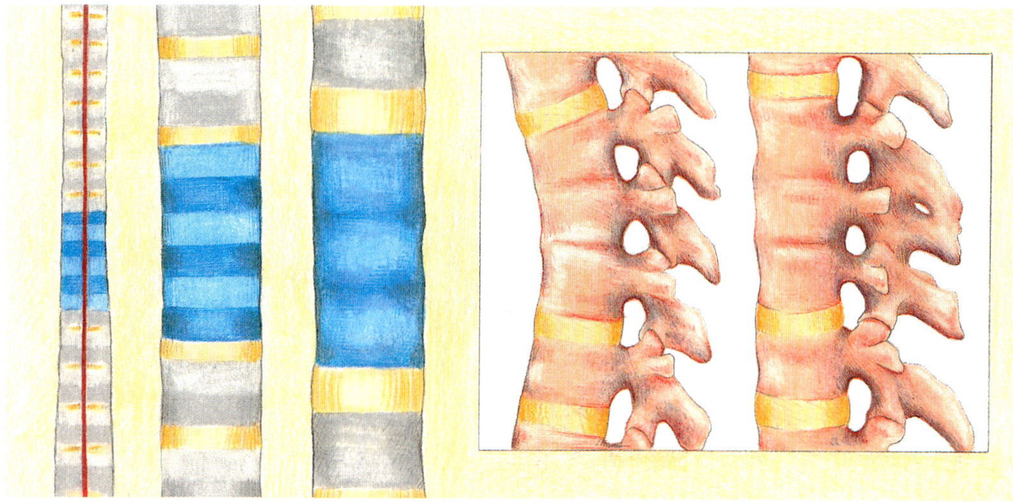

Figure 10.2 Schematic drawing to illustrate the formation of block vertebrae during early development. The intervertebral disc normally develops from the central portion of the cartilaginous somite, whereas the vertebral body develops from the fusion of adjacent somites (see Section 1, Chapter 4). Note that in the usual case, where both the vertebral bodies and the posterior arches are fused, the affected segment is relatively straight. However when only the vertebral bodies are involved, there may be increased kyphosis.

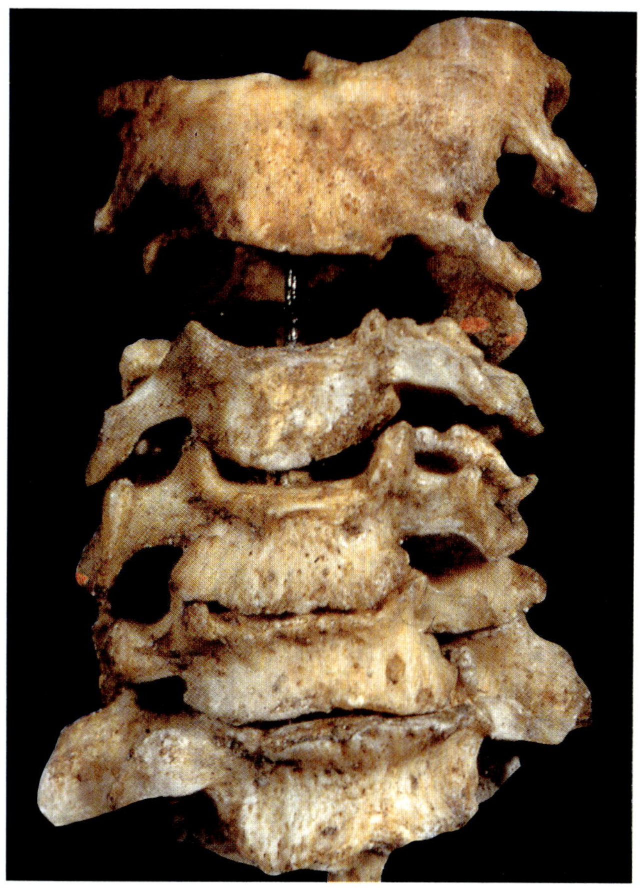

Figure 10.3 Photograph of a macerated specimen of the cervical spine to demonstrate fusion of C-1 to C-3. (Courtesy of the Royal College of Surgeons of England)

KLIPPEL-FEIL SYNDROME

The classic case of Klippel-Feil syndrome results from a failure in segmentation of the cervical spine. It is characterized by:

1. A reduction in the number of cervical vertebrae
2. Severe restriction of neck motion due to fusion of some of the cervical vertebrae
3. A short neck, and consequently a low posterior hairline (Fig. 10.6)

This syndrome often is associated with scoliosis and other congenital anomalies involving the auditory, nervous, cardiopulmonary, and genitourinary systems. Most cases of Klippel-Feil syndrome are not discovered radiographically until the patient is fully grown (Fig. 10.7). Although the cervical spinal defect is usually asymptomatic during childhood, the concentration of all movement within one or two unfused spinal segments may lead to structural instability with cord or nerve root compression, especially if movement is restricted further by the presence of an accessory omovertebral bone.

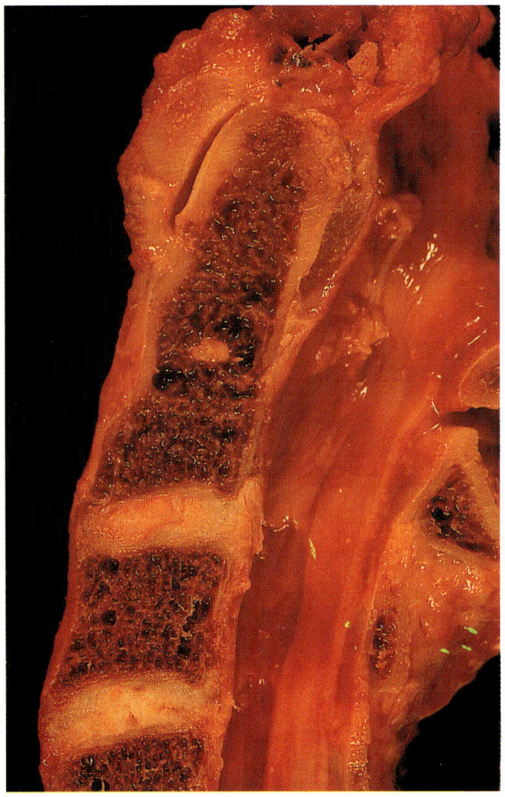

Figure 10.4 Photograph of a sagittal section of the upper cervical spine to demonstrate fusion of C2-3. A small remnant of disc is present. The posterior elements are not fused.

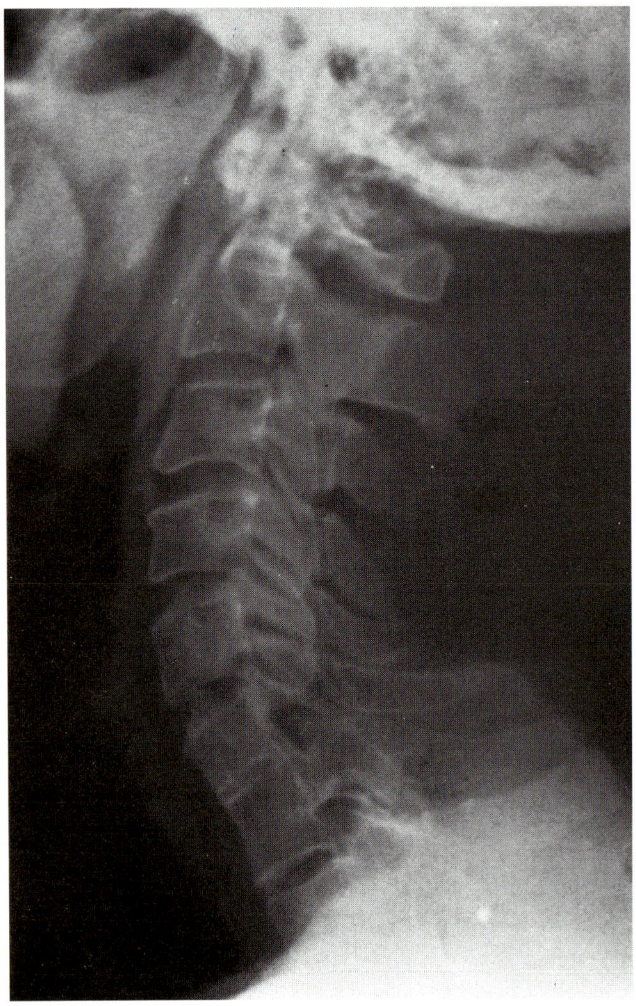

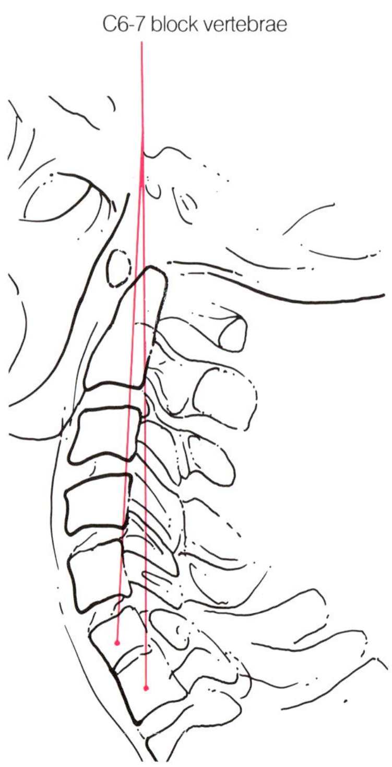

Figure 10.5 Lateral radiograph of the cervical spine in a 35-year-old man showing block vertebrae of C6-7. The articular processes also are fused.

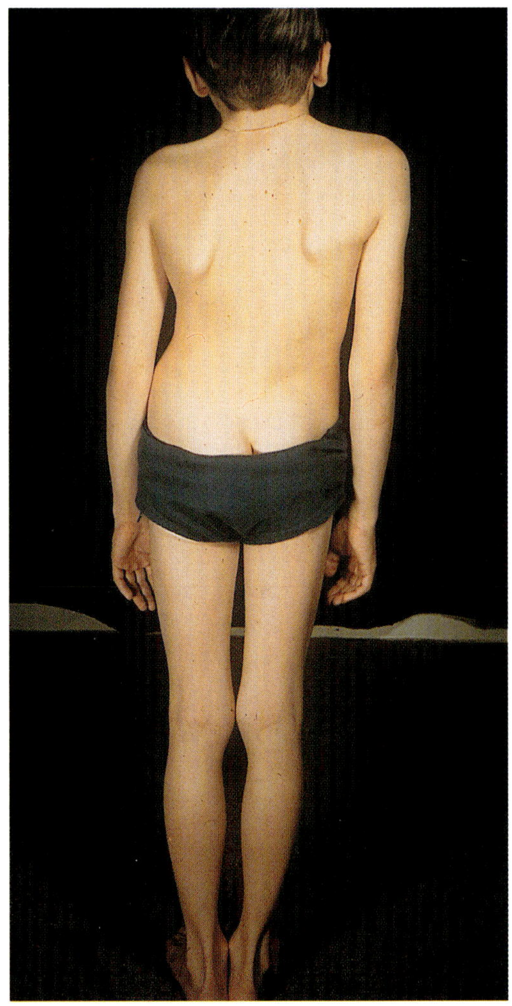

Figure 10.6 Clinical photograph of a 7-year-old boy with Klippel-Feil syndrome. Note the short neck, low hairline, and elevation of the right shoulder and scapula. Note also the lateral trunk shift associated with mild spinal curvature. (Courtesy of Dr. David Levine)

Vertebral Body Malformations

HEMIVERTEBRA

Hemivertebrae result from a failure in the formation of a part of the vertebral body during early development (Fig. 10.8). The hemivertebra may be solitary, or there may be multiple hemivertebrae adjacent to one another or scattered in several areas of the spine, with varied patterns of spinal deformity and clinical significance.

Hemivertebra results from failure either of cartilage development or ossification of one lateral half of the vertebral body. They may be classified into three types:

1. Fully segmented with open disc spaces on both sides
2. Semi-segmented with an open disc on one side and a fused disc on the other
3. Incarcerated or unsegmented with fused discs on both sides

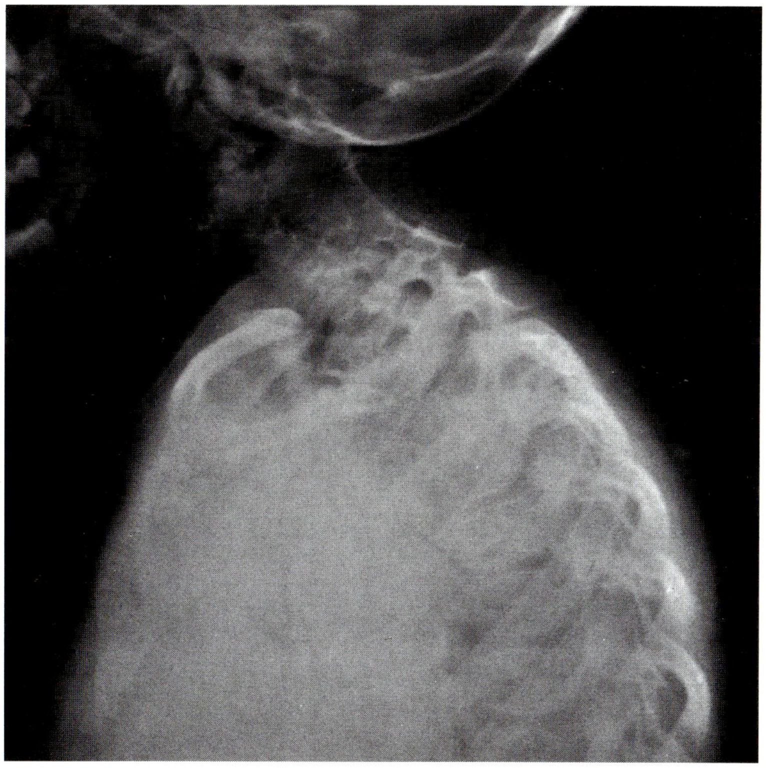

Figure 10.7 Lateral radiograph of the head and upper body of a patient with Klippel-Feil syndrome. Note the short neck and fusion of the hypoplastic cervical vertebral bodies and posterior elements.

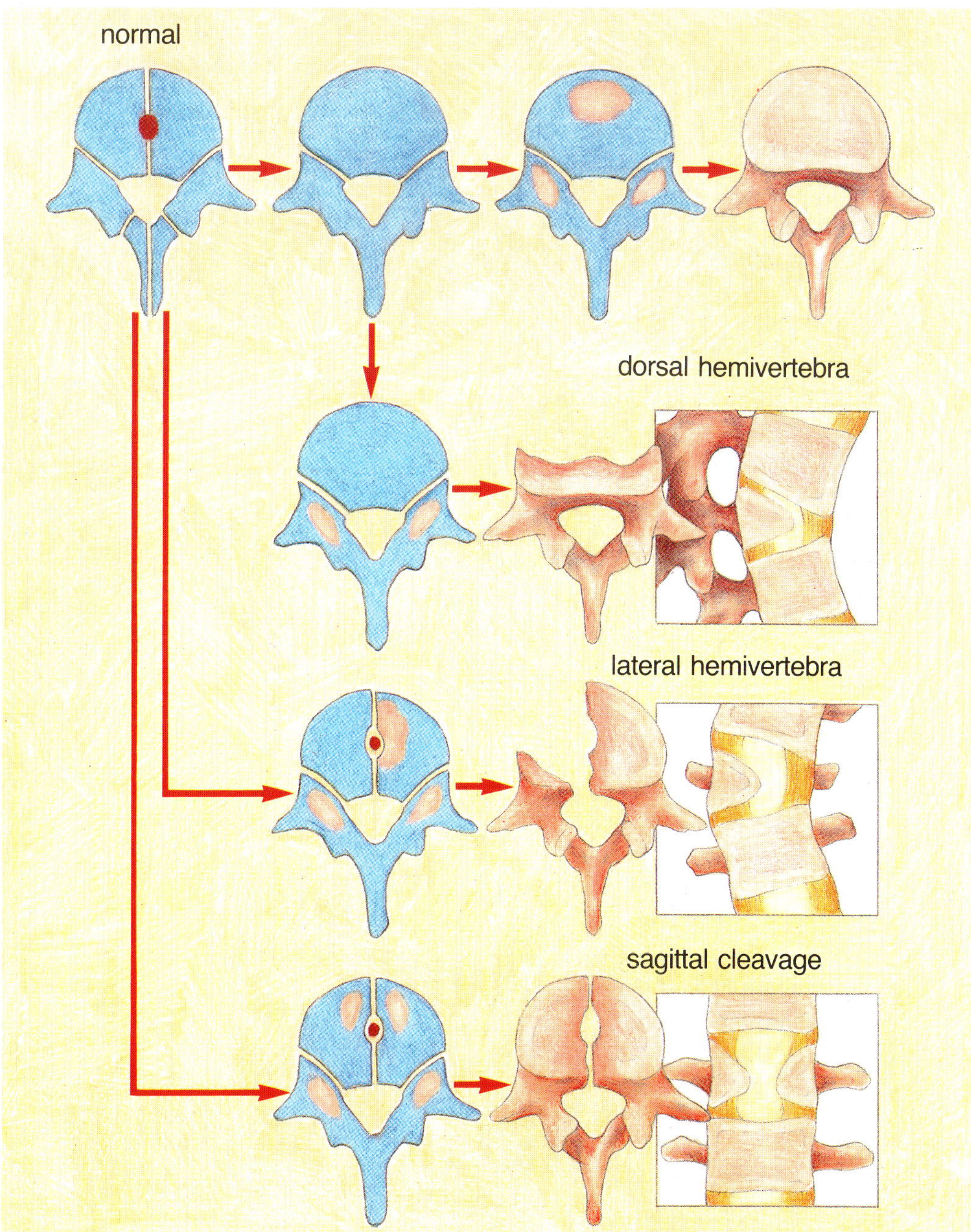

Figure 10.8 Schematic drawing to illustrate the formation of hemivertebrae. A dorsal hemivertebra will result in the development of an anterior angular or gibbus deformity; a lateral hemivertebra will result in the development of scoliosis; sagittal cleavage will result in the development of a "butterfly" vertebra.

The potential for deformity is *least* for the unsegmented type and *greatest* for the fully segmented type (Fig. 10.9). A dorsal hemivertebra will result when the anterior cartilaginous anlage of the body fails to develop or fails to ossify (Fig. 10.10). This usually results in an angular kyphosis (gibbus). Dorsal hemivertebrae are localized mostly in the upper lumbar region and may present clinically as the sole spinal deformity in association with a more generalized disease such as hypothyroidism, achondroplasia, or other chondrodystrophy.

Cleft vertebra may develop as a result of a failure of the cartilaginous somites to fuse together, with delayed regression of the notochord and subsequent failure of the ossification center to fuse across the midline. During early development the affected vertebral body assumes a butterfly shape (Fig. 10.11).

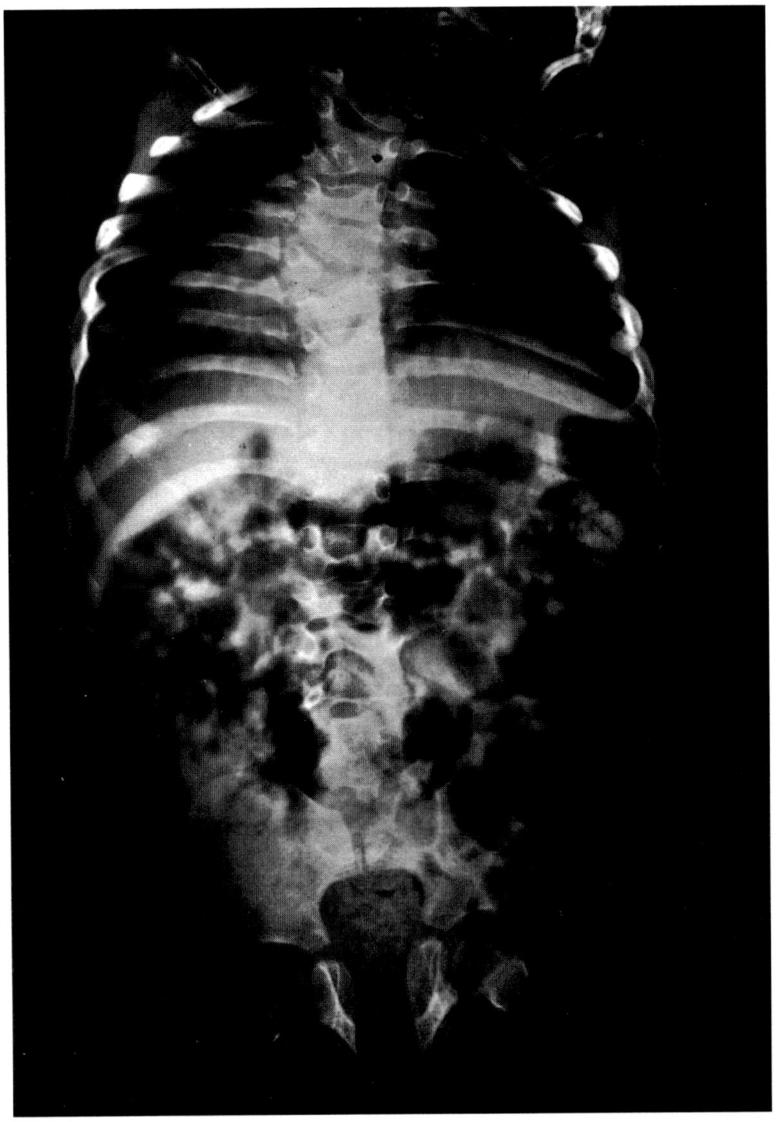

Figure 10.9 AP radiograph of the spine in a 6-year-old boy with multiple congenital abnormalities of the vertebral bodies, including lateral hemivertebrae at several levels in the thoracic spine. In addition, there is spina bifida at several levels in the lumbar spine.

DIASTEMATOMYELIA

Diastematomyelia is a congenital malformation of the neural canal that involves a splitting of the spinal cord or, more commonly, of the cauda equina by a fibrocartilaginous or bony septum that protrudes from the posterior midline portion of one or two vertebral bodies, most commonly L-1, L-2, or L-3. This defect probably results from a failure of the notochord, which arises from the endoderm, to separate completely from the neuroectodermal plate at the affected level. The septum indents the dura, splitting the spinal cord either partially or completely (Fig. 10.12). Particularly when the septum is bony, a neurologic deficit may result, requiring removal of the septum and release of the tethered cord.

Since most of the differential growth of the cord and spine is completed at 2 months of age, the pathogenesis of the neurologic damage in diastematomyelia is not believed to be due to traction during developmental ascent of the cord. Rather, it is believed that the relative immobilization of the lower cord by the septum leads to neural damage, especially with flexion and extension, as the child becomes more active. In most cases, diastematomyelia has been found to be associated with spina bifida occulta, while in about half of cases it is associated with hemivertebra. A high percentage of patients have associated scoliosis.

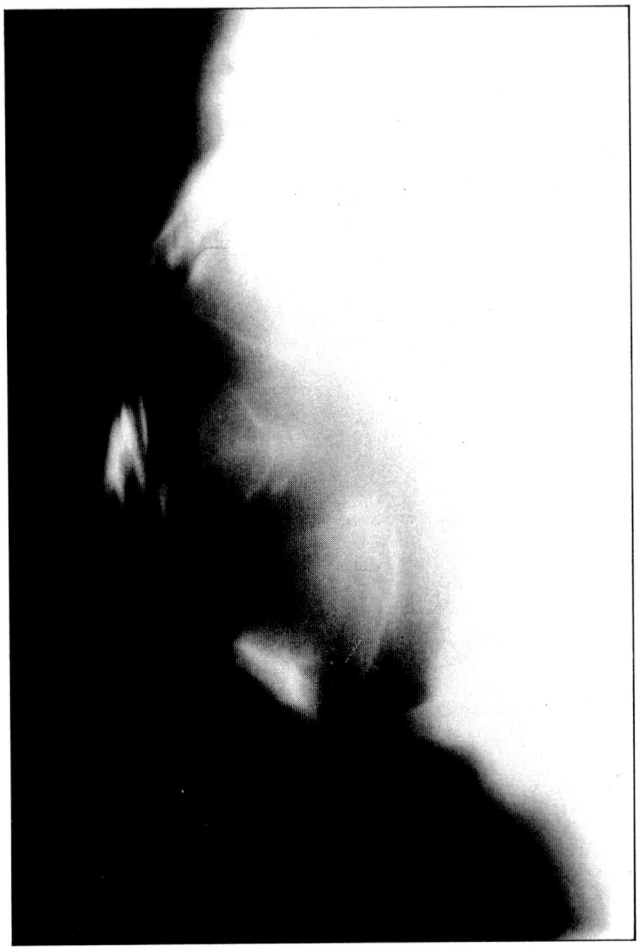

Figure 10.10 Lateral radiograph to illustrate a dorsal lumbar hemivertebra with angular kyphosis.

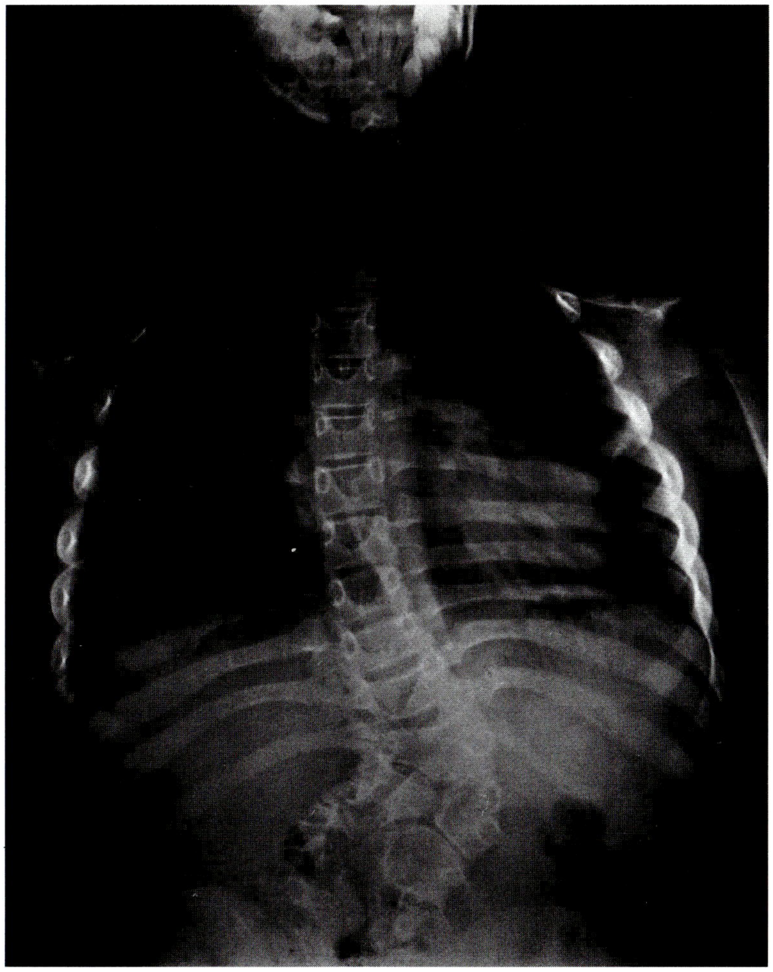

Figure 10.11 AP radiograph of the lumbar spine in a child with lumbar congenital scoliosis, due to butterfly vertebrae and other vertebral anomalies.

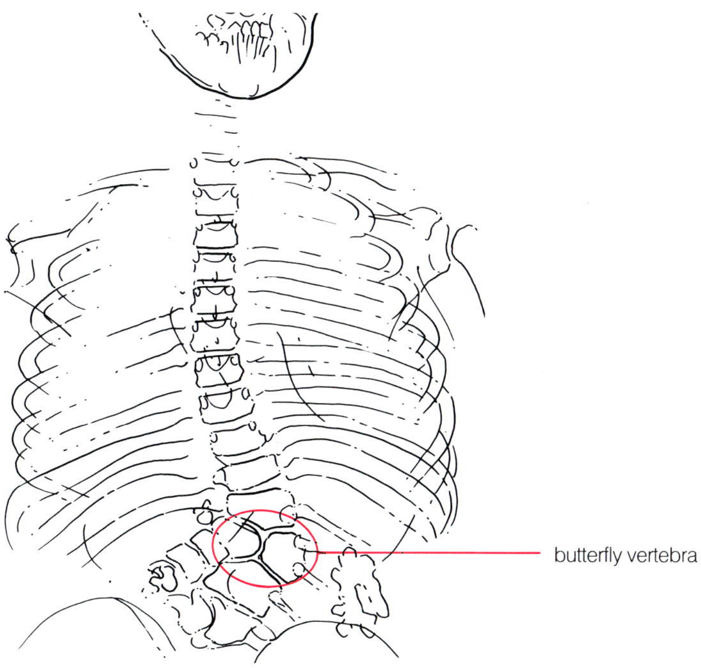

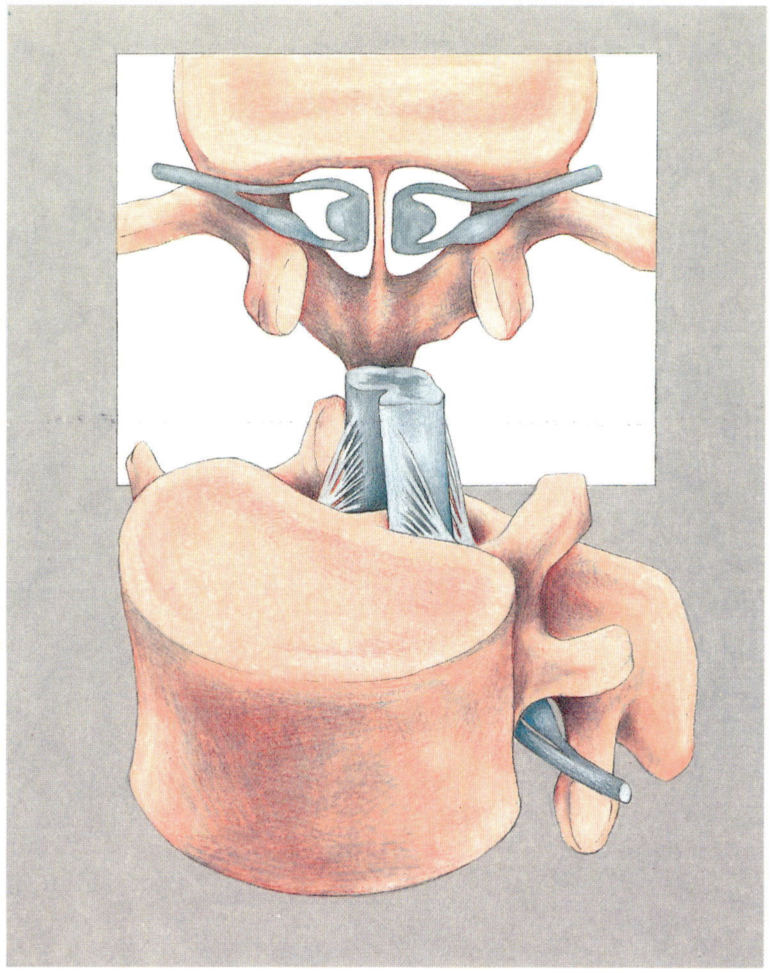

Figure 10.12 Schematic drawing of diastematomyelia. The septum, which arises from the vertebral body, may fuse to the posterior arch or, more commonly, it may be incomplete. In either case, cleavage of the spinal cord results. It may be associated with a hemivertebra or with spina bifida.

Radiographic findings in diastematomyelia include a widened interpedicular distance at the affected level and an abnormal posterior arch. Myelography and CT scan are useful in confirming and better delineating the lesion of diastematomyelia (Fig. 10.13).

SACRAL CYSTS

In the sacral region, approximately 0.5% of the population will be found to have cysts that may extend posteriorly or anteriorly. Generally, these cysts are closed by a fibrous membrane, and are filled with fluid (Figs. 10.14 and 10.15).

VERTEBRAL ARCH MALFORMATION

As previously discussed, the formation of the vertebral body is dependent on the notochord, whereas the development of the vertebral arch is influenced greatly by the neural tube. While failure of formation of the posterior neural arch is very rare, when it occurs it results in severe lordotic deformity and pulmonary compromise (Fig. 10.16). Posterior cleavage of the vertebral arch is commonly referred to as spina bifida. When only the bony elements are involved, which occurs in 5 to 10% of the population, the condition is referred to as spina bifida occulta; where the

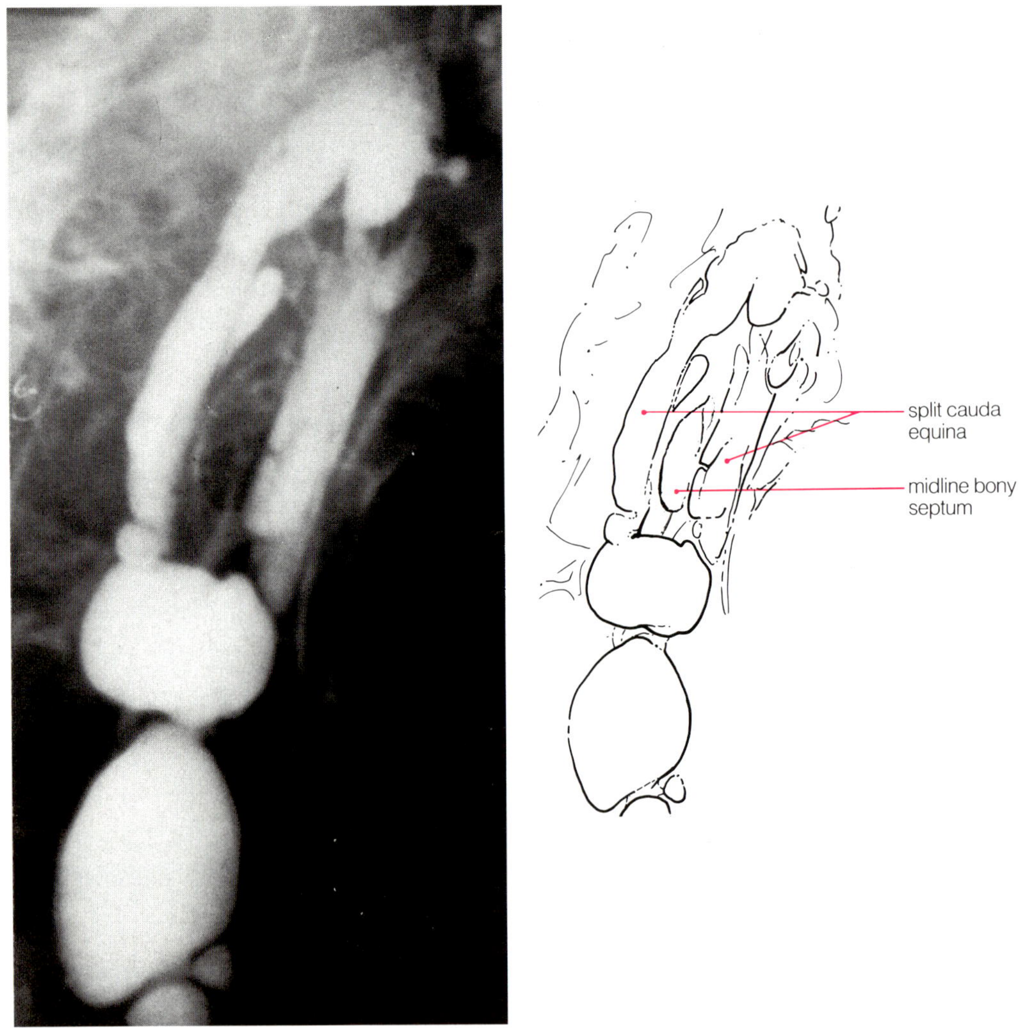

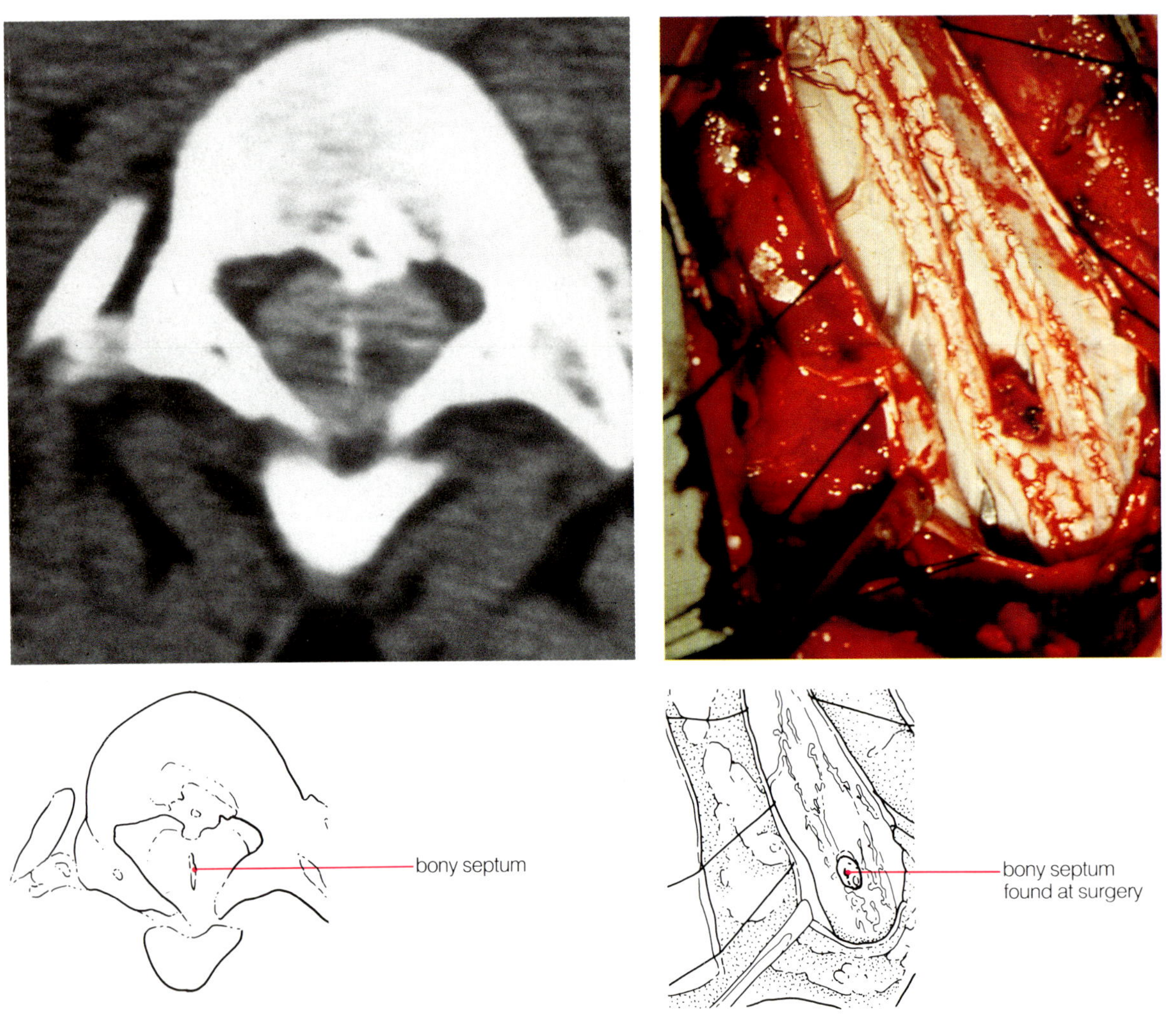

Figure 10.13 Myelogram (*top*) of a patient with diastematomyelia. The bony septum, which is in the lower lumbar spine, in this case was associated with both hemivertebra and spina bifida. The split in the cauda equina is clearly visible. A CT scan (*bottom left*) demonstrates the bony septum. An intraoperative photograph (*bottom right*) demonstrates the bony septum and the split in the cord. (Courtesy of Dr. David S. Bradford)

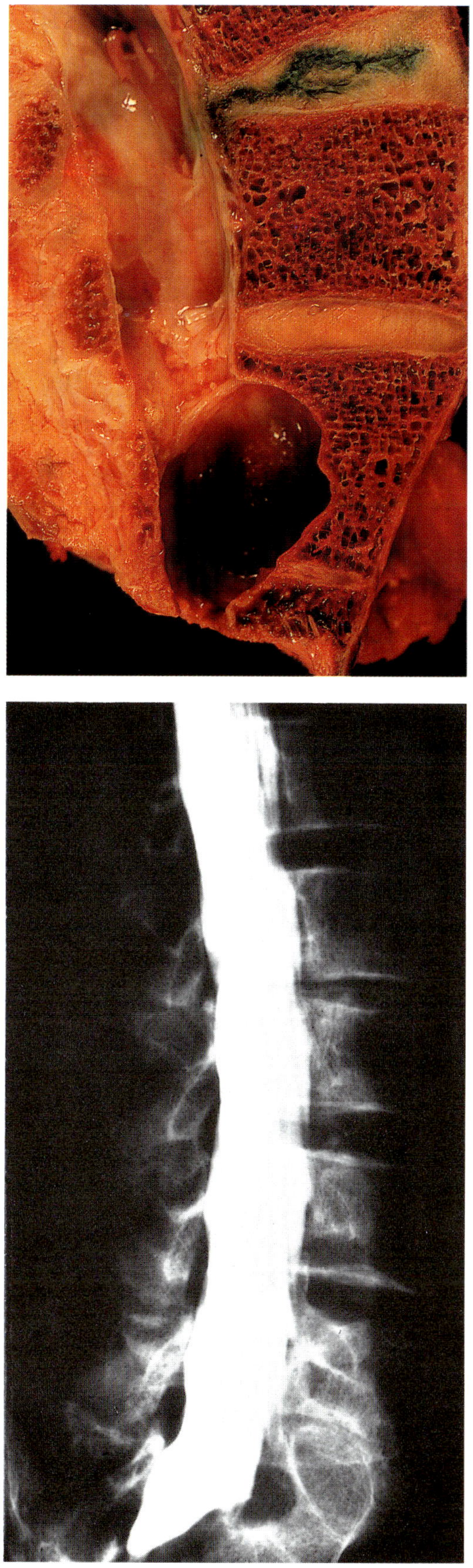

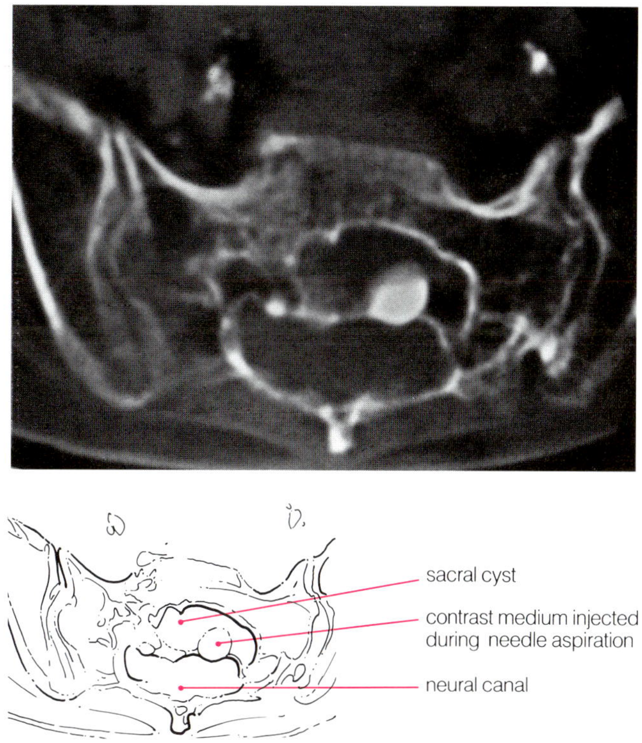

Figure 10.15 CT myelogram of a 79-year-old female with an incidental finding of a posterior sacral cyst.

Figure 10.14 Photograph (*top*) of a sagittal section through the lumbosacral junction, in which the posterior wall of S-1 and a portion of S-2 have been eroded by the anterior protrusion of a meningeal cyst. The cyst has replaced much of the osseous substances of S-1. Oblique myelogram (*bottom*) of the same specimen demonstrates that there is no communication between the neural canal and the sacral cyst.

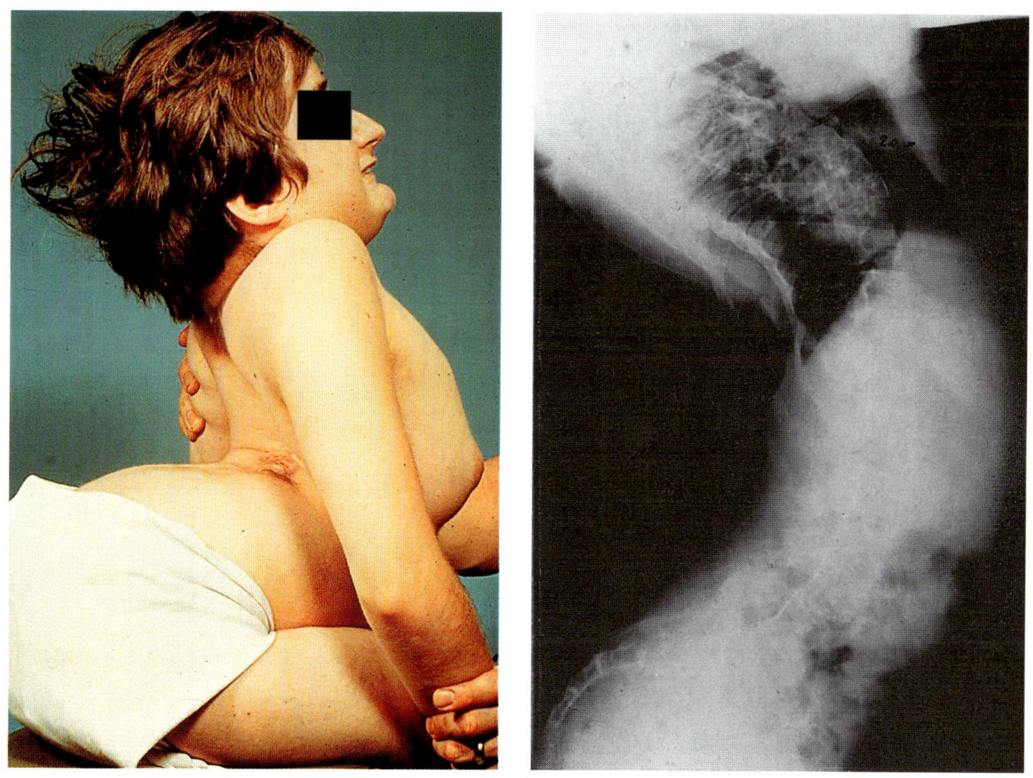

Figure 10.16 Clinical photograph (*left*) of a patient with hyperlordosis due to absence of the posterior arches of the thoracolumbar spine. A lateral radiograph (*right*) demonstrates the absence of the posterior arches. Note the severe reduction of the AP diameter of the thoracic cage. (Courtesy of Dr. David S. Bradford)

meninges and/or the spinal cord are affected, which occurs in approximately 0.2% of the population, the condition is known as spina bifida cystica (myelodysplasia), and it usually affects several levels.

PATHOGENESIS

During normal embryonic development, the mesoderm comes to surround the neural tube separating the ectoderm from the endoderm. The meninges form from the mesoderm at the time of separation of the neural tube from the ectoderm (Fig. 10.17). Nonfusion of the vertebral arch while the spinal cord and meninges remain in their normal position results in spina bifida occulta (Figs. 10.18 and 10.19). It is believed that during development, at the time that the outlets are forming for the cerebrospinal fluid, a brief period of hydrocephalus occurs. It has been proposed that the resultant increase in spinal fluid pressure may lead to a rupture of the neural tube, with damage to the overlying mesoderm and ectoderm. This occurs most commonly in the lower lumbar spine. The resulting abnormalities may be subdivided into meningoceles and myeloceles (see Fig. 10.18).

PRESENTATION

Meningoceles show herniation of both dura and arachnoid out of the spinal canal, with the cord remaining in its normal position. The meninges may be exposed extracutaneously, or they may be covered by skin and subcutaneous tissue, or sometimes by lipoma. In myeloceles, in addition to the vertebral arch deformity, the neural plate fails to close. The exposed neural plate may become infected, with resulting fibrosis and scarring. Neurologic disturbances may result from excessive fluid or infection. Hydrocephalus, the most serious complication, is also the most common. There is no sex predilection for meningoceles. Myeloceles in contrast have a female preponderance of 1:1.25 (male to female) suggesting that the female embryo is more likely to form this malformation. Spinal deformities such as scoliosis, lordosis, and kyphosis usually accompany myelodysplasia (Fig. 10.20). In rare instances, one encounters cases of dysplasia of the pars, which leads to congenital spondylolisthesis (see Fig. 10.31).

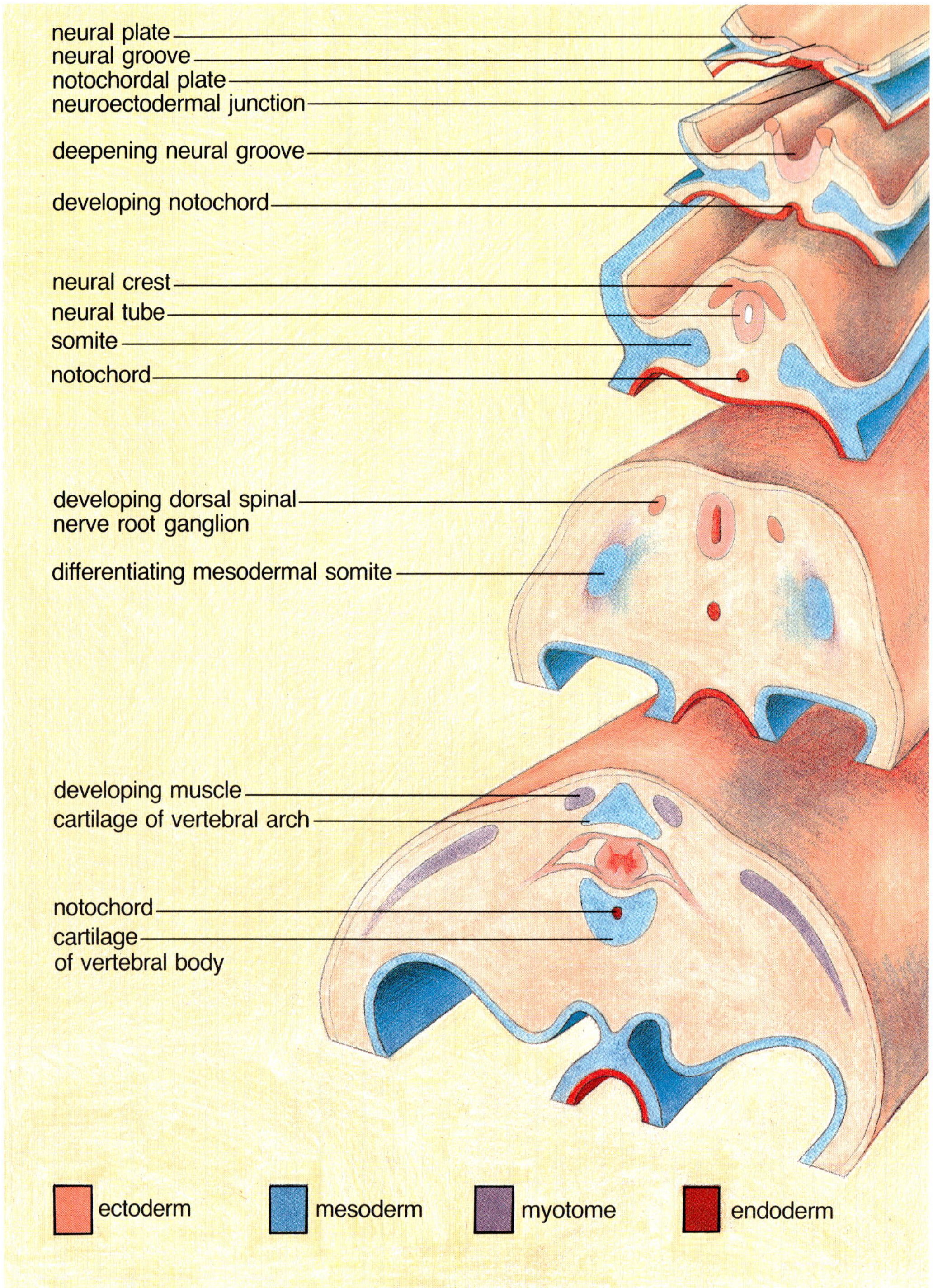

Figure 10.17 Schematic drawing to show the development of the spinal cord, the notochord, and the cartilaginous vertebral column. In this series, the various malformations of the vertebral arch and the neural tube may be comprehended.

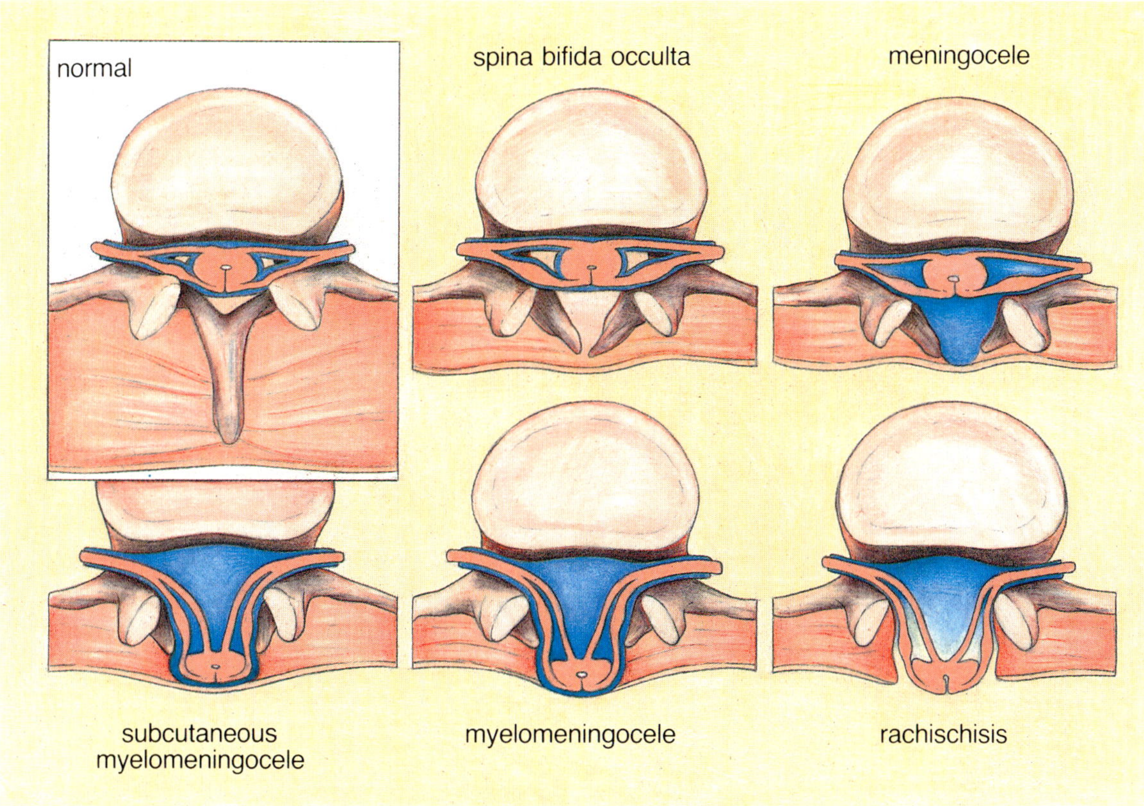

Figure 10.18 Schematic drawing to illustrate the various malformations of the neural arch and its contents, shown in ascending order of severity.

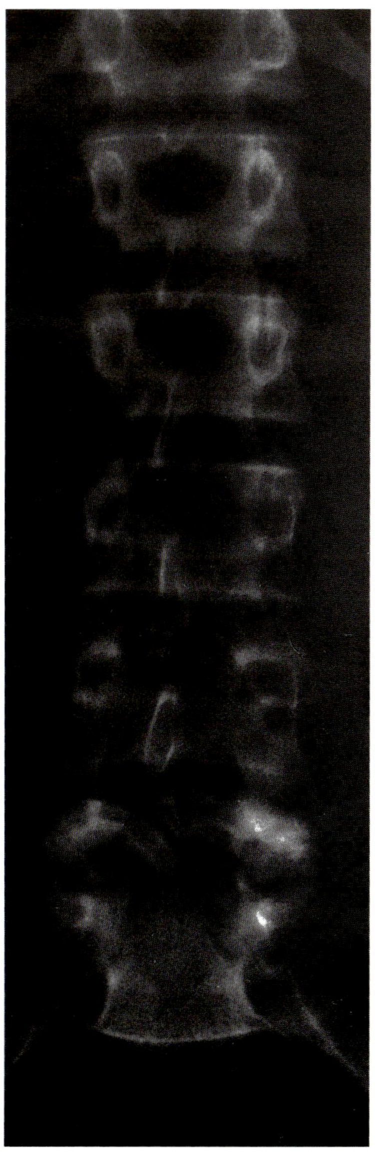

Figure 10.19 Radiograph of spina bifida occulta at L-5.

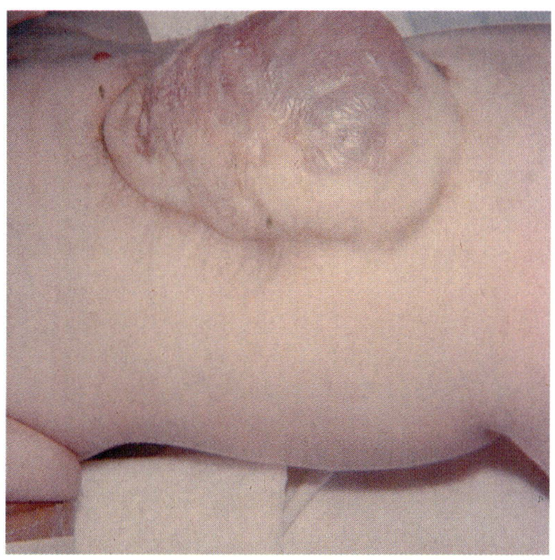

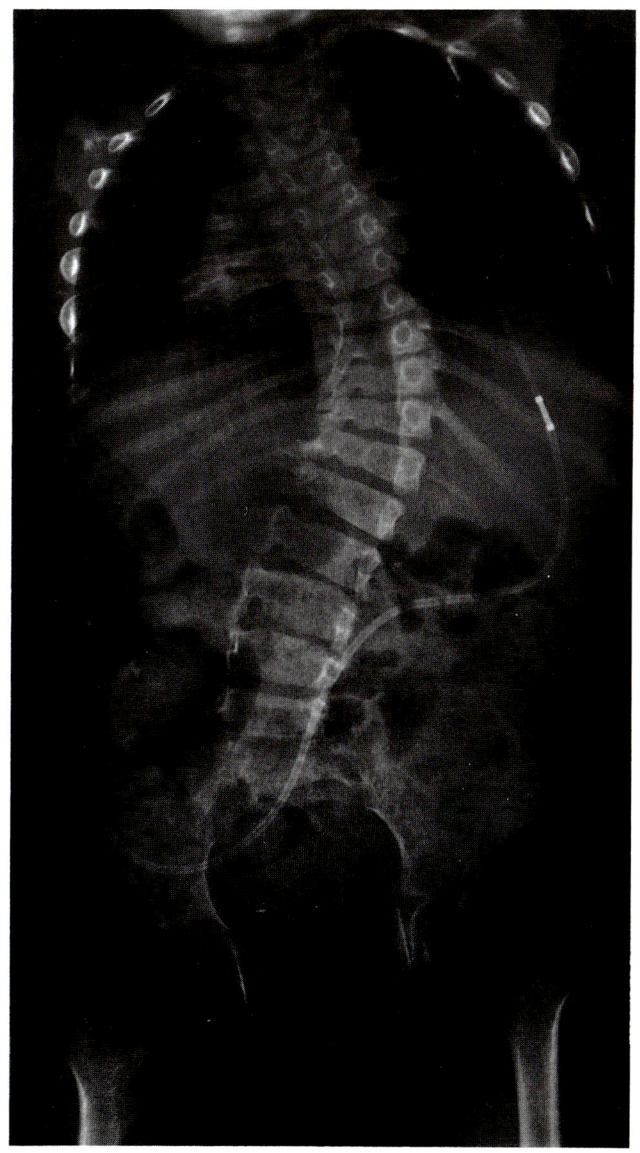

Figure 10.20 Clinical photograph (*left*) of a newborn with myelodysplasia and exposed dura. AP radiograph (*right*) of an 8-year-old girl with severe myelomeningocele and hydrocephalus, who has been treated with a ventriculoperitoneal shunt. Note the spina bifida at multiple levels, with associated scoliosis and subluxation of the right hip. (Left-hand photograph courtesy of Dr. James W. Ogilvie)

DEVELOPMENTAL ABNORMALITIES IN THE CARTILAGINOUS END PLATE

DWARFISM

A reduced rate of cartilage growth and endochondral ossification may be seen in various forms of dwarfism, both congenital and acquired, including hypothyroidism, hypopituitarism, and the congenital dyschondroplasias. Achondroplasia is an autosomal dominant inherited condition characterized by short-limbed dwarfism beginning in early fetal life (Fig. 10.21). Despite pronounced shortness of the extremities, the trunk is relatively normal in length (Fig. 10.22). However, often there is an excessive thoracolumbar kyphosis, with a compensatory lordosis that often is associated with the presence of hemivertebrae (Fig. 10.23). The kyphotic curvature of the thoracolumbar region and the excessive lordotic curvature of the lumbosacral area may be present even in the newborn. Also in the newborn, the vertebral bodies may be of normal dimensions although they consist largely of cartilage. The delay in ossification and the failure in endochondral ossification generally lead to premature fusion of the vertebral bodies with their arches, with resultant short thick pedicles leading to reduction in the dimensions of the spinal canal, both in AP and lateral diameters.

SCHEUERMANN'S DISEASE

Scheuermann's disease, which has its clinical onset in adolescence, also is known as juvenile kyphosis. It is characterized by an abnormal increase in the dorsal convexity of the thoracic spine (Fig. 10.24). Although the etiology of the disease is unknown, it is generally believed to result from an abnormality in the cartilaginous end plate. The reported incidence of Scheuermann's disease varies between 0.4% and 8%, depending on whether radiographic or clinical criteria are employed. There is a slight female preponderance. In the classic and most common form of the disease, the apex of the curve is around T7–9, while in the less common form the apex is at T11–12.

Lateral radiographs are most helpful in clinical diagnosis and classification. Anterior wedging of the thoracic vertebrae exceeding 5 degrees is characteristic, while irregularities of the vertebral end plates constitute a prominent feature (Fig. 10.25). Schmorl's nodes are characteristic, and in the late stage of the disease narrowing of the intervertebral disc space occurs, and interbody

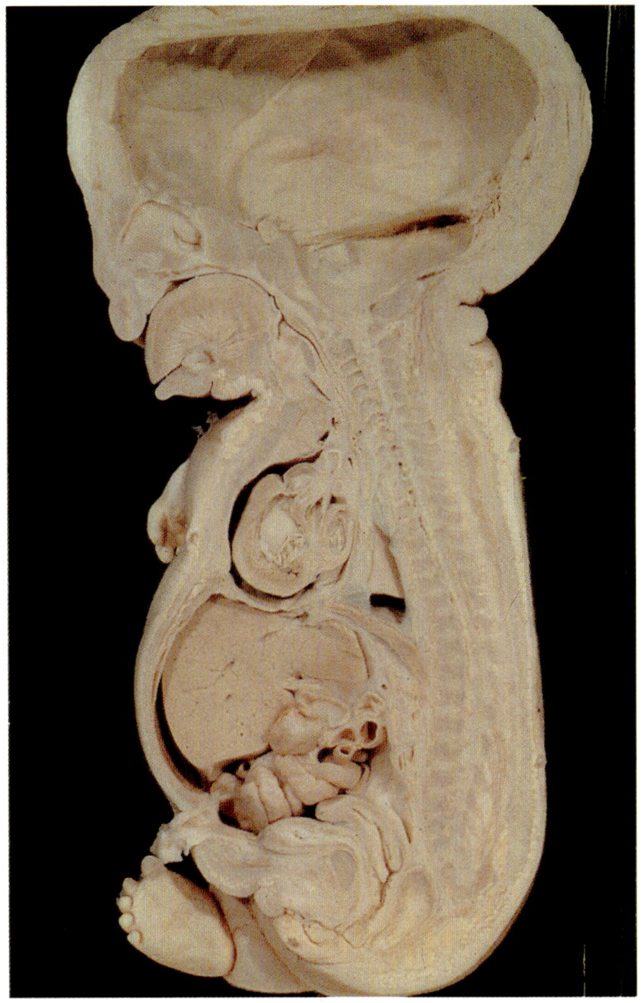

Figure 10.21 Photograph of a sagittal section through a female stillborn with achondroplasia. The limbs are stunted and the base of the skull is shortened. Even at this stage, there is some thoracolumbar kyphosis. (Courtesy of the Royal College of Surgeons of England)

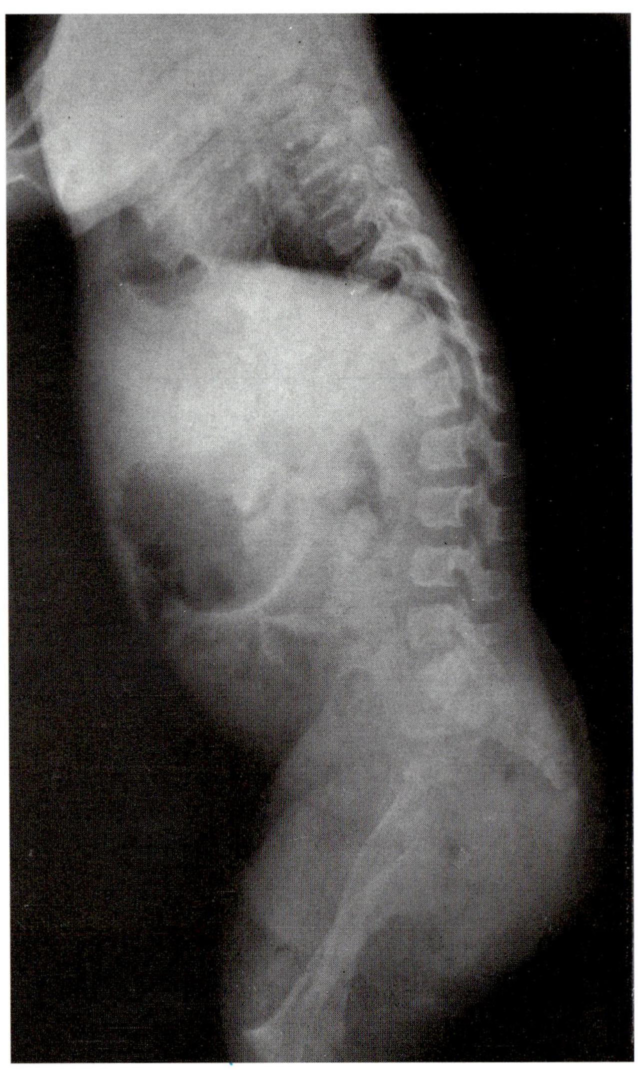

Figure 10.22 Lateral radiograph of an adolescent boy with achondroplasia. Note the disproportionate lengths of the femora and the trunk, and the thoracolumbar kyphosis.

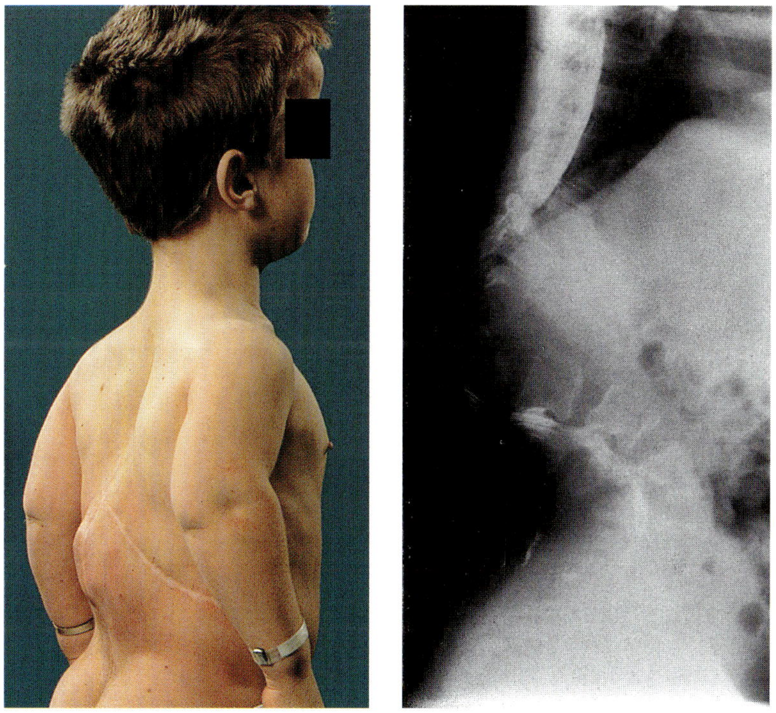

Figure 10.23 Clinical photograph (*left*) of an adolescent boy with achrondroplasia and thoracolumbar kyphosis, who presented with signs of spinal cord compression. Note the increased lumbar lordosis and the presence of surgical scars following stabilization. A lateral radiograph (*right*) of the same patient demonstrates the thoracolumbar kyphosis due to multiple hemivertebrae. Note the obstruction of dye in the thecal sac at the apex of one curve. (Courtesy of Dr. David S. Bradford)

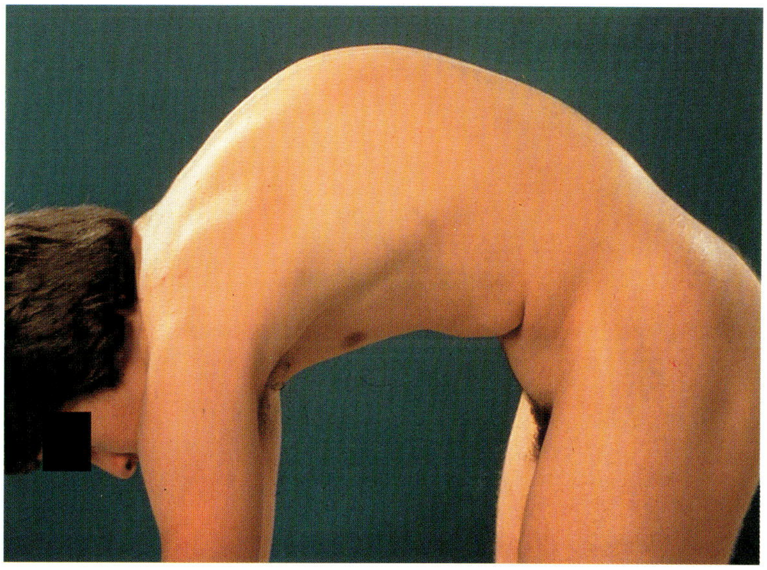

Figure 10.24 Clinical photograph of a 16-year-old boy with adolescent kyphosis. In this case, significant thoracic kyphosis has occurred as a result of Scheuermann's disease. (Courtesy of Dr. David S. Bradford)

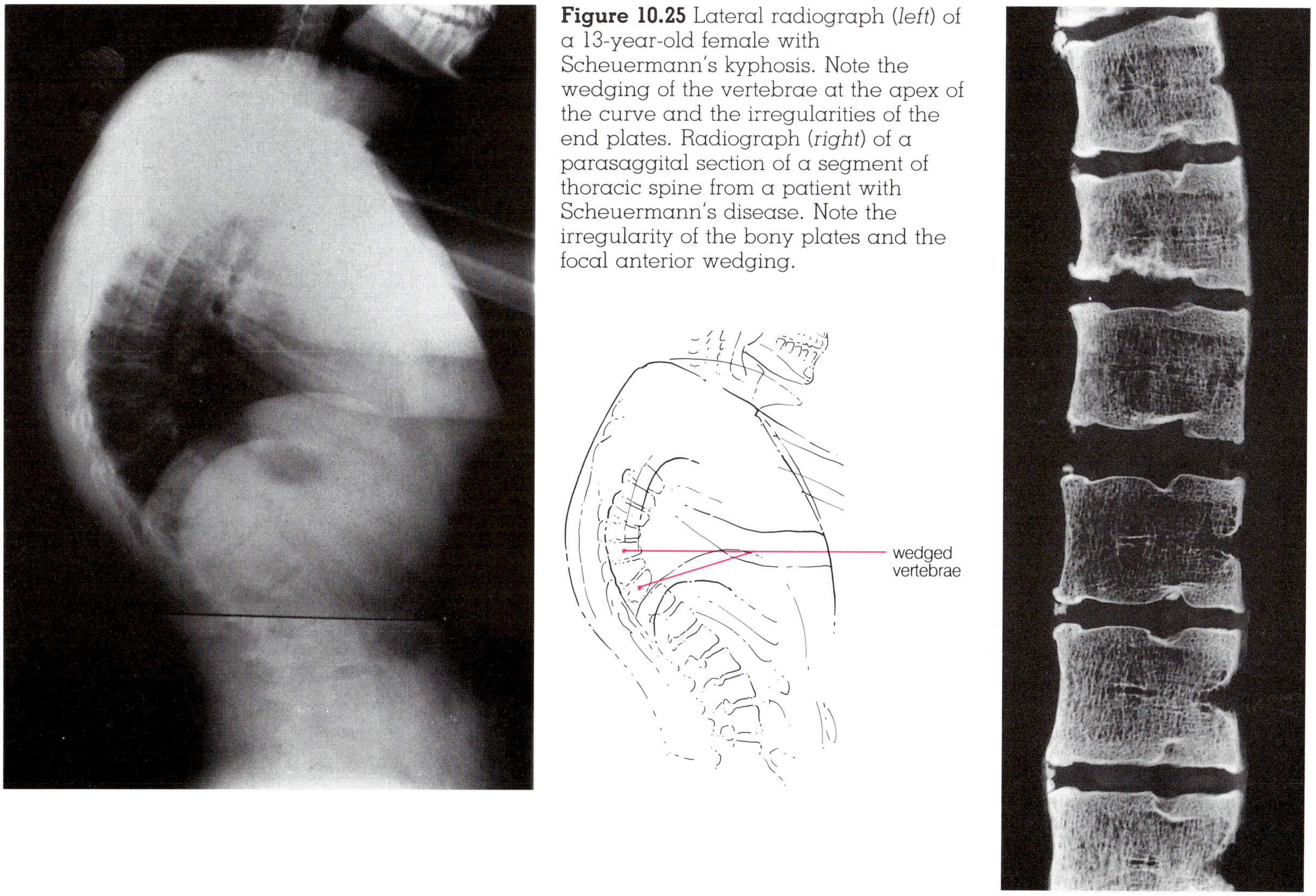

Figure 10.25 Lateral radiograph (*left*) of a 13-year-old female with Scheuermann's kyphosis. Note the wedging of the vertebrae at the apex of the curve and the irregularities of the end plates. Radiograph (*right*) of a parasaggital section of a segment of thoracic spine from a patient with Scheuermann's disease. Note the irregularity of the bony plates and the focal anterior wedging.

fusion may result (Fig. 10.26). Concomitant with the above changes is an increase in the thoracic kyphosis (beyond 40 degrees), the magnitude of which is probably related to the extent of the disc prolapse and vertebral wedging.

Characteristic anatomical findings in Scheuermann's disease include alterations in the intervertebral disc, cartilaginous growth plates, and vertebral bodies. The intervertebral discs are narrowed and the cartilaginous end plates are irregularly thinned, with focal attenuations through which herniations of the intervertebral disc tissue extend into the adjacent vertebral body (Fig. 10.27). The narrowing of the disc is usually more pronounced anteriorly than it is posteriorly, resulting in interference with growth of the vertebral ring epiphysis.

Defects of the Pars Interarticularis

Spondylolysis, a defect in the pars interarticularis, in most cases is probably traumatic in origin. It is not present at birth and therefore does not constitute a congenital lesion. Spondylolysis more commonly is a lesion of childhood and early adult life, and often it is asymptomatic (Fig. 10.28). The reported incidence is 4 to 7%. A higher incidence among

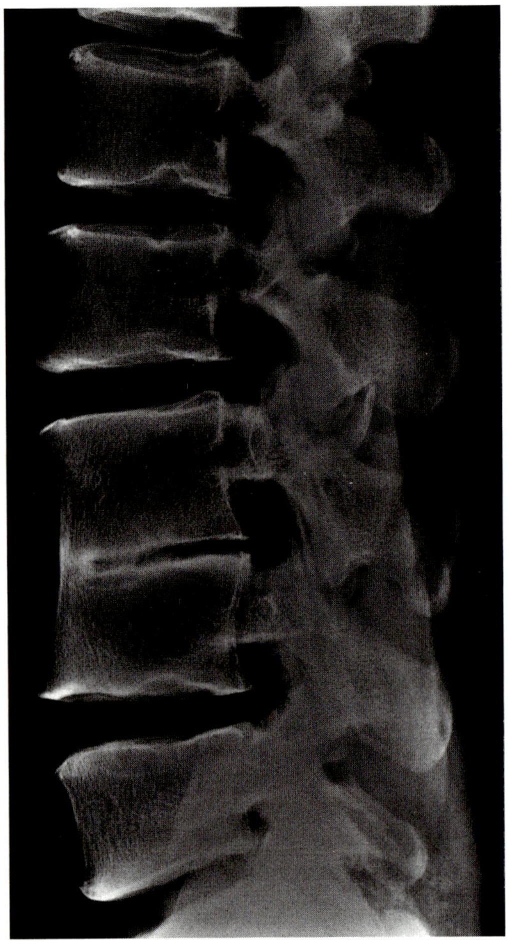

Figure 10.26 Lateral radiograph of the lumbar spine from the same case in Figure 10.25 shows anterior interbody fusion of L3-4.

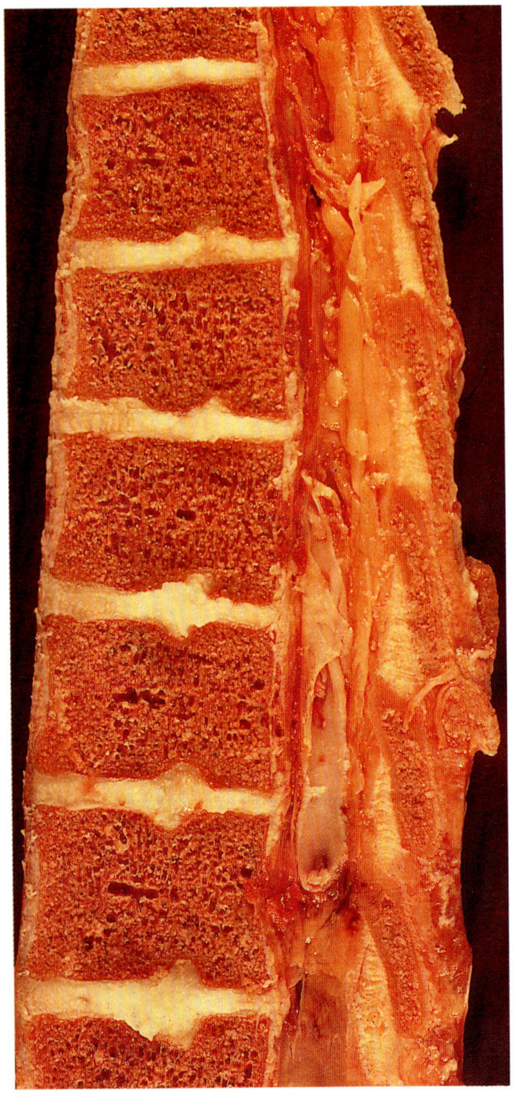

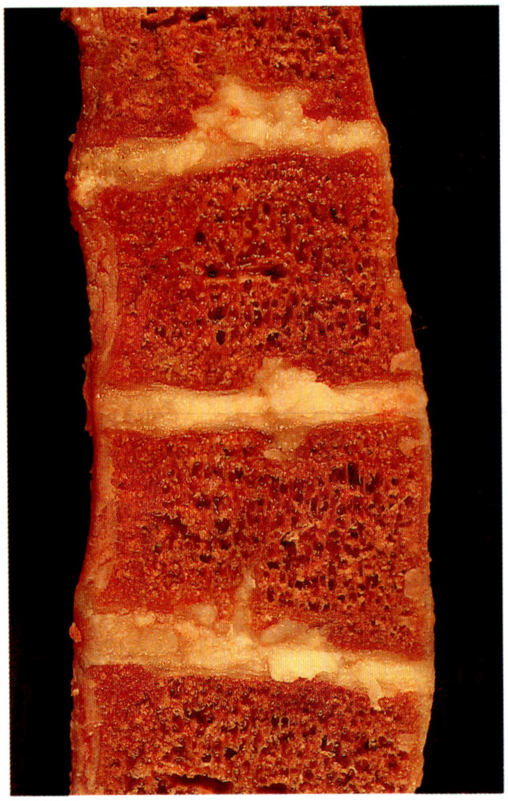

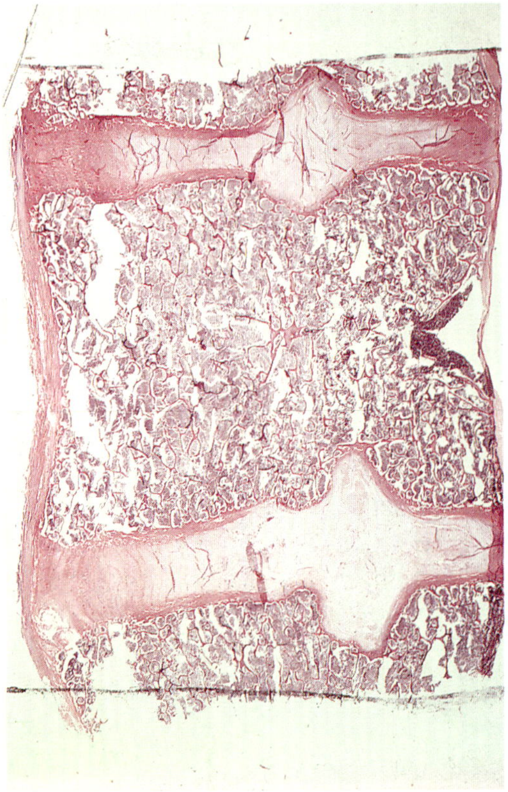

Figure 10.27 Photograph (*left*) of a sagittal section of the thoracic spine illustrated in Figures 10.25 and 10.26. Note the multiple Schmorl's nodes. An enlarged view (*center*) of a segment of the same spine demonstrates end-plate irregularities as well as herniation of the disc tissue into the adjacent vertebral bodies. A photomicrograph (*right*) of a histologic section from this specimen shows disc displacement into the adjacent bone. While the end plate is attenuated, it appears to be continuous around the displaced disc tissue. This appearance is in contrast to the isolated Schmorl's nodes seen in older individuals, in which the end plate is violated.

family members (26%) was reported by Wiltse (1962). However, this may be due to environmental factors such as the occurrence of spondylolysis in athletic children of athletic parents. A high incidence is reported among the Eskimos (18 to 56%), in whom a rugged icy terrain and numerous falls have been implicated as significant causative factors.

The lesion of spondylolysis may be unilateral or bilateral, with the highest incidence at L-5. Almost all of the remaining cases may be accounted for by L-4 and L-3. Its preponderance in the lowest lumbar level supports the notion that gravity, the upright posture, lordosis, and transition from mobility to fixity are factors in the etiology of this disease. It is interesting to note that spina bifida is found to be six times more common in patients with spondylolysis than in the general population. It is possible that spina bifida, with its concomitant ligamentous inadequacy, contributes to excessive local pivotal strains across the pars of the affected vertebra.

The presence of callus has been demonstrated in unilateral cases, suggesting that the remaining intact pars provides a certain measure of stability. On the other hand, bilateral defects generally show fibrous union or pseudarthroses. Radiographically, oblique projections of the lumbar spine are most useful in identifying a defect or callous formation, which in such views is seen as the collar of the "Scottie dog" (Fig. 10.29). Occa-

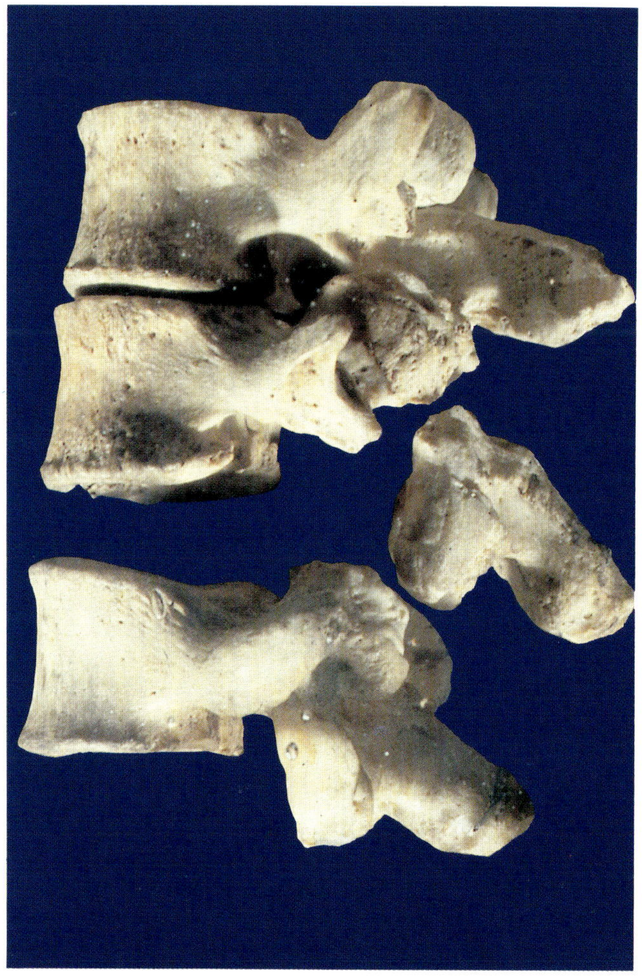

Figure 10.28 Photograph of a lateral view of a macerated segment of lumbar spine to show a defect of the pars interarticularis of the middle vertebra. (Courtesy of the Royal College of Surgeons of England)

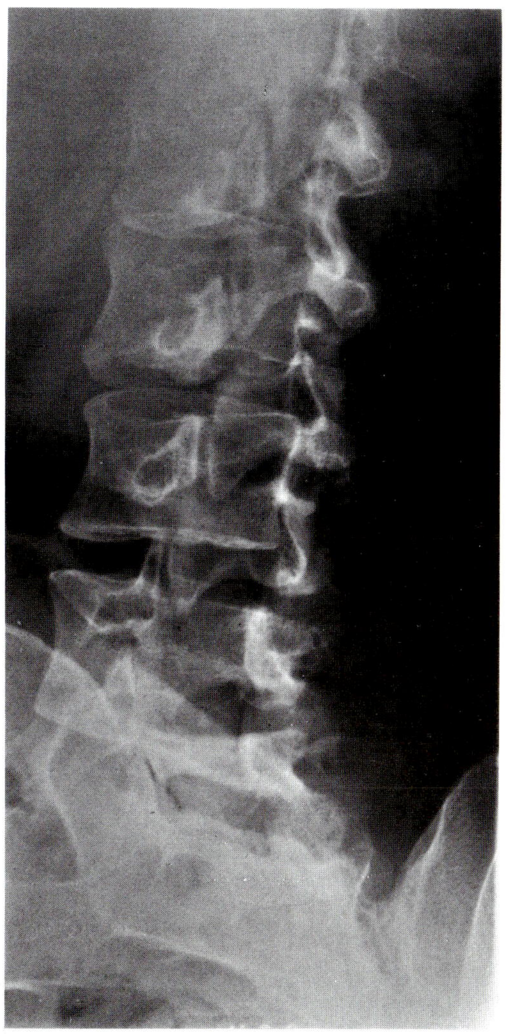

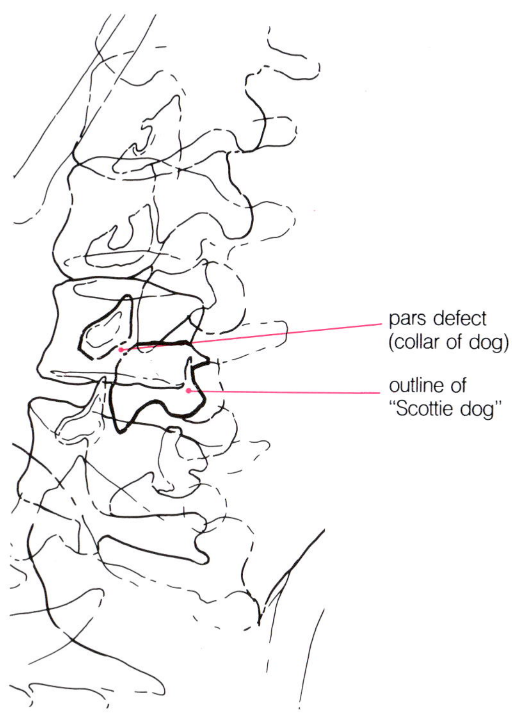

Figure 10.29 Clinical radiograph of an oblique projection of the lumbar spine of a young adult to demonstrate a pars defect at L-3. The projection of the "Scottie dog" is shown in the accompanying line drawing.

sionally, the defect in the pars may lead to instability, with degenerative changes in the intervertebral disc and slippage of one vertebra on the subjacent one (true spondylolisthesis). The resulting spondylolisthes is can be graded as follows:

Grade 1: 0 to 25%
Grade 2: 25 to 50%
Grade 3: 50 to 75%
Grade 4: 75 to 100%

When the slippage is complete (spondyloptosis), severe deformity and neurologic deficit may result (Figs. 10.30 through 10.32).

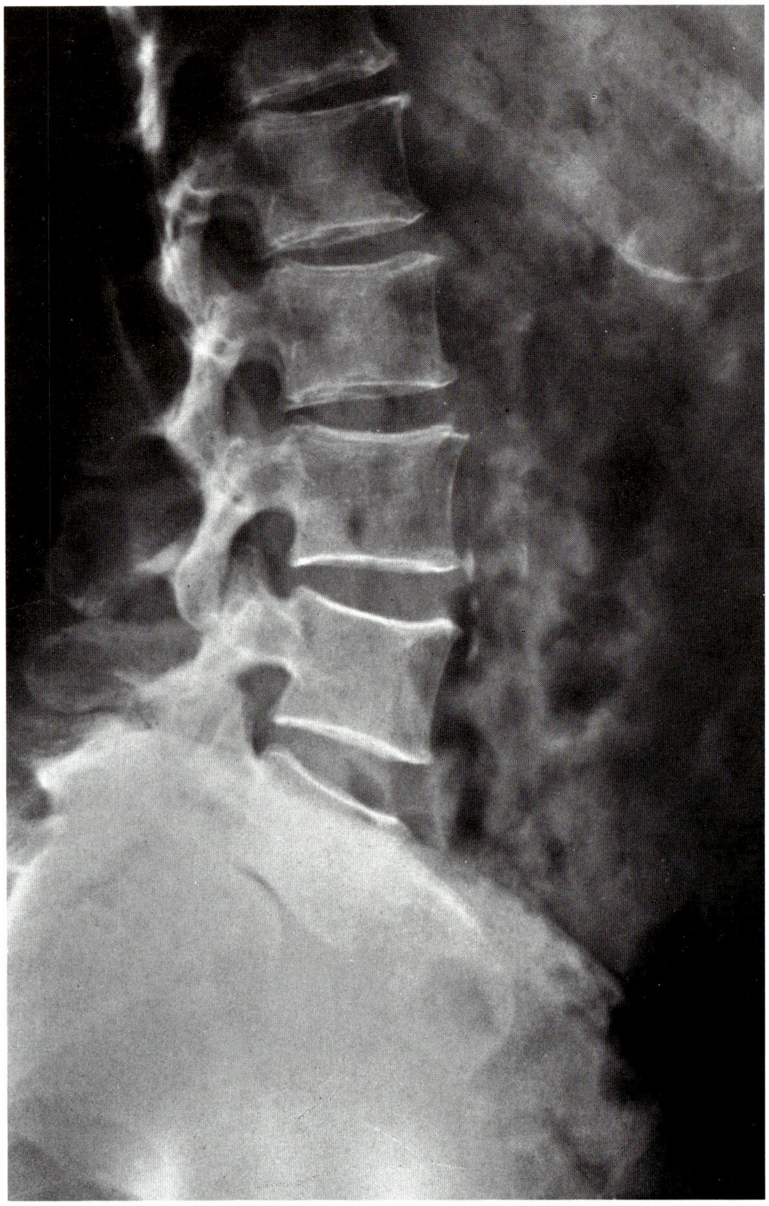

Figure 10.30 Lateral radiograph (*top*) of the lumbar spine to demonstrate spondylolytic spondylolisthesis at L-5 to S-1. This is grade-2 spondylolisthesis. A table (*bottom*) illustrates the four different grades of spondylolisthesis.

GRADES OF SPONDYLOLISTHESIS*

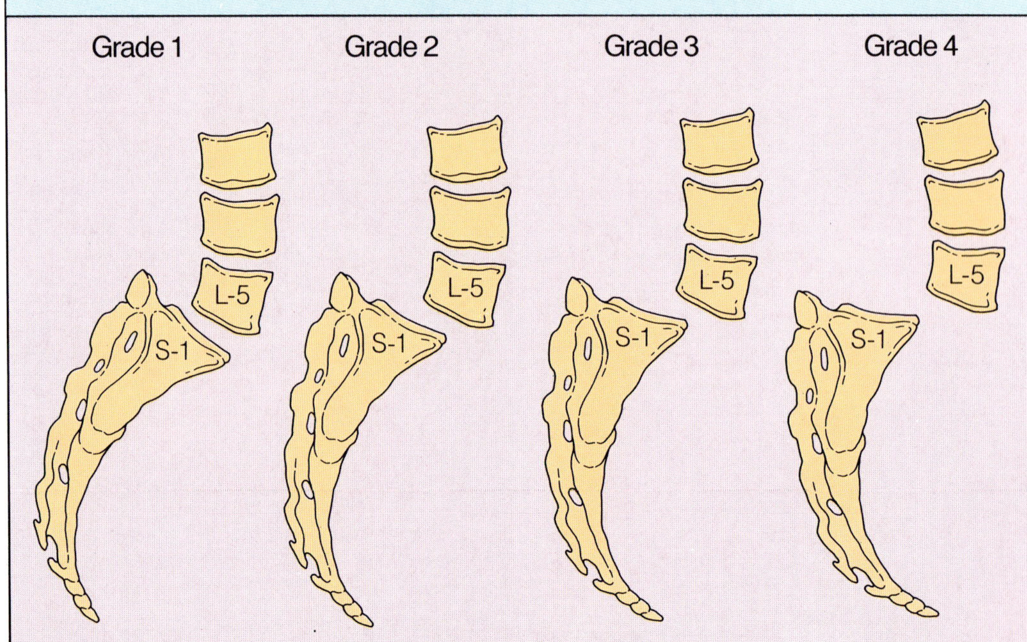

*Note the vertical disposition of the sacrum (sacral inclination) with progressive slippage.

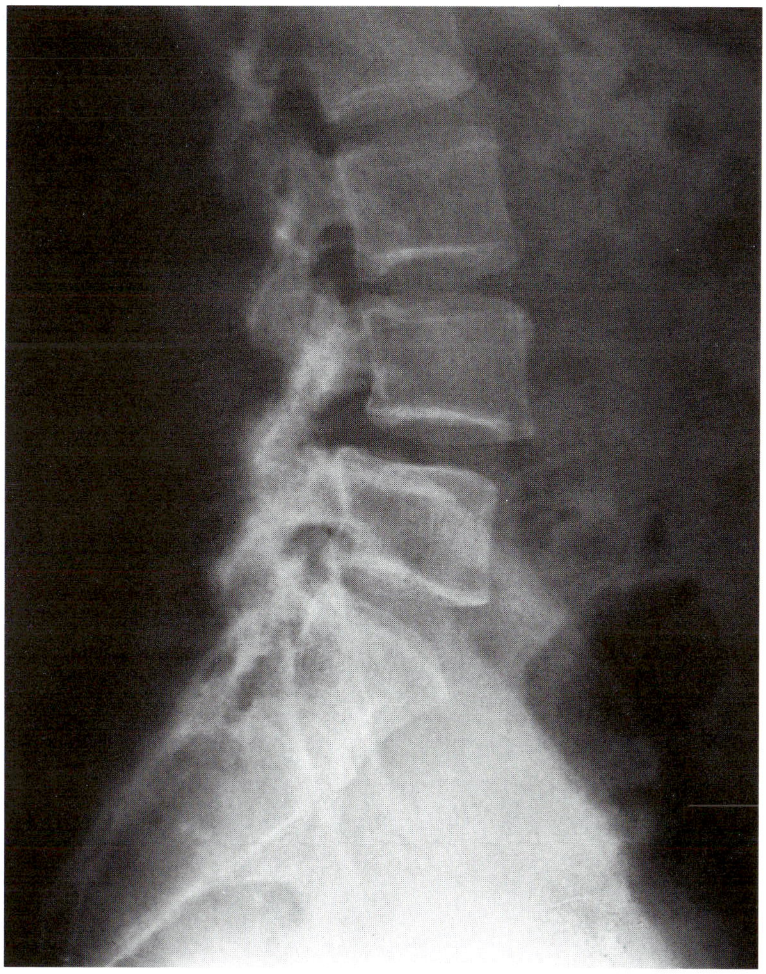

Figure 10.31 Lateral radiograph of the lumbosacral spine to demonstrate L4-5 spondylolisthesis.

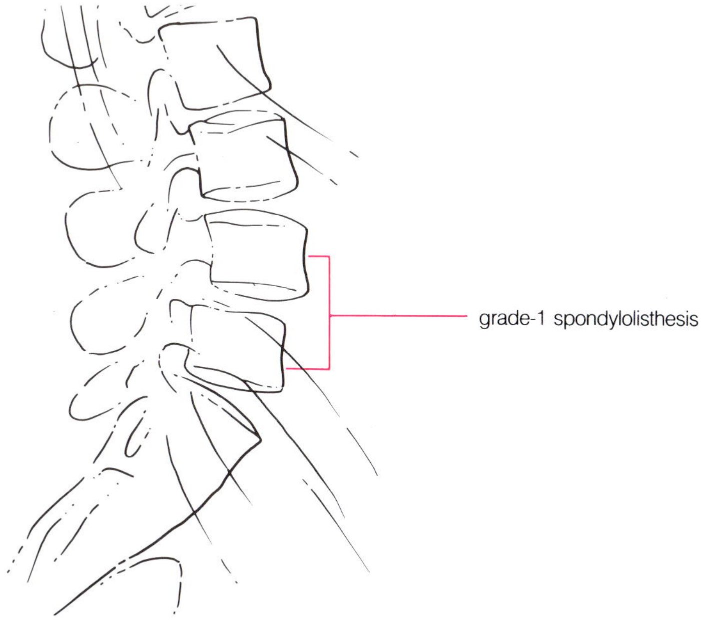

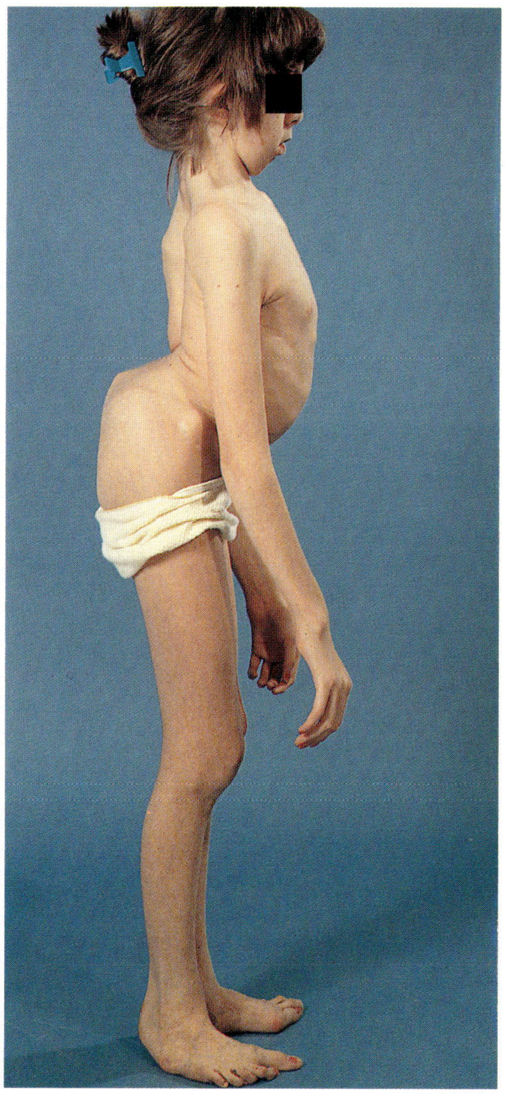

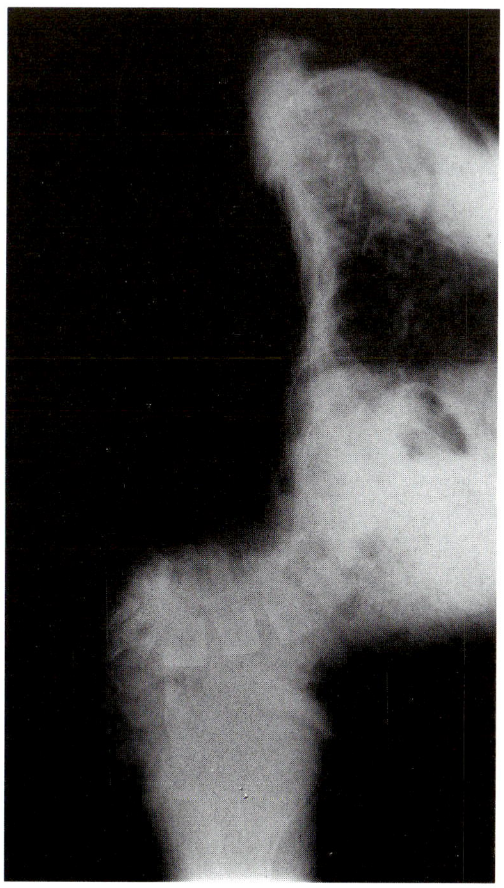

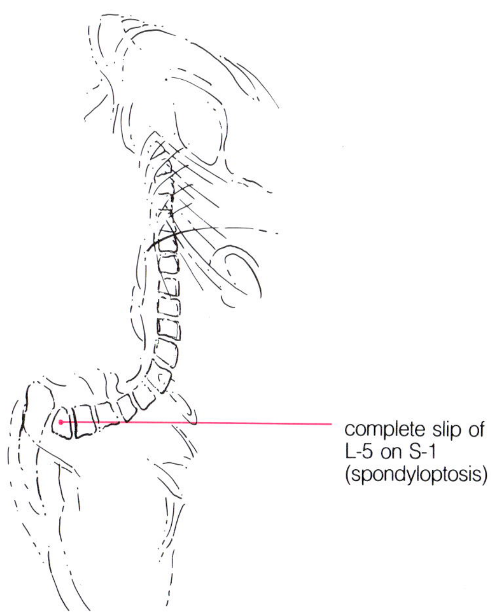

Figure 10.32 Clinical photograph (*left*) of a 17-year-old female with severe spondylolisthesis. The trunk has moved forward and downward in relation to the pelvis. In the lateral radiograph (*right*), there is a complete slip of L-5 on S-1. The thoracolumbar spine shows hyperlordosis and the sacrum is vertical. (Courtesy of Dr. David S. Bradford)

11

CHAPTER

METABOLIC AND HEMATOLOGIC DISEASES OF THE SPINE

INTRODUCTION

The skeleton serves two purposes. Its first purpose is a mechanical one, providing support and movement (see Section 1, Chapter 3); its second purpose is the central role that it plays in the maintenance of calcium homeostasis. Since its mechanical and supportive functions depend on the presence of an organized matrix, it is evident that the formation and deposition by the cells of an adequate amount of collagen, proteoglycan, and calcium are essential. Calcium homeostasis, which is under the control of the endocrine system (in particular, through the actions of parathormone, calcitonin, and vitamin D), requires not only the normal functioning of the endocrine system but also of its target organs, especially the intestines, kidneys, and bone.

Disturbances in bone structure may result from the formation of a defective matrix, as occurs with disturbances in collagen synthesis, proteoglycan synthesis, or calcium deposition; or, they may result from disturbances in the rates of bone formation and/or resorption, as occurs in hyperparathyroidism, osteoporosis, and Paget's disease.

Bone formation is effected by the osteoblasts, which synthesize the organic matrix made up of type I collagen and an assortment of noncollagenous proteins, including sulfated mucopolysaccharides. The osteoblasts also control calcification of the organic matrix. Bone resorption, on the other hand, is effected by the osteoclasts, cells which are able to digest the calcified matrix of the bone. The physiologic maintenance of a normal skeleton depends on the balanced activity of these two cell types. Both osteoblasts and osteoclasts are under the influence of feedback mechanisms, which maintain a mechanically functioning skeleton as well as calcium homeostasis. When one of these systems is affected by a pathologic process, the other is likely to be affected also. In Paget's disease, for example, an increase in osteoclast activity primarily affects structural homeostasis. However, in addition, there also is an increased amount of calcium released into the bloodstream. Similarly, in primary hyperparathyroidism, which results in a disturbance of calcium homeostasis, the skeleton also is structurally weakened because of the increased bone resorption and remodeling.

Since the hematopoietic tissue is lodged in the bone, bone disease also may result from conditions that primarily affect the hematologic system. In thalassemia for example, because of the hemolysis, there is a marked increase in the amount of bone marrow, as a result of erythroid hyperplasia. This results in displacement of the cancellous bone by the bone marrow and in secondary osteoporosis, which in turn, is likely to manifest clinically as fractures.

In the present chapter, we will discuss firstly those diseases that occur as a result of a structurally defective matrix; secondly, those that result from disturbances in bone remodeling; and, finally, those that are the result of hematologic disturbances.

DISEASES RESULTING FROM A STRUCTURALLY DEFECTIVE MATRIX

THE MUCOPOLYSACCHARIDOSES

The mucopolysaccharidoses are a group of conditions that occur as a result of abnormalities of mucopolysaccharide metabolism. They have been divided into various types, numbered I to VII, depending on the particular enzyme deficiency involved. In many of the mucopolysaccharidoses, a defect in the metabolism of the particular substance involved results in its widespread deposition and storage in histiocytes throughout the body. Since the mucopolysaccharides are widely distributed throughout the body, it is not surprising that these diseases are characterized by multi-organ involvement.

The mucopolysaccharides play a particularly important role in the composition and thus in the structural integrity of cartilage. Therefore, since most of the skeleton is preformed in cartilage, many of the mucopolysaccharidoses are marked by developmental abnormalities in the skeleton, particularly disproportionate growth and misshapen bones. The two common forms of mucopolysaccharidosis seen in the spine are Morquio's disease (MPS IV) and Hurler's syndrome (MPS I).

In Morquio's disease, children show characteristic deformities of the vertebral bodies, with occasional hemivertebrae giving rise to spinal deformities (Figs. 11.1 and 11.2). In addition, there are marked abnormalities at the epiphysial ends of the long bones, which, later in life, lead to arthritic changes. In contrast, Hurler's syndrome is characterized chiefly by mental retardation, dermatologic, and cardiovascular disease. Although there may be some retardation of skeletal growth, rarely is it severe. The vertebral bodies appear relatively normal, although patients frequently have a kyphotic deformity resulting from a malformation of at least one vertebral body, usually T-12 or L-1 (Fig. 11.3). In Hurler's syndrome, the vertebral column does not show a general wedging of the vertebral bodies, as it does in Morquio's disease. Also, unlike Morquio's disease, patients with Hurler's syndrome progress rapidly, and most die within the first decade of life.

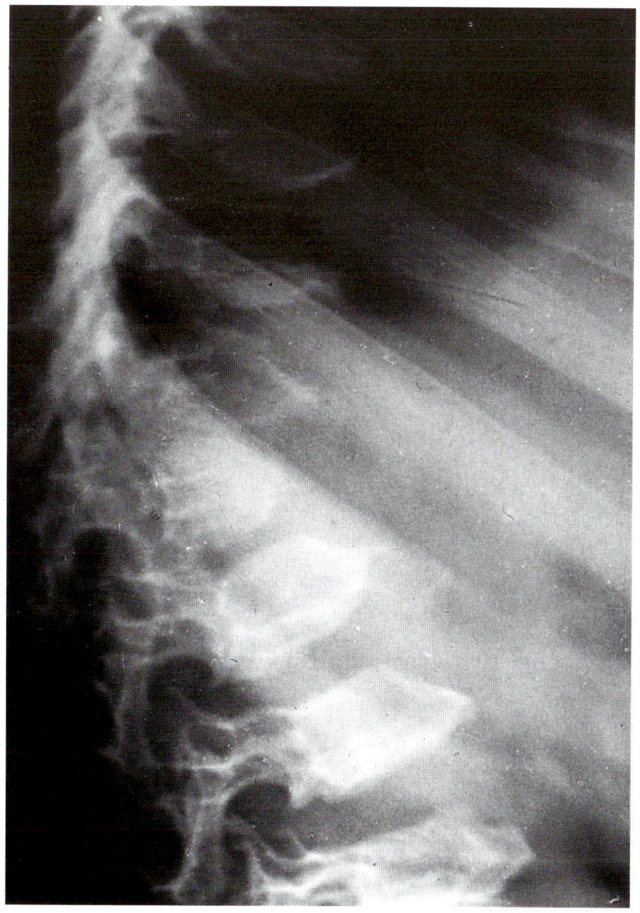

Figure 11.1 Lateral radiograph of the thoracolumbar spine in a 17-year-old girl with Morquio's disease, showing the typical tongue-like extensions of the anterior margins of the vertebral bodies. There also is a hemivertebra, which in this case has given rise to a thoracolumbar kyphosis—a typical occurrence in these patients.

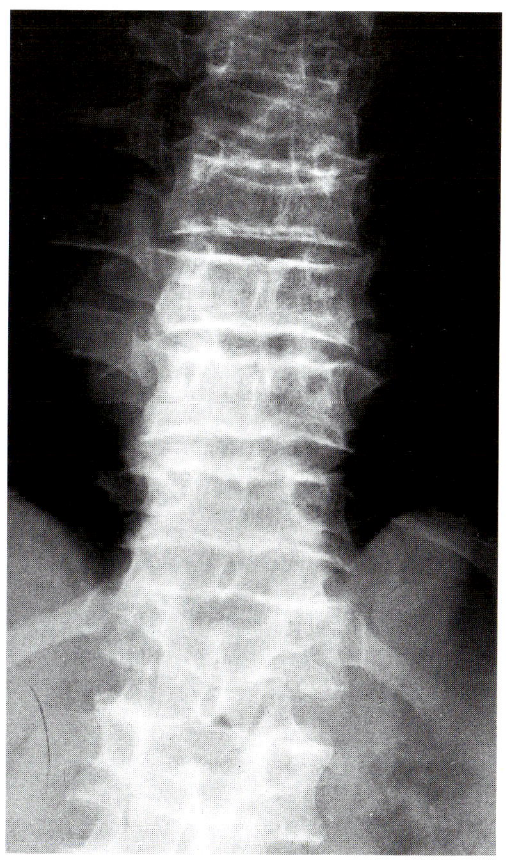

Figure 11.2 AP radiograph of the thoracolumbar spine in a young adult with Morquio's disease. Note the flattening of the vertebral bodies and early degenerative changes in the discs.

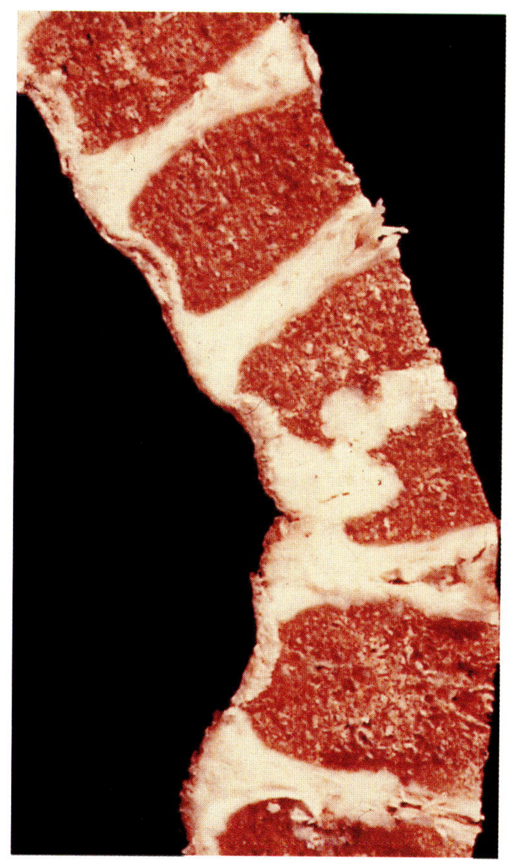

Figure 11.3 Photograph of a portion of the thoracolumbar spine in a patient with Hurler's syndrome showing a hemivertebra at the level of T-12. The vertebra above is also slightly deformed on its inferior surface, though the remaining vertebrae in this photograph appear to be within normal limits. (Courtesy of Dr. James W. Milgram)

COLLAGEN DISEASES

Disturbances in collagen synthesis and in collagen fiber formation may either be genetically determined, as in osteogenesis imperfecta, Ehlers-Danlos syndrome, and Marfan's syndrome, or they may be acquired, as in scurvy and lathyrism. The genetic disturbances in particular are likely to give rise to profound structural abnormalities and diffuse osteoporosis.

The most common genetically determined disturbance in collagen production is that seen in osteogenesis imperfecta. In this disease, there is a quantitative deficiency in collagen production, and very possibly a qualitative disturbance in the organization of the collagen molecule itself. The condition is seen either as a severe crippling disease without family history, or, more commonly, as a familial disease of varying severity. In any case, patients generally are severely osteoporotic and almost all show some degree of spinal deformity due to multiple fractures secondary to osteoporosis (Figs. 11.4 through 11.8).

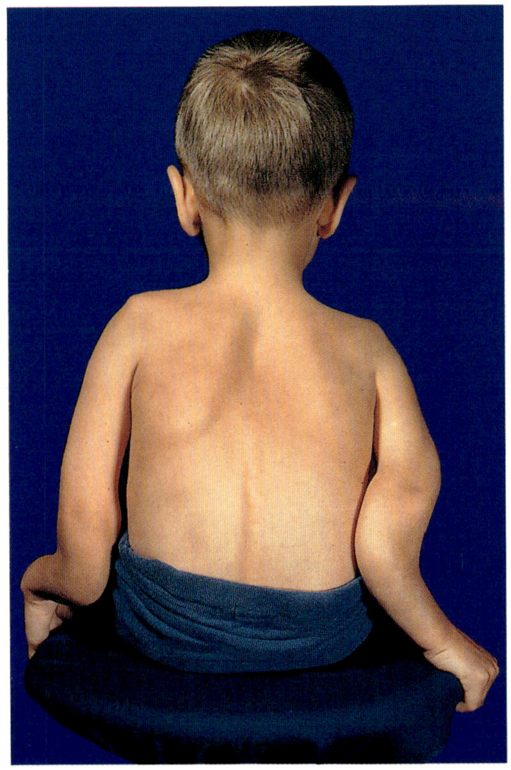

Figure 11.4 Clinical photograph of a young child with a congenital form of osteogenesis imperfecta. This photograph shows severe deformities of both arms, and a mild scoliosis with increased kyphosis at the thoracolumbar junction. In general, although all children with osteogenesis imperfecta have some spinal deformities, rarely are they severe on clinical examination.

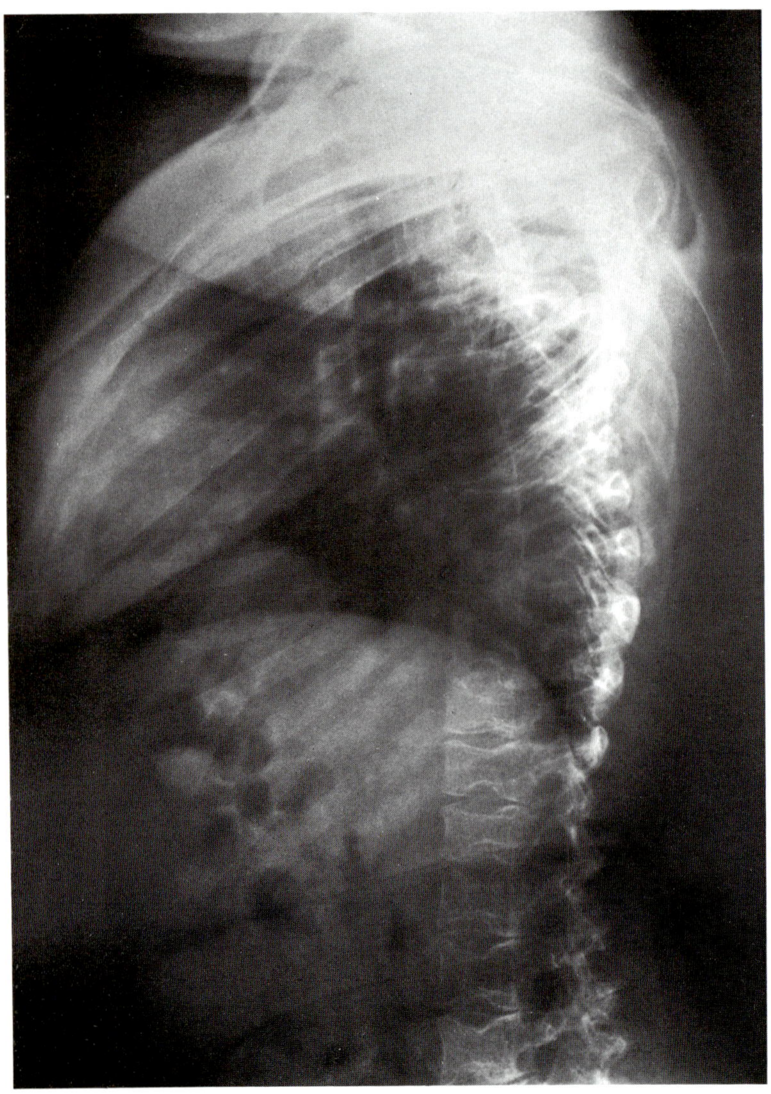

Figure 11.5 Lateral radiograph of a patient with the tarda form of osteogenesis imperfecta, showing generalized osteoporosis and collapse of most of the vertebral bodies leading to fish-mouth deformities. The spine is hypokyphotic.

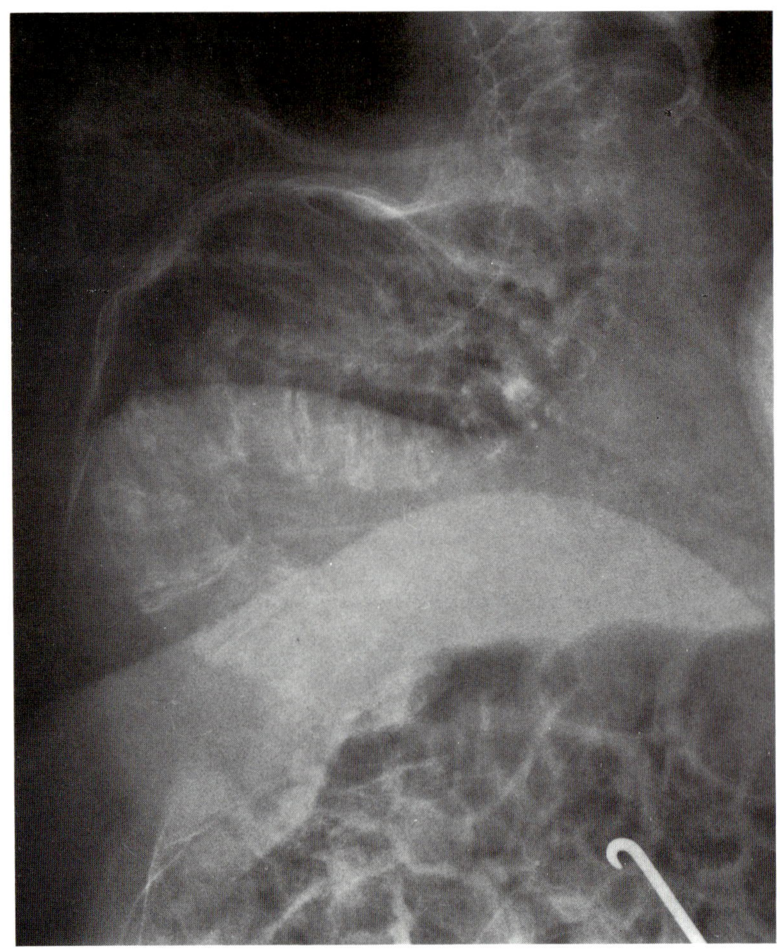

Figure 11.6 AP radiograph of an adolescent girl with severe osteogenesis imperfecta. There is a severe spinal deformity and marked osteopenia.

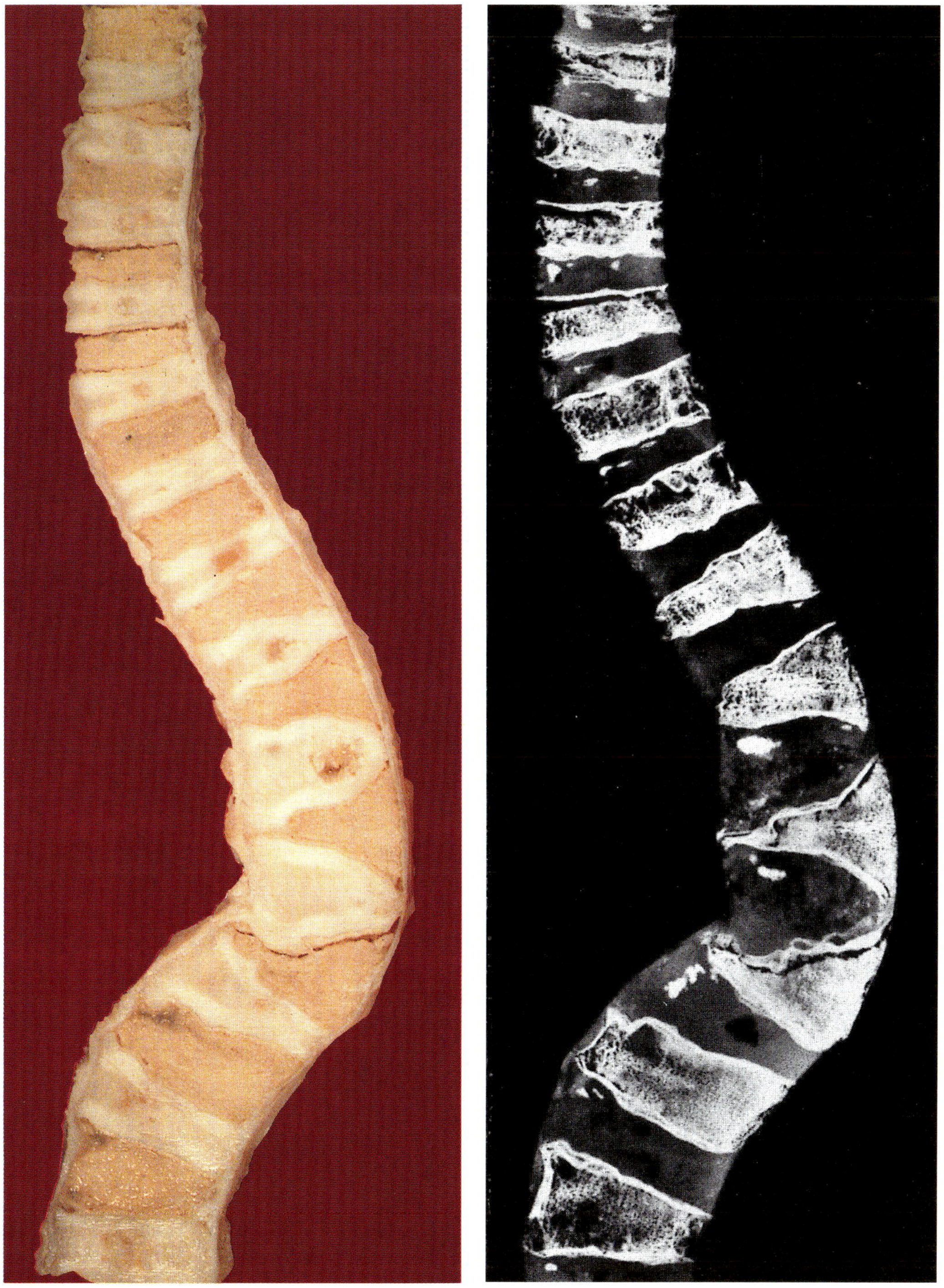

Figure 11.7 Photograph (*left*) of a coronal section through the spine of a patient with osteogenesis imperfecta, showing some scoliosis secondary to multiple compression fractures. The compression fractures, resulting in vertebral wedging, can be seen in the accompanying specimen radiograph (*right*).

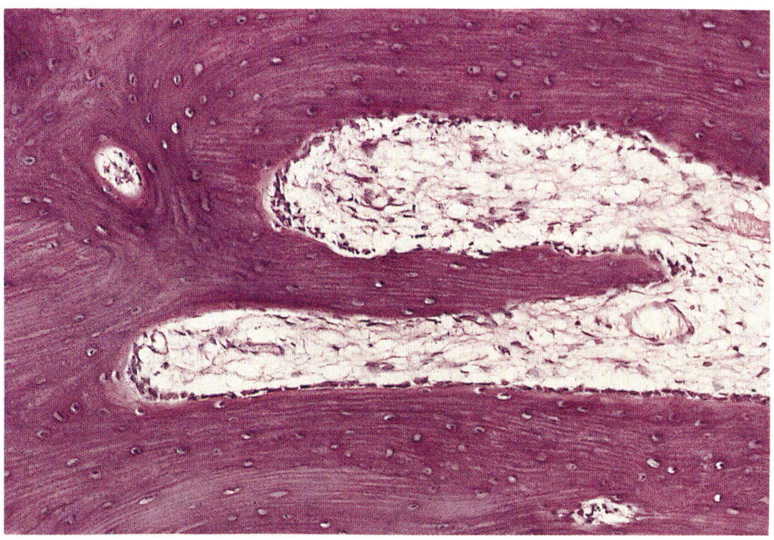

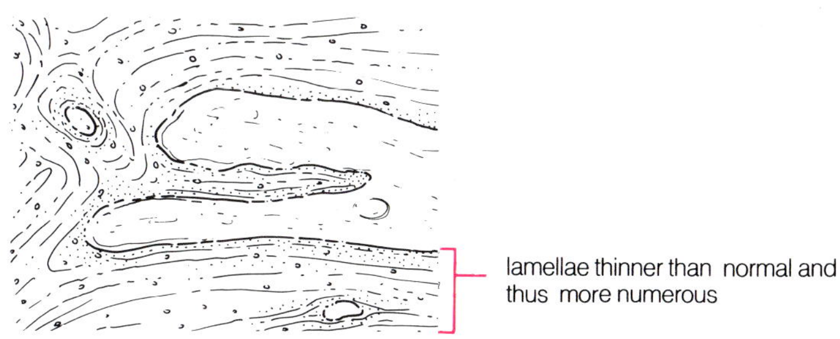

Figure 11.8 Photomicrograph of a specimen from a patient with osteogenesis imperfecta. Note the increased number of osteocytes per unit area of bone, together with a fine lamellar pattern. This appearance of hypercellularity and finely packed lamellae is characteristic of osteogenesis imperfecta.

In type VI Ehlers-Danlos syndrome, which is due to a lysyl hydroxylase deficiency that results in a disturbance in collagen fibril formation, there is severe osteoporosis as well as ligamentous laxity of a severe degree (Fig. 11.9). As a result, patients have a kyphoscoliosis, which worsens during adolescence and ends in severe spinal curvature with pulmonary embarrassment (Fig. 11.10). In Marfan's syndrome, the fundamental defect is unknown, although it almost certainly involves an abnormality of collagen production. Here, the severe ligamentous laxity that characterizes the disease frequently leads to severe scoliosis (Figs. 11.11 and 11.12).

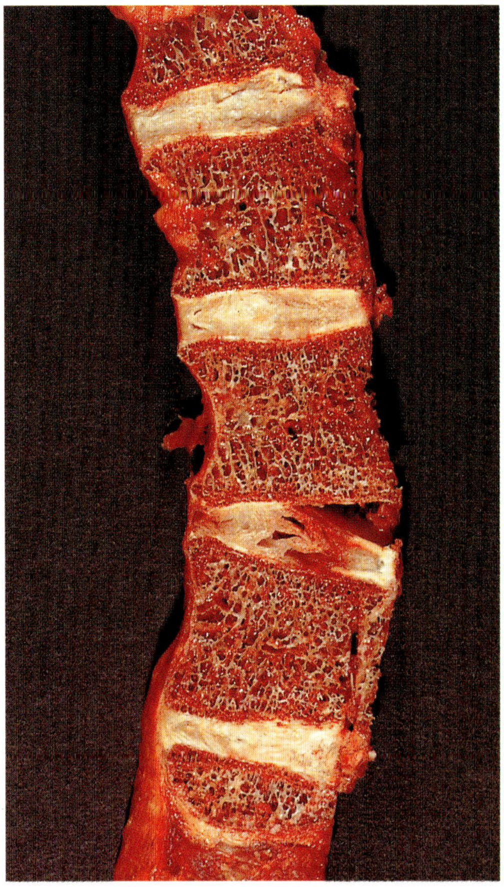

Figure 11.9 Photograph of a coronal section through a segment of lumbar spine from a 30-year-old male with Ehlers-Danlos syndrome. Severe osteoporosis is seen, with accentuation of the vertebral trabeculae.

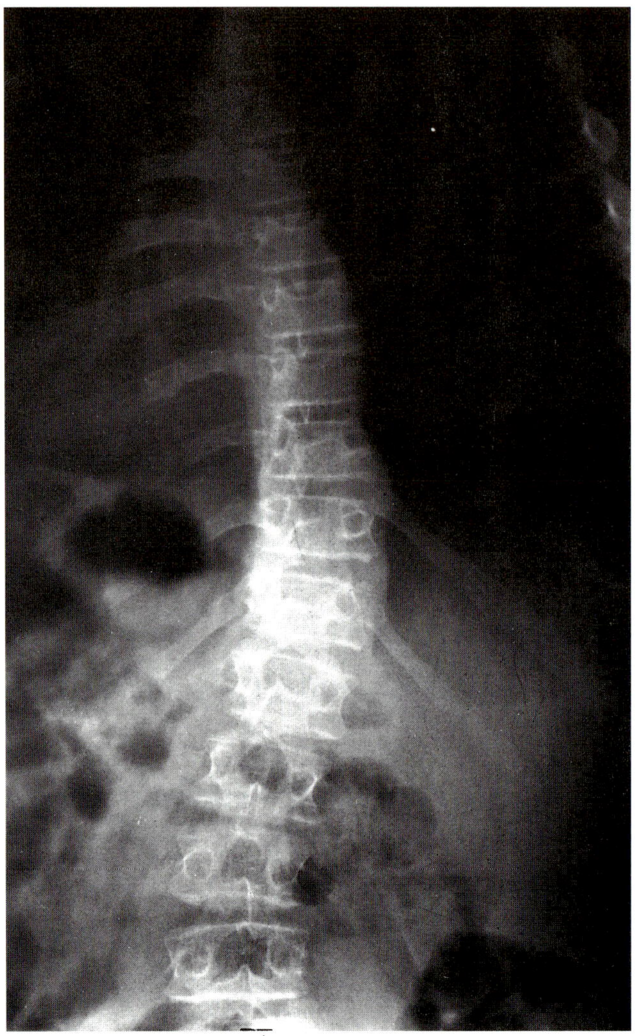

Figure 11.10 AP radiograph of a young adult with Ehlers-Danlos syndrome. The bone is markedly osteopenic, and there is a mild scoliosis with some rotational deformity.

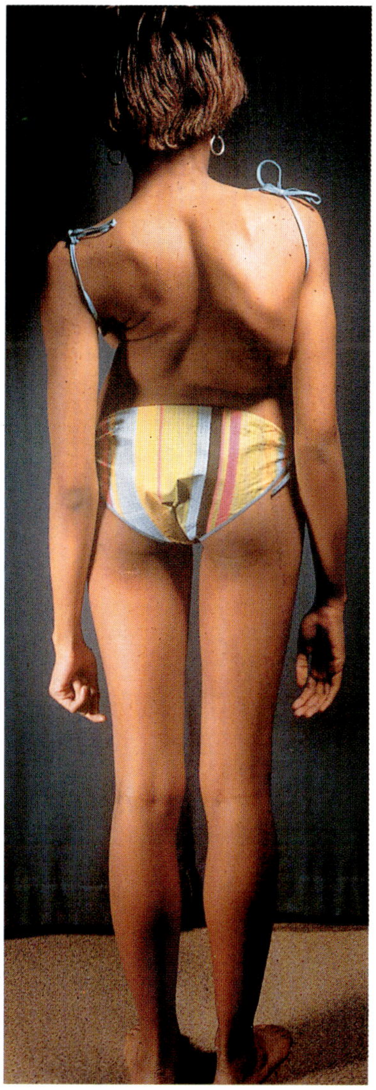

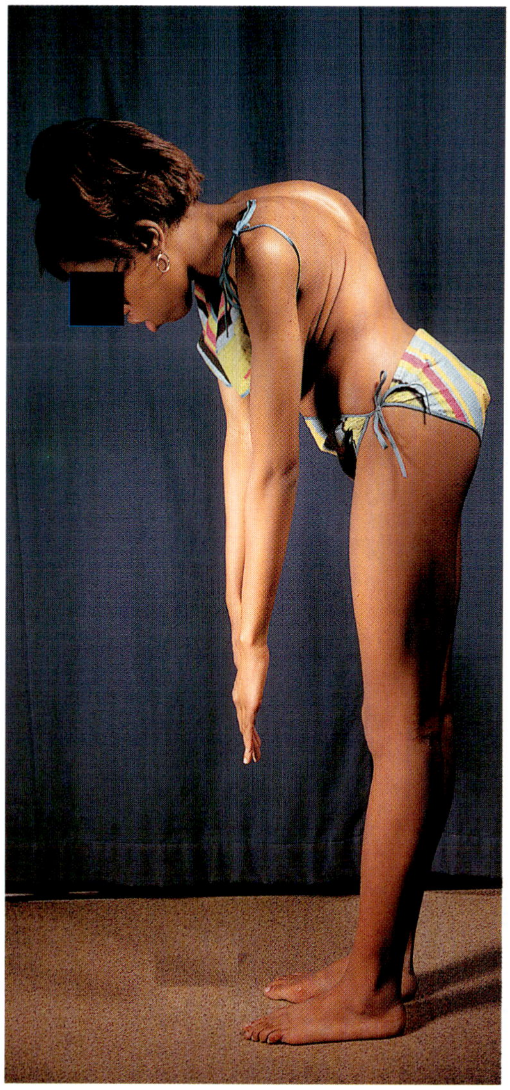

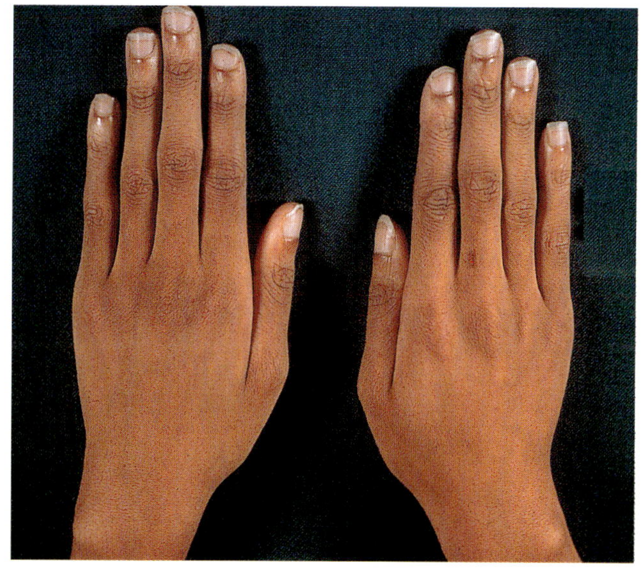

Figure 11.11 Clinical photograph (*left*) of an adolescent female with Marfan's syndrome in posterior view, showing a severe spinal deformity. In profile (*center*), the severity of the kyphosis becomes apparent. The hands in this patient (*right*) show the typical elongated fingers (arachnodactyly) associated with Marfan's syndrome. (Courtesy of Dr. David Levine)

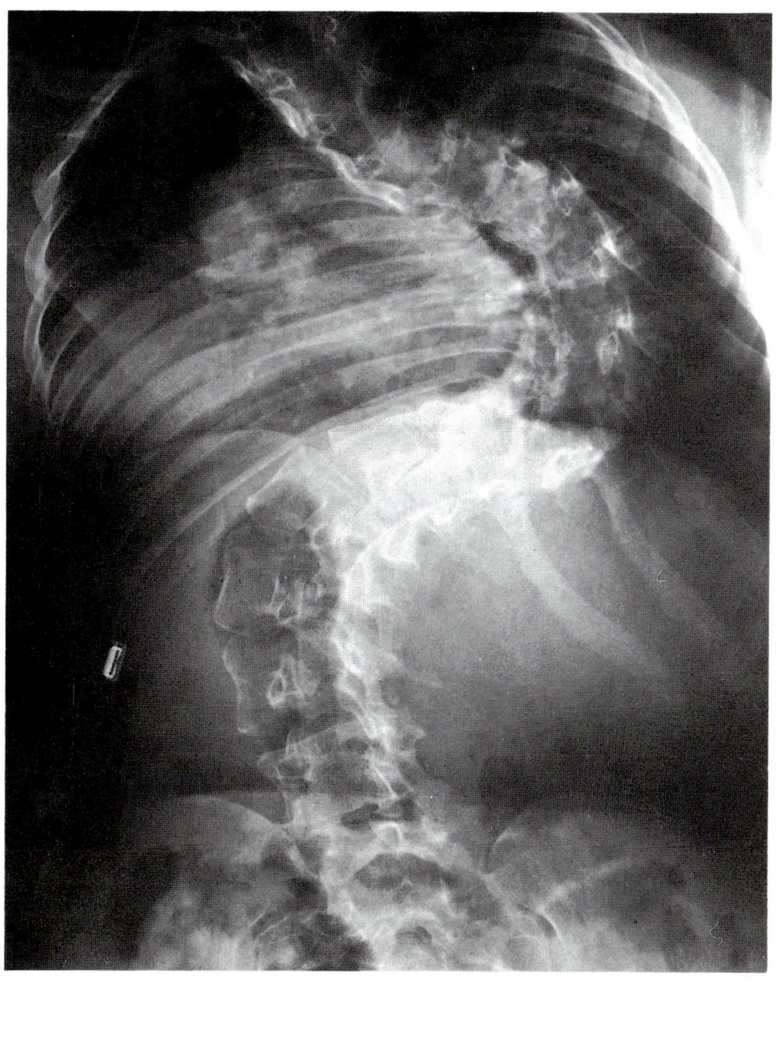

Figure 11.12 AP radiograph of the patient in Figure 11.11 demonstrates the severity of the spinal deformity.

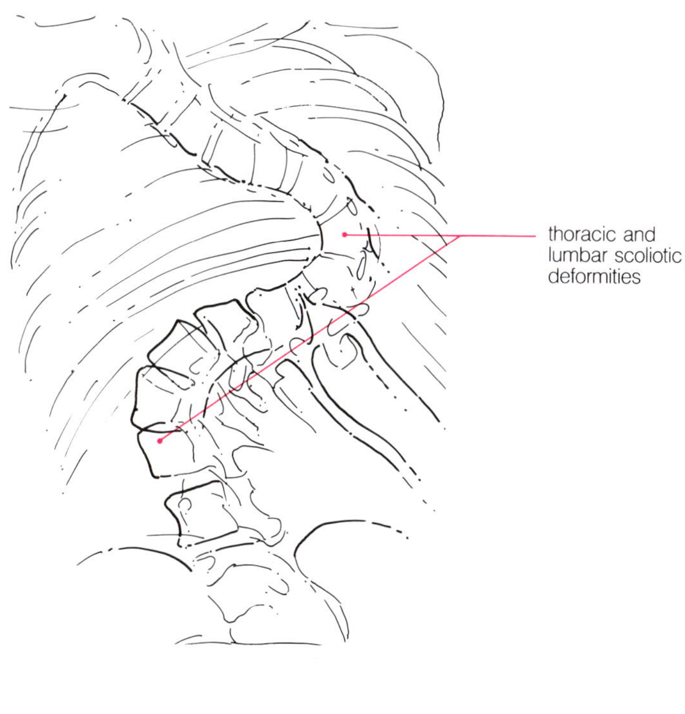

DISTURBANCES IN CALCIFICATION

Disturbances in calcification may be inherited or acquired. An example of an inherited calcification disturbance is that of hypophosphatasemia, in which there is an inborn deficiency of the enzyme alkaline phosphatase. Children with hypophosphatasemia fail to calcify their skeletons adequately, and thus present with clinical manifestations resembling those seen in rickets (Figs. 11.13 and 11.14). Very rarely, individuals are seen who have hyperphosphatasemia, with an overabundance of alkaline phosphatase, and in such cases the skeleton is overabundant and shows a fluffy excessive calcification. This appearance has been referred to as juvenile Paget's disease, though mistakenly, since the mechanisms in hyperphosphatasemia are totally different from those seen in adult Paget's disease.

The most common cause of an acquired disturbance in calcification, leading to inadequately mineralized bone tissue, is that of disturbed calcium metabolism due to a deficiency in active vitamin D (1,25-dihydrocalciferol). Such a deficit may be nutritional or it may be metabolic, due to a disturbance in the pathway of vitamin D metabolism in the liver or kidney (Fig. 11.15). A lack of dietary calcium, or the presence of bowel dysfunction leading to defective calcium absorption, may lead to the same condition. In children, the disease is generally referred to as rickets (Fig. 11.16), while in adults it is referred to as osteomalacia. Spinal deform-

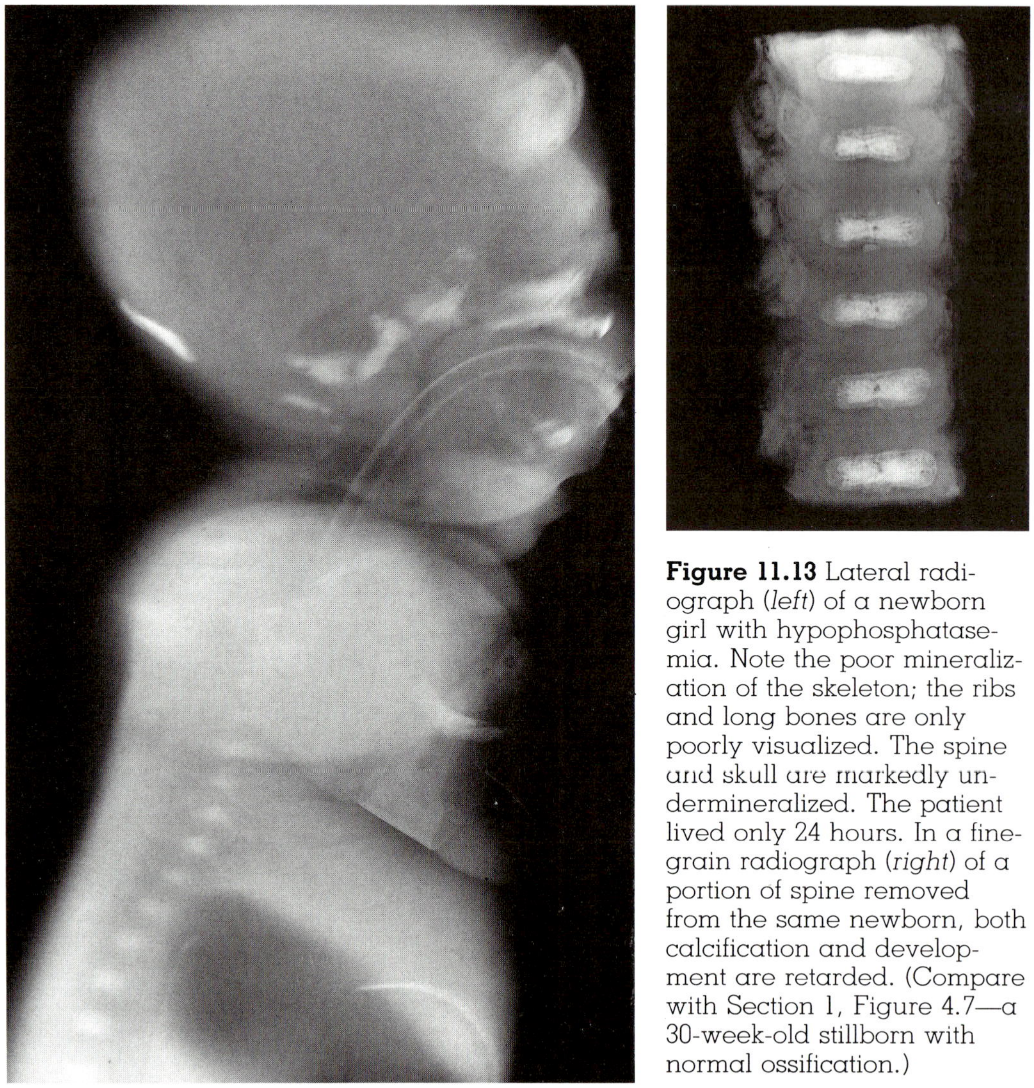

Figure 11.13 Lateral radiograph (*left*) of a newborn girl with hypophosphatasemia. Note the poor mineralization of the skeleton; the ribs and long bones are only poorly visualized. The spine and skull are markedly undermineralized. The patient lived only 24 hours. In a fine-grain radiograph (*right*) of a portion of spine removed from the same newborn, both calcification and development are retarded. (Compare with Section 1, Figure 4.7—a 30-week-old stillborn with normal ossification.)

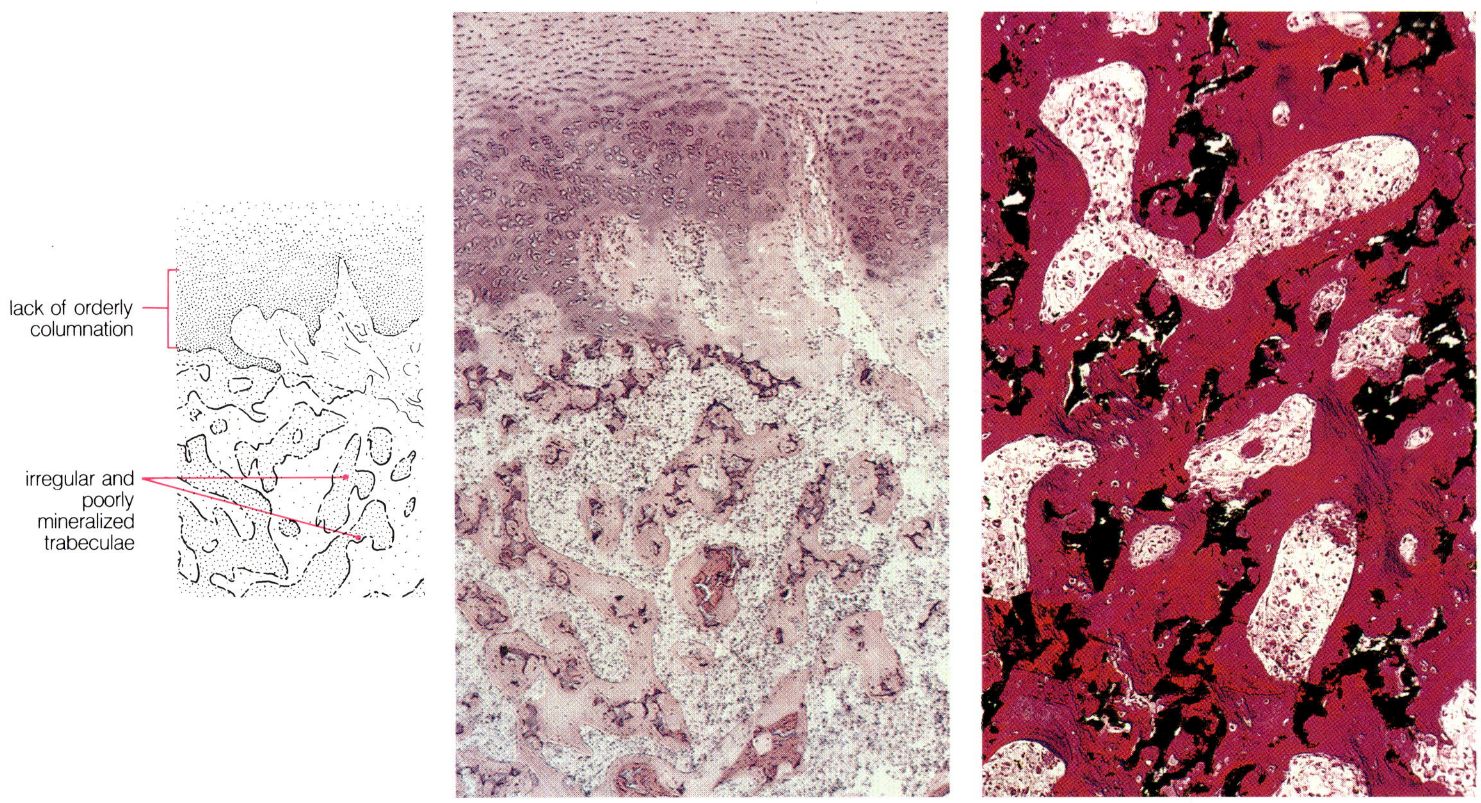

Figure 11.14 A photomicrograph (*left*) of a cross section of a vertebral body from the same patient seen in Figure 11.13 demonstrates disturbed endochondral ossification. A photomicrograph (*right*) with the von Kossa stain shows the poor mineralization of the bone, which is being formed. Only the areas stained black are mineralized.

ities in rickets and osteomalacia usually are minimal, though in severe osteomalacia stress fractures in the thoracic spine, particularly at the levels of T-8 and T-9, may lead to hyperkyphosis.

Disturbances in calcification also may result from the deposition of aluminum and possibly of other elements in the mineralization front (Fig. 11.17). This is seen particularly in association with renal dialysis or with ingestion of aluminum gels. In such cases, patients do not respond either to vitamin D or to parathyroidectomy. However, they do respond dramatically to treatment with chelating agents, which remove or inhibit the effect of aluminum on the osteoblast and at mineralization fronts.

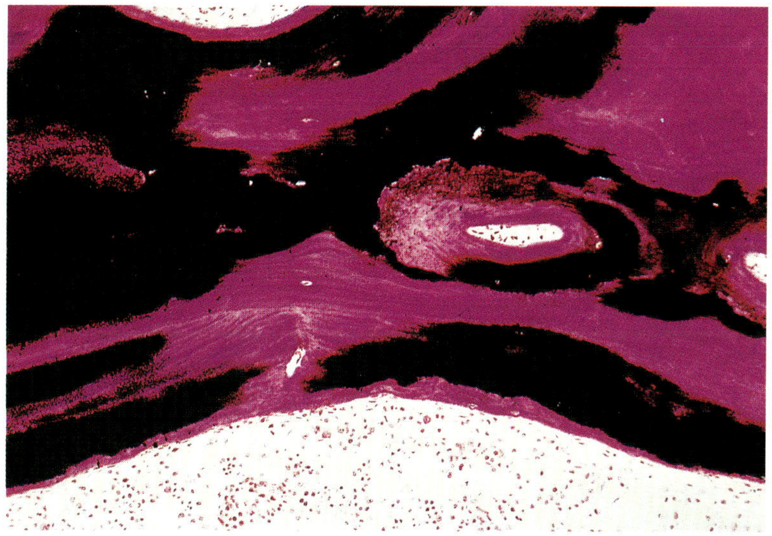

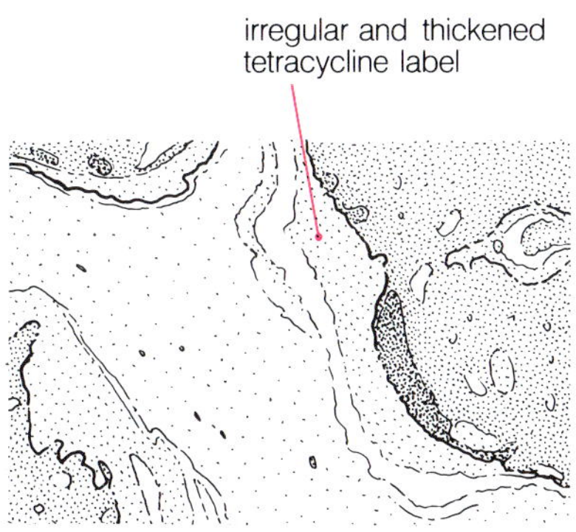

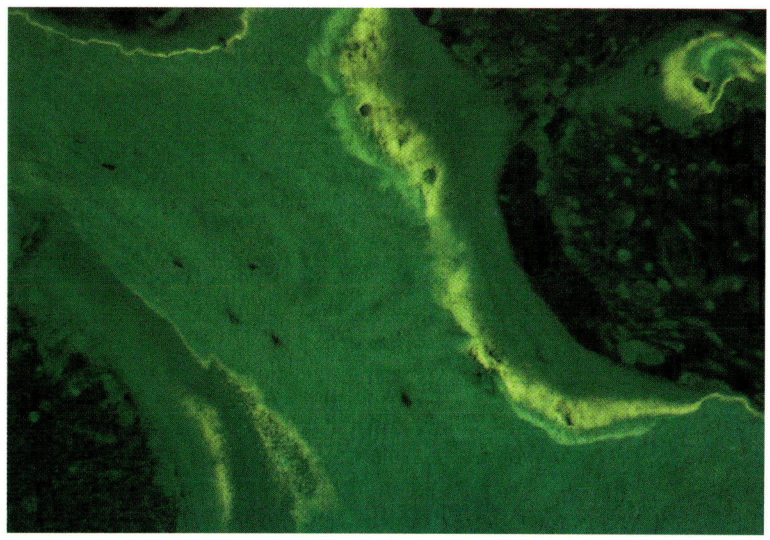

Figure 11.15 Photomicrograph (*top*) of bone to demonstrate the lack of mineralization that occurs in vitamin D deficiency. A thick band of unmineralized bone, in this preparation stained red, covers all of the bony surfaces. The mineralized bone, stained black, has an irregular border with the unmineralized osteoid, which is characteristic of osteomalacia. (von Kossa stain, × 4 objective) The defect in calcification is demonstrated by the diffuse uptake of tetracycline at the mineralization front as seen in this photomicrograph (*bottom*). (Tetracycline label, fluorescent light, × 10 objective)

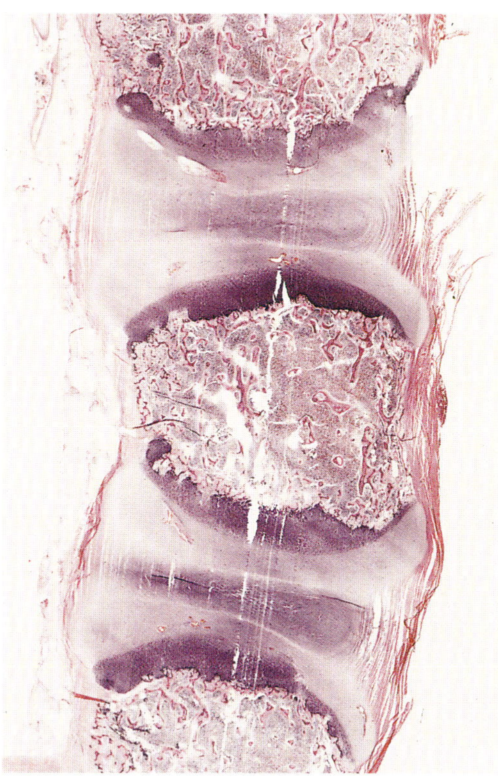

Figure 11.16 Photomicrograph of a seg ment of spine removed from an infant with rickets. Note the thick growth cartilage seen in this casę, and the irregularity of the bone-cartilage junction. (Courtesy of Dr. Howard Dorfman)

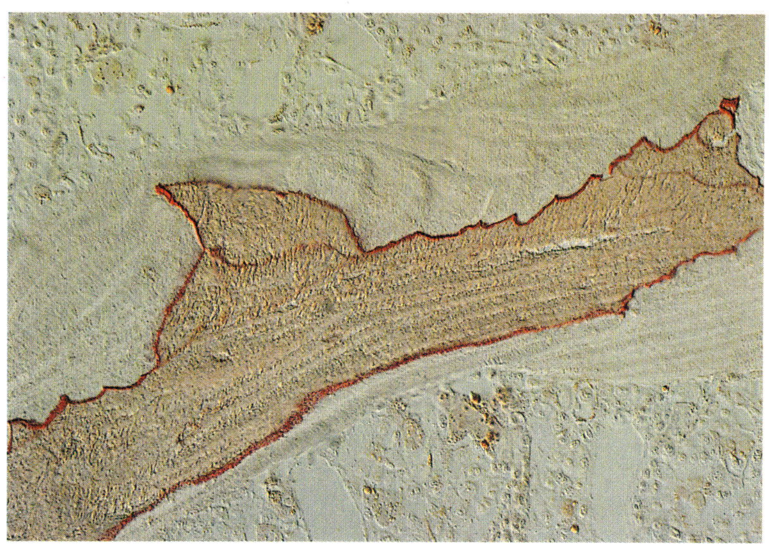

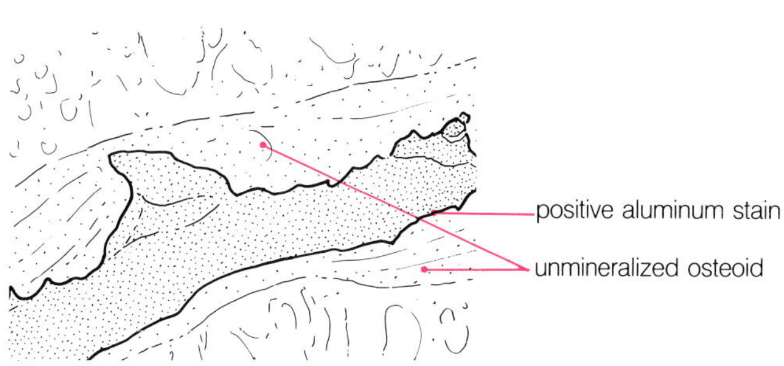

Figure 11.17 Photomicrograph of a section of bone with increased osteoid, stained with aurine tricarboxylic acid stain, which stains aluminum bright red. The red stain is seen to be concentrated at the mineralization front; it has been proposed that the presence of aluminum at this site blocks further mineralization of the bone. (Nomarski optics, × 10 objective)

DISEASES RESULTING FROM DISTURBANCES IN BONE REMODELING

HYPERPARATHYROIDISM

Hyperparathyroidism may be primary, due to an adenoma, a carcinoma, or a primary hyperplasia of the parathyroid glands, or it may be secondary, related to renal disease. This latter form of disease, which is usually referred to as renal osteodystrophy, is today perhaps the more common of the two.

In primary hyperparathyroidism, the bones generally are osteopenic, due to the excessive bone resorption characteristic of the disease (Fig. 11.18), which histologically is associated with the presence of numerous osteoclasts. Usually there is some paratrabecular fibrosis, and characteristically there is dissection of bone trabeculae by groups of osteoclasts that leave typical tunnels inside the bone—so-called *tunneling resorption* (Fig. 11.19). Although the spine in particular is not usually singled out, in rare instances a brown tumor, i.e., a localized area of massive bone resorption associated with giant cells and hemorrhage, may give rise to local symptoms (Figs. 11.20 and 11.21). Very rarely,

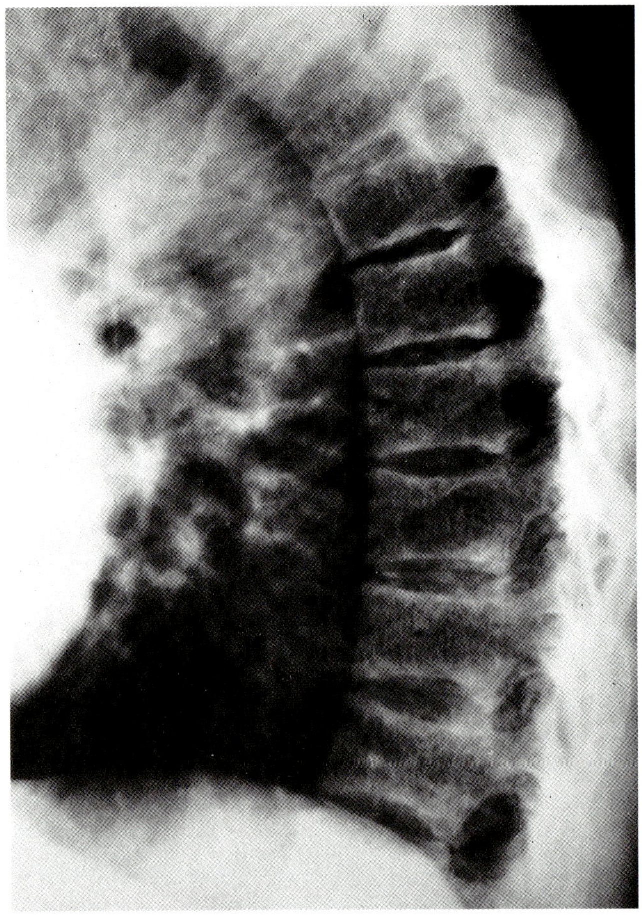

Figure 11.18 Lateral radiograph of the thoracic spine of a 20-year-old female, who presented with severe hypercalcemia due to a parathyroid adenoma. There is osteopenia of the spine, together with some irregularity of the bone end plates and focal collapse of the vertebral bodies. Note the disc calcifications in the lower thoracic spine.

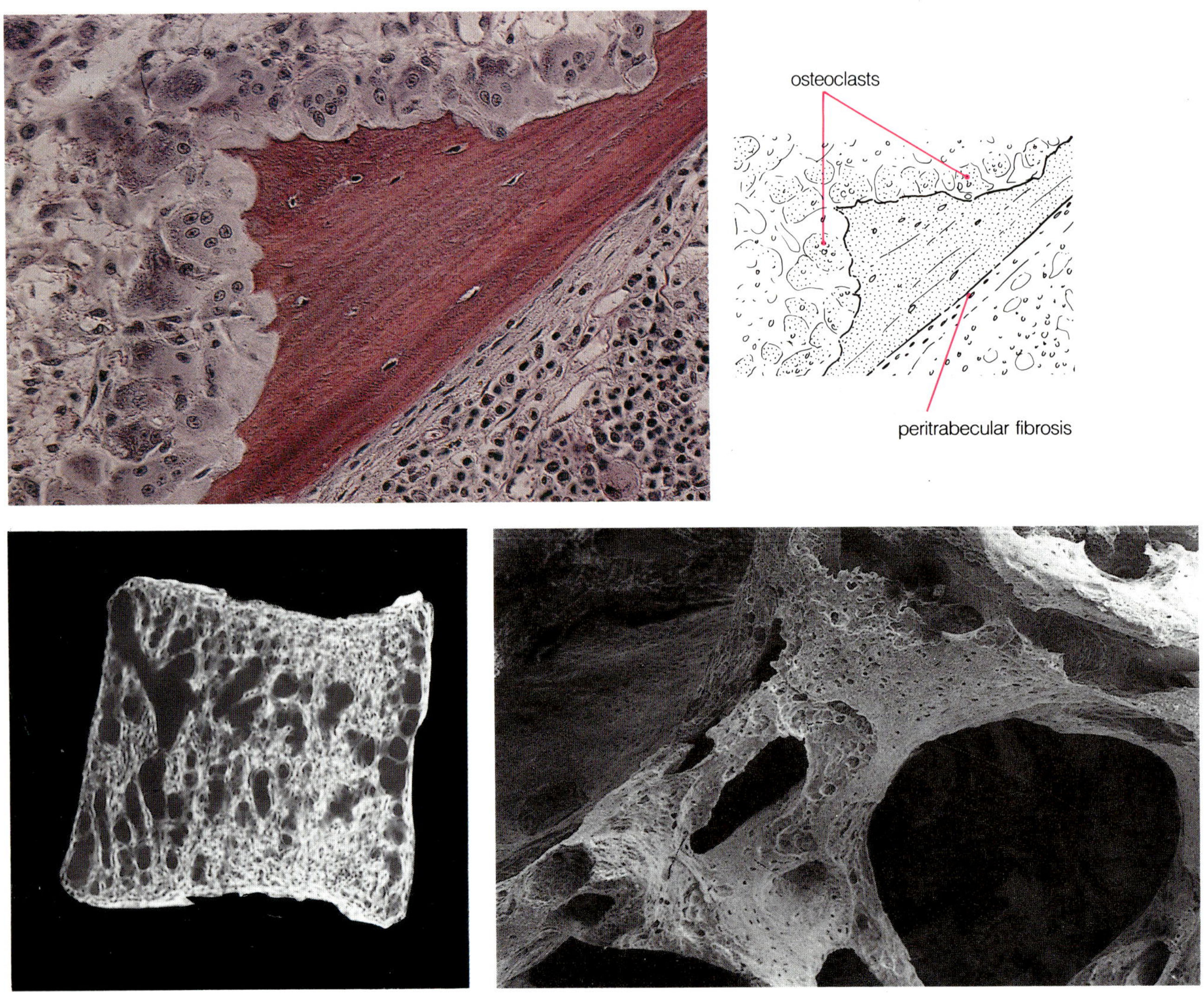

Figure 11.19 Photomicrograph (*top left*) to show severe osteoclastic bone resorption in a patient with primary hyperparathyroidism. Note the mild peritrabecular fibrosis on the inferior bone surface. (H & E, × 25 objective) In a specimen radiograph (*bottom left*) of a slice of vertebral body affected with primary hyperparathyroidism, the trabeculae contain lytic lines within them, due to the dissecting resorption characteristic of this condition. Note the partial resorption of the end plates. A scanning electron micrograph (*bottom right*) of the cancellous bone demonstrates numerous irregular erosions on the bone surface, due to osteoclastic resorption.

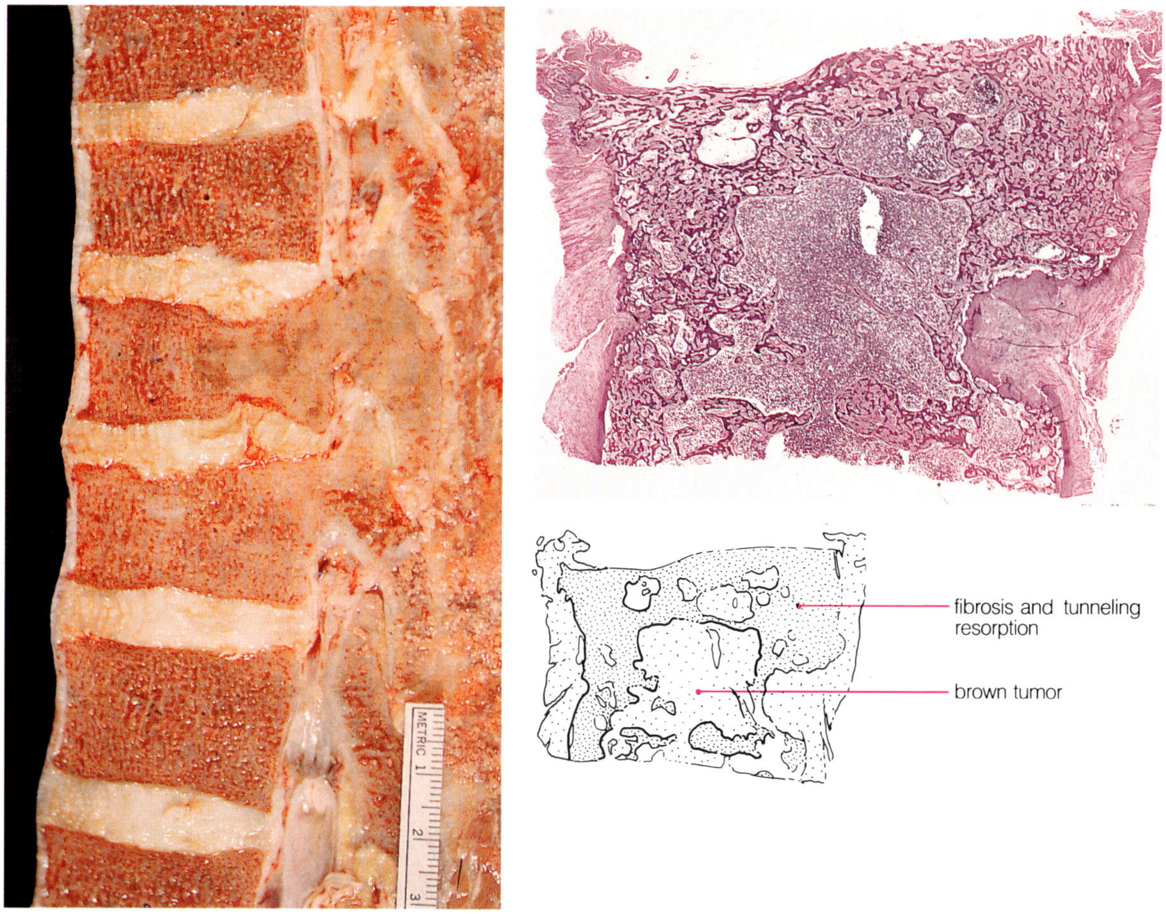

Figure 11.20 Photograph (*left*) of a sagittal section through a segment of thoracolumbar spine in a patient with primary hyperparathyroidism resulting from a parathyroid carcinoma. One of the vertebral bodies shows a large destructive lesion, which is extending posteriorly into the spinal canal and is filled with brownish-tan tissue. On microscopic examination, this proved to be a brown tumor. A photomicrograph (*right*) of one of the brown tumors found in this case shows an extensive area of bony lysis in the central part of the vertebral body. The resultant space is filled by a cellular giant cell lesion. Note that in the surrounding bone there is extensive fibrosis of the bone marrow, with irregular and thinned trabecular bone. This photograph should be compared with the specimen radiograph in Figure 11.19. (Courtesy of Dr. Howard Dorfman)

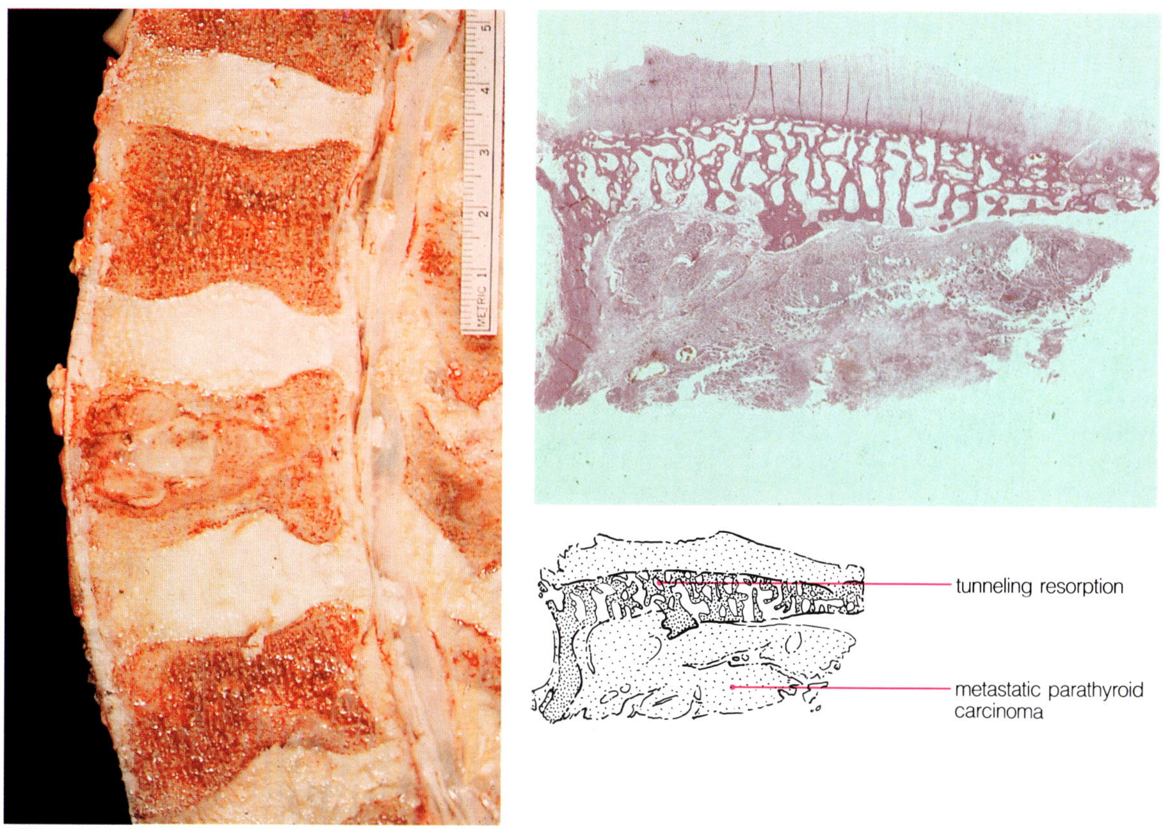

Figure 11.21 Photograph (*left*) of a metastatic lesion from the parathyroid carcinoma described in Figure 11.20. A histologic preparation (*right*) demonstrates the metastatic parathyroid carcinoma. (Courtesy of Dr. Howard Dorfman)

back pain secondary to vertebral compression fractures has been seen as a presenting symptom in primary hyperparathyroidism.

With regard to secondary hyperparathyroidism, chronic renal failure is usually accompanied by bone disease, and lesions include both increased bone resorption and a failure of the bone to mineralize properly. With the introduction of hemodialysis, bone disease has come to constitute a major problem; in many patients there is an increased radiodensity in the skeleton, which, in the spine, gives rise to a typical banded appearance referred to as a *rugger-jersey* spine (Fig. 11.22). This appearance, on occasion, may be confused with that of Paget's disease, although unlike Paget's disease, the sclerosis associated with chronic renal failure generally appears to be confined to the bone adjacent to the vertebral end plates; it does not involve the anterior and posterior cortices (window-frame vertebrae) in the way that it does in Paget's disease (Fig. 11.23).

OSTEOPOROSIS

Although increased radiolucency of bone (osteopenia) is associated with a variety of conditions (including osteogenesis imperfecta, Ehlers-Danlos syndrome, osteomalacia, hyperparathyroidism, and neoplasia), perhaps the most common clinical presentation of osteopenia in the spine is that associated with postmenopausal or senile osteoporosis. Osteoporosis is perhaps best defined as a normally calcified but quantitatively deficient bone (Fig. 11.24), which has resulted in clinical disability. It is a generalized disease that occurs following an imbalance in the rates of bone formation and resolution. While all individuals experience some bone loss with advancing age, the term osteoporosis should be confined to those patients in whom there is symptomatology referrable to the condition. Even so, the number of older individuals who will complain of back pain and/or deformities secondary to osteoporosis is considerable. In a radiologic

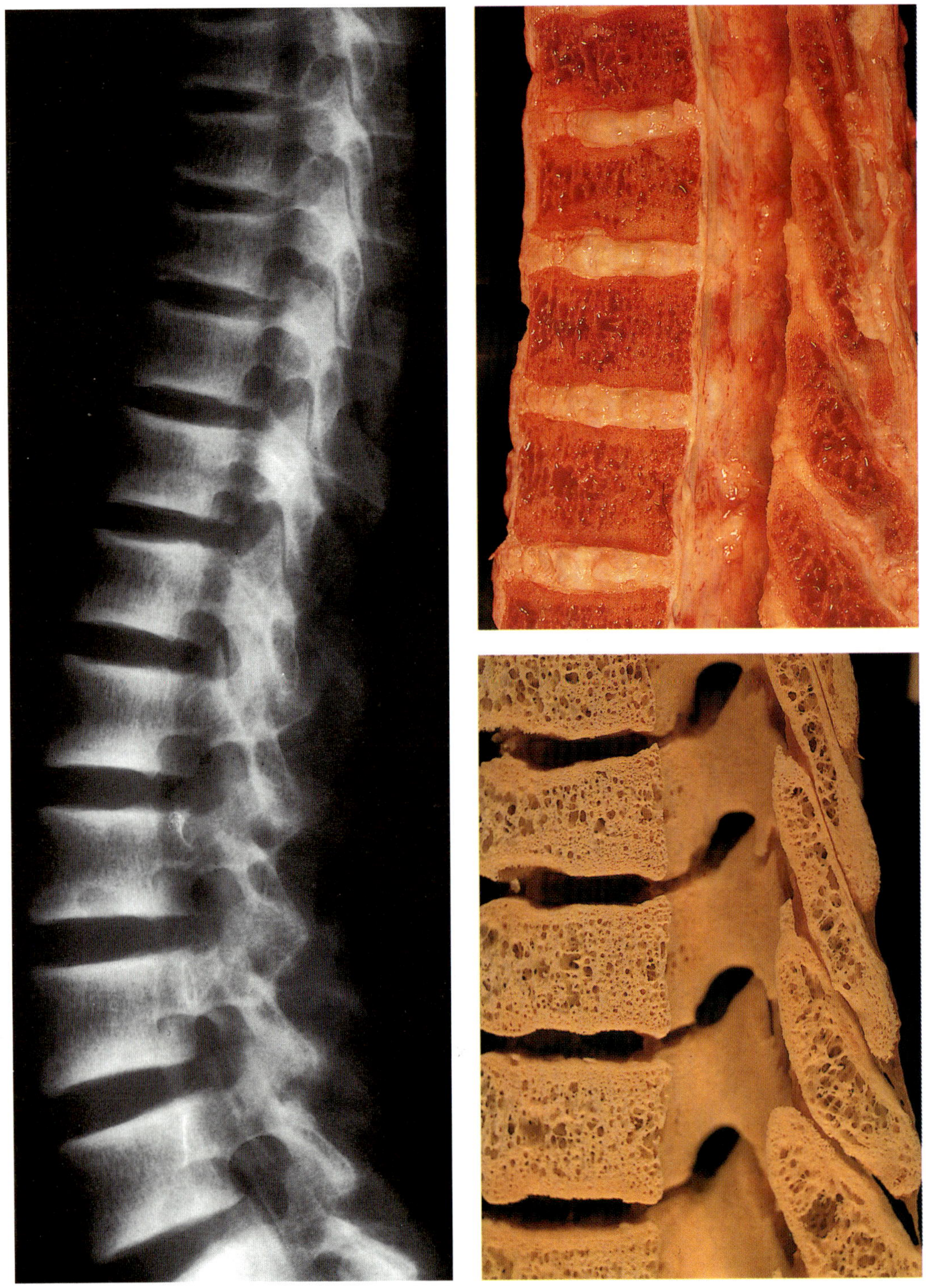

Figure 11.22 Specimen radiograph (*left*) of the spine from a patient with renal osteodystrophy. The cancellous bone has a blurred pattern and there is irregular thickening of the bone concentrated at the end plates, particularly in the lower thoracic and lumbar spine. A sagittal section (*top right*) through this spine demonstrates sclerosis of the bone beneath the end plates. The striped appearance of the bone is sometimes referred to as a "rugger jersey" spine. The macerated preparation (*bottom right*) of this same specimen is demonstrated.

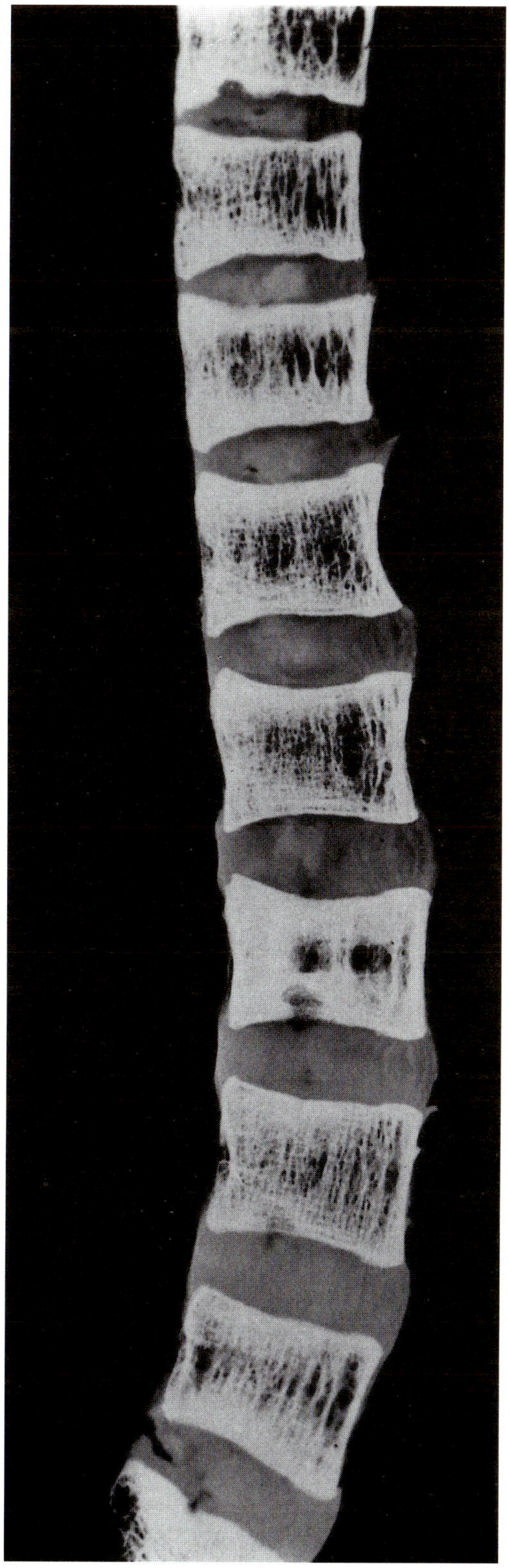

Figure 11.23 Radiograph of a sagittal slice of spine removed from a patient with renal osteodystrophy. In this case, the bony sclerosis is very exaggerated and in some of the vertebral bodies a picture-frame appearance is seen, simulating Paget's disease. However, in Paget's disease, it would be unusual for all of the vertebral bodies to be involved, as they are here.

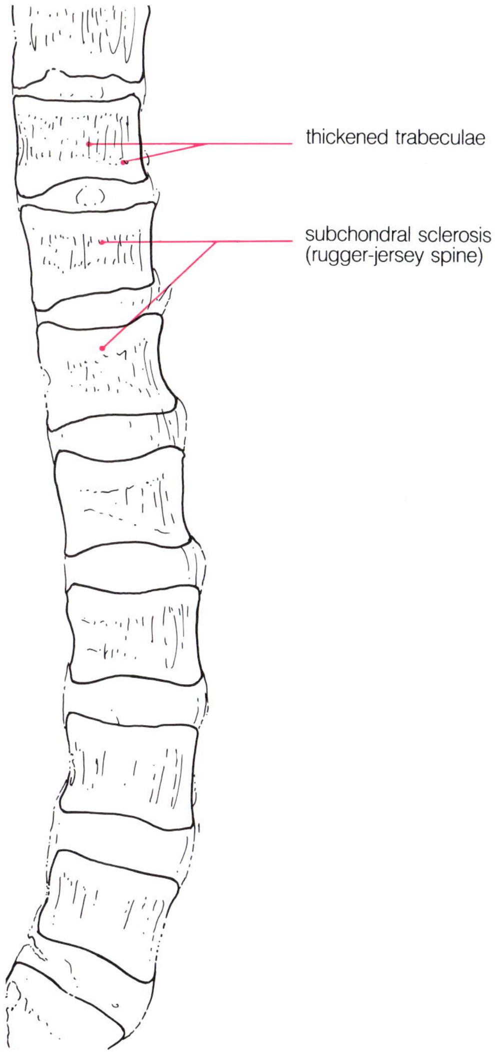

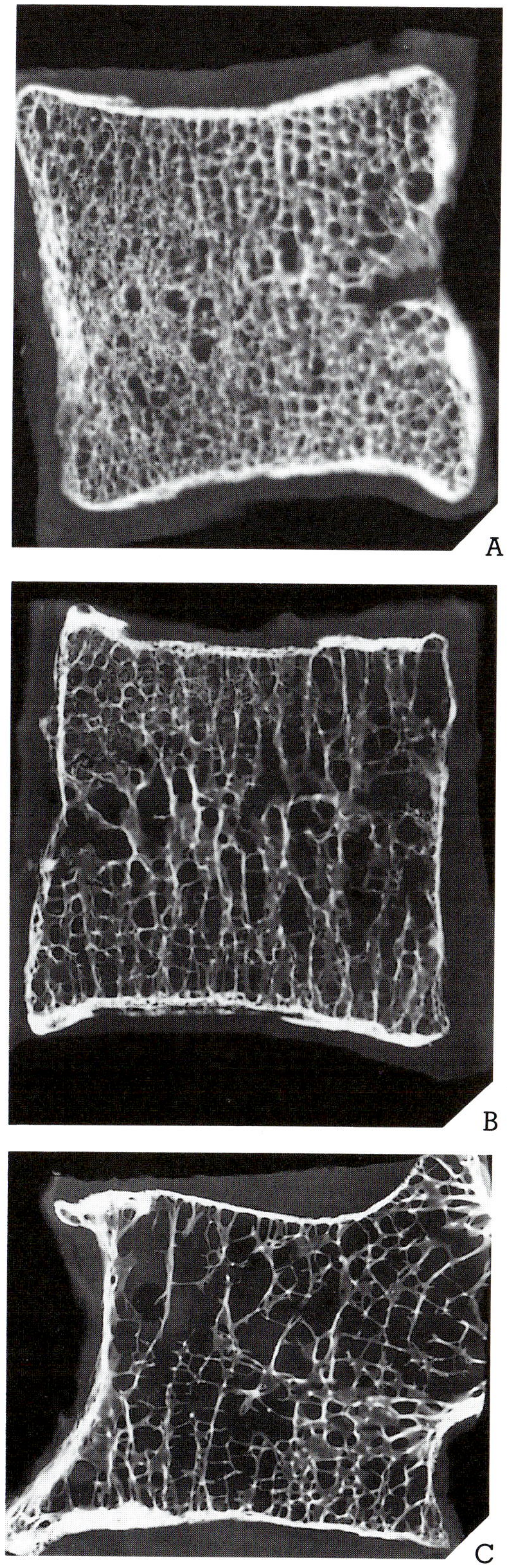

Figure 11.24 Specimen radiographs of 2-mm slices through the vertebral body of T-2. **A** The first specimen represents normal bone texture, density, and pattern. **B** The second specimen shows a moderate degree of osteopenia, with accentuation of the vertical trabeculae and a selective loss of the horizontal trabeculae. **C** The third specimen shows severe osteoporosis, with irregular pin trabeculae and partial central collapse of the superior end plate.

survey, 20% of men and 29% of women over age 60 showed compression fractures of the vertebral bodies. Back pain, associated with loss of height due to vertebral compression and increased thoracic kyphosis, is a common manifestation (Figs. 11.25 and 11.26). Neurologic complications are unusual in osteoporosis.

The radiographic diagnosis of osteoporosis in the spine is based on bone porosity, a change in trabecular pattern, and a change in vertebral body shape. It should be noted that from 30 to 50% of the bone must be lost before a recognizable abnormality can be seen on routine spinal radiographs (Fig. 11.27). However, by use of more sensitive techniques, like quantitative CT scanning (Fig. 11.28) and dual-beam densitometry, a much more accurate assessment of bone loss can be made. In using these techniques, one should be aware that with vertebral compression, porosity may be masked, owing to compaction of the trabeculae and to formation of fracture callus (Fig. 11.29). In the vertebral bodies, it has been observed that there is a selective loss of the horizontal trabeculae, with a consequent accentuation of the vertical trabeculae. This leads to the presence of rather prominent, vertical radiodense striations or bars (Fig. 11.30). The loss of bone in the vertebral bodies may be such that radiographically it is difficult to discern any difference in density between the intervertebral disc and the vertebral body, with the end plate being the only portion of the body

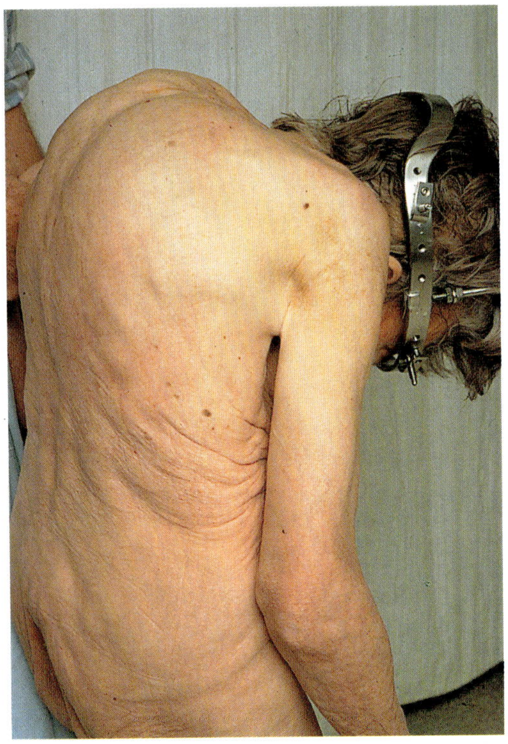

Figure 11.25 Clinical photograph of a 67-year-old female with postmenopausal osteoporosis and a progressive kyphotic deformity, with inability to lift her chin more than one inch off her sternum. (Courtesy of Dr. David S. Bradford)

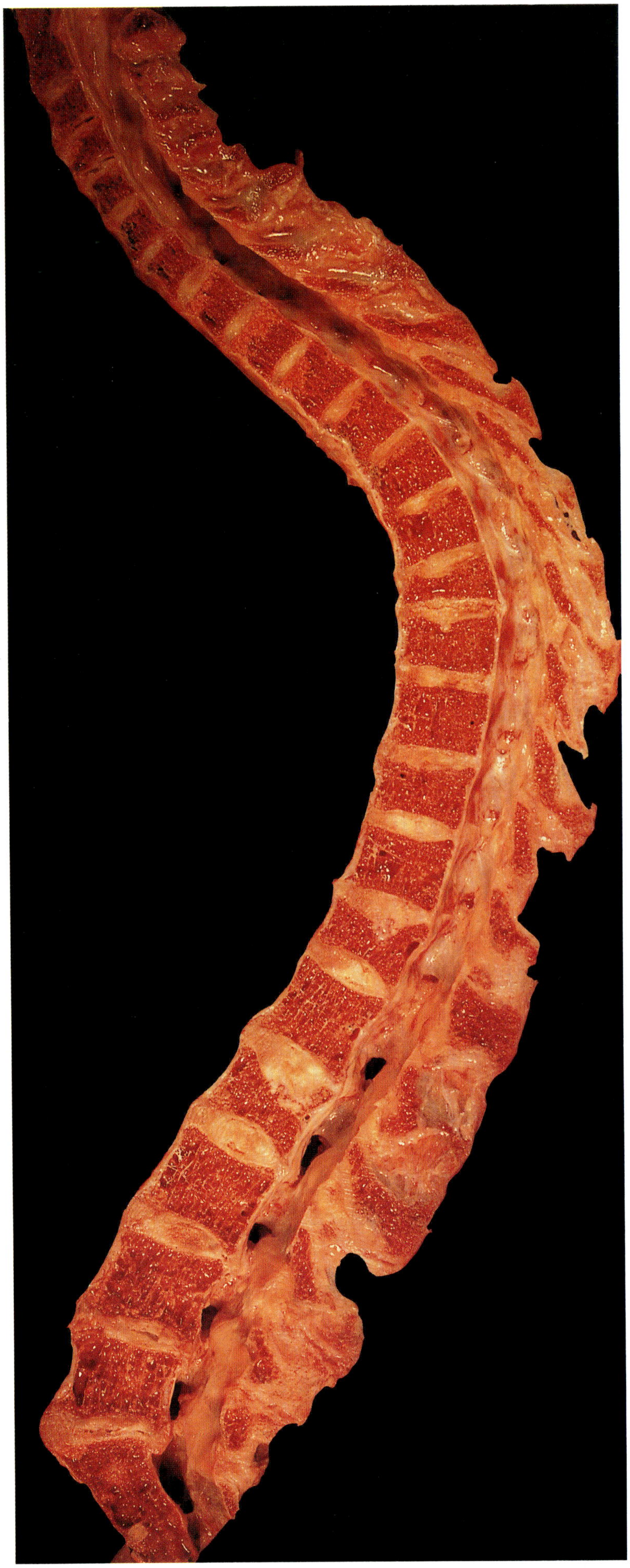

Figure 11.26 Sagittal section of the spine removed from a patient with severe osteoporosis and thoracic kyphosis that had developed rapidly following menopause. Note the wedge-shaped collapse of T-7, and the biconcave collapse in T-12 and L-2.

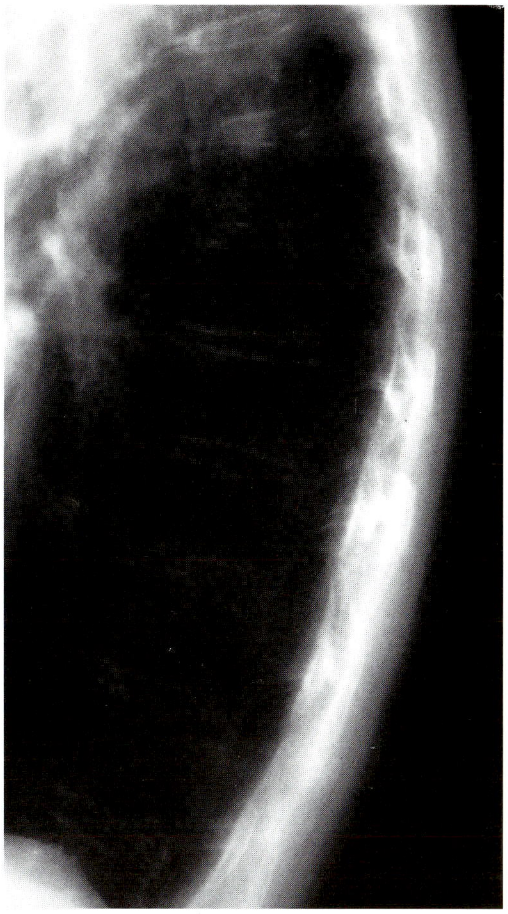

Figure 11.27 Lateral radiograph of the thoracic spine in a 72-year-old woman with back pain. In addition to diffuse osteopenia, note that the only radiologically recognizable structure in this radiograph is the end plate of the vertebral body.

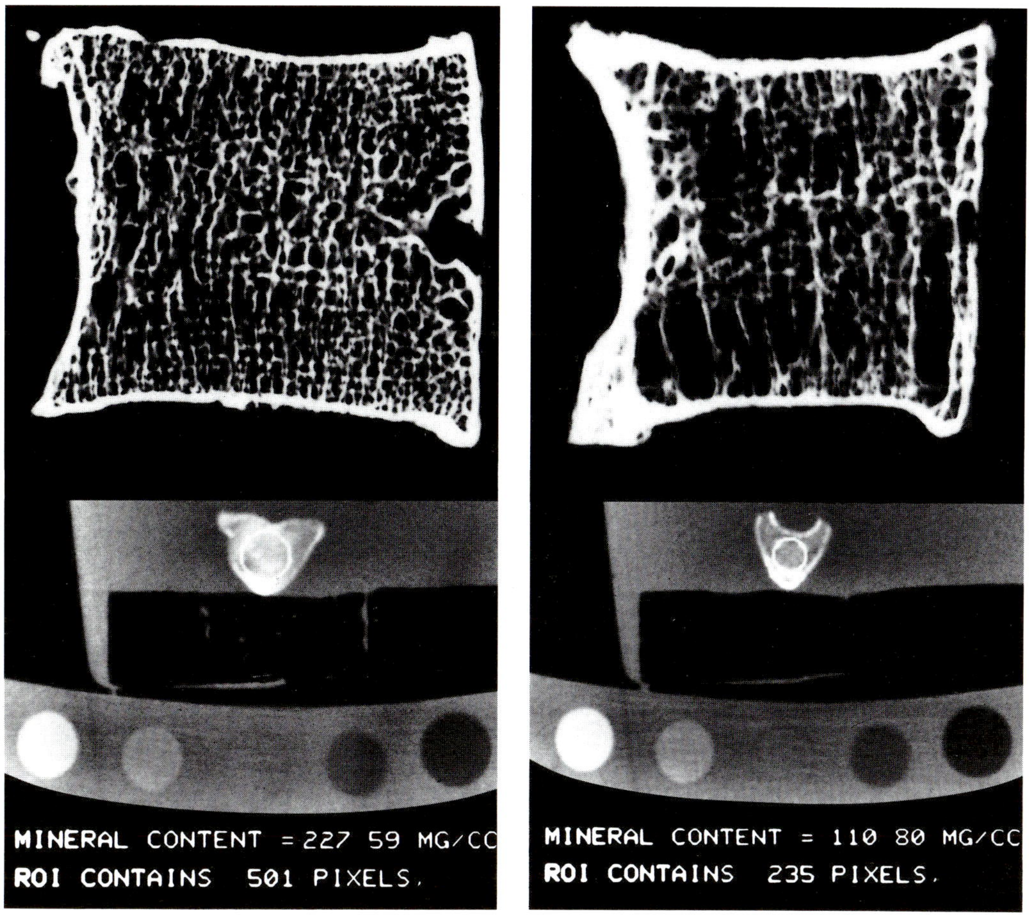

Figure 11.28 Specimen radiographs and CT scans comparing a relatively normal second thoracic vertebra (*left-hand views*) with an osteopenic one (*right-hand views*). The specimen radiographs are of a 2-mm sagittal slice of bone; the quantitative CT scans are through a midsection of the whole body. The phantom below is for standardization. In the "normal" specimen (*left*) the CT scan gives a reading of 227.59 milligrams of calcium per milliliter. In the osteopenic specimen (*right*), the reading is 110.80 mg/mL.

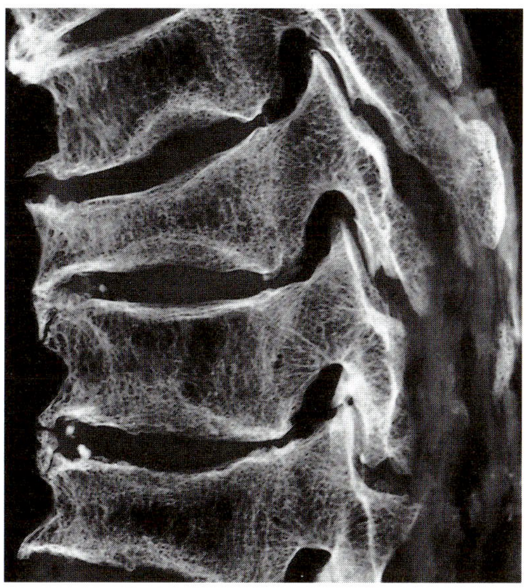

Figure 11.29 Specimen lateral radiograph to demonstrate how compression secondary to fracture may result in an apparent increase in density, especially when bone from vertebral bodies similar to these is used for dual-beamed densitometry or quantitative CT scanning.

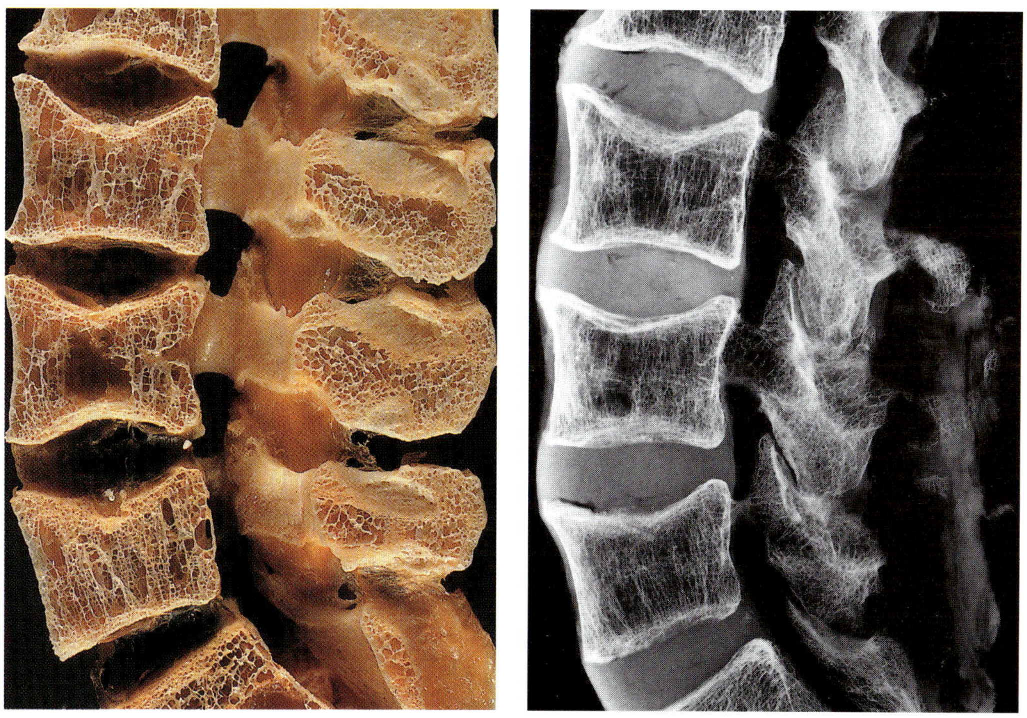

Figure 11.30 Photograph (*left*) of a sagittal section through the macerated spine of an elderly patient with severe osteoporosis. Note the central collapse of the end plates in the four lumbar vertebrae, along with accentuation of the vertical trabeculae and marked central porosity of the vertebral bodies. A specimen radiograph (*right*) of this patient emphasizes the uniform biconcavities of the end plates in addition to the patchy nature of the osteoporosis.

visible on the film (Fig. 11.31). Highly characteristic of osteoporosis is a change in vertebral shape, and such changes include flattening of the vertebral body, anterior wedging of the vertebra, and a biconcavity of the vertebra that is sometimes referred to as a fish-mouth vertebra (Fig. 11.32). All of these deformities are due to compression fractures within the vertebral body, with the type of deformity seen depending on the local mechanical situation, as determined mainly by location. Wedge fractures, for example, are more typical in the midthoracic spine, whereas biconcave fish-mouth vertebrae are more common in the lower thoracic and lumbar spine. Fish-mouth vertebrae also may be seen in association with other diseases like Paget's, renal osteodystrophy or even neoplasms, although additional characteristics of the underlying disease processes usually are discernible. Schmorl's nodes are a common accompaniment of osteoporosis and generally are more common on the lower cartilaginous plate than on the upper plate (see Chapter 7).

PAGET'S DISEASE

Paget's disease, a condition common in individuals of northern European descent, is reported to occur in approximately 4% of individuals over age 40. In the majority of these cases, the disease is restricted to a few bones; often, only one bone or part of a bone is affected. Generally, there are no clinical complaints. The basis of the disease appears

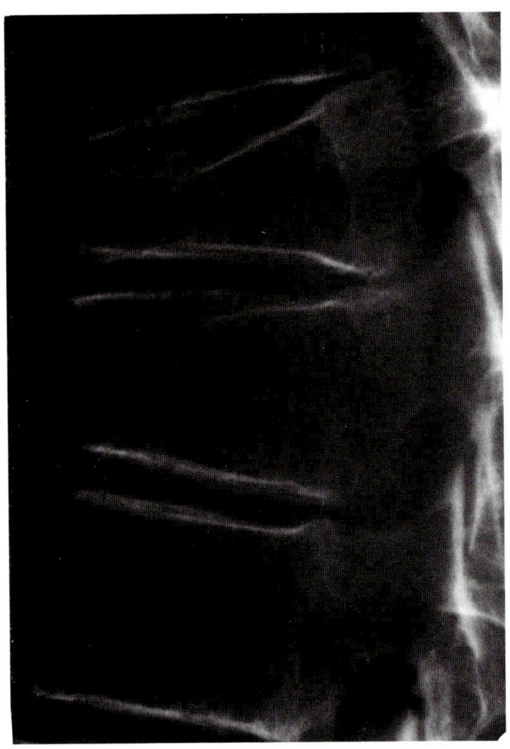

Figure 11.31 Specimen radiograph to show that in osteoporosis, the density of the vertebral body and the density of the intervertebral disc may become so similar that no differentiation can be made; it is only the presence of the bony end plates that allows visualization of the vertebral bodies.

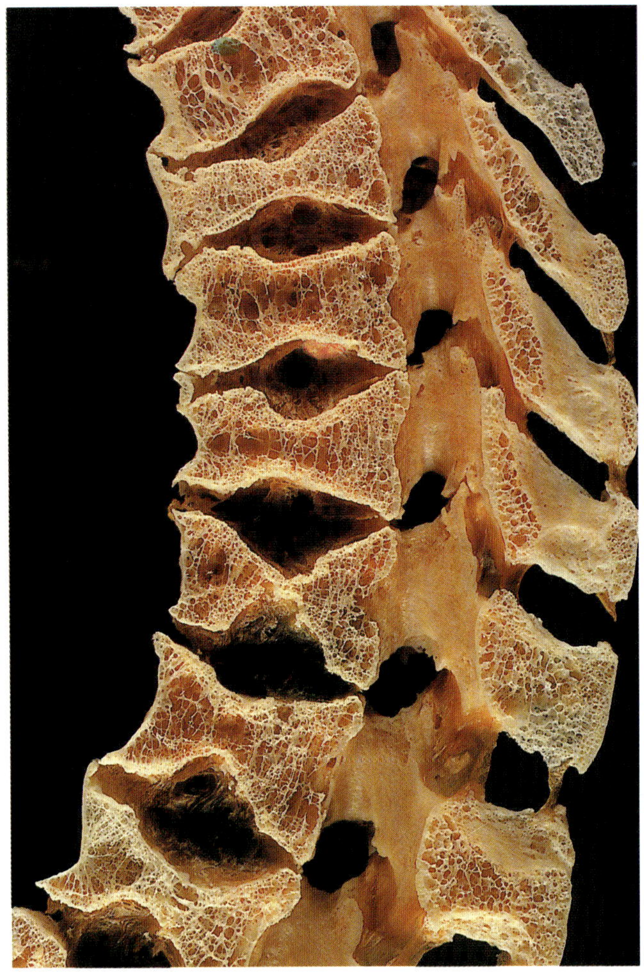

Figure 11.32 Photograph of a sagittal section of the macerated thoracic spine of the patient seen in Figure 11.30. This specimen demonstrates the various patterns and degrees of collapse that may be seen within the vertebral bodies. In the upper part of the segment, flattening of the vertebral bodies with some anterior wedging is seen. In the lower part of the segment, the more typical biconcave compression fractures of the central end plates are seen, which give rise to so-called fish-mouth vertebrae.

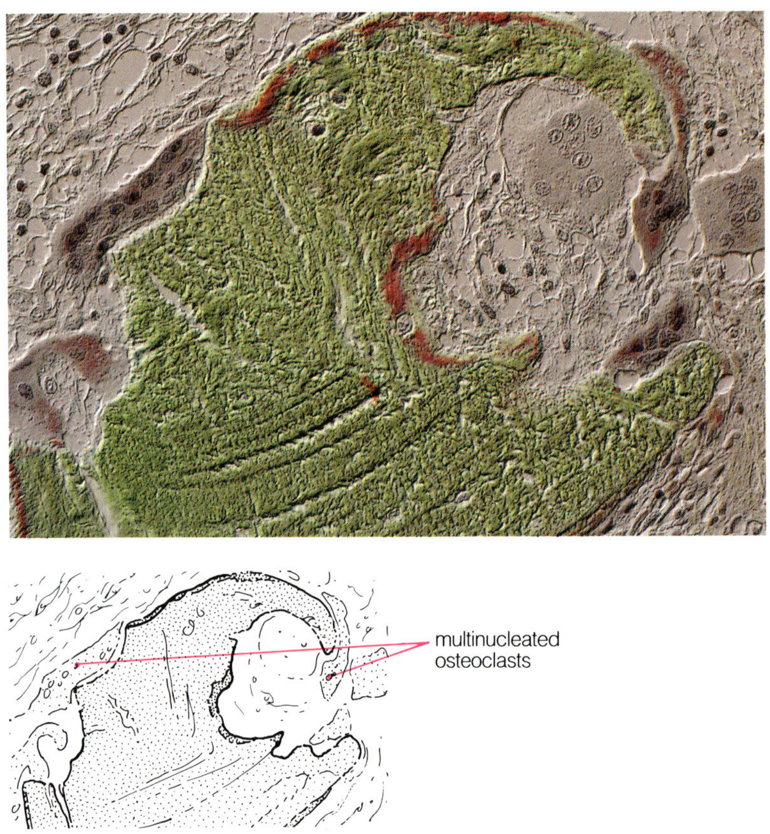

Figure 11.33 Photomicrograph of Paget's disease in the active phase, to demonstrate the marked osteoclastic bone resorption typical of this disease as well as the large size of the osteoclasts, which here show up to 20 nuclei. (Goldner stain, × 10 objective)

to be an unrestricted hyperactivity of osteoclasts in the affected areas of bone (Fig. 11.33). It has been suggested that this hyperactivity is brought on by a virus. As a secondary response to increased osteoclastic resorption, there is increased osteoblastic bone deposition, with a subsequent disturbance in the normal bone architecture. This is marked by irregular trabeculae, numerous cement lines, and, in the early stage of the disease, a considerable proportion of woven bone. The marrow space is frequently fibrotic and hypervascular (Fig. 11.34).

In advanced cases of Paget's disease the vertebral column is usually involved, and often extensively so, with the lumbar vertebrae and pelvic bones affected most commonly (Fig. 11.35). In the spine, the changes seen in the vertebral body are more conspicuous than those seen in the arch, although both often are involved. It is not unusual for the vertebral bodies to show peripheral sclerosis, together with a reduction in height and an increased AP and transverse diameter. The vertebral body thus assumes the shape

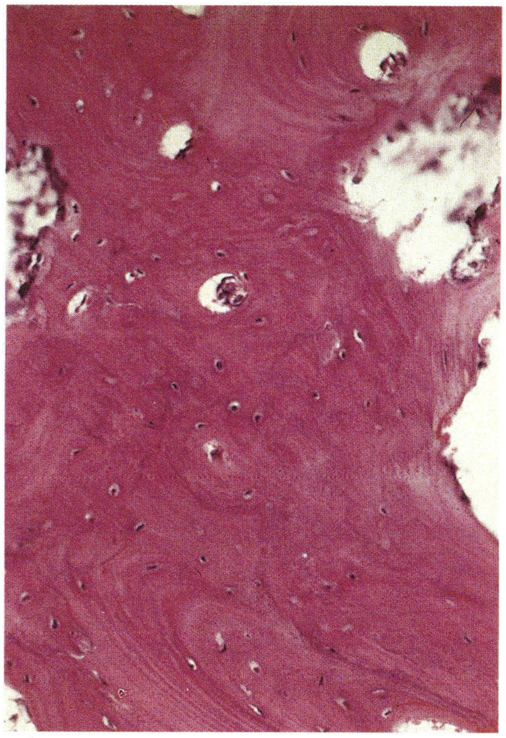

Figure 11.34 Photomicrograph showing the late stages of Paget's disease. The osteoblastic and osteoclastic reaction may be much less evident and the mosaic pattern difficult to appreciate, because the tissue has been overdecalcified or the staining not adequate enough to show the basophilic lines clearly. (H & E, × 10 objective)

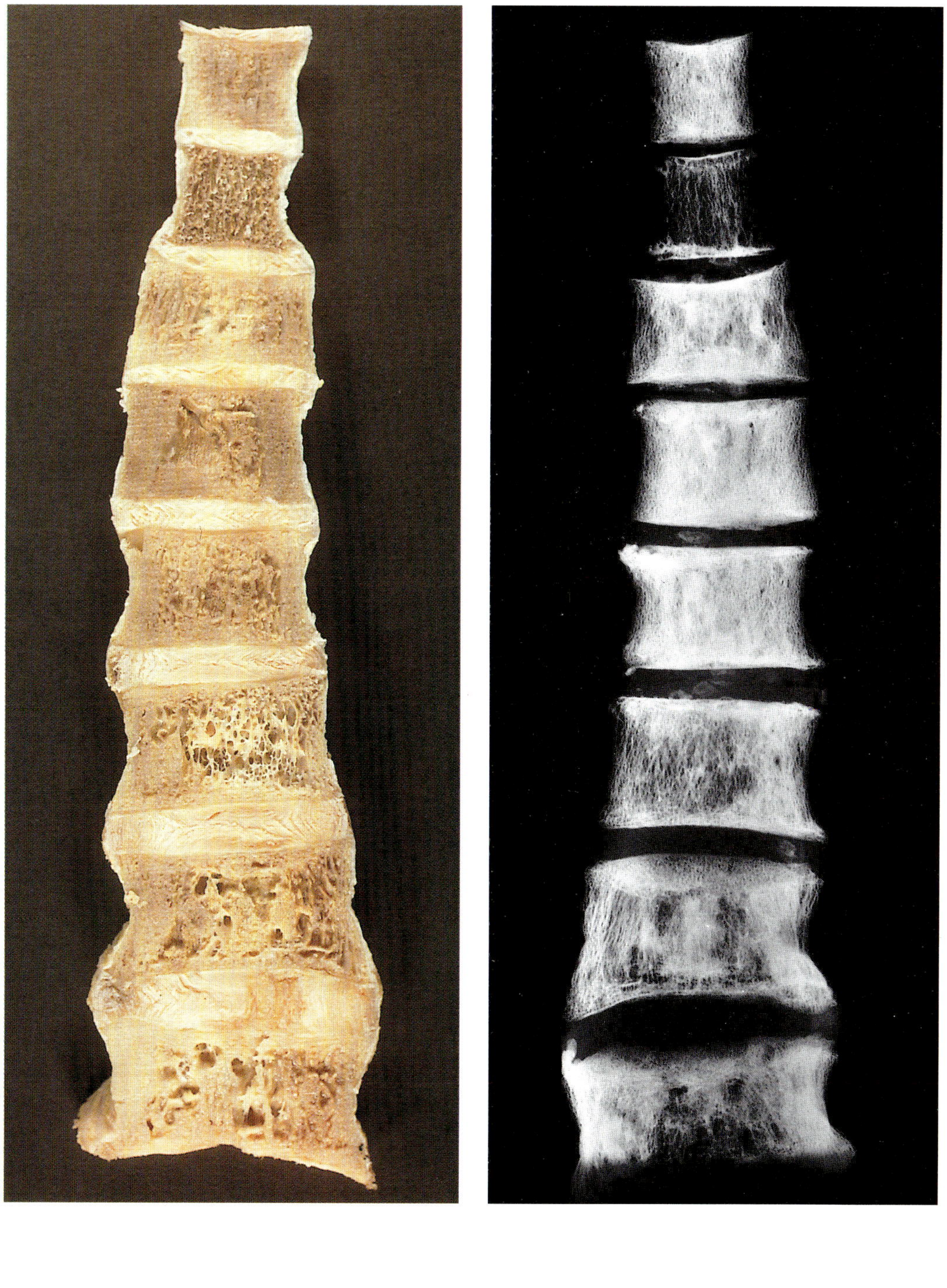

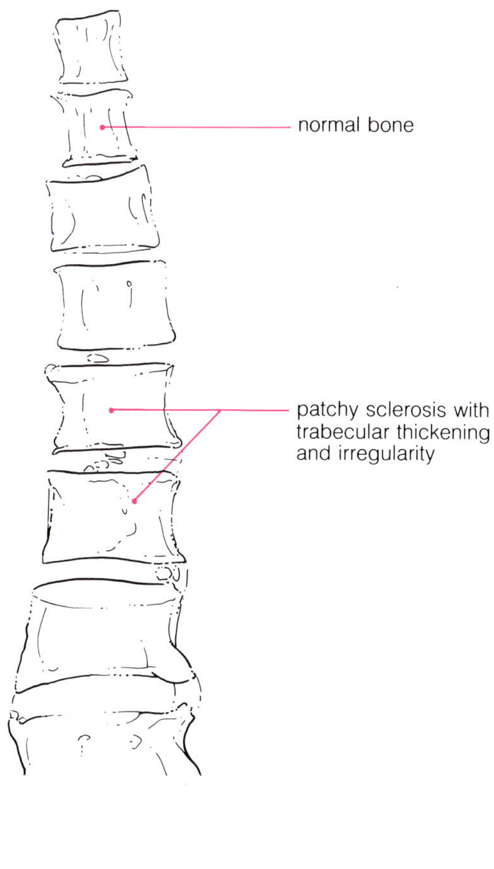

Figure 11.35 Photograph (*left*) of coronal section through the lower thoracic and lumbar spine of a patient with generalized Paget's disease. In this specimen, only T-11 remains uninvolved by the process. The other vertebrae show marked coarsening of the trabeculae, especially at the periphery. This is particularly apparent in L-1, L-2, and L-3, giving a so-called picture-frame appearance to these bones. Specimen radiograph (*right*) of the same segment of spine demonstrates the varying radiographic appearances of the affected vertebrae. The coarse trabeculation is best seen here in T-12, L-4, and L-5. In addition, there is patchy sclerosis.

of a window frame (Fig. 11.36). Disc degeneration may be associated, and through the formation of marginal osteophytes the vertebral bodies may become fused. These changes may lead to a kyphotic or kyphoscoliotic deformity of the vertebral column. Usually there are few clinical complaints, apart from mild pain. However, spinal cord and cauda equina compression is a recognized albeit rare complication of Paget's disease in the vertebral column.

Monostatic disease may be seen in a younger age group, and sometimes the lesions may present as a purely sclerotic or ivory vertebra, giving rise to problems in differential diagnosis with lymphoma or metastatic disease (Fig. 11.37). The diagnosis may be particularly problematic if an unusual site such as the cervical spine is involved. On occasion, giant cell tumors or sarcomas also may develop in association with Paget's disease, and in such cases the initial clinical presentation may be neurologic. Sarcomatous degeneration may occur in monostatic forms of the disease and is not confined only to the generalized form of the disease (Fig. 11.38).

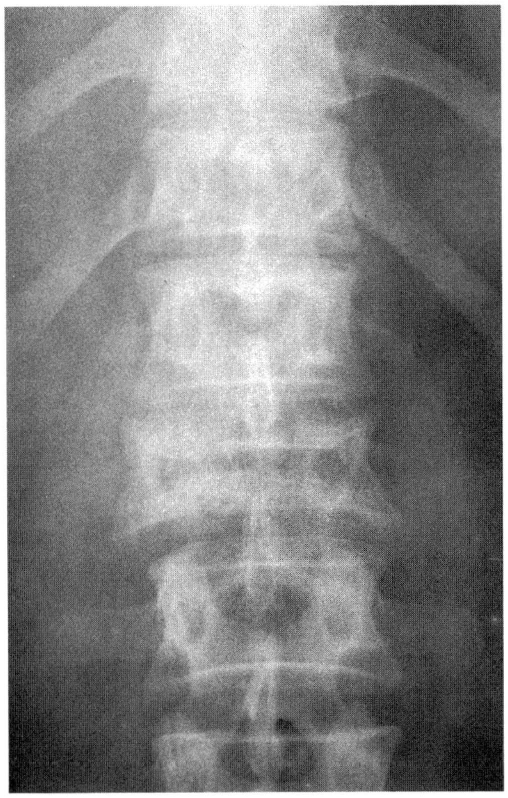

Figure 11.36 Clinical radiograph of the spine of a 50-year-old male with complaints of back pain. A solitary focus of Paget's disease is seen in L-2. Note the increased width of the vertebral body, the loss of height, and the coarse trabeculation around the periphery, which gives it a picture-frame appearance.

OSTEOPETROSIS

Osteopetrosis is a rare disorder characterized by a marked increase in the density of the skeletal tissue as seen on radiographic examination (Fig. 11.39). In addition, the long bones usually are short, and frequently show a modeling defect, which is apparent as a loss of the normal metaphysial flare. The disease often is complicated by multiple

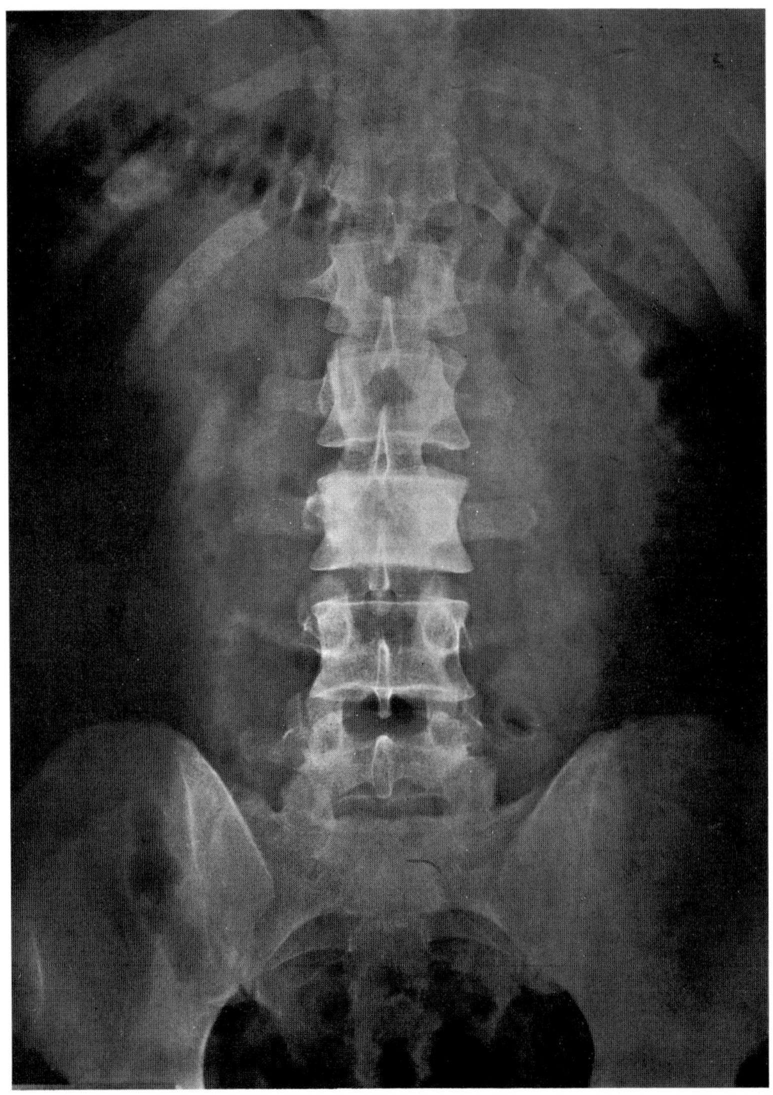

Figure 11.37 Clinical radiograph of a 38-year-old patient, who presented with complaints of vague back pain. In this radiograph, a rather uniform sclerosis is seen in the body of L-3; the initial radiographic diagnosis was of lymphoma. Because of the sclerosis, a needle biopsy was obtained with difficulty but clearly demonstrated the mosaic-pattern marrow fibrosis and increased osteoclastic resorption typical of Paget's disease.

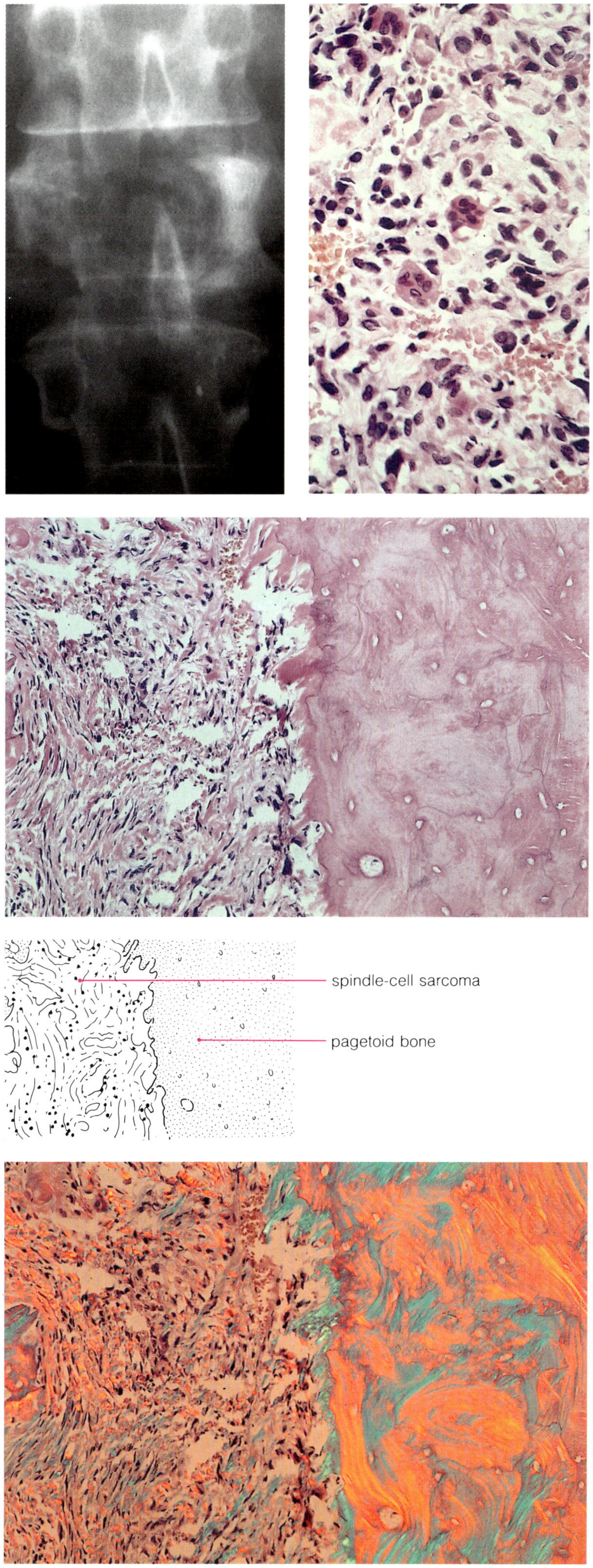

Figure 11.38 Spinal radiograph (*top left*) of a 58-year-old female with a two-month history of low back pain. Fourteen years earlier she had undergone a hysterectomy for cervical carcinoma. A patchy sclerotic and lytic appearance was noted, which was interpreted to be consistent with metastatic disease. However, there is some widening of the body, which is unusual in metastasis. A needle biopsy (*top right*) showed an anaplastic tumor with many giant cells consistent with Paget's sarcoma; foci of bone obtained with this biopsy showed the typical mosaic pattern of Paget's. The patient died approximately 4 months later. Autopsy revealed local extension of the tumor, which involved T-12 and L-2, and compression and encasement of the vena cava. Extensive lung metastases had the pattern of a Paget's sarcoma. An H & E section (*center*) of a portion of bone adjacent to the tumor shows increased numbers of cement lines within the bone. In the polarized section (*bottom*) of the same field, the disorganized bony architecture is obvious. This case is significant as it demonstrates that even in monostatic Paget's disease, a sarcoma may rarely occur as a complication.

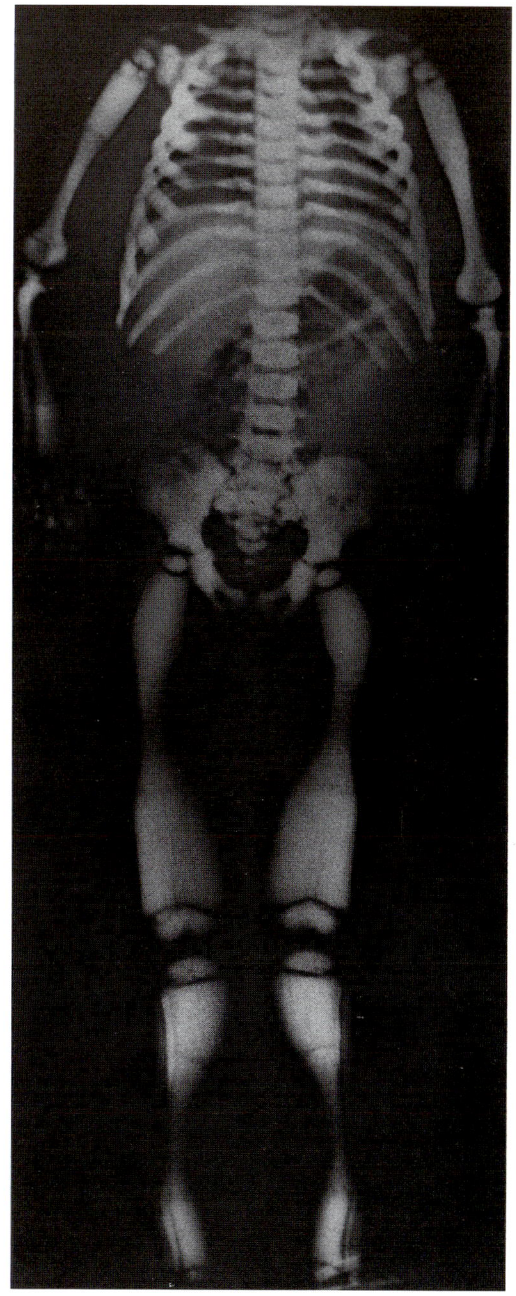

Figure 11.39 Whole body radiograph of a young child with osteopetrosis shows a marked increase in the density of the bones. In addition, there is the typical metaphysial flaring, which is particularly prominent around the knees, hips, and upper humerus. The trabecular pattern of the bone is lost.

fracture as well as by anemia. The spine usually shows fairly pronounced changes, most markedly in the vertebral body. In the newborn, the vertebral bodies, though largely radiodense, may already show some central clearing (Fig. 11.40). However, in older individuals, this central clearing becomes much more pronounced, giving rise to a sandwich-like or rugger-jersey appearance, similar to that seen in hyperparathyroidism (Fig. 11.41). Histologic sections show an extremely irregular bony architecture and many of the bone trabeculae will be seen to have coarse calcified cartilage within them (Fig. 11.42). Although osteoclasts can be observed in the tissue section, they do not appear to be resorbing the bone. Consequently, it has been proposed that there is an enzymatic defect rendering the osteoclasts nonfunctional.

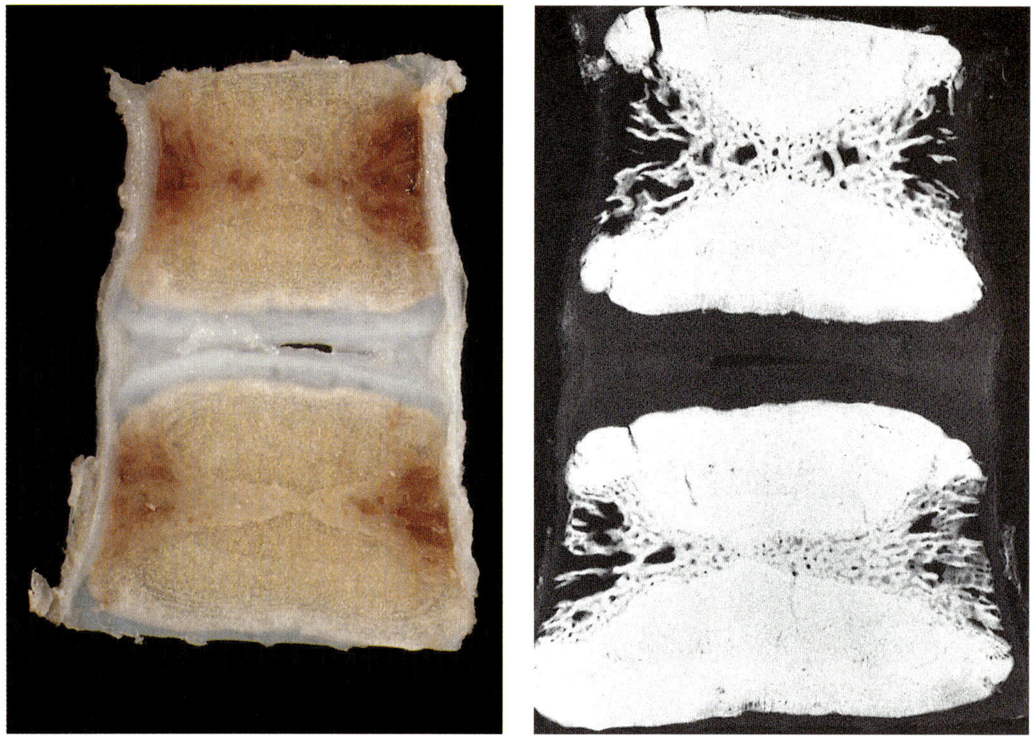

Figure 11.40 Photograph (*left*) of a frontal section through two vertebrae of a newborn with osteopetrosis shows the extremely dense bone, with marrow tissue confined to the central peripheral portions only. In the specimen radiograph (*right*), the density is seen in the metaphysial end-plate regions.

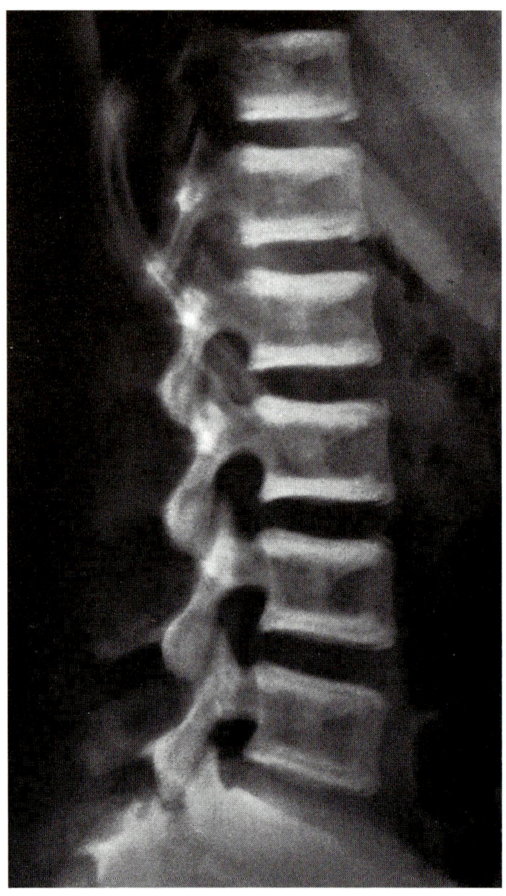

Figure 11.41 Lateral radiograph of an adult with osteopetrosis. Note the markedly increased density of the proximal and distal thirds of the vertebral bodies, with central clearing giving a sandwich-like appearance. This is somewhat reminiscent of the rugger-jersey spine seen in renal osteodystrophy.

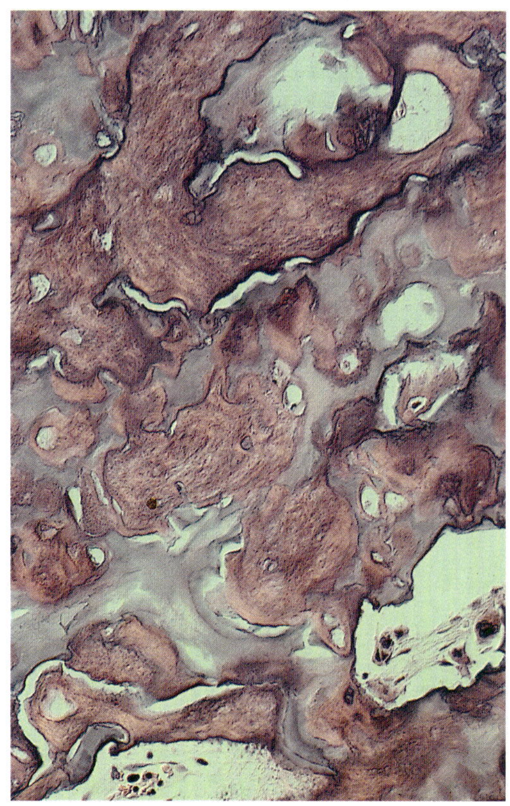

Figure 11.42 Photomicrograph to demonstrate the disturbed architecture of osteopetrosis. Note the residual calcified cartilage and the cracking along the cement lines (a source of structural weakness). Some osteoclasts are seen on the lower right. (H & E, × 10 objective)

Diseases Resulting from Hematologic Disturbances

MYELOFIBROSIS

Myelofibrosis is a relatively uncommon disease that is characterized by fibrosis of the bone marrow, extramedullary hematopoiesis, and in approximately 50% of cases involving the bones (particularly, the axial skeleton) a diffuse but occasionally patchy sclerosis (Fig. 11.43). The disease occurs about equally in men and women, and is more common among older individuals. The involved bones are not expanded and there is no change in their contour (Fig. 11.44). The differential diagnosis generally is not difficult, due to the diffuse sclerosis that occurs in this condition. Rarely, it may be closely mimicked by some cases of metastatic carcinoma and the rare osteosclerotic form of myelomatosis; however, histologic studies will resolve the differential diagnosis (Fig. 11.45). Rare cases of spinal cord compression resulting from an extradural mass of hematopoietic tissue have been reported. Many patients with myelofibrosis eventually will develop a myelogenous leukemia.

SICKLE CELL DISEASE

A number of hematologic conditions result from the abnormal formation of hemoglobin, and these conditions are known collectively as the hemoglobinopathies. In sickle cell disease, a substitution of one of the amino acids in the beta hemoglobin chain results in an increased hemolysis of the blood under low oxygen tension, and in a crystallization of the hemoglobin molecule that results in formation of the abnormal sickle-shaped red cell. The hemolytic anemia results in bone marrow hyperplasia, and consequent to this there is some associated osteoporosis, which at times is associated with vertebral collapse, wedge-shaped deformities, and ky-

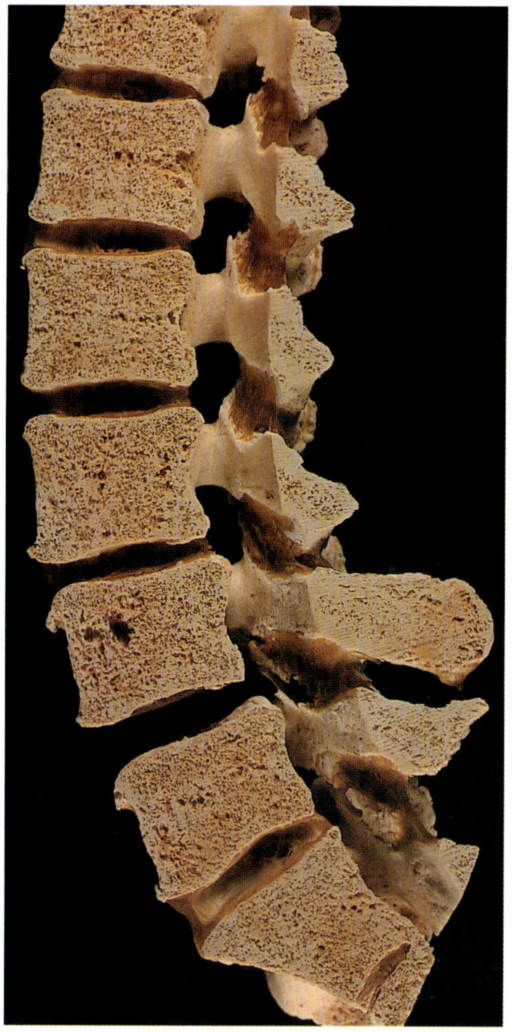

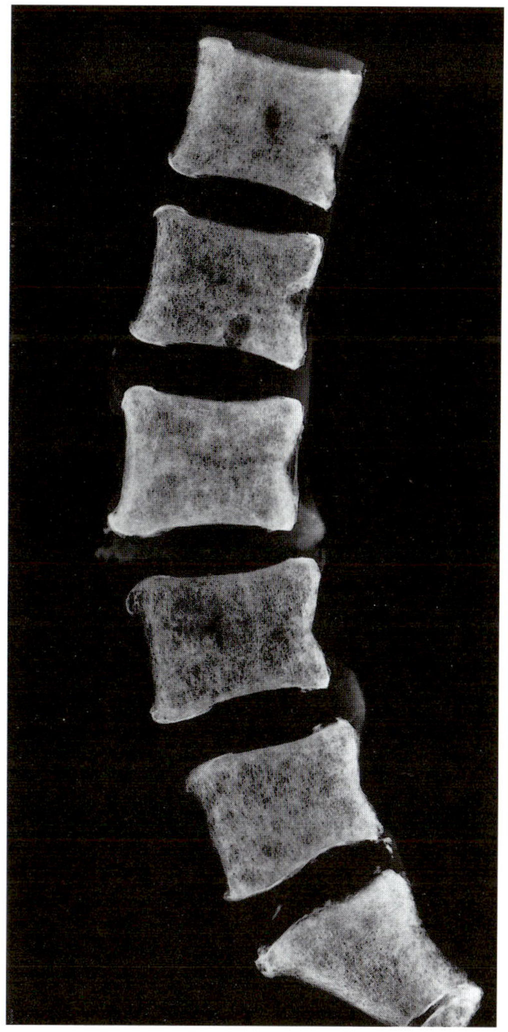

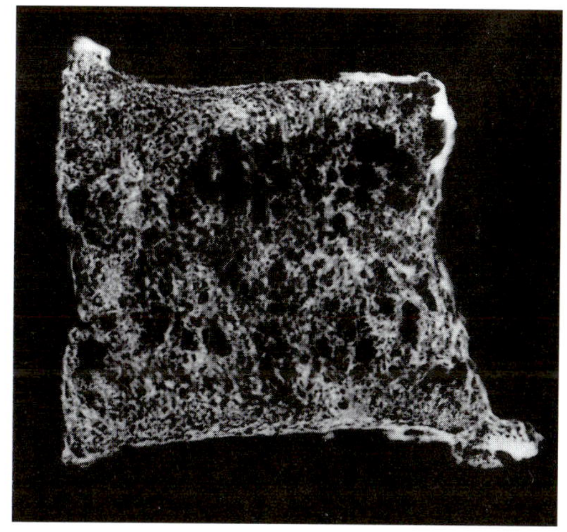

Figure 11.43 Photograph (*left*) of a sagittal section through the macerated lumbar spine of a patient with myelofibrosis. Note the extremely sclerotic bone associated with this condition. A radiograph (*center*) of the same specimen shows patchy osteosclerosis, with a complete loss of the normal trabecular pattern. A specimen radiograph (*right*) of a 2-mm slice through one of the vertebrae demonstrates the sclerosis and loss of trabecular pattern seen in this condition.

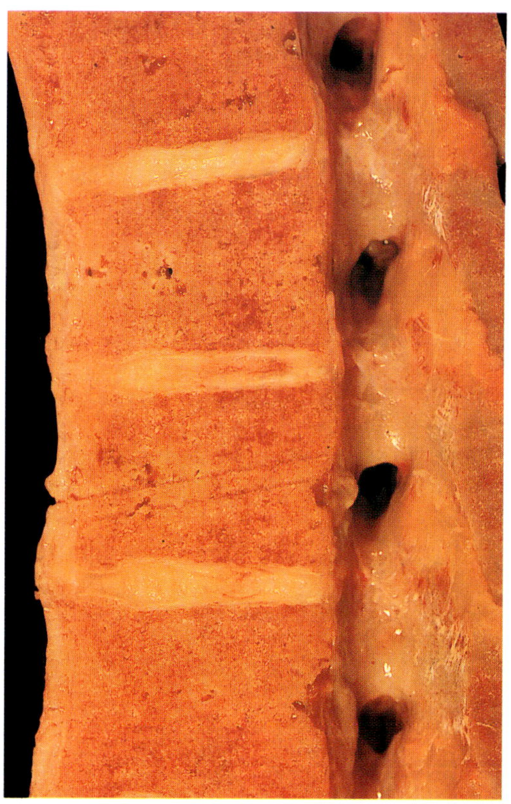

Figure 11.44 Close-up photograph of a portion of the lower thoracic spine to show the pale appearance due to the fibrotic replacement of the bone marrow. Note the lack of any deformity in the contours of the vertebral bodies.

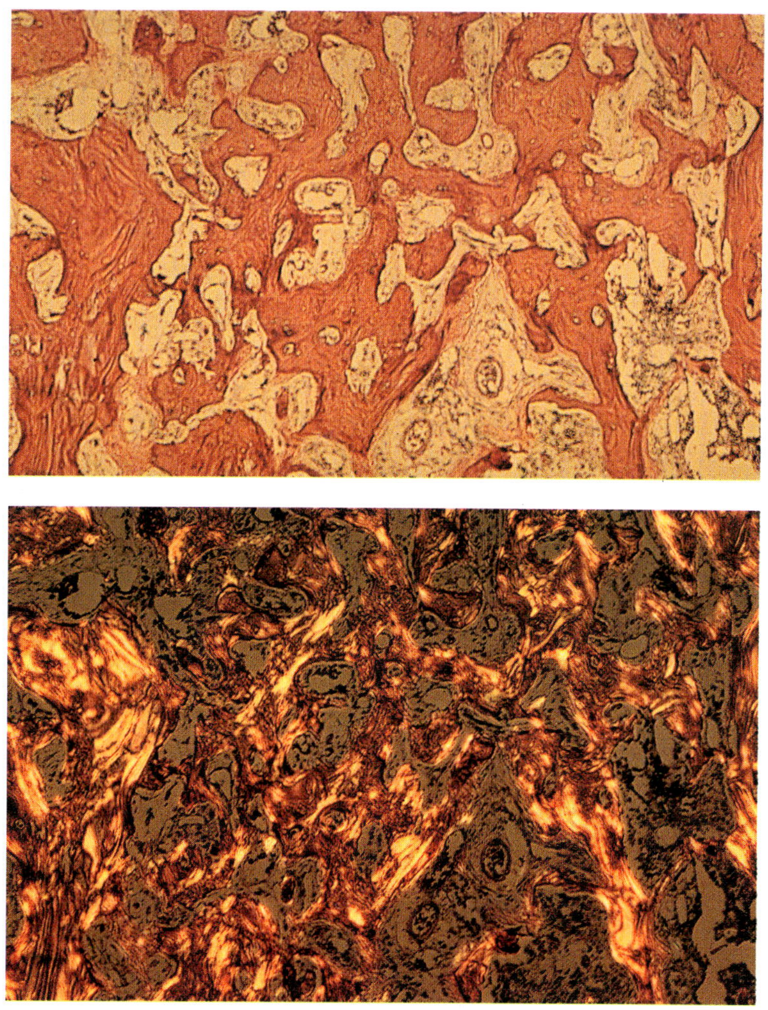

Figure 11.45 Photomicrograph (*top*) showing a section of bone from a patient with myelofibrosis. Note that there is extensive new bone formation, as well as fibrosis of the marrow space with displacement of the hematopoietic tissue. The same specimen photographed with polarized light (*bottom*) shows that the extensive new bone formation has an immature or woven pattern. (× 10 objective)

phoscoliosis (Fig. 11.46). However, the most severe problem in sickle cell disease is the development of infarctions. These may result in sudden pain located anywhere in the back, though usually in the lower back, which may awaken the sleeping patient. Initial radiographs will be normal, with infarction-related changes developing only after some months. In addition to compression fractures and wedging fractures, one also may see in the spines of affected children a double concavity, due to collapse of the central portion of the vertebral body under the hyaline growth plate. Rather than being compression fractures due to mechanical failure, it has been suggested that these lesions are the result of a relative ischemia in this region of the vertebral body. Osteomyelitis is a well-recognized complication of sickle cell disease, and when it occurs it may be due to infection with the salmonella organism (Fig. 11.47).

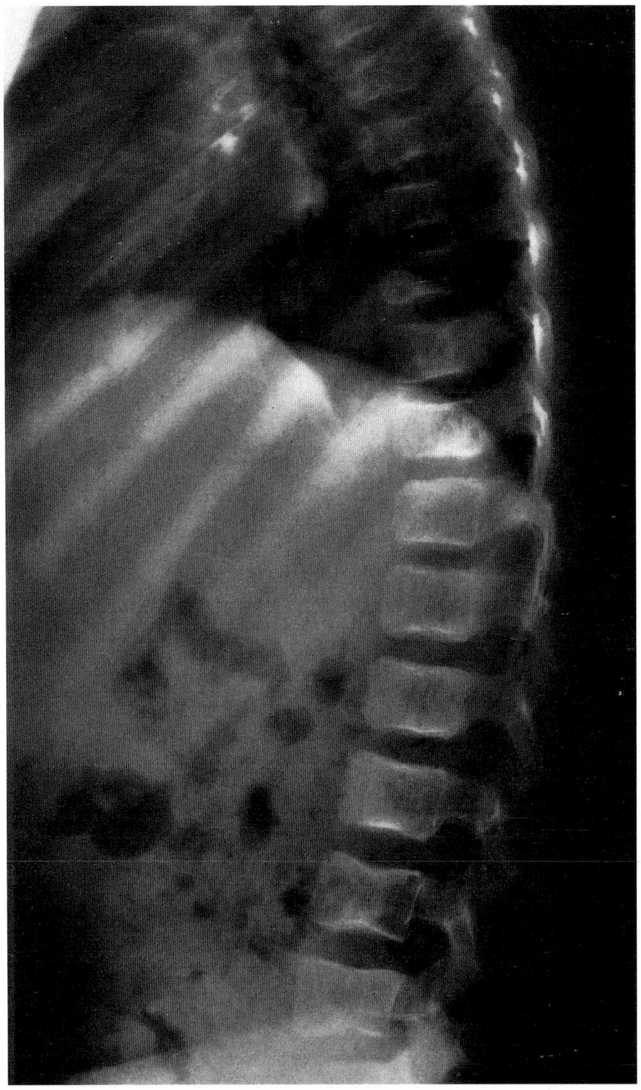

Figure 11.46 Lateral radiograph of an adolescent male with sickle cell disease. Note the osteopenia, with accentuation of the vertical trabeculae, and the central collapse of the vertebral bodies in the upper and midthoracic spine.

THALASSEMIA

In the thalassemias, the hemoglobin abnormality is due to a deletion of one of the amino acid chains, which results in a profound hemolytic anemia and consequently in a severe marrow hyperplasia (mainly, erythroid hyperplasia) that is associated with a profound osteoporosis (Figs. 11.48 and 11.49). In severe cases, some kyphoscoliosis may be apparent from vertebral collapse. Occasionally, thalassemia is seen in association with sickle cell disease, and in such a case infarction may be superadded.

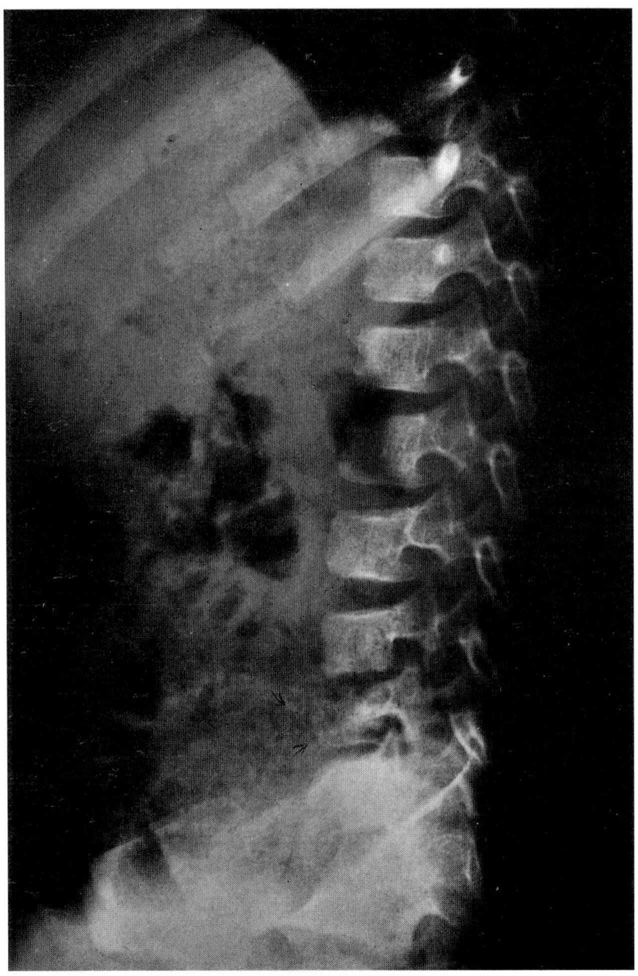

Figure 11.47 Lateral radiograph of a young child with sickle cell disease, who developed severe pain in the lower back, associated with fever and chills. A destructive process is seen in L-5, with loss of the superior end plate and patchy lysis within the body. A needle biopsy of this lesion demonstrated acute osteomyelitis and the culture grew *Salmonella typhi*.

GAUCHER'S DISEASE

Gaucher's disease is an inherited condition in which there is an abnormality in the metabolism of the glucocerebrosides, due to a deficiency in the activity of the enzyme glucosylceramide beta glucosidase. As a result of this deficiency, there is an accumulation of lipid material in histiocytes in the liver, spleen, lymph nodes, and bone marrow (Fig. 11.50). Osteopenia, infarction, and a modeling defect, seen most frequently at the rapidly growing ends of the long bones (e.g., the Erlenmeyer flask deformity of the lower femur), may result. The spine generally shows a loss of density, and frequently one or more of the vertebrae show collapse, with a wedge-shaped deformity, platyspondyly, or, occasionally, fish-mouth deformities (Fig. 11.51). Radiographically, in addition to osteopenia, some osteosclerotic lesions occasionally are present. These appearances are probably the result of the replacement of bone marrow by Gaucher's cells as well as of infarction within the bone.

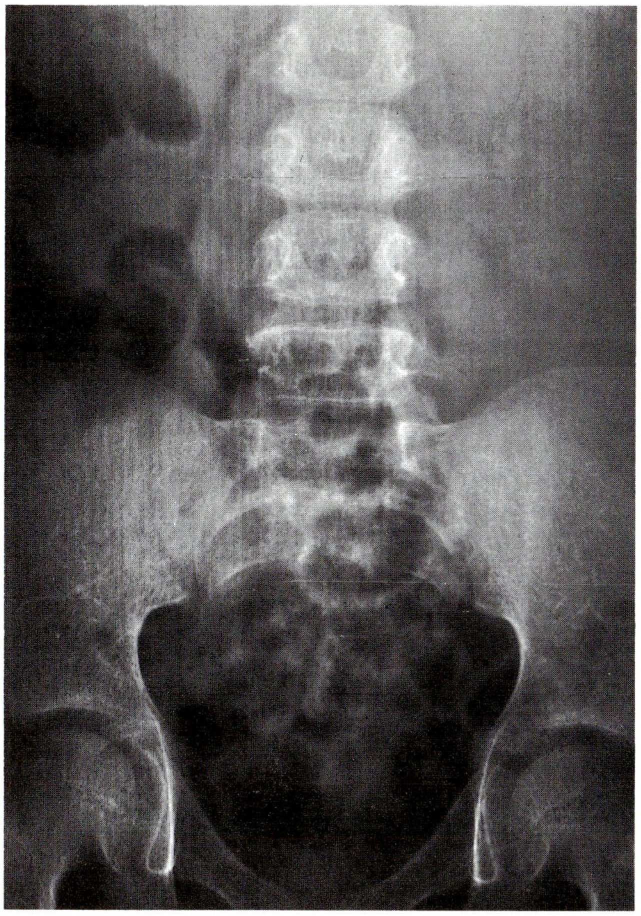

Figure 11.48 AP radiograph of a young adolescent with thalassemia major. There is profound osteoporosis with marked accentuation of the vertebral trabeculae of the spine. No obvious deformity is seen in this radiograph.

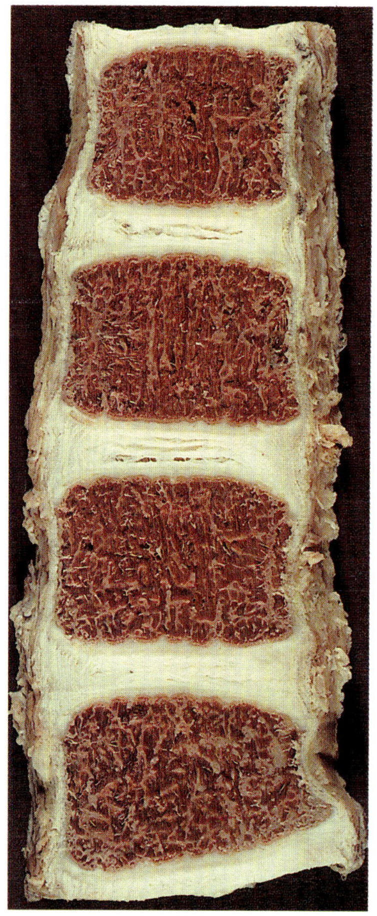

Figure 11.49 Photograph of a frontal section through the lower thoracic and upper lumbar spine of a patient with thalassemia, who came to autopsy. Note the mahogany brown color, secondary to severe hyperplasia and hemosiderosis of the bone marrow, together with loss of bone substance and partial collapse of the lower vertebra.

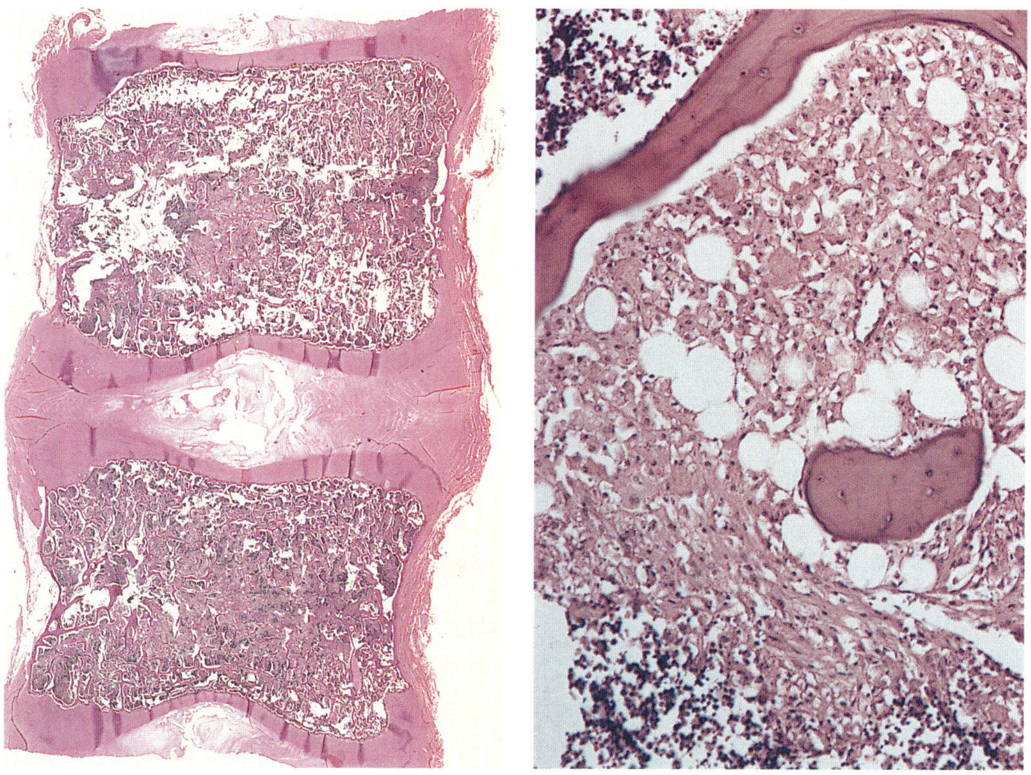

Figure 11.50 Photomicrograph (*left*) of a section of two vertebrae, showing extensive replacement by pale pink tissue. (Courtesy of Dr. Krishnan K. Unni) At higher power (*right*), the Gaucher cells are seen to be swollen histiocytes with a rather typical foamy cytoplasm and a crinkled appearance. This histiocytic infiltrate is replacing the normal bone marrow.

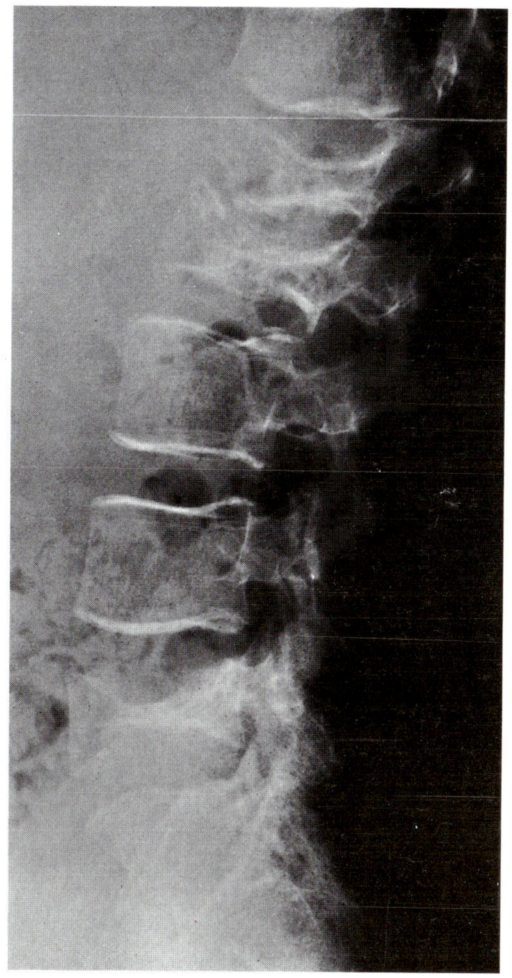

Figure 11.51 Lateral radiograph of a patient with Gaucher's disease. Osteopenia and collapse of L-1, L-2, and L-5 are seen. There is a kyphotic deformity in the thoracolumbar region.

12 CHAPTER

SPINAL INFECTIONS

Introduction

Infection of the spine has become rare in the western world and therefore may not always be considered when a patient complains of back pain. In certain groups of individuals however, including debilitated elderly patients, diabetics, immunocompromised patients, and drug addicts, infection should always be considered in evaluating back pain.

Infection of the spine usually is secondary to a primary focus elsewhere and it is hematogenous in spread. Generally it starts in the vertebral bone, although in both pyogenic and granulomatous infections the discs and surrounding soft tissues eventually become involved in the process. Neurologic complications are common. Before the advent of chemotherapeutic agents, spinal infection had a high incidence of both morbidity and mortality.

Pyogenic Spondylitis

Pyogenic spondylitis has been reported by most recent investigators to be rare in comparison to infections of the appendicular skeleton, and constitutes less than 1% of all cases of osteomyelitis. In previous times it was children who were most commonly affected by pyogenic spondylitis. Nowadays, although the disease may be seen at any age, it is most common after the sixth decade of life.

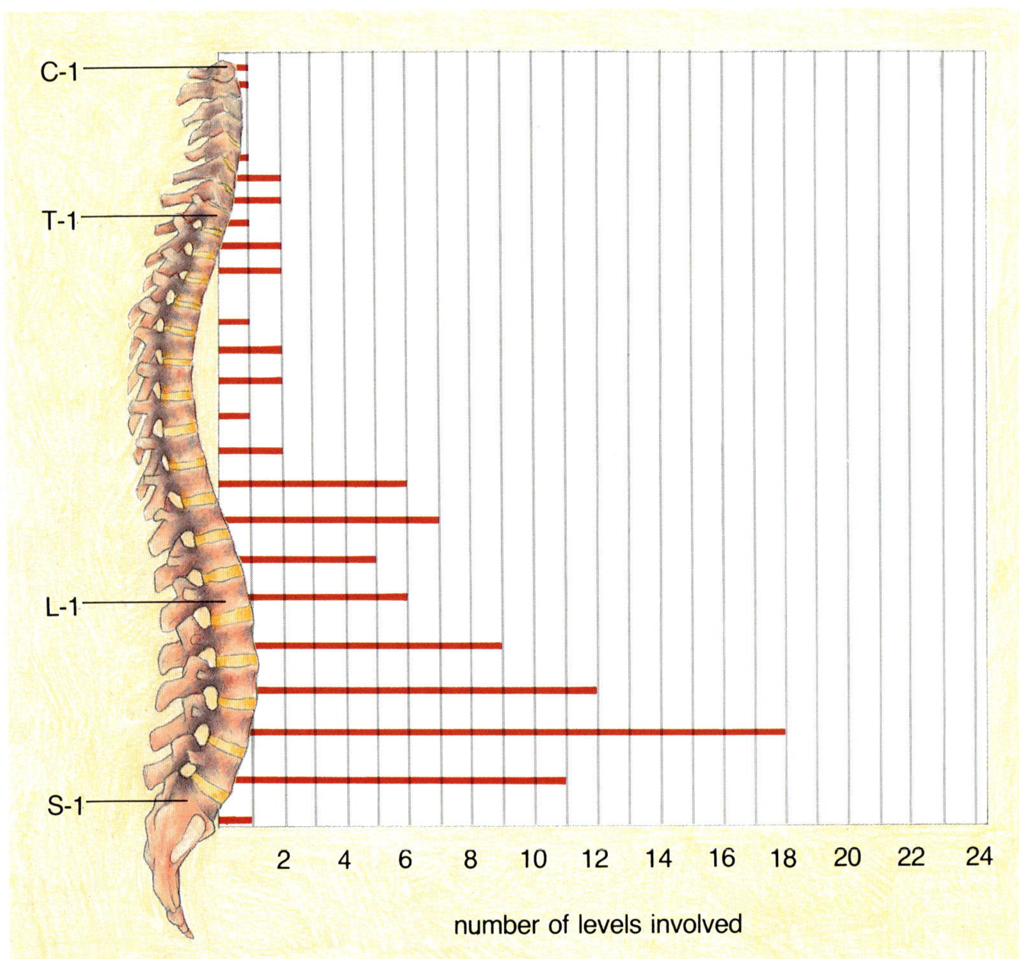

Figure 12.1 Schematic drawing to show the frequency of involvement at various levels of the spine in 40 cases of pyogenic spondylitis. In half of the cases there was an associated abscess, and in all of the cases more than one vertebral body was involved.

Predisposing factors include systemic urinary tract infection, diabetes, and IV drug addiction. The lumbar spine is involved twice as frequently as is the thoracic spine, and the cervical spine is only rarely involved (Fig. 12.1). Depending on the virulence of the infectious agent, pyogenic spondylitis may present with back pain, radiculopathy, and/or systemic signs of acute infection. Generally however, the patient presents with only vague localizing symptoms and a general malaise. An untreated infection may lead to significant deformity of the spine and to severe neurologic deficit.

RADIOGRAPHIC FEATURES

The earliest conventional radiographic findings usually manifest 4 to 6 weeks after onset of the disease (Fig. 12.2). These findings include local destructive changes within the affected vertebral body, increased paravertebral shadows from soft-tissue edema or abscess, and progressive narrowing of the disc space with blurring of the subchondral bony end plate of the adjacent vertebral bodies (Fig. 12.3). Progressive destruction of the vertebral body leads to its collapse. The development of paravertebral abscesses in the neck may cause an increase in the retropharyngeal space; in the thorax, in displacement of the parietal pleura; and, in the lumbar region, in indistinct psoas definition.

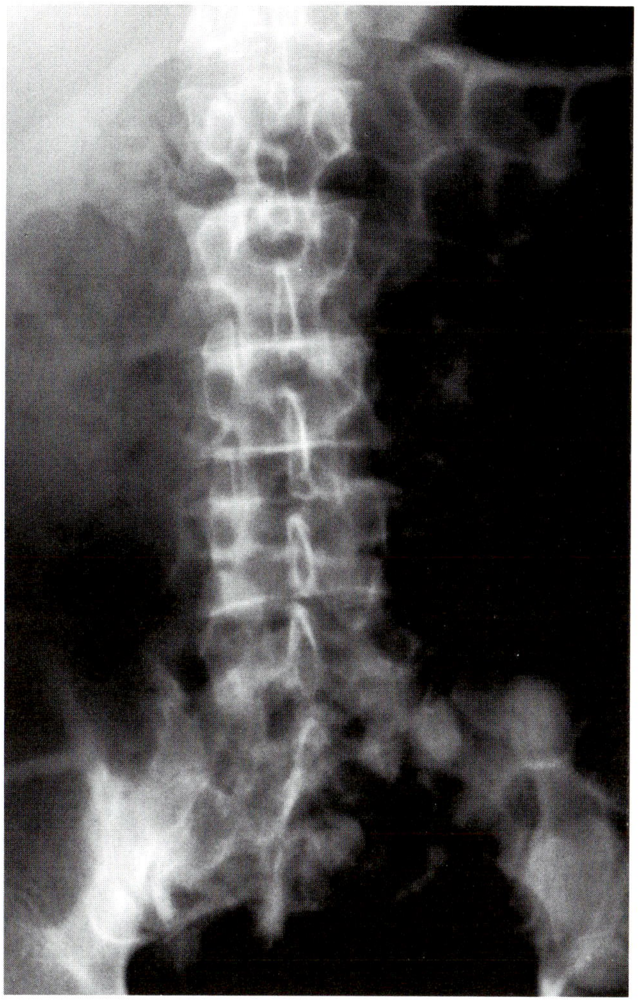

Figure 12.2 AP radiograph of a 55-year-old male with a history of chronic intravenous drug abuse. The outline and bone texture of the body of L-5 are blurred. The bony end plates are not well visualized.

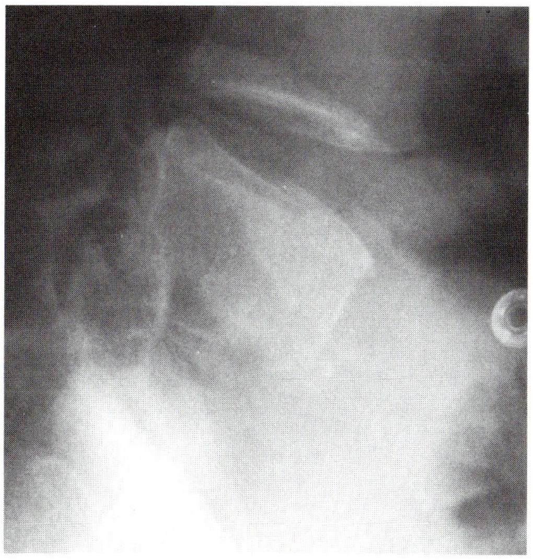

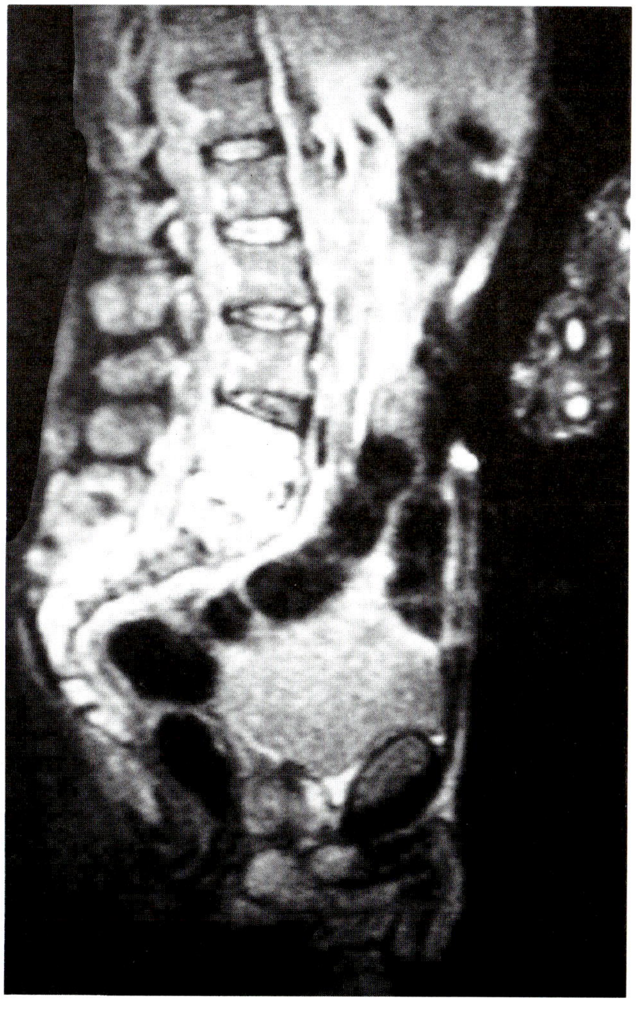

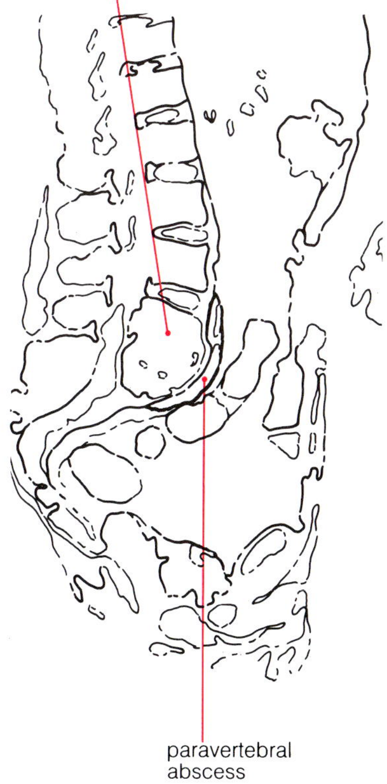

Figure 12.3 Lateral radiograph (*left*) of the lumbosacral region of the patient illustrated in Figure 12.2. The L-5 to S-1 disc space is poorly visualized, and the end plates are indistinct. In a sagittal MRI (*right*) of the same patient, an increased signal is seen in L-5 to S-1, with a paravertebral mass displacing the colon anteriorly. An aspirate from this area produced pus, from which grew *Staphylococcus aureus*.

Even before the earliest radiographic changes are obvious on plain films, CT scans may be helpful in identifying both early vertebral destruction (Fig. 12.4) and the presence of a paravertebral mass. Radioisotope bone scan also may help in identifying and localizing the septic focus.

Radiographic features suggestive of infection also may occur (Figs. 12.5 through 12.7) with osteochondrosis.

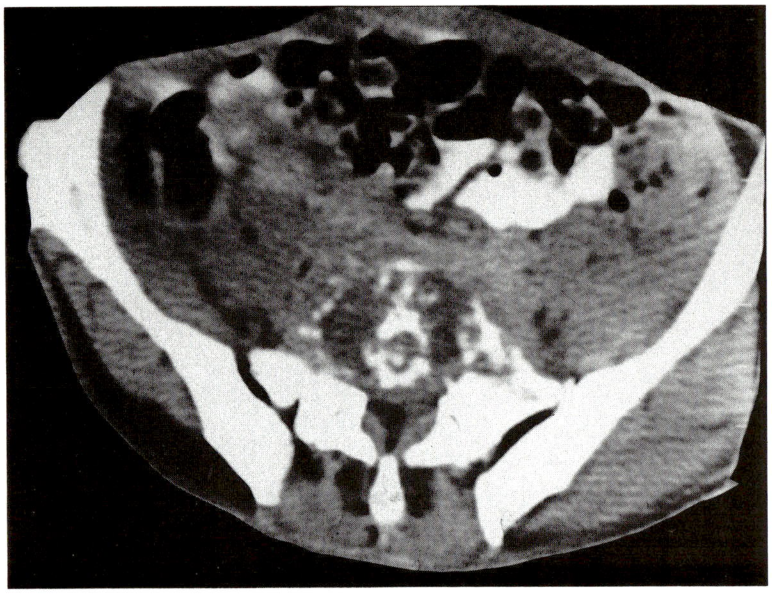

Figure 12.4 CT scan of S-1 and the pelvis of the patient illustrated in Figures 12.2 and 12.3. Note the extensive peripheral destruction of the vertebral body.

PATHOPHYSIOLOGY

Definitive diagnosis depends on recovery of the responsible organism, either by blood culture or by local aspirate. However, the latter in some cases may be difficult to procure, leaving open surgery as the only means of establishing a definitive bacteriologic diagnosis.

The most commonly isolated organism is *Staphylococcus aureus*. However, gram-negative organisms, especially *Escherichia coli*, have been recovered in association with lower urinary tract infections. Among drug addicts pseudomonas is likely to be isolated, and in sickle cell patients salmonella may be implicated.

In the majority of cases, the organism is introduced into the bone by the hematogenous route. In hematogenous vertebral osteomyelitis, either the vertebral body or the neural arch may be involved first. The intervertebral disc becomes secondarily involved, with ultimate involvement of the end plates and subsequent destruction of the disc tissue. Wiley and Trueta (1959) have shown by their injection studies that the arterial route is almost certainly the most important one in the spread of infection to the spine, although in the past both arterial and venous dissemination have been implicated. The vertebral metaphysis is richly supplied by the peripheral arterioles and by the main nutrient artery entering posteriorly, and these provide for the arterial route of dissemination. The venous route of dissemination to the vertebral bone is of particular importance in urinary tract and other pelvic organ infections. It is effected through Batson's plexus of interconnecting valveless veins; increased intraabdominal pressure allows retrograde hematogenous spread from the pelvis and abdominal organs to the vertebral column.

An abscess in the vertebral body may spread posteriorly to involve the posterior arch, or it may violate the anterior cortex and ligamentous structures to form paravertebral soft-tissue abscesses. Likewise, retropharyngeal abscesses may form from cervical infections, and abscess in the paraspinal muscle may form from thoracic infections. In the lumbar region, an abscess in the psoas sheath may spread to the groin or even to the popliteal fossa. The central nervous system may become contaminated by the spread of infection into the neural canal, resulting in meningitis. The adjacent vertebrae often are

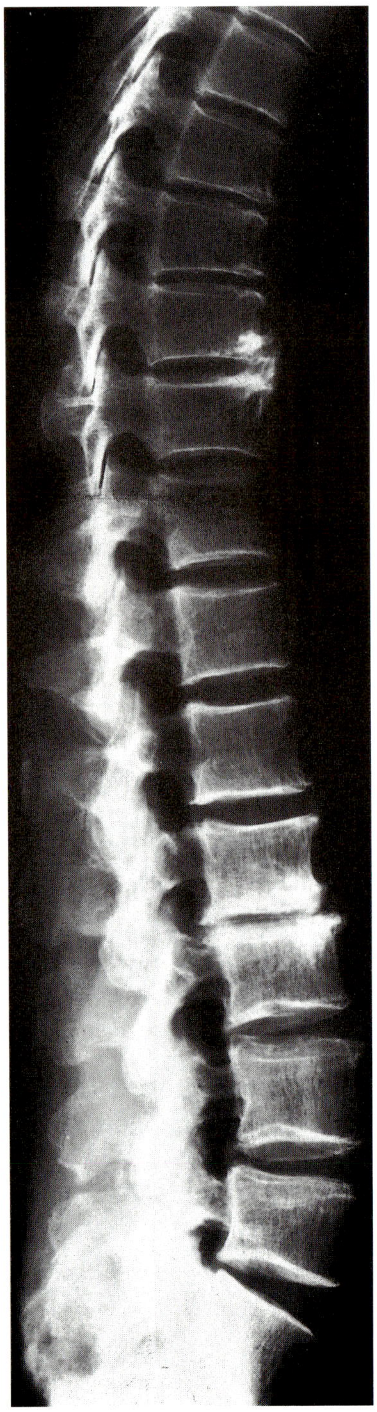

Figure 12.5 Specimen radiograph of the lumbar spine from a 72-year-old male who was immunocompromised. At autopsy, there were multiple sites of infection, including the spine. The organism recovered was *Pseudomonas aeruginosa*. At the L1-2 space, there is paradiscal sclerosis and anterolateral peripheral hypertrophy. The disc space is narrowed. At T8-9, a similar process is noted, though less severe in degree.

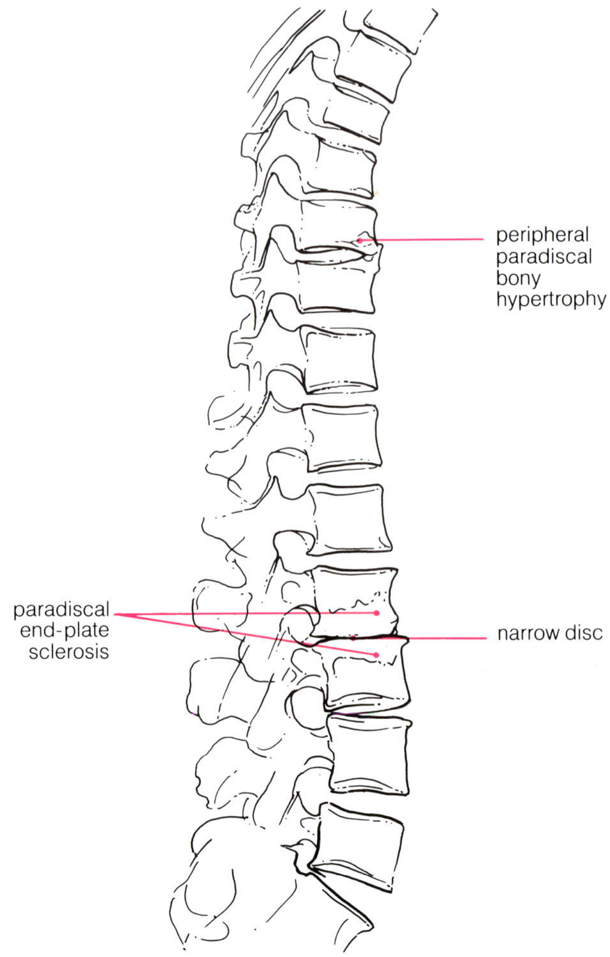

infected by spread along the vertebral ligaments, and the intervertebral disc becomes sequestered and eventually may be destroyed. The affected vertebral body may subsequently collapse, resulting in a kyphotic deformity (Fig. 12.8). In the case of organisms of low virulence, hypertrophic changes with bony sclerosis and osteophyte formation may result in eventual bony an-

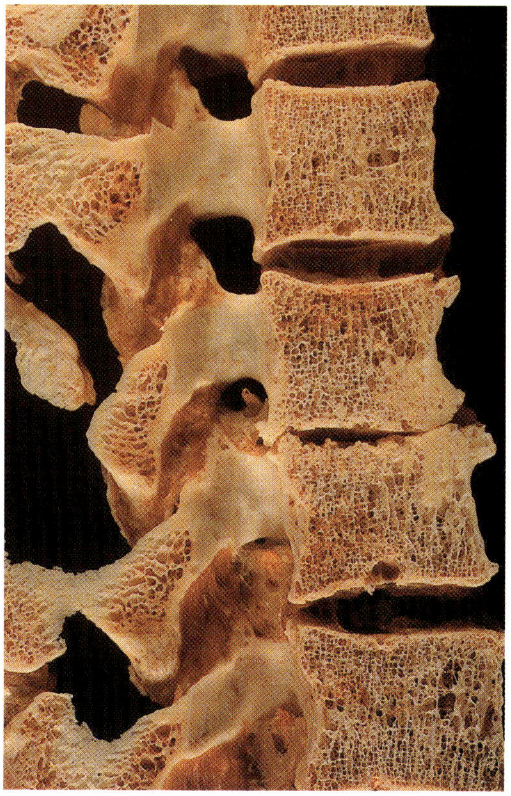

Figure 12.6 Photograph of a sagittal section of T-12 to L-3 of the macerated specimen of the same case shown in Figure 12.5. Note especially the irregularity of the end plates, as well as the marked sclerosis of the bone.

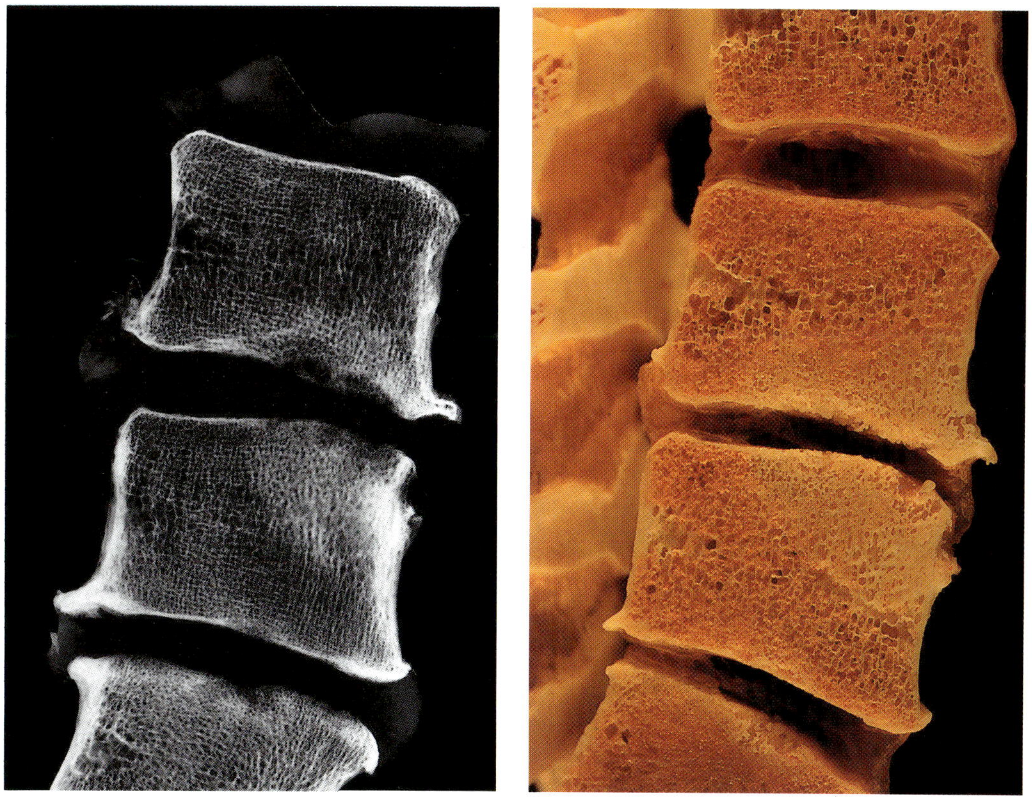

Figure 12.7 Specimen radiograph (*left*) of a section of the lower lumbar spine from a patient with osteochondrosis and *no* evidence of infection, to demonstrate discogenic sclerosis at both L4-5 and L-5 to S-1 for comparison with Figure 12.6. Note the irregularity of the end plates anteriorly, and in L4-5, the associated anterior narrowing of the disc. Posteriorly, the end plates are preserved. In L-5 to S-1, the lesion is central and confined mostly to the superior surface of S-1. Photograph (*right*) of the macerated specimen.

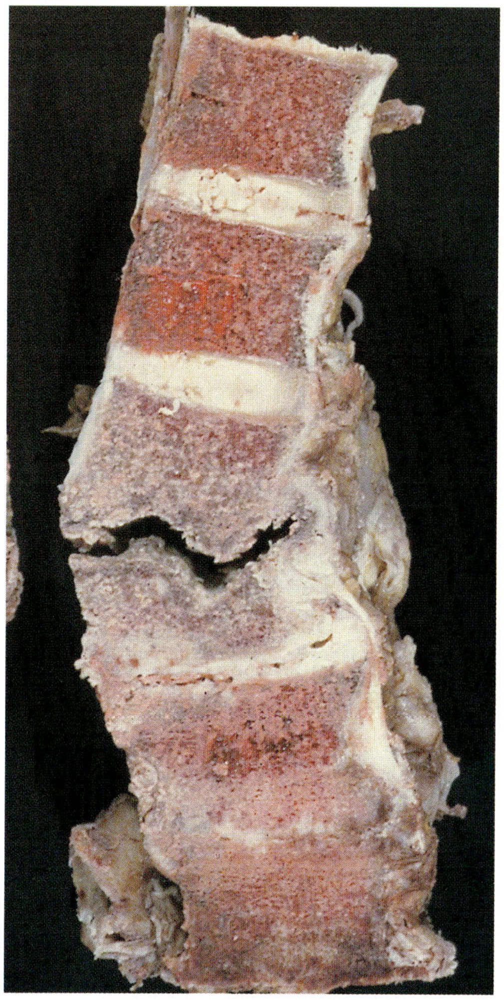

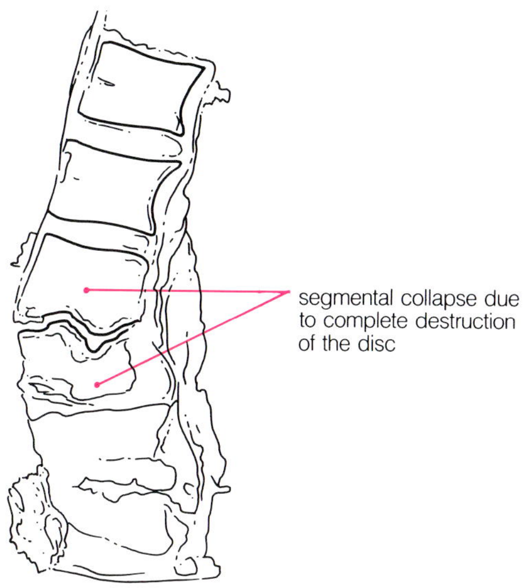

Figure 12.8 Photograph of a sagittal section through the thoracolumbar spine of a patient with pyogenic spondylitis to show involvement of few vertebral segments. A mild kyphotic deformity is apparent. Note the complete destruction of the disc by the disease process. (Courtesy of Dr. Krishnan K. Unni)

kylosis. Microscopic changes will depend on the duration of the disease (Fig. 12.9).

In children, pyogenic spondylitis is modified by the anatomy of the developing vertebral body. With the presence of an active epiphysial growth plate and of growth cartilage, extension of the infection to the disc space appears to occur more readily than it does in adults. The most common location of disease is in the lumbar spine, and in only about one-third of patients can a positive culture be obtained by aspiration of the primary lesion. In a quarter of affected children, spontaneous fusion may occur.

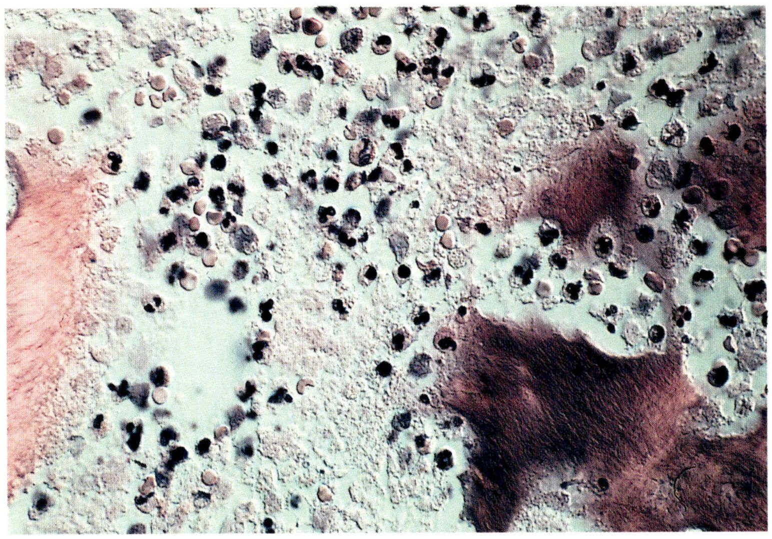

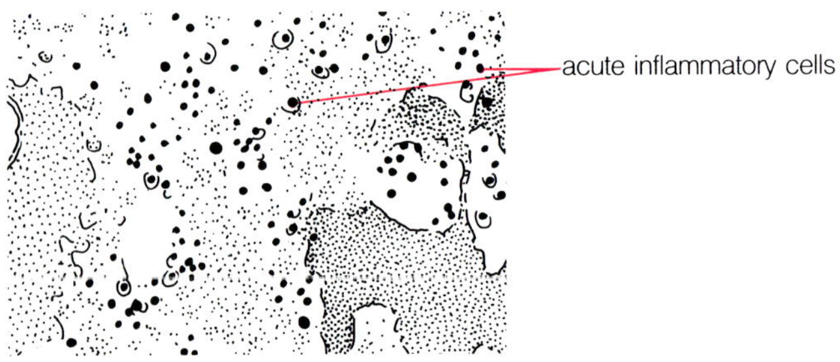

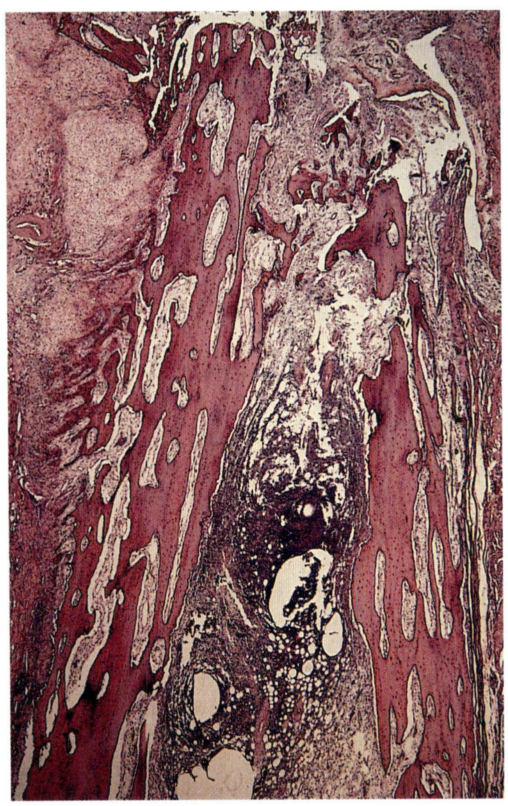

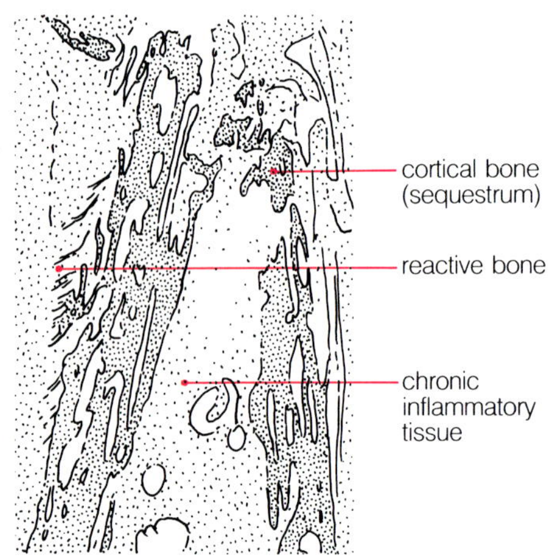

Figure 12.9 Photomicrograph (*top*) to show acute inflammation of the marrow space in early osteomyelitis. (H & E, × 25 objective) Photomicrograph (*bottom*) to show chronic inflammatory cells, fibrosis, and reactive bone formation in chronic osteomyelitis. (H & E, × 2.5 objective)

Tuberculous Spondylitis (Pott's Disease)

GENERAL FEATURES

The most common form of spinal infection is that associated with tuberculosis (Fig. 12.10). Approximately 1% of patients with tuberculosis develop musculoskeletal complications and the most common site of skeletal involvement is the spine. In 1779, Pott described the classic presentation of angular kyphotic deformity and paraplegia now known to result from tuberculous spondylitis.

In the underdeveloped world, tuberculous spondylitis remains a very common disease affecting mainly children. In western developed nations, it is on the decline. However, in the past decade, there has been no significant decrease in the number of cases in the United States. Although spinal tuberculosis affects primarily the elderly and immunocompromised, it also remains the most common cause of vertebral infection in the young.

In most patients, the onset of symptoms is likely to be insidious, and includes local pain as well as systemic signs of chronic debilitating illness. At the time of initial presentation, the patient may complain of persistent back pain, of months to years duration; however, with the passage of time, signs of nerve root compression with radiculopathy, meningitis, or other neurologic deficits, such as lower extremity weakness, loss of reflex, or paraplegia, may develop. Other findings upon physical examination and history are subcutaneous flank mass, dysphagia, night sweats, and kyphosis, frequently involving the thoracic region.

Other patients may present because of a cold abscess in the groin or elsewhere (Fig. 12.11). Paraplegia is the most serious complication of tuberculous spondylitis, and it results from extension of the disease process into the peridural space, with resultant cord compression; this may be accentuated by the development of a gibbus deformity. Moreover, dislocation may lead to sudden paraplegia.

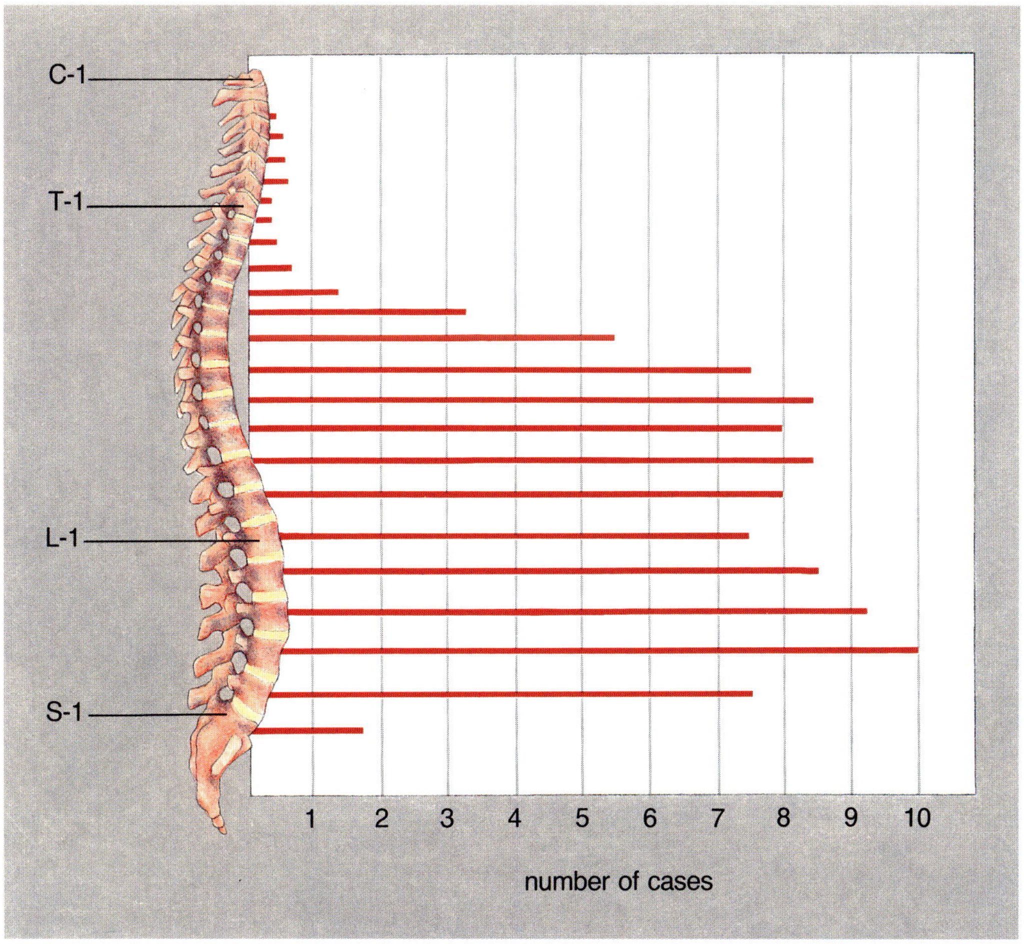

Figure 12.10 Schematic drawing to show the distribution of cases of spinal tuberculosis at various spinal levels. (Adapted from Schmorl)

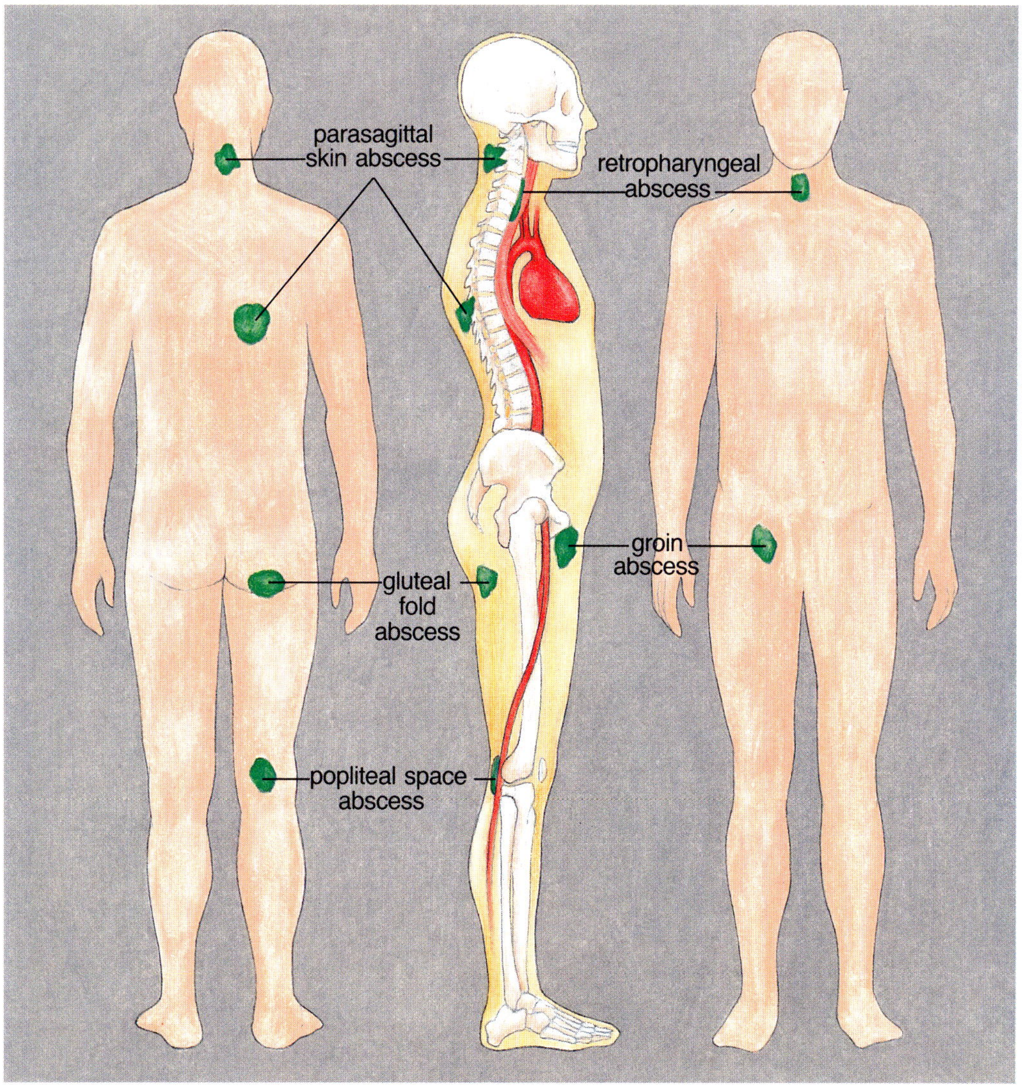

Figure 12.11 Schematic drawing to show the distribution of soft-tissue abscesses associated with tuberculous spondylitis. (Adapted from Schmorl)

RADIOGRAPHIC FEATURES

CT scan and plain radiographs are the best way to assess bone destruction and extension of a tuberculous process. Investigators have found the CT scan to be better than conventional radiographic techniques for early detection of tuberculous spondylitis, and some have found soft-tissue lesions and calcifications easier to visualize with this technique.

The CT criteria for spinal tuberculosis include:

1. Vertebral destruction
2. Paravertebral soft-tissue mass
3. Soft-tissue calcification
4. Two vertebrae imaged simultaneously at different planes of inclination

Other related findings are a preserved spinal canal and surrounding sclerotic changes (possibly indicating a healing phenomenon). In addition, the CT scan can further aid in differentiating between tuberculosis and pyogenic infection: tuberculosis results in narrowing of the intervertebral disc space late in the course of disease and pyogenic infection early in the course of the disease; large calcified paraspinal masses are seen rarely with pyogenic infections.

CT scan also is useful in determining the optimal site from which to obtain a specimen for histologic study. Gallium scintiscans and ultrasound are additional imaging tools for assessing soft-tissue mass and for guiding needle aspirations.

On plain radiographs, the classical appearance for tuberculosis in the vertebral body is the "paint brush" image, in which hypodensity of the involved vertebral body and disc is seen. Common radiographic findings include central collapse, adjacent vertebral destruction, "ivory" vertebrae, and soft-tissue abscess formation (Fig. 12.12). Even so, a spine infected with tuberculosis may sometimes have a relatively normal appearance. If the tuberculosis is limited to the vertebral body center or to a small area, the process may easily be confused with a pyogenic or a fungal infection on conventional radiographs. Often on plain film, the number of involved vertebrae may be underestimated. The diagnosis may be made even more difficult if the intervertebral disc is uninvolved, and if the cancellous bone is involved only by a productive lesion rather than a destructive lesion with an exudative process. In addition, some lesions on conventional radiography may be difficult to recognize, because of interference by heart shadow or bowel gas.

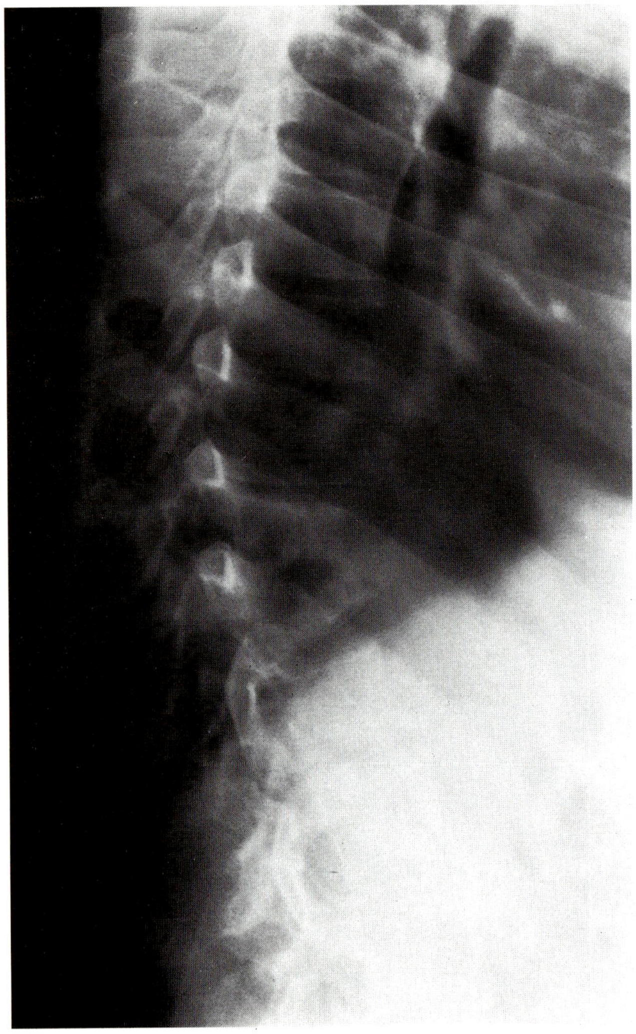

Figure 12.12 Lateral radiograph demonstrating a destructive lesion involving T-9 and T-10 and the intervening disc space. Note the absence of bony sclerosis and osteophytes, which helps to distinguish tuberculosis from pyogenic infection. A kyphotic deformity has developed.

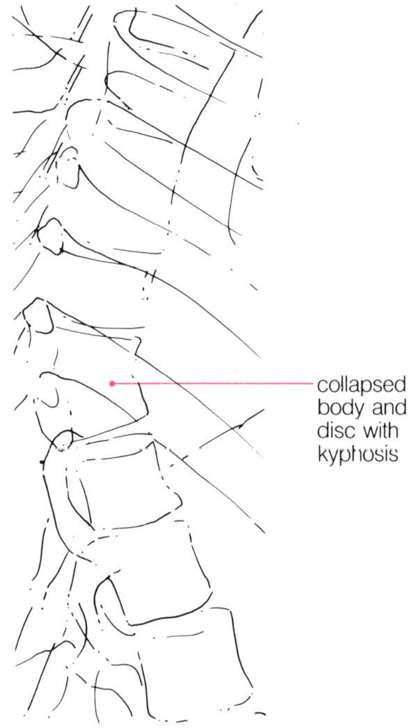

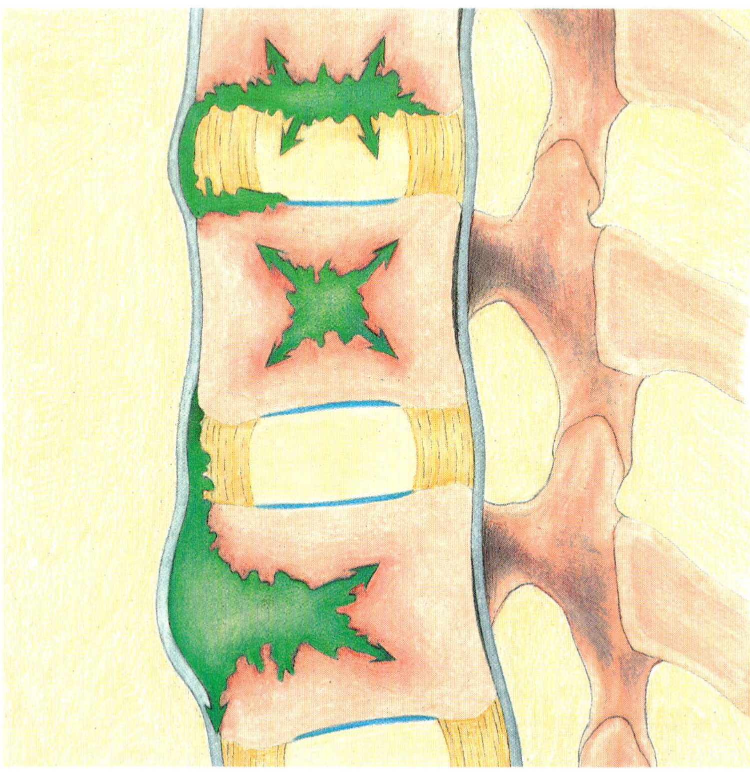

Figure 12.13 Schematic drawing to show three possible locations of the primary focus of tuberculous infection in the vertebral body. Each will result in a characteristic radiographic presentation. (Adapted from Schmorl)

PATHOLOGIC FEATURES

The primary granulomatous abscess in tuberculous spondylitis may be located in the vertebral body either anteriorly, paradiscally or centrally, giving rise to three characteristic presentations (Fig. 12.13); the vertebral arch is rarely involved. The anterior lesion, which accounts for approximately 20% of cases, usually leads to cortical bone destruction under the anterior longitudinal ligament. As the ligament lifts off the vertebral margin, there is spread of infection to the adjacent vertebral segment (Fig. 12.14).

The paradiscal lesion, which accounts for over half of cases, begins in the vertebral metaphysis and erodes through the cartilaginous end plate, extending around and sequestering the disc, to extend into the adjacent vertebra. Disc-space narrowing, bone destruction with subsequent kyphotic deformity, and eventual interbody fusion usually occur after 1 to 2 years (Fig. 12.15).

The central lesion, which accounts for the remaining cases, begins in the mid-portion of the vertebral body. It then spreads to involve the whole vertebral body, leading to collapse. This generally leads to development of the pronounced gibbus deformity described by Pott. A characteristic radio-

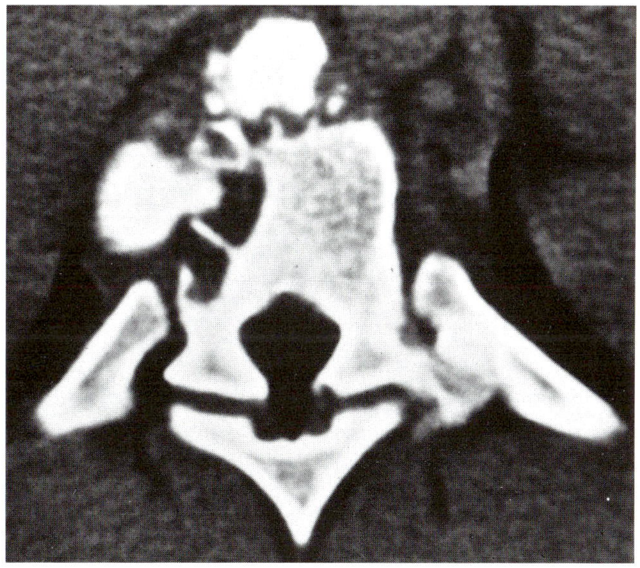

Figure 12.14 CT scan to demonstrate an anterolateral focus of infection by tuberculosis, with cortical erosion and elevation of the anterior longitudinal ligament by abscess. The abscess was injected with contrast agent at the time of diagnostic aspiration.

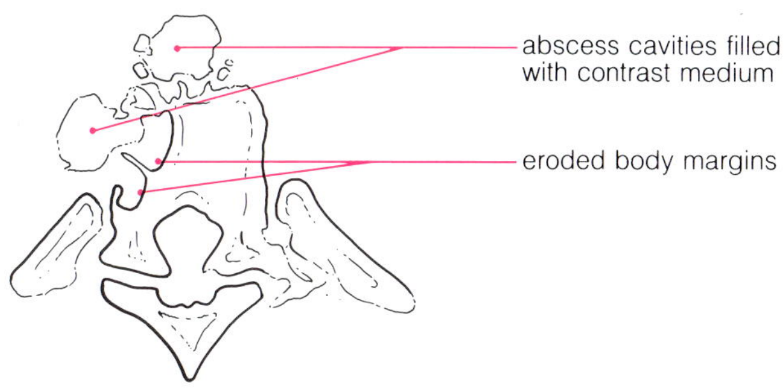

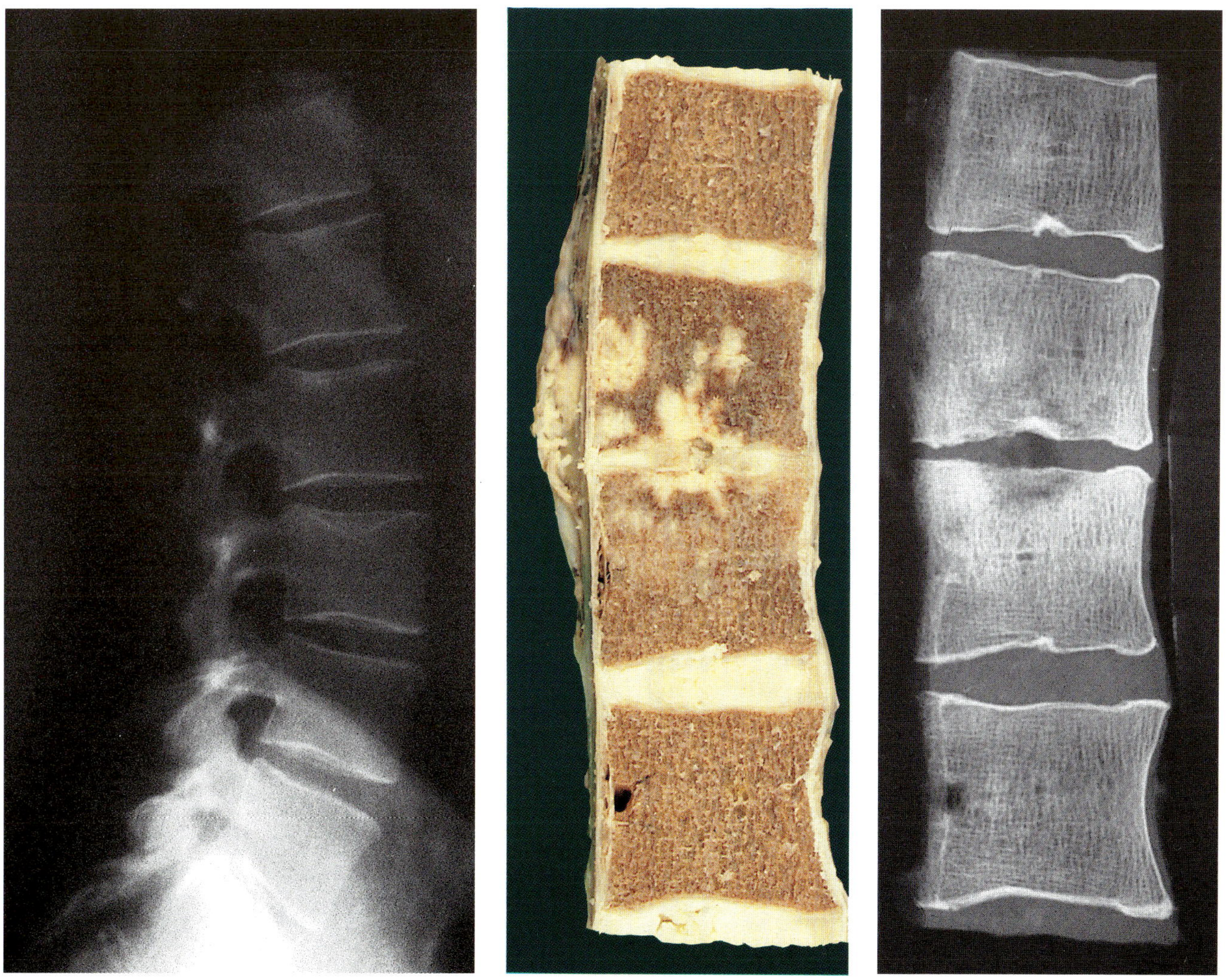

Figure 12.15 Clinical radiograph (*left*) of a patient with tuberculosis of T-11 to T-12. At this early stage of the disease, there is some irregularity of the vertebral end plates as well as disc narrowing. Photograph (*center*) of a sagittal section of the thoracolumbar spine obtained at autopsy in the same case. There is paradiscal involvement by the disease process, which has extended posteriorly to elevate the dura. The specimen radiograph (*right*) shows minimal bone destruction, with central irregularity of the bony end plates. (Courtesy of Dr. V. Fornasier)

graphic feature is that of a soft-tissue paravertebral shadow (Fig. 12.16).

Tuberculosis of the bones and joints, including the spine, occurs mostly as a result of secondary hematogenous and lymphatic spread from the lungs. However, the spine also may become involved by direct extension from adjacent visceral lesions. The lower thoracic spine is the most frequent site of tuberculous spondylitis in both children and adults, and involvement of several vertebral bodies occurs in 50% of cases.

The vertebral body usually is involved in tuberculous spondylitis with relative sparing of the posterior neural arch. Overall progressive bone loss is more prominent than are proliferative bone changes (Fig. 12.17). Posterior extension frequently leads to a neurologic deficit (Figs. 12.18 and 12.19).

The gross pathologic picture of tuberculosis is the finding of exudative granulation tissue studded with small abscesses. When the abscesses are confluent, the resulting lesion is referred to as a focus of caseation necrosis, and, associated with this, often there is secondary calcification. The affected tissue will appear yellow on gross examination, and frequently it has an opaque cheesy appearance. Ten percent of patients with tuberculous spondylitis have been reported to have noncontiguous vertebral body involvement, i.e., skip lesions.

Microscopic examination shows focal chronic inflammation with a nodular (i.e., granulomatous) appearance and central necrosis of the granulomas (Fig. 12.20). High-power examination will reveal typical Langerhans giant cells, with peripherally disposed nuclei. Definitive diagnosis depends on demonstration of acid-fast bacilli (Fig.

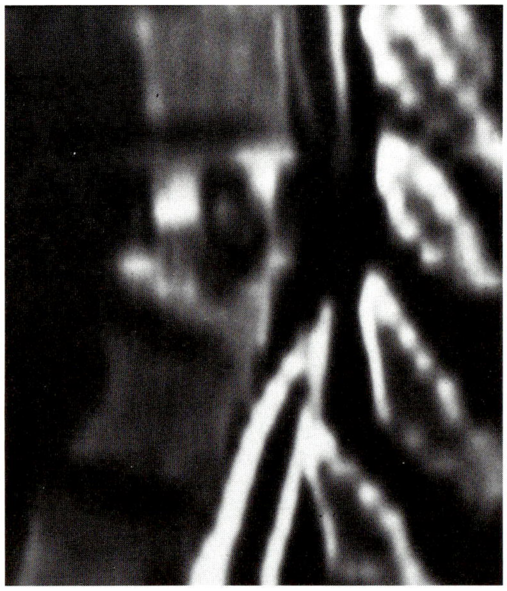

Figure 12.16 Sagittal CT scan (*top*) with myelogram to demonstrate a central tuberculous lesion with a partial block of the neural canal. An AP myelogram (*bottom*) of the same case demonstrates vertebral collapse and bilateral paravertebral shadow.

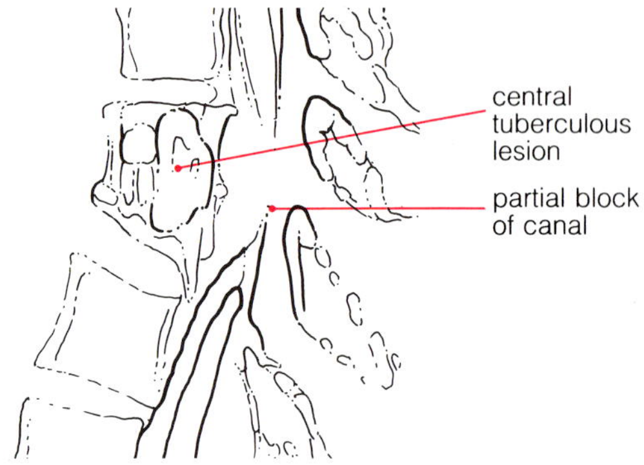

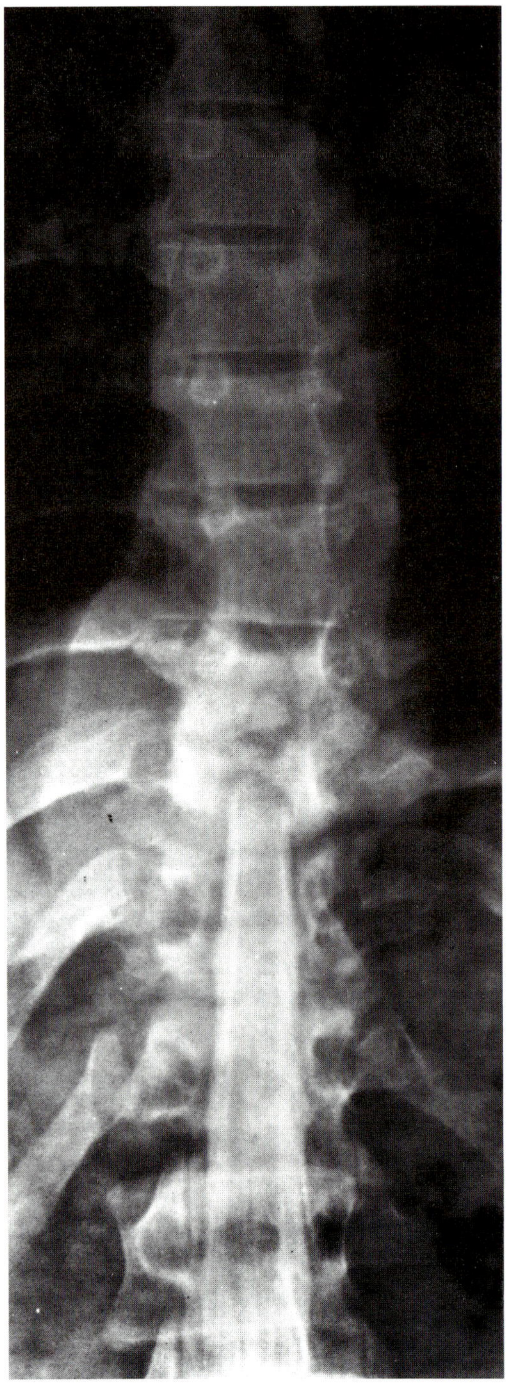

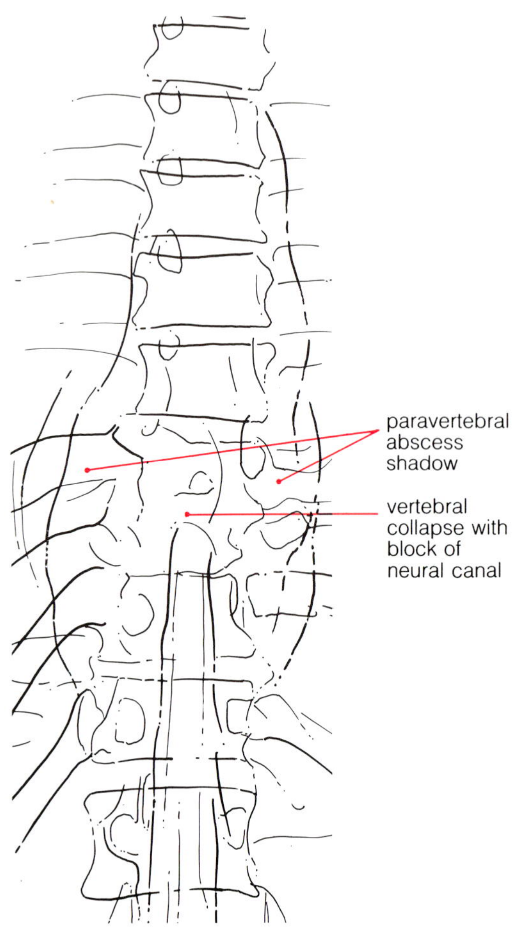

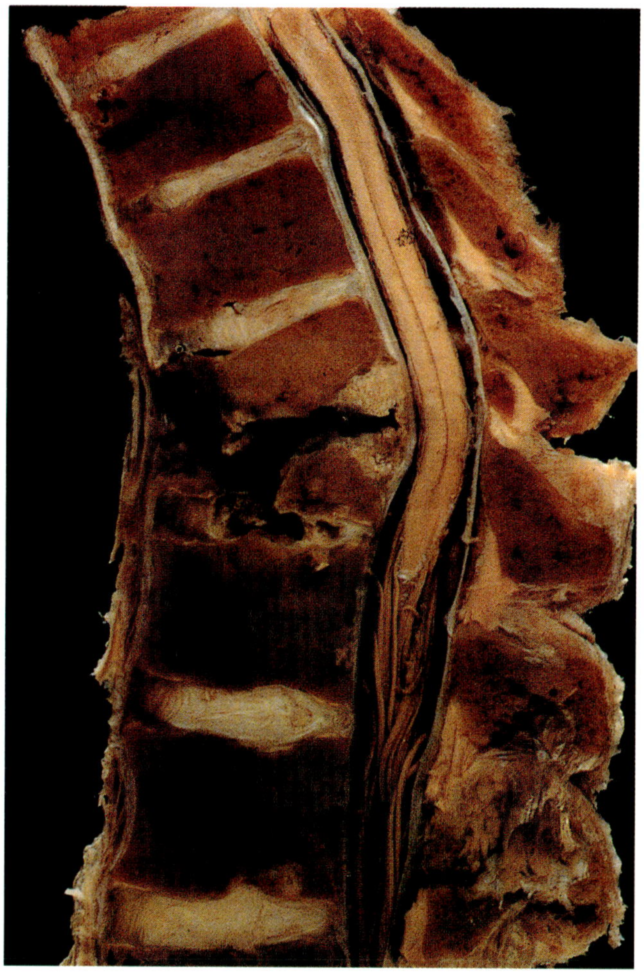

Figure 12.17 Photograph of a sagittal section of the thoracolumbar spine of a 52-year-old man showing extensive destruction of two of the vertebral bodies by cavitating caseous necrosis. The damaged bone bulges posteriorly into the spinal canal, compressing the cord. The patient was known to have had pulmonary tuberculosis for the preceding 4 years. During the last 6 months of his life, he had developed back pain associated with gradual loss of power and sensation in the legs. Toward the end of this period, he was completely paraplegic, with loss of excretory sphincter control. (Courtesy of the Royal College of Surgeons of England)

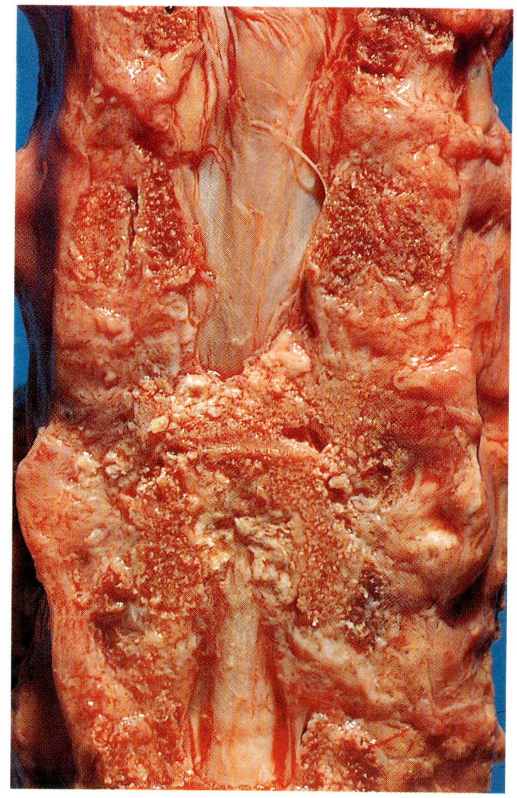

Figure 12.18 Photograph of a posterior view of a spine from a patient with tuberculosis, to demonstrate the severe cord compression that may occur in this disease.

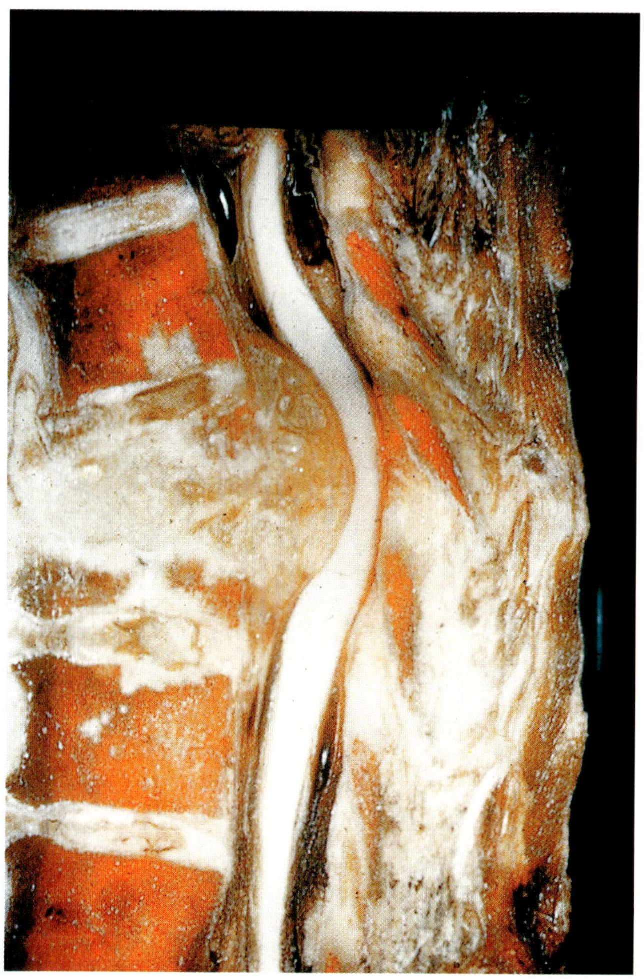

Figure 12.19 Photograph of a sagittal section of spine from a patient with tuberculosis. There is almost complete destruction of two of the vertebral bodies as well as of the intervertebral discs. The abscess has extended both anteriorly and posteriorly, resulting in severe cord compression.

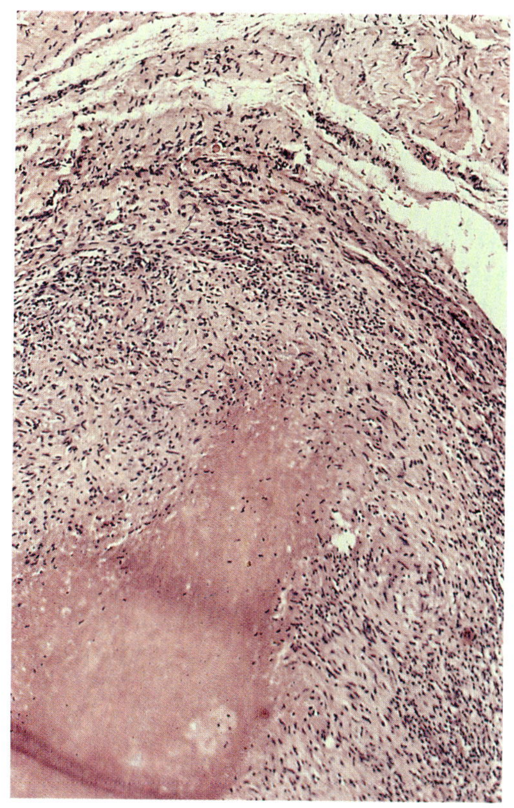

Figure 12.20 Photomicrograph of a tuberculous granuloma demonstrating central caseation necrosis surrounded by chronic inflammatory tissue. (H & E, × 80)

12.21). However, in many sections it may be difficult to demonstrate the bacilli, and obtaining positive cultures without open surgery also may be difficult.

DIFFERENTIAL DIAGNOSIS

Tuberculous spondylitis runs a longer course than does pyogenic spondylitis and results in more significant bony destruction and deformity (Figs. 12.22 and 12.23). Eventually, fusion and healing of the involved segment may occur (Fig. 12.24). A pyogenic infection has an acute onset and is of shorter duration than tuberculosis, where the onset is insidious. Like tuberculosis, pyogenic infections may be associated with abscess formation, vertebral collapse, gibbus formation, ankylosis, and proliferative marginal reactions. Disc-space involvement occurs early in pyogenic infection, whereas in tuberculosis the vertebral interspace is maintained for a long time, due to the inability of the mycobacteria to produce proteolytic enzymes. In addition, metastatic involvement of the spinal meninges and neural tissue is frequent in pyogenic infection, but is an uncommon complication of tuberculosis. While metastatic neoplasms also can mimic tuberculosis infections, usually they occur in an older age group.

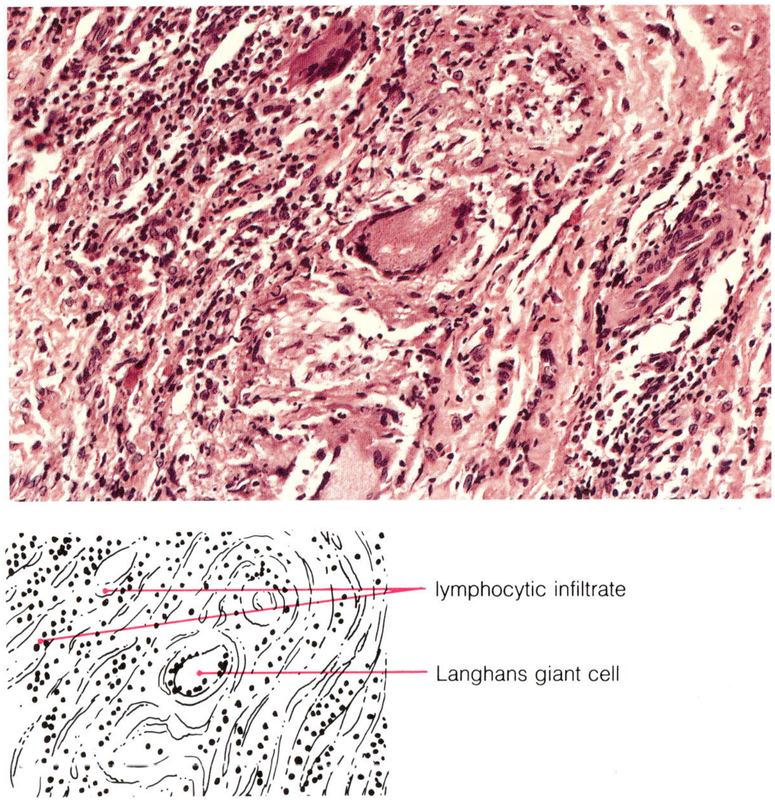

Figure 12.21 A high-power view of the chronic inflammatory tissue shown in Figure 12.20 demonstrates a histiocytic (epithelioid cell) lymphocytic infiltrate, with three typical Langhans giant cells. Note that these changes are not specific for tuberculosis, and definitive diagnosis requires demonstration of acid-fast bacilli, which in bone tissue specimens may be difficult to find. (H & E, × 450)

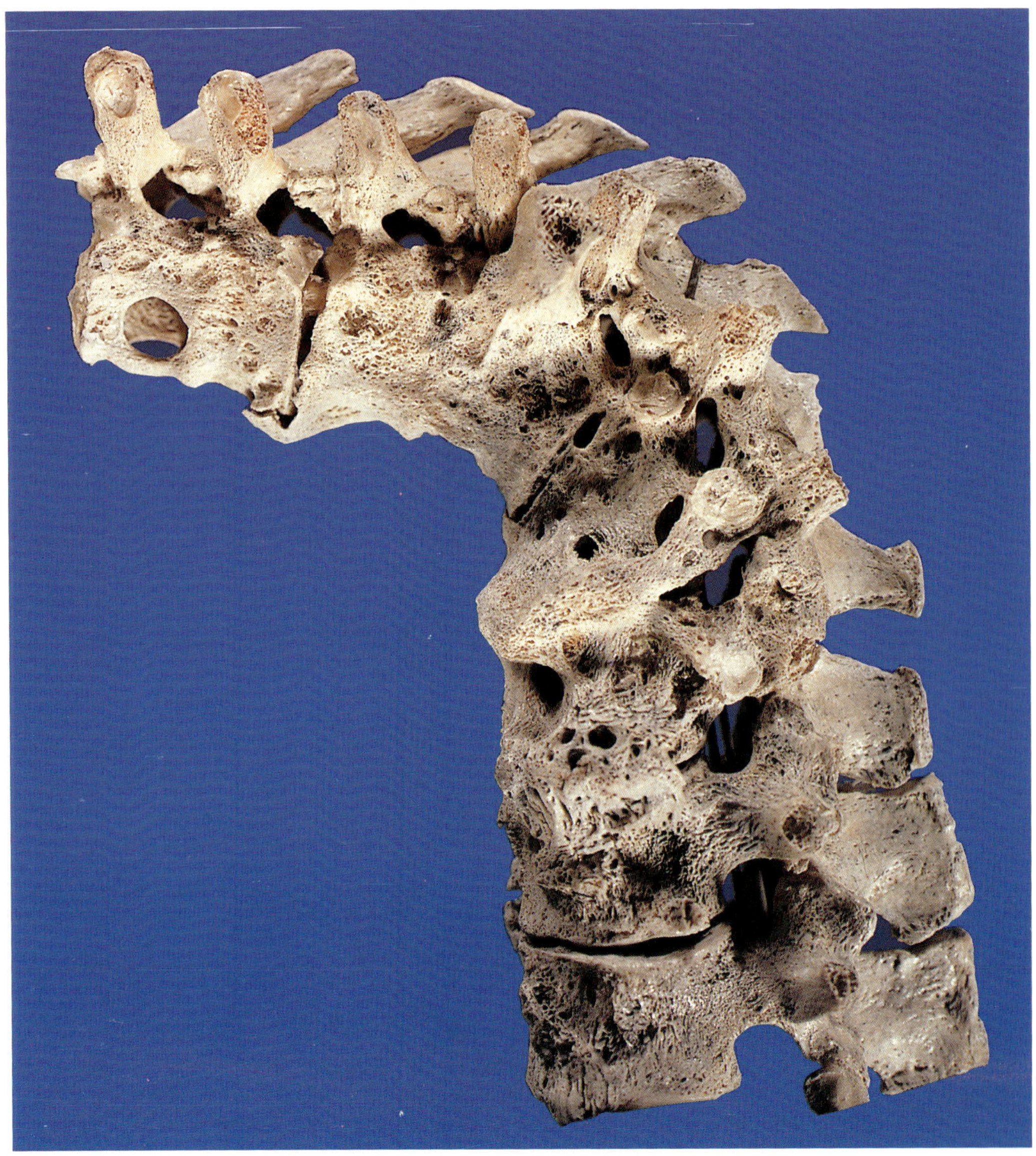

Figure 12.22 Photograph of a macerated specimen of spine obtained from a case of tuberculosis before the antibiotic era. Extensive bony destruction with fusion and gibbus deformity is apparent.

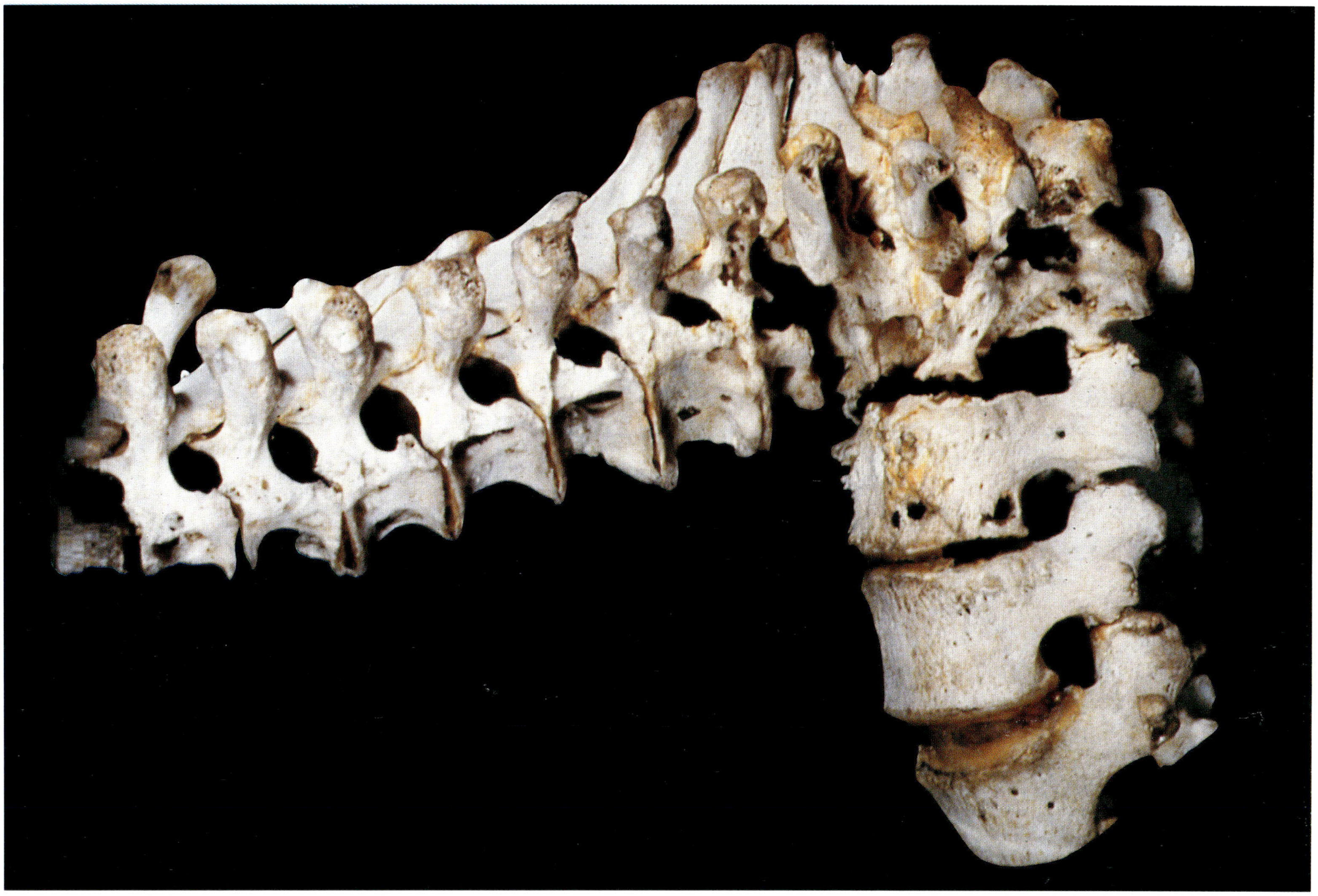

Figure 12.23 Photograph of a macerated postmortem specimen from a 26-year-old male, who for two years was known to have a tuberculous "cold abscess" in the lumbar region. At autopsy, the abscess was seen to extend into the posterior mediastinum. This spine shows extensive tuberculous destruction of five adjacent vertebral bodies, leading to gross angulation. Superiorly, where the anterior surfaces of the vertebrae have been in contact with the "abscess," they are eroded. (Courtesy of the Royal College of Surgeons of England)

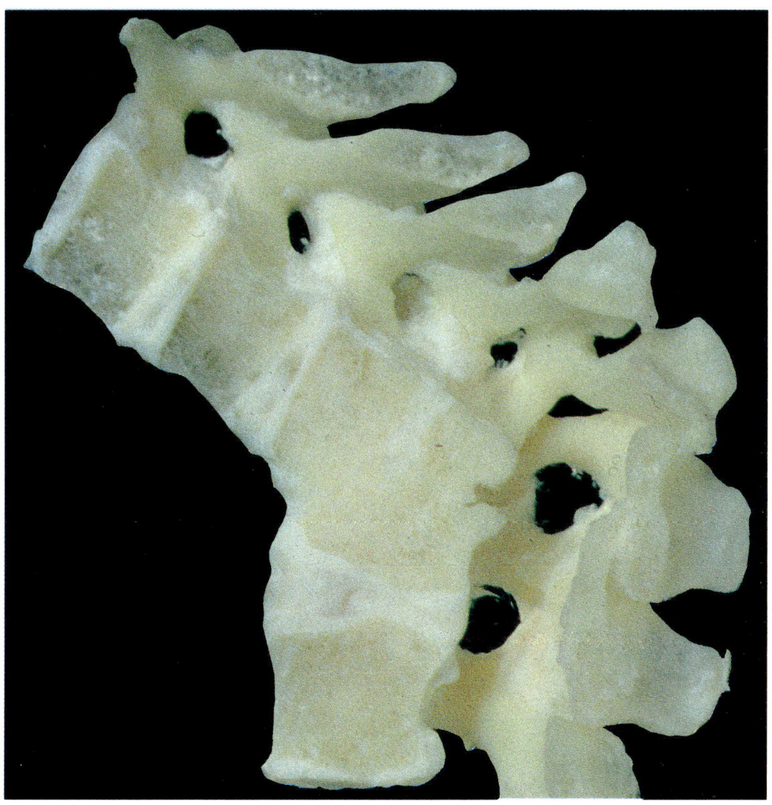

Figure 12.24 Photograph of a partially macerated specimen of spine from a child with tuberculosis. A sharp angular curvature is seen, due to tuberculous destruction of the three lower thoracic and first lumbar vertebrae. The caseous process has healed, resulting in bony ankylosis. The vertebral canal appears normal. (Courtesy of the Royal College of Surgeons of England)

Mycotic Infection of the Spine

The spine, as well as other bones and joints, may be involved by mycotic infections, most commonly actinomycosis, blastomycosis, and coccidiomycosis (Figs. 12.25 and 12.26). The radiographic and pathologic features are similar to those of tuberculosis, although the disc or neural canal is rarely affected. The lesion may involve single spinal segments, or, as a result of spread of paravertebral abscesses, multiple spinal segments, especially in the lumbar region. The lesions usually are lytic, with indiscriminate involvement and destruction of vertebral bodies, neural arches, and contiguous ribs (Fig. 12.27). Late changes of vertebral collapse may render differentiation from tuberculous spondylitis difficult.

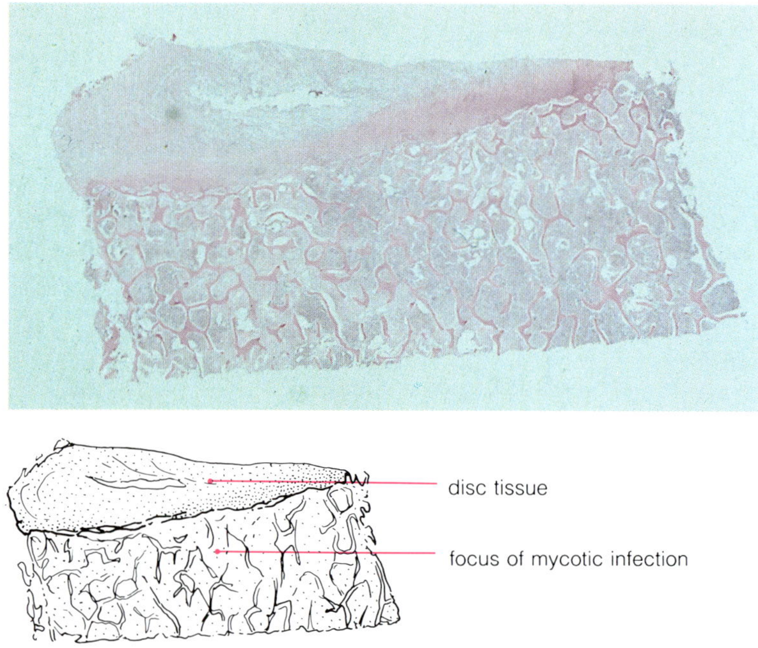

Figure 12.25 Photomicrograph of a histologic section of a portion of spine extensively involved by coccidioidomycosis. Note the sparing of the disc tissue in this section.

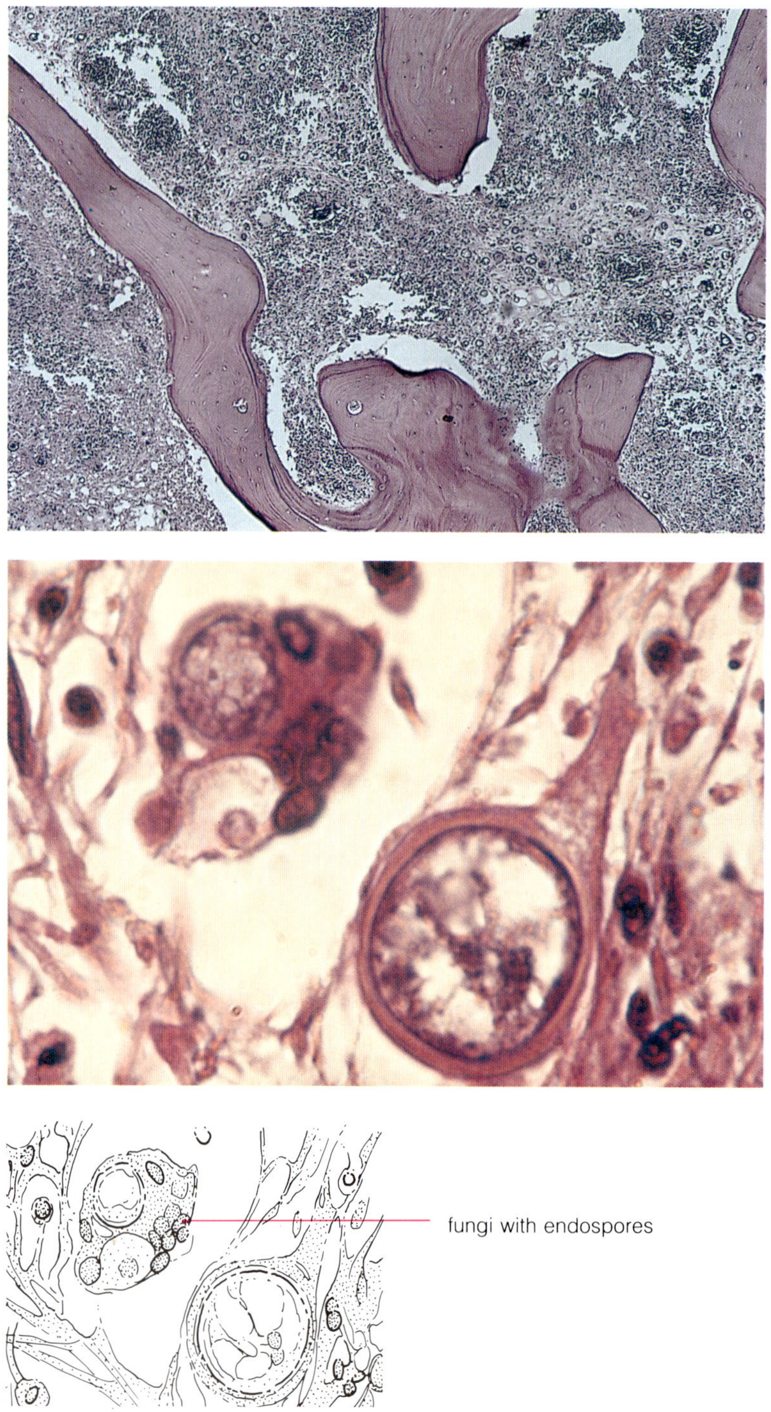

Figure 12.26 Photomicrograph (*top*) of tissue obtained from a patient with chronic spinal disease, resulting from infection with *Coccidioides immitis*. The marrow space is infiltrated by chronic inflammatory tissue. A high-power view (*bottom*) shows two round, thick-walled fungal organisms containing endospores.

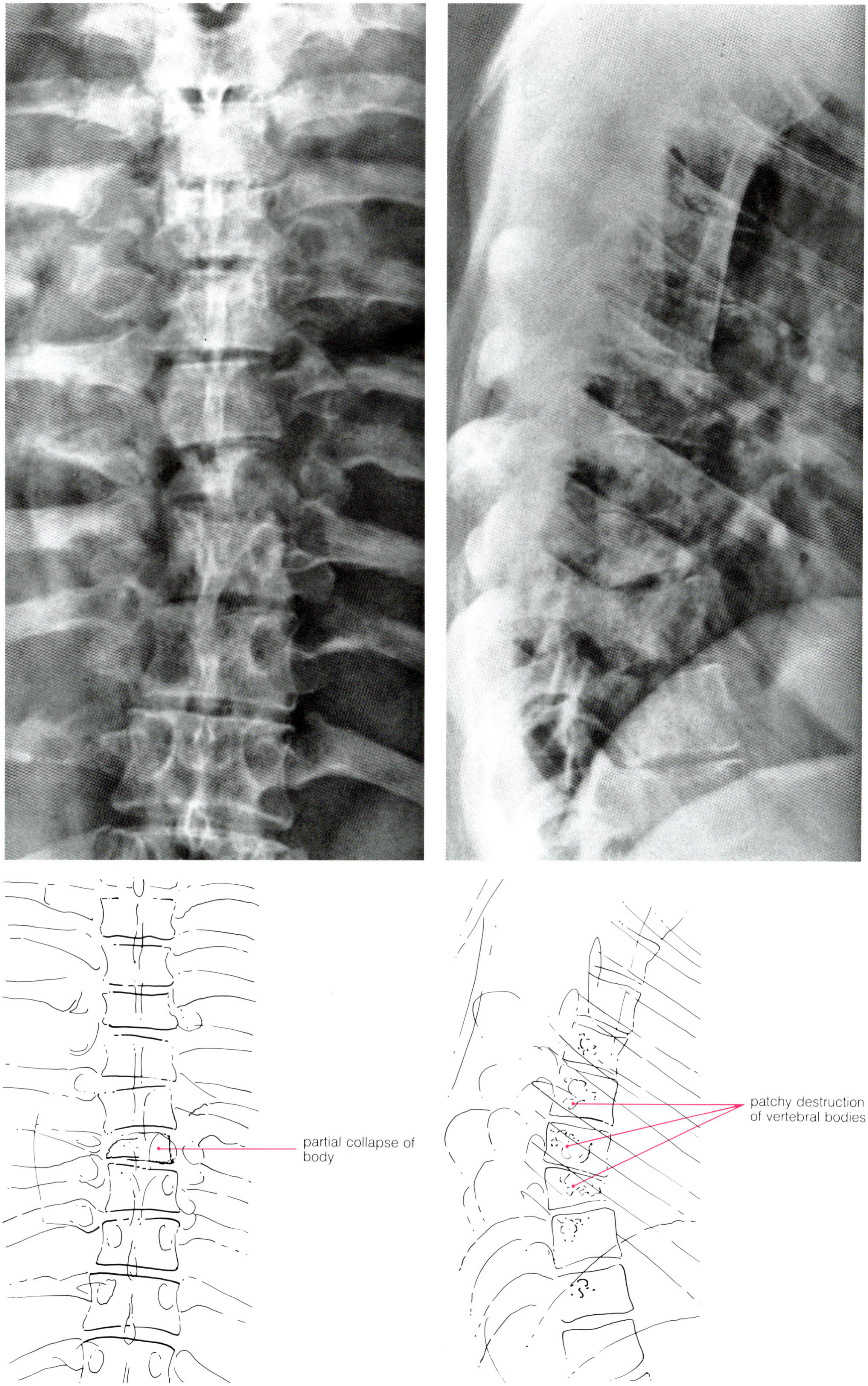

Figure 12.27 AP (*left*) and lateral (*right*) radiographs of a thoracic spine to demonstrate multiple destructive lesions. Several vertebral bodies are involved, some of which are partially collapsed. Biopsy proved this to be the result of blastomycosis.

13 CHAPTER

SPINAL TUMORS: BENIGN

General Features of Spinal Tumors

In clinical practice, far and away the most common tumor encountered in the skeleton is metastatic cancer, and it is the spine that is most likely to be involved. On the other hand, primary tumors of the spine are decidedly rare. In Dahlin's series of 1,447 surgically diagnosed benign skeletal tumors, approximately 7.7% were in the vertebral column with one-third being in the sacrum. In Dahlin's series of 4,774 primary malignant tumors in the skeleton, 15% were in the vertebral column, of which just under half were in the sacrum. The three most common surgically diagnosed benign tumors of the spine, in order of frequency, are giant cell tumor, aneurysmal bone cyst, and osteoblastoma. These are followed closely by hemangioma, osteochondroma, osteoid osteoma, and eosinophilic granuloma. The two most commonly diagnosed malignant tumors are myeloma and chordoma, each of which is approximately three times more common than are the other four malignant tumors commonly found in the spine, namely, chondrosarcoma, lymphoma, osteosarcoma, and Ewing's sarcoma.

Because of their location, the diagnosis and treatment of spinal tumors may be difficult. A careful history is important. The age of the patient is particularly significant in the diagnosis of bone tumors of the spine; in general, benign tumors are seen more commonly in young people, whereas malignant tumors are more common in adults. The patient with a symptomatic tumor (benign or malignant) is likely to complain of constant pain that is not relieved by rest. In addition, encroachment on the structures in the spinal canal may produce neurologic deficits, as well as symptoms of urinary, bowel, or sexual dysfunction.

In some cases, laboratory tests may be useful in diagnosis: for example, serum pro-

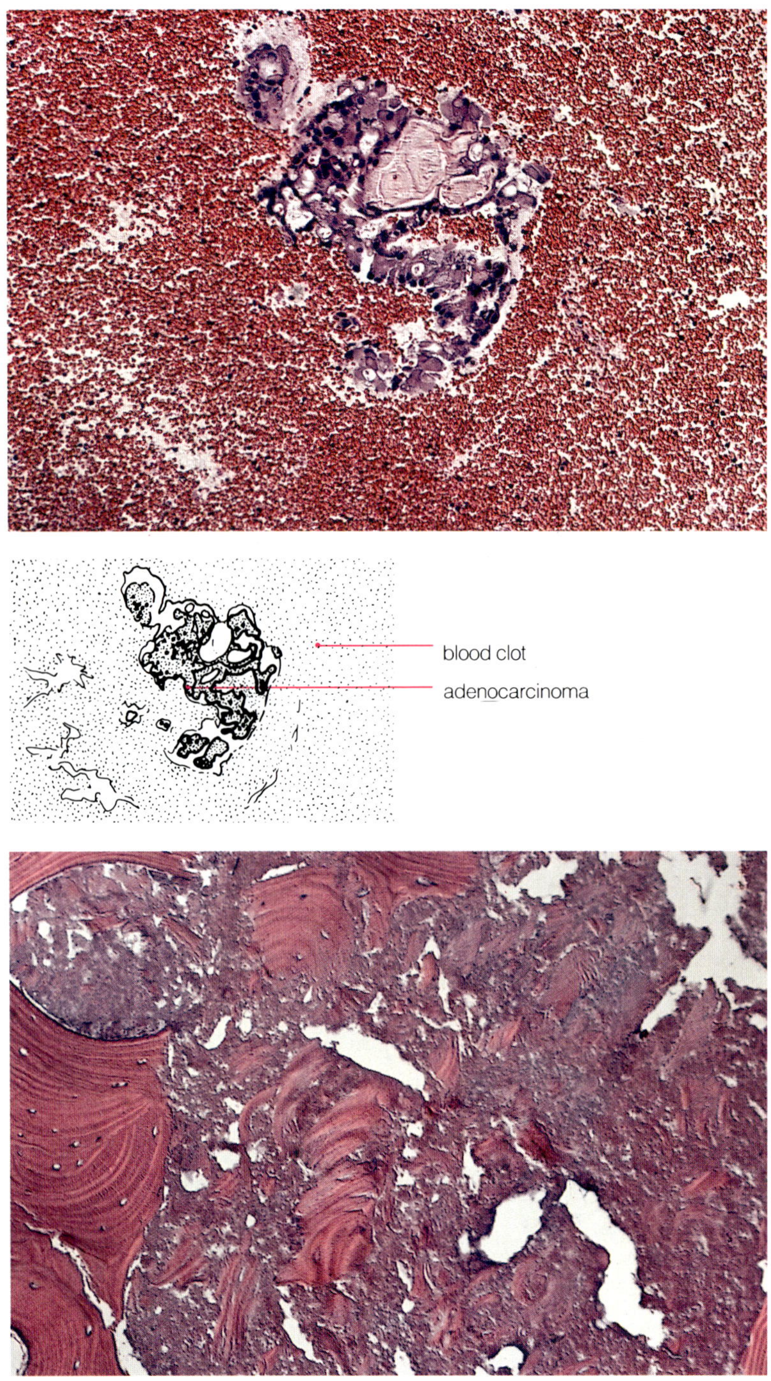

Figure 13.1 Photomicrograph *(top)* of a blood clot obtained by aspiration from a sclerotic lesion in a vertebral body. A well-preserved focus of mucus-secreting adenocarcinoma is present. In the blood specimen *(bottom)* obtained from the same case, there is such a degree of crush artifact that no tumor could be recognized. (H & E, × 10 objective)

tein electrophoresis where myeloma is suspected; acid phosphatase where metastatic prostatic carcinoma is suspected; urinary vanillylmandelic acid (VMA) where metastatic neuroblastoma is suspected; alkaline phosphatase where osteogenic sarcoma is suspected; and a complete blood count in cases of suspected lymphoma.

In all suspected cases of bone tumor, malignant or benign, AP, lateral and oblique radiographs, together with radioisotopic scanning, are necessary; once the lesion has been localized, CT scanning (with myelography, where indicated) usually will better define the lesion.

With regard to the histologic diagnosis of vertebral lesions, many authors have stressed the usefulness of needle biopsy in which, using biplanar imaging, biopsies can be obtained safely at almost all spinal levels. With aspiration biopsy, one is likely to obtain a blood clot as well as a piece of bony tissue. In our laboratory, we have made it a policy to examine the fixed blood clot and smears obtained from it, in addition to sections obtained from the decalcified bone specimen. We have found the blood clot to be particularly useful in diagnosis, since the bone specimen is likely to be crushed (Fig. 13.1). Needle biopsy will not serve in all cases, and open biopsy may be necessary. It cannot be overemphasized that consultation between the surgeon, radiologist, and pathologist is essential for accurate diagnosis and optimal management.

In the present chapter, we will briefly review the most common benign tumors found in the spine.

Giant Cell Tumor

The incidence of giant cell tumor in the spine has been reported to be approximately 5% of the total number of giant cell tumors. Although giant cell tumor may occur anywhere in the spine, it is most common in the sacrum and lumbar spine. Clinically these lesions are likely to present with neurologic disturbances, the extent of which depends on both the aggressiveness of the tumor and its location.

Radiographically, giant cell tumors of the spine and sacrum, unlike those in long bones, have no recognizable diagnostic characteristics (Fig. 13.2). They tend to erode and replace the bone partly or completely, and they may extend into the pedicles and neural arches (Fig. 13.3) or penetrate into adjacent soft tissue. Because giant cell tumors tend to be highly vascular, it is important to distinguish them microscopically from an-

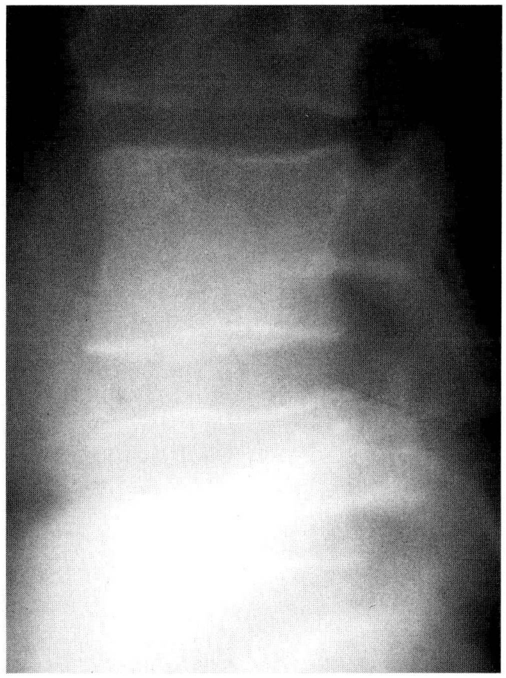

Figure 13.2 Lateral radiograph of a portion of the lumbar spine in a middle-aged woman. L-3 is largely replaced and expanded by a lytic tumor, which on biopsy proved to be a giant cell tumor of bone.

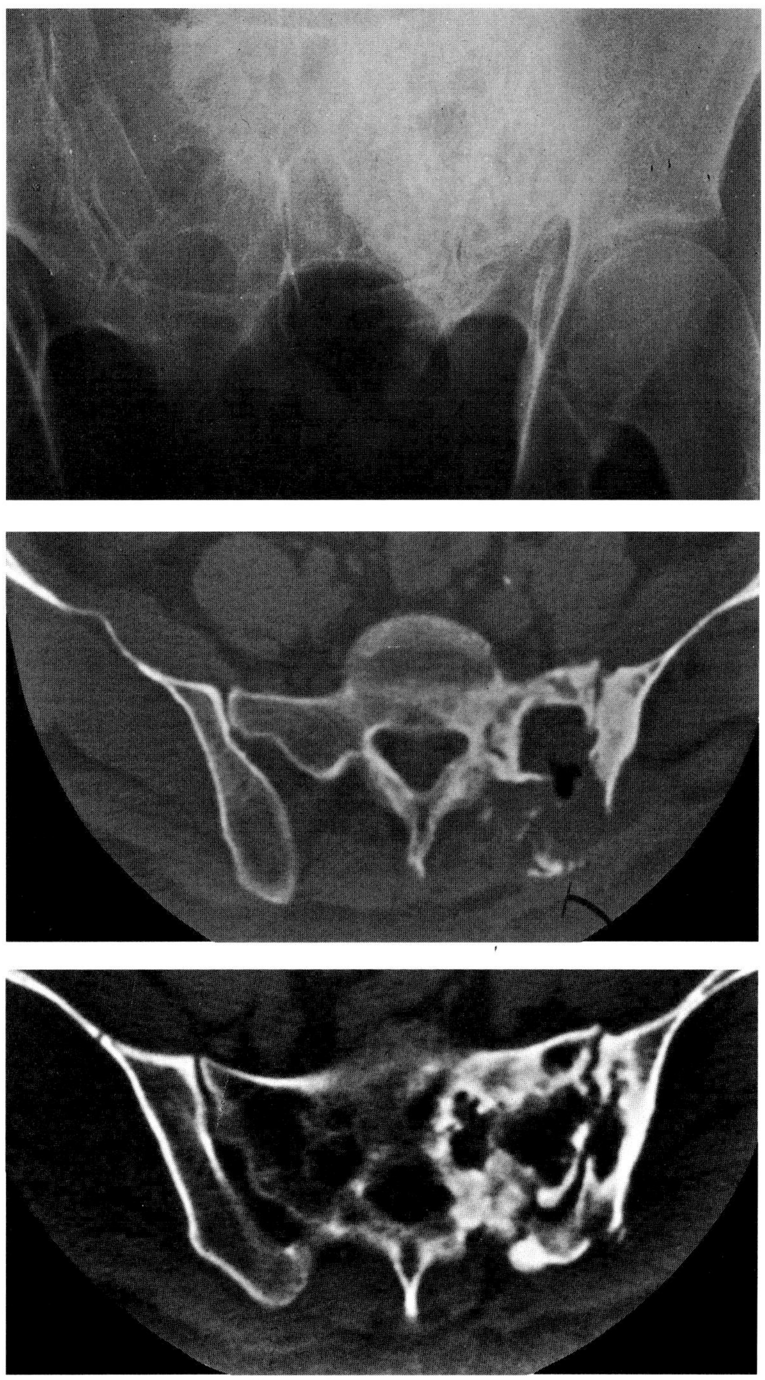

Figure 13.3 AP radiograph *(top)* of the pelvis of a patient with giant cell tumor of the pelvis showing a large sclerotic lesion involving the body of S-1 and S-2 and extending into the pedicles and across the sacroiliac joint, into the adjacent wing of the ilium. In CT scans of this lesion, a cut through S-1 *(center)* shows extensive involvement of the transverse process of S-1 and of the posterior wing of the ilium, the cortex of which has been breached. The intense sclerosis about this lesion results from reactive new bone formation secondary to fracture around the periphery. A cut through S-2 *(bottom)* again shows the extent of the lesion and the involvement of both the sacrum and the ilium.

other common lesion of the spine, aneurysmal bone cyst. Accordingly, the histologic finding of giant cells should not be regarded as the sole criterion for a diagnosis of giant cell tumor. The typical polygonal stromal cells must be seen, with giant cells evenly distributed throughout the lesional tissue (Fig. 13.4). The finding of islands of reactive bone formation in giant cell tumor is not unusual and should not be overdiagnosed. Very rarely, giant cell tumors may complicate cases of Paget's disease, and cases of multiple giant cell tumor in Paget's disease also have been reported (Fig. 13.5).

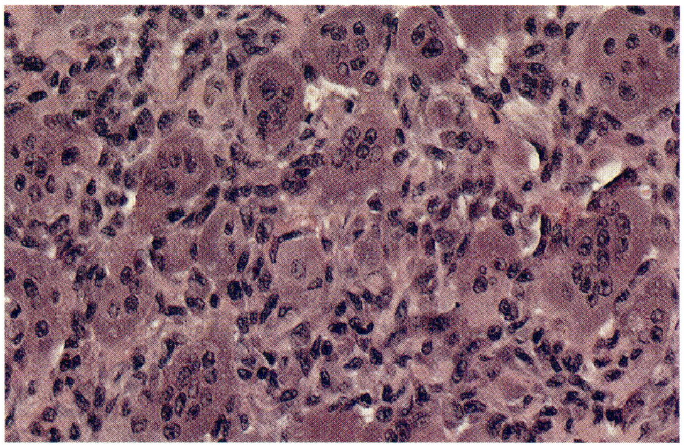

Figure 13.4 Photomicrograph of a conventional giant cell tumor to demonstrate the evenly spaced and crowded giant cells, with intervening polygonal stromal cells. (H & E, × 25 objective)

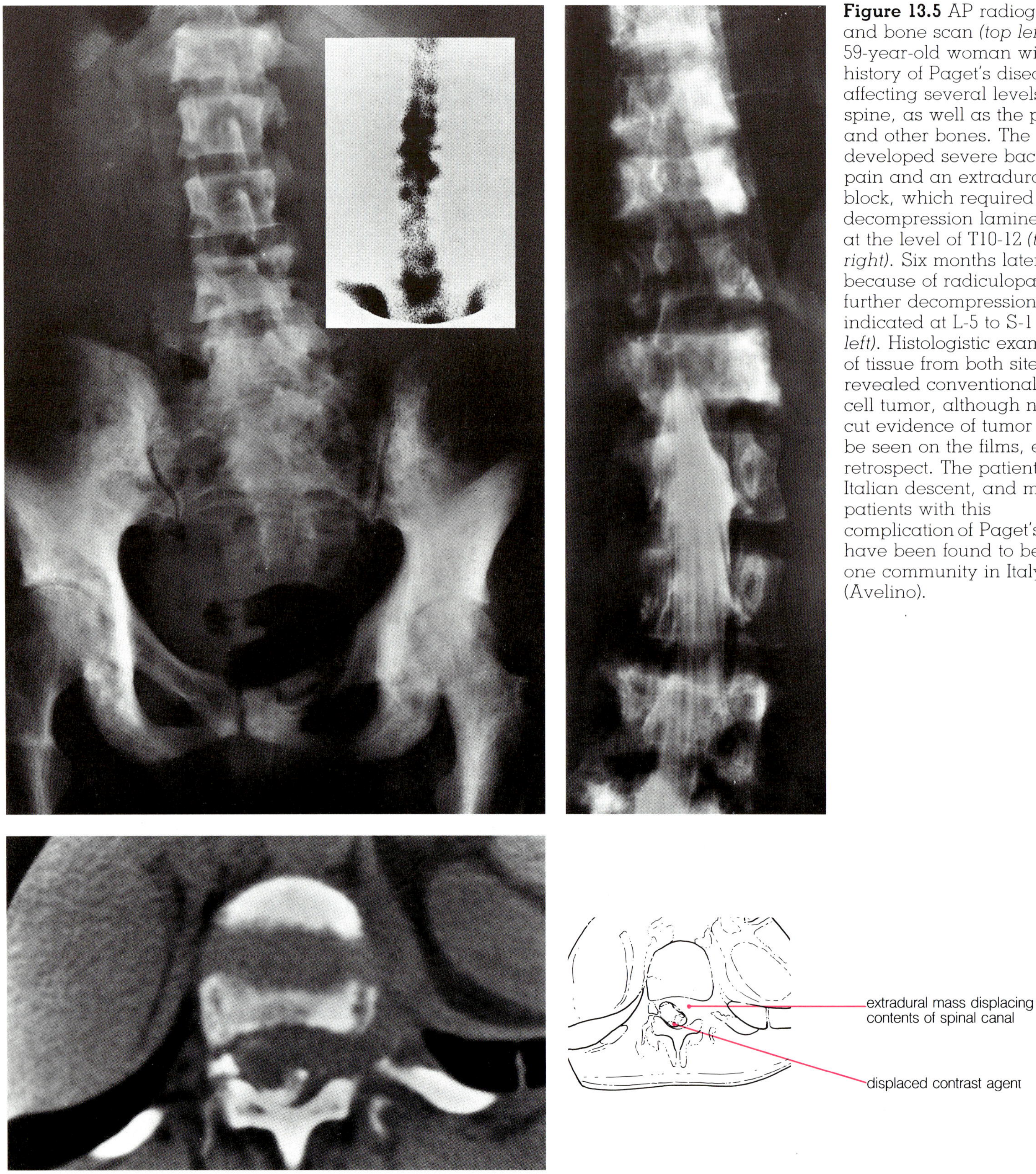

Figure 13.5 AP radiograph and bone scan *(top left)* of a 59-year-old woman with a history of Paget's disease affecting several levels in the spine, as well as the pelvis and other bones. The woman developed severe back pain and an extradural block, which required decompression laminectomy at the level of T10-12 *(top right)*. Six months later, because of radiculopathy, a further decompression was indicated at L-5 to S-1 *(bottom left)*. Histologistic examination of tissue from both sites revealed conventional giant cell tumor, although no clear-cut evidence of tumor could be seen on the films, even in retrospect. The patient was of Italian descent, and many patients with this complication of Paget's disease have been found to be from one community in Italy (Avelino).

Aneurysmal Bone Cyst

Approximately 15% of all aneurysmal bone cysts occur in the spine. They may occur at any spinal level except for the coccyx, and multiple vertebrae occasionally are affected. Although these tumors mainly involve the vertebral arches, they sometimes extend into the vertebral bodies (Fig. 13.6). Extradural cord compression is fairly common, and may cause neurologic complications.

Unlike giant cell tumors, aneurysmal bone cysts have a characteristic radiographic presentation. Radiographically, they appear as expanded "blow-out" osteolytic lesions, with an indistinct periphery and generally a trabeculated appearance. Occasionally, a spinous process may become so large as to result in a mild kyphotic deformity (Fig. 13.7).

On gross examination, the wall of the aneurysmal bone cyst is usually soft and fibrous. However, once it is opened, separated spaces containing friable brownish blood clot usually become apparent (Fig. 13.8).

Histologically, the tissue consists of fibrous septa containing giant cells, frequently with hemosiderin pigment and foci of reactive woven bone (Fig. 13.9). Occasionally, the lesion is seen in association with another lesion, most frequently as osteoblastoma. In such a case, multiple sections of the lesion are required, for identification of the underlying lesion.

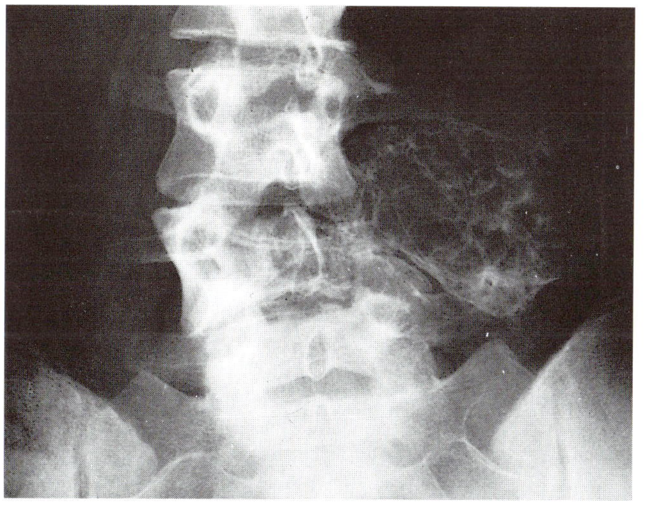

Figure 13.6 AP radiograph of the lumbar spine of a woman in her mid twenties with complaints of low back pain. Examination revealed a scoliotic deformity and slight local tenderness. This film shows collapse of the L-4 body, with a huge expansion of the transverse process. The cortex is intact and the bone has a honey-combed trabeculated appearance; the pedicle is not seen on the affected side. The mild scoliotic deformity has developed as a result of the lesion.

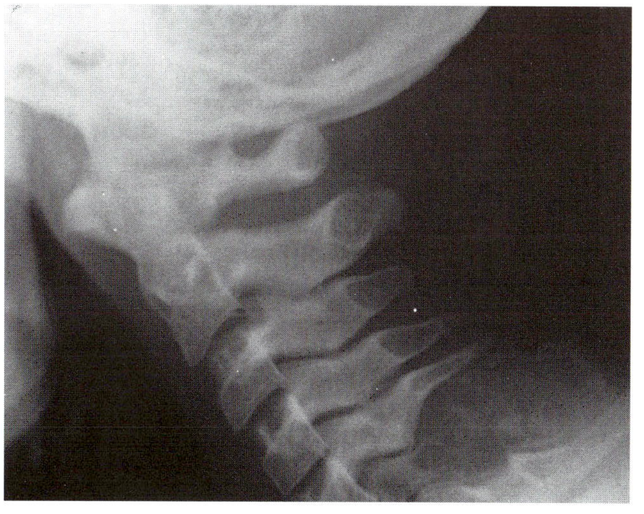

Figure 13.7 Lateral radiograph of the cervical spine in a 19-year-old male complaining of neck pain. A large lytic, expanded lesion is seen in the spinous process of C-6, and has the typical features of an aneurysmal bone cyst—a thin cortical shell and a trabeculated honey comb appearance to the bone tissue.

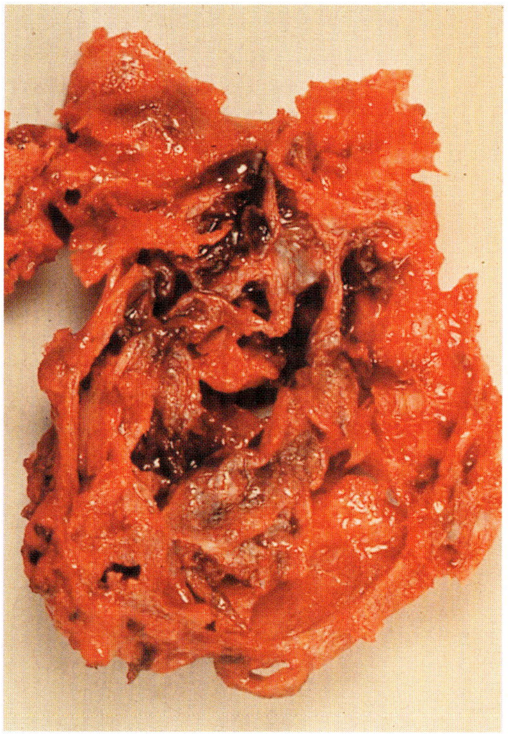

Figure 13.8 Photograph of an aneurysmal bone cyst resected from the neural arch of C-2. This lesion measured approximately 5 cm in diameter, and its gross appearance is typical. Fibrous septa, often containing some gritty bone, separate large blood-filled spaces. (Courtesy of Dr. Krishnan K. Unni)

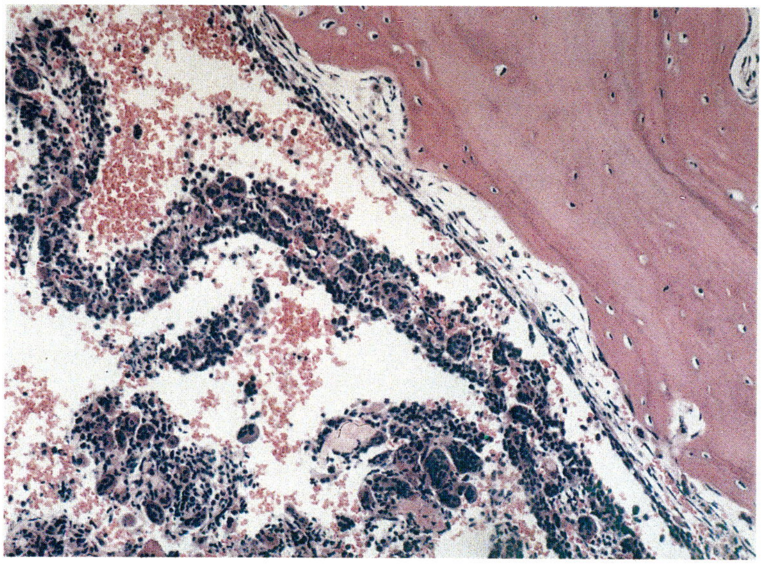

Figure 13.9 Photomicrograph of a portion of an aneurysmal bone cyst to demonstrate the septate pattern and giant cells that generally line the septa. In addition, one may see scarring, hemosiderin pigment, and foci of immature bone within the lesional tissue. (H & E, × 10 objective)

Benign Osteoblastoma

Benign osteoblastoma, though rare, is the only benign tumor of bone that favors the vertebral column; approximately 30% of osteoblastomas occur in the spine. The clinical presentation may include both myelopathic and/or radicular symptoms, and so may suggest either an intraspinal tumor or a herniated disc. Progressive scoliosis also may appear, and, if the cervical spine is affected, the lordotic curve may be reversed and torticollis may be prominent. Benign osteoblastomas occur about equally in the cervical and lumbar regions, with the thoracic region being less frequently involved. Occasionally, they may be found in the sacrum (Fig. 13.10).

The radiologic picture is not entirely characteristic. The tumor may be ill-defined and thus difficult to distinguish from an aneurysmal bone cyst or a giant cell tumor (Figs. 13.11 and 13.12). The lesions affect the vertebral arch, occurring in the spinous and transverse processes and in the laminae and pedicles. In only a few cases does the lesion seem to originate within the vertebral bodies.

On gross examination, the tissue comprising the osteoblastoma is compact and soft, with a gritty consistency (Fig. 13.13). Often it has a dark, reddish color. Histologically, the tumor is formed of mesenchymal cells, which show osteoblastic differentiation and immature bone formation (Fig. 13.14).

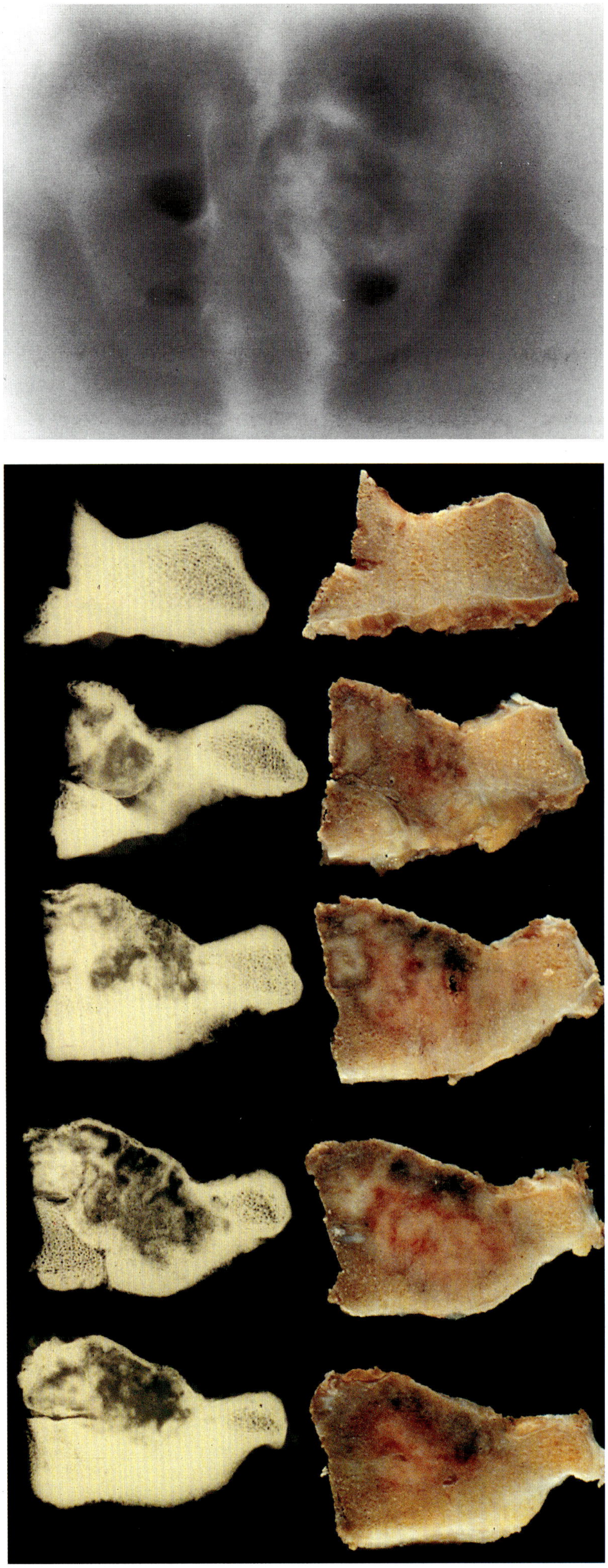

Figure 13.10 AP tomogram *(top)* of the sacrum of a young male, demonstrating a well-circumscribed lytic and blastic lesion, involving both the body and transverse processes of one half of the sacrum. A series of slices *(bottom)* have been made through the lesion. When matched with fine-grain radiographs, they demonstrate the mixed lytic and sclerotic areas seen in this osteoblastoma. (Courtesy of Dr. Alberto G. Ayala)

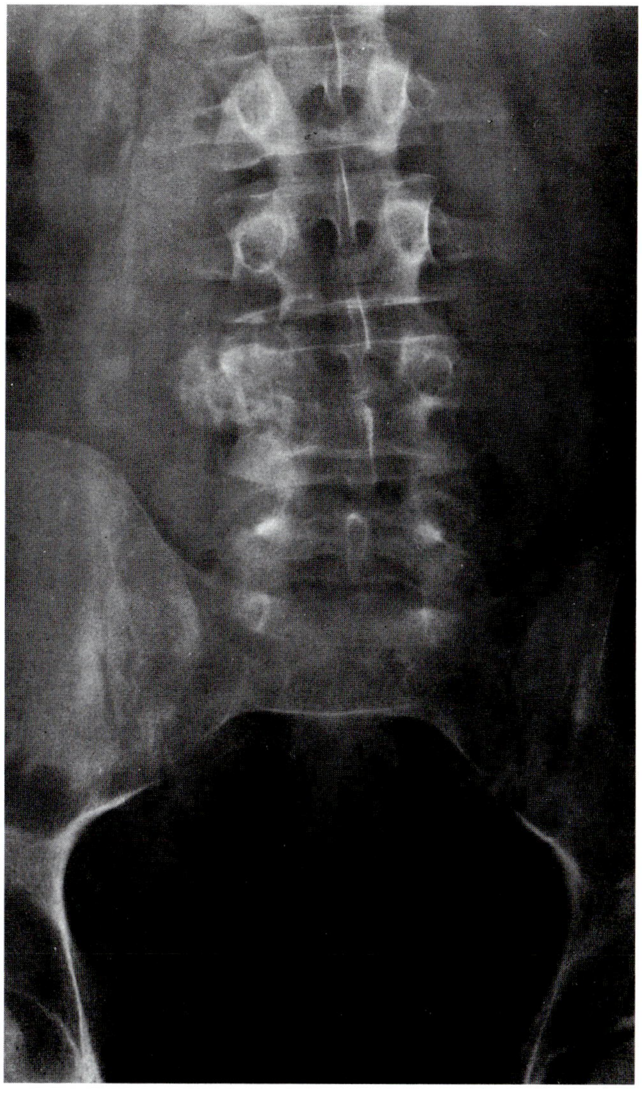

Figure 13.11 AP radiograph of the lumbar spine of a 20-year-old female complaining of low back pain. The radiograph shows a lesion involving the pedicle and transverse process of L-4, which, histologically, proved to be an osteoblastoma. The lesion shows an irregular ossification, but the margins are well defined. This view should be compared with the aneurysmal bone cyst shown in Figure 13.6.

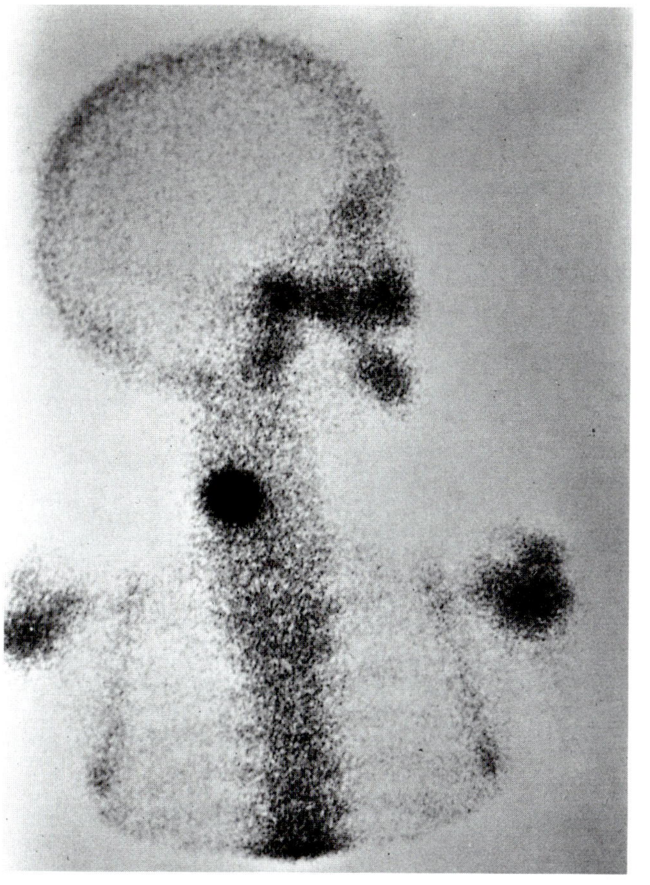

Figure 13.12 Radioisotope scan of an osteoblastoma in the transverse process and pedicle of C-5. The intense uptake is typical of that seen in association with both osteoblastomas and osteoid osteomas. In this case, the size of the lesion would indicate that this is an osteoblastoma.

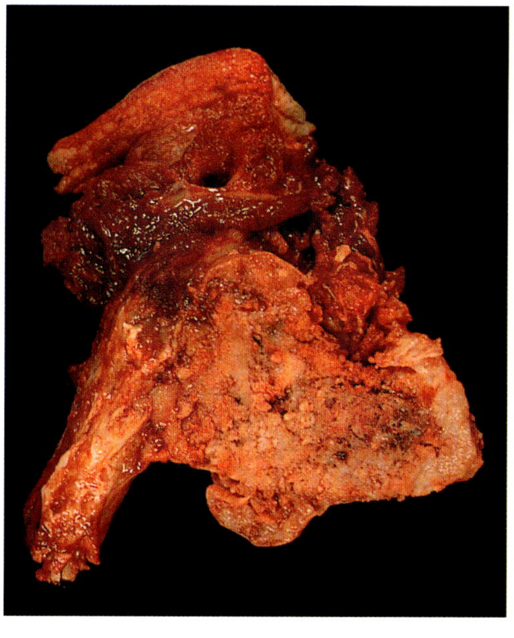

Figure 13.13 Photograph of an osteoblastoma affecting the pedicle and transverse process of T-4, which has been resected with a portion of involved rib and overlying muscles and skin. The typical gritty appearance of an osteoblastoma can be seen. (Courtesy of Dr. Krishnan K. Unni)

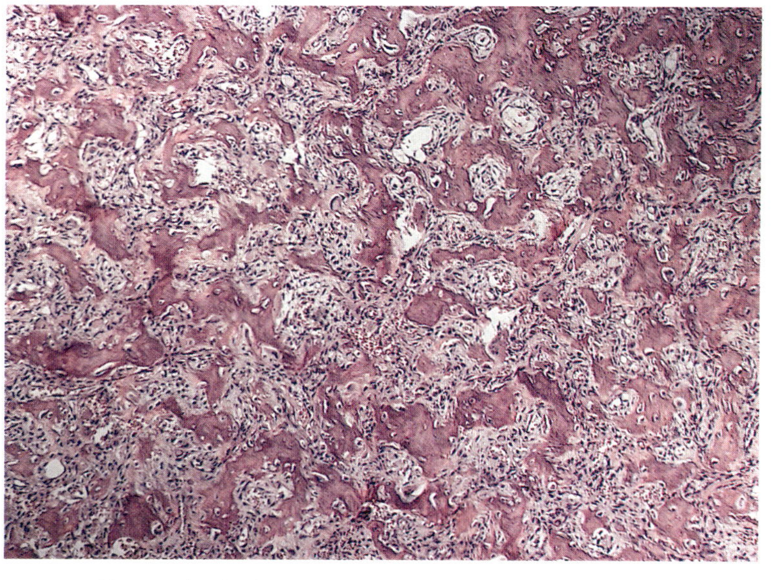

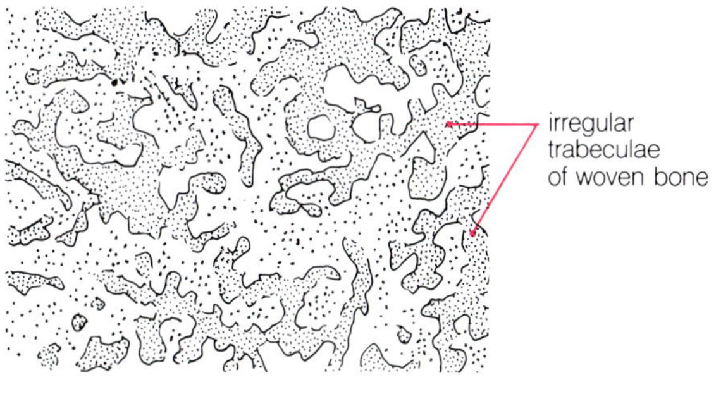

Figure 13.14 Photomicrograph of an osteoblastoma to show the usual pattern of disorganized trabeculae of immature bone set in a cellular vascular stroma. (H & E, × 4 objective)

The stroma is likely to be extremely vascular, and osteoclastic activity may be prominent (Fig. 13.15).

Very occasionally, some osteoblastomas may demonstrate an unexpectedly aggressive clinical course. In these cases, the microscopic appearance of the tumor tissue generally is atypical. The osteoblasts may form sheets of cells, and, furthermore, the bone matrix that is formed also may have an atypical appearance. In such a case, the differential diagnosis with osteosarcoma may be difficult. However, whereas osteosarcoma is likely to pursue a rapidly fatal course, aggressive osteoblastoma is a problem only in terms of local recurrence; metastases are not likely.

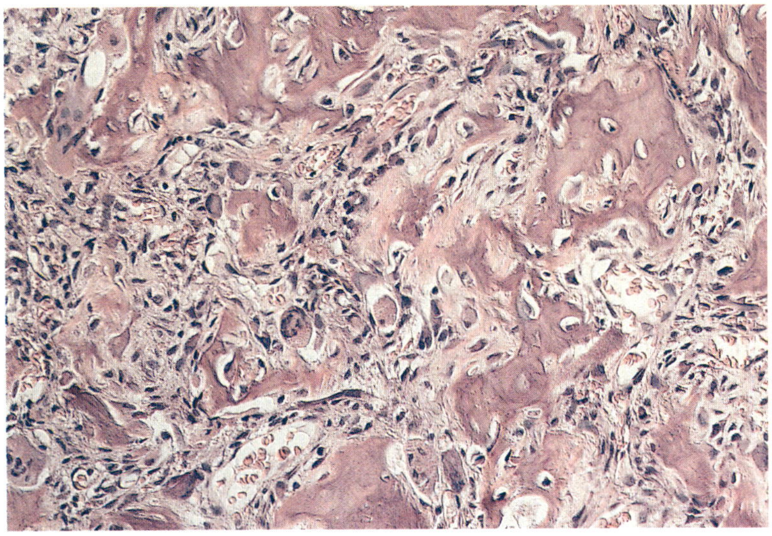

Figure 13.15 Photomicrograph of an osteoblastoma at a higher magnification to show the marked osteoblastic and osteoclastic activity at the bone surfaces. (H & E, × 25 objective)

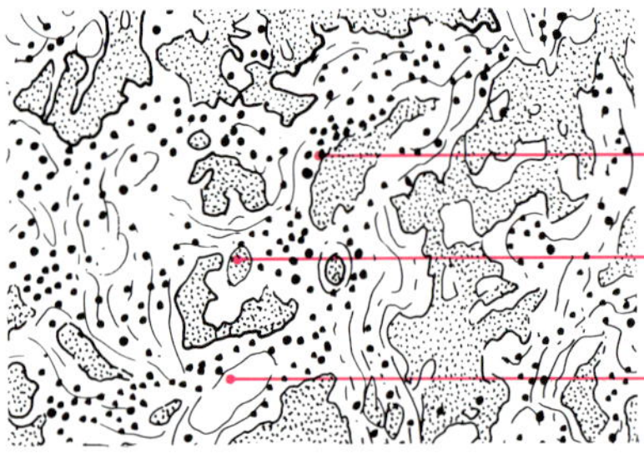

HEMANGIOMA

Hemangiomas are vascular tumors, composed of vessels of varying sizes with well-differentiated endothelium. They are among the most frequently occurring spinal tumors, although in general they are found only incidentally on a radiographic survey or following careful autopsy studies. Clinically, they constitute only about 2 to 3% of spinal tumors, often presenting with neurologic symptoms following extension of the angiomatous tissue into the epidural space (Fig. 13.16). They are found most commonly in the lower thoracic vertebrae, somewhat less frequently in the lumbar spine, and infrequently in both the cervical spine and in the sacrum. Erosion of the horizontal trabeculae of the vertebral bodies leads to the typical radiographic appearance of accentuated, somewhat thickened, vertical trabeculae (Fig. 13.17). When hemangiomas are seen in children, the bone may have a stippled or mottled appearance, radiographically. The lesion usually is confined to the vertebral body, though on occasion the arch may be affected (Figs. 13.18 and 13.19). Thinning of the vertebral body cortex frequently is present, and on occasion there may be bulging of the vertebral margins. Multiple hemangiomas also may be seen, leading to problems in differential diagnosis with metastatic cancer or myeloma, and on rare occasions they may be sclerotic rather than lytic (Figs. 13.20 through 13.22).

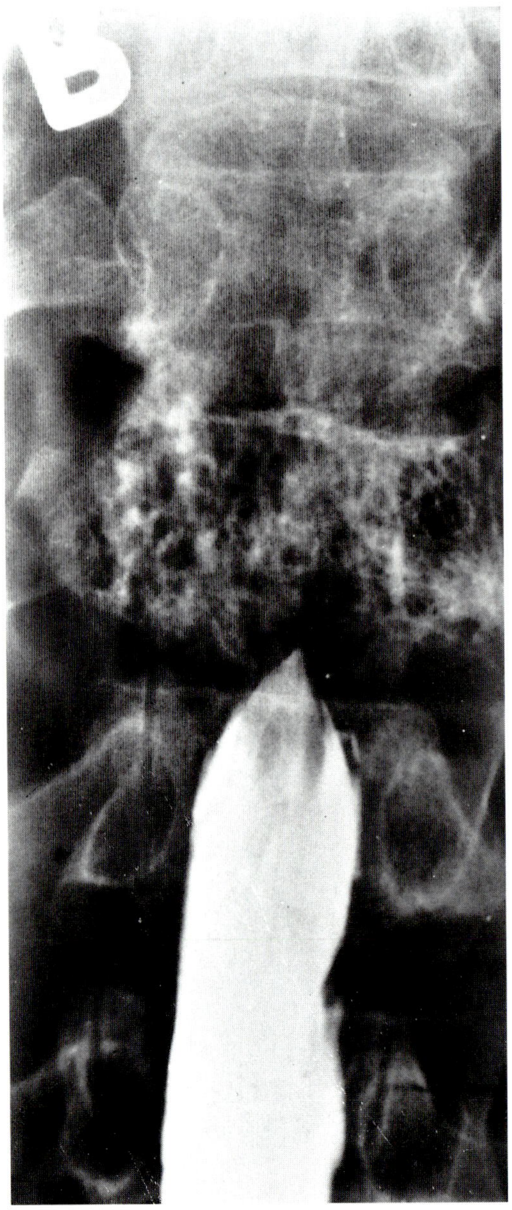

Figure 13.16 AP myelogram showing a block at the level of T-12, the body of which shows an exaggerated trabecular pattern. The pedicles are obscured. This accentuated coarse trabecular pattern is typical of hemangioma.

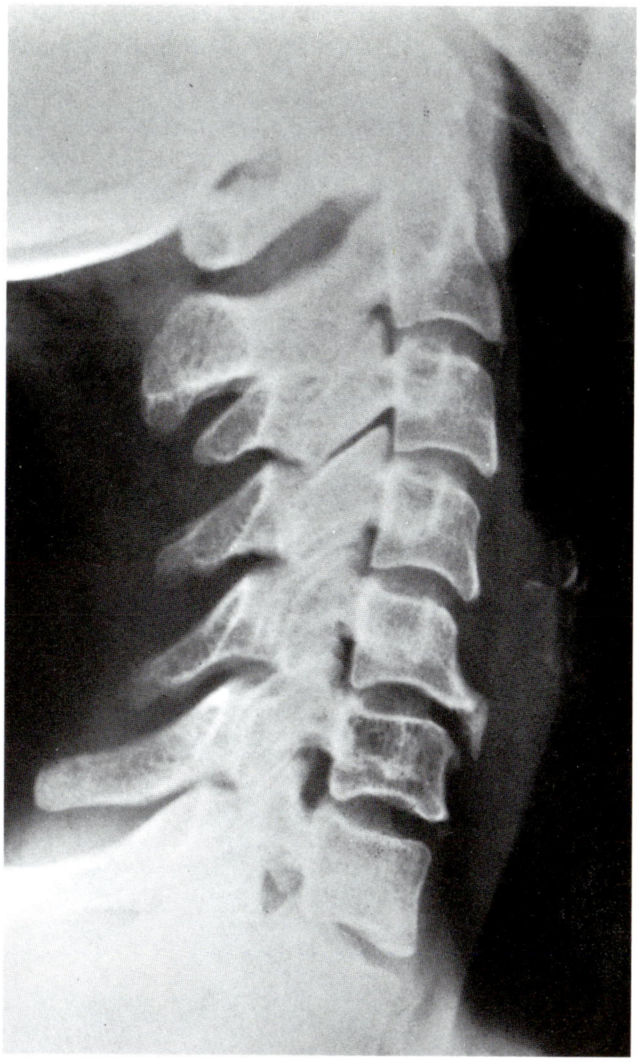

Figure 13.17 Lateral radiograph of the cervical spine showing an accentuated trabecular pattern in the body of C-6 due to a hemangioma. Hemangiomas are frequent in the cervical spine but may occur anywhere within the vertebral column. Note the prediscal ossifications at C5-6 and C6-7, indicative of early DISH.

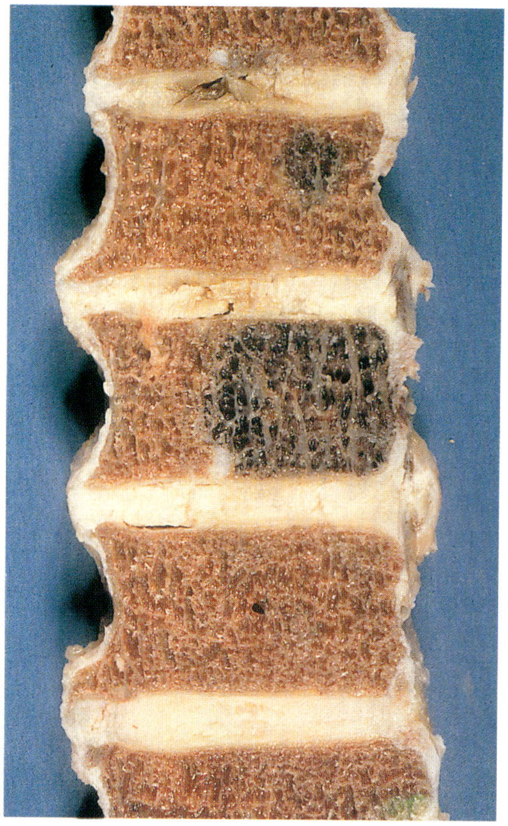

Figure 13.18 Photograph of a coronal section through a portion of the thoracolumbar spine. A small hemangioma is seen in one vertebra; in the adjacent vertebra, a hemangioma involving almost two-thirds of the vertebral body is present.

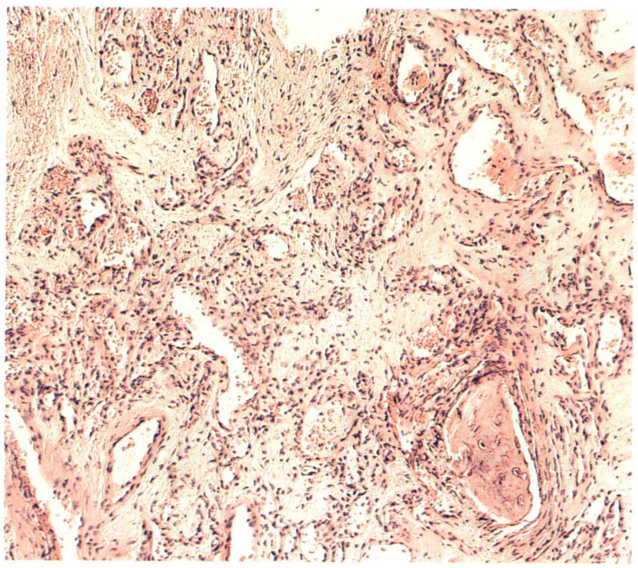

Figure 13.19 Photomicrograph of a hemangioma in the bone shows irregular vascular channels separated by loose fibrous tissue, which replaces the marrow spaces and focally displaces the bony tissue. (H & E, × 4 objective)

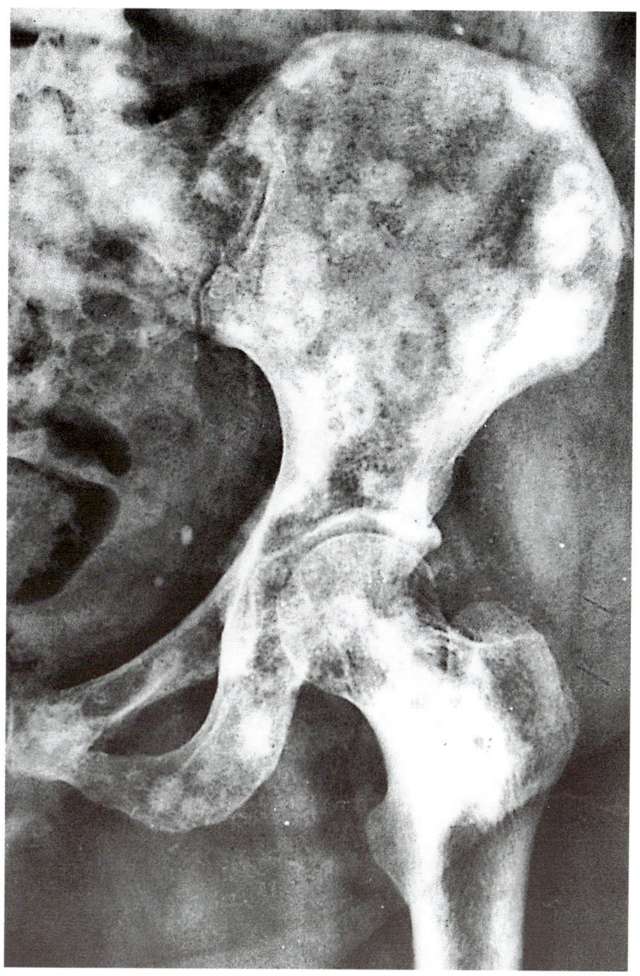

Figure 13.20 Clinical radiograph of a patient with hemangiomatosis showing multiple densities, some with cleared centers, present throughout the skeleton. This appearance may be confused with that of a malignant bone-forming metastatic tumor.

Massive osteolysis, or disappearing bone disease (Gorham's disease), is a rare condition in which there is extensive osteoclasis, with associated benign vascular proliferations; on occasion the spine may be involved, and thoracic involvement has been reported most frequently (Fig. 13.23). The disease is relentlessly progressive, resulting in the eventual radiographic disappearance of the bone; hence the name "disappearing bone disease." Fatalities have been reported from hemorrhage, especially in cases with spinal involvement.

OSTEOCHONDROMA

Although solitary osteochondromas occur rarely in the spine in comparison to other sites, the frequency with which they are found in the spine is equal to that of other benign tumors in this site. For example, whereas only 3% of osteochondromas occur in the spine in comparison to 30% of osteoblastomas, the overall incidence of these tumors in the spine is approximately equal. Most reported osteochondromas have been described as being of large size, often palpable, generally confined to the posterior elements, and associated at times with neurologic symptoms. Occasionally, spinal lesions also will be seen in patients with multiple hereditary exostosis. CT scanning is probably the best means of imaging for this lesion, since it delineates the tumor matrix precisely and defines the extent of the lesion (Fig. 13.24).

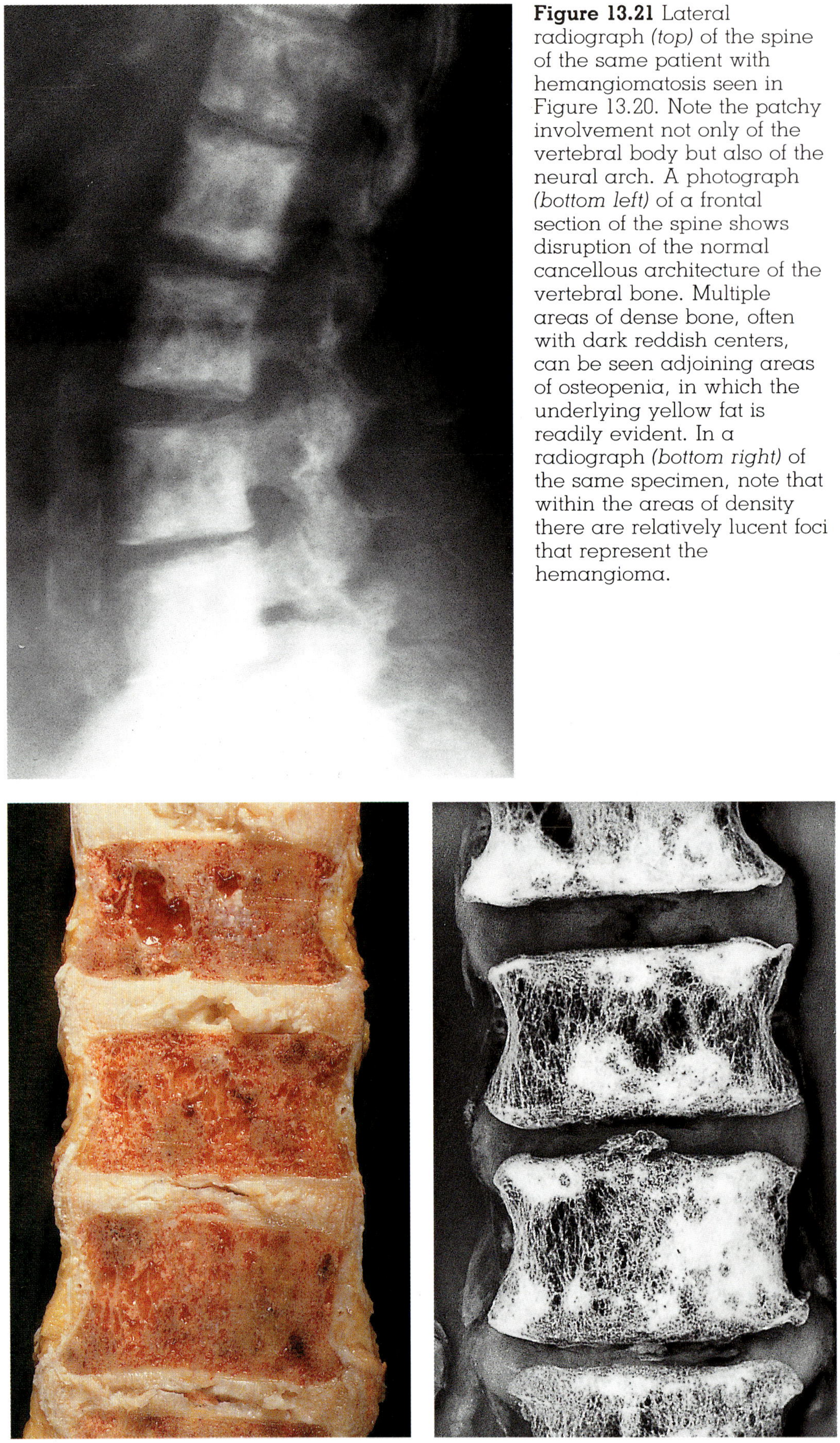

Figure 13.21 Lateral radiograph *(top)* of the spine of the same patient with hemangiomatosis seen in Figure 13.20. Note the patchy involvement not only of the vertebral body but also of the neural arch. A photograph *(bottom left)* of a frontal section of the spine shows disruption of the normal cancellous architecture of the vertebral bone. Multiple areas of dense bone, often with dark reddish centers, can be seen adjoining areas of osteopenia, in which the underlying yellow fat is readily evident. In a radiograph *(bottom right)* of the same specimen, note that within the areas of density there are relatively lucent foci that represent the hemangioma.

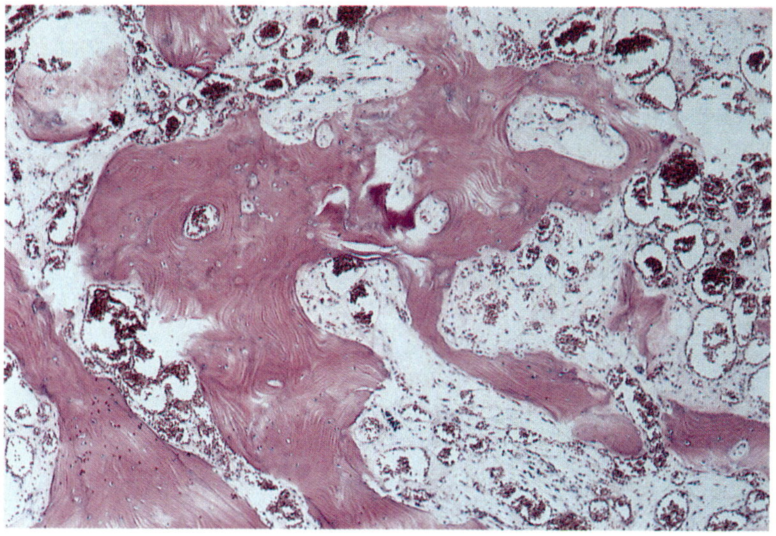

Figure 13.22 Photomicrograph of one of the dense hemangiomatous lesions illustrated in Figure 13.21. Vascular channels of varying sizes and shapes can be seen. The thickened bone appears immature, with increased cellularity and irregular architecture.

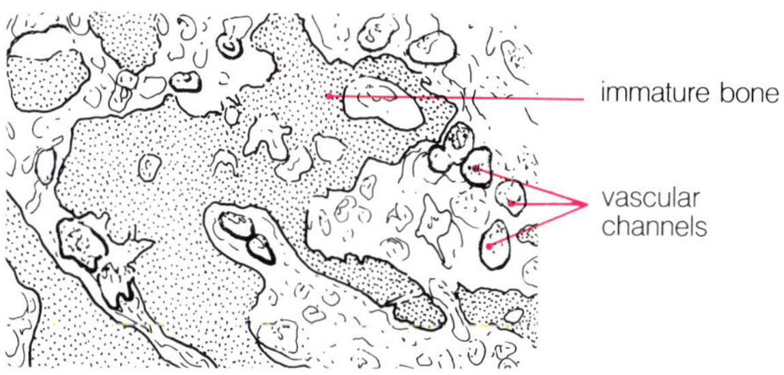

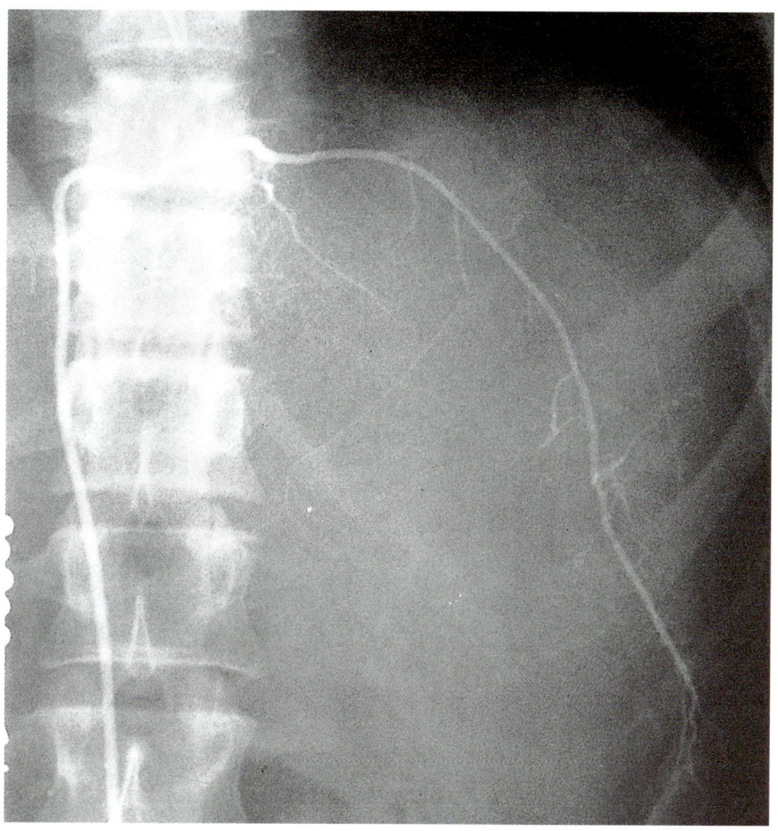

Figure 13.23 AP angiogram of the thoracolumbar spine showing early disappearance of the tenth and eleventh ribs posteriorly, with poor visualization of the structures in the tenth and eleventh thoracic vertebral bodies. The angiogram shows some increased vascularity in the affected portions of the skeleton.

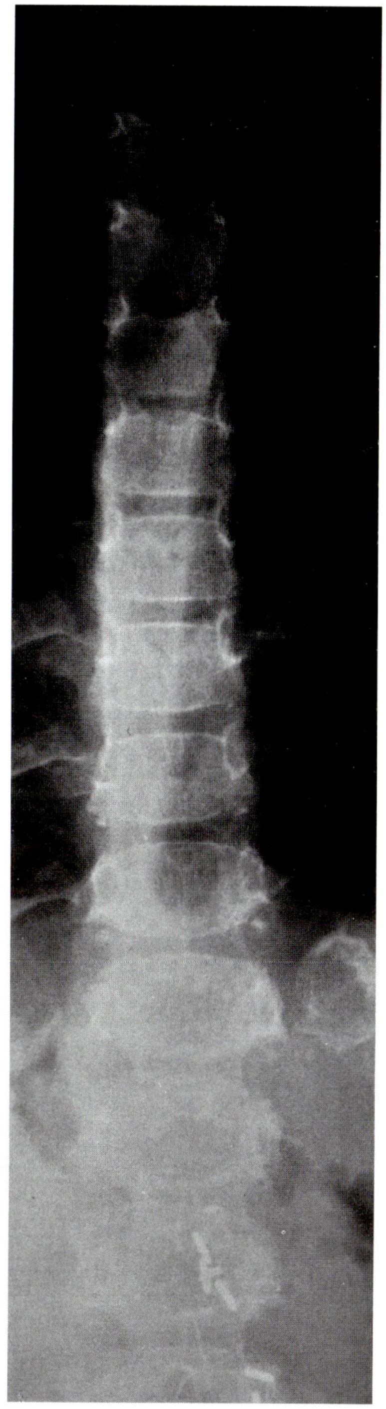

Figure 13.24 AP radiograph *(top)* of the thoracic spine in a 7-year-old boy with a mature bony mass lateral to T-12. An oblique tomogram *(bottom)* of this lesion demonstrates the continuity of this lesion with the vertebral arch, as is typical of osteochondrosis.

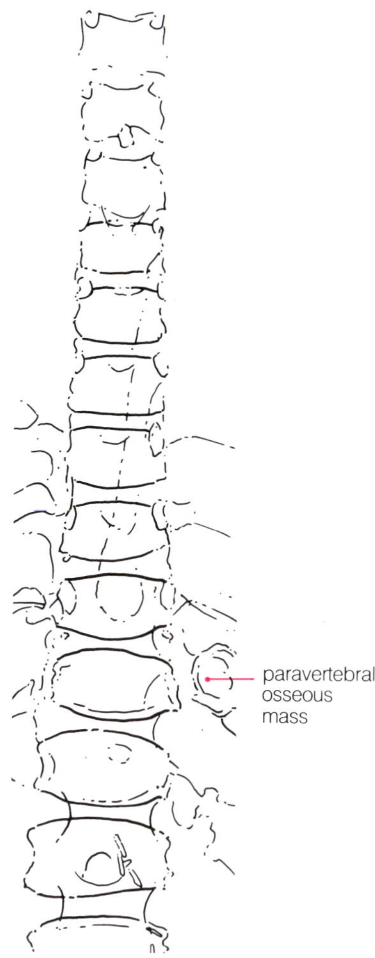

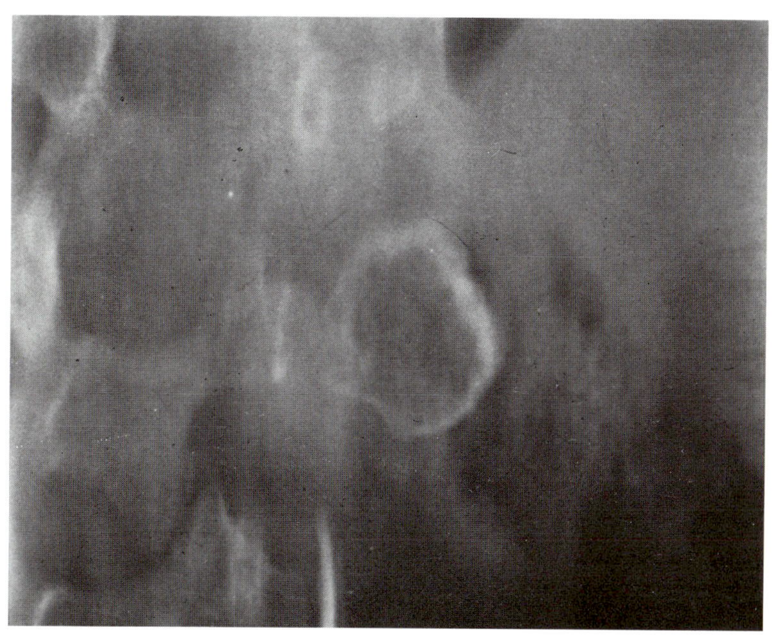

On gross examination, the bony stalk of the exostosis is seen to be continuous with the underlying cortex of the bone (Fig. 13.25). Normally, the cartilaginous cap in the child is generally thick and active, resembling growth plate; however, after adolescence, it becomes thin and relatively inactive. The finding of a thick and proliferating cartilage cap in an adult should lead one to the consideration of peripheral chondrosarcoma.

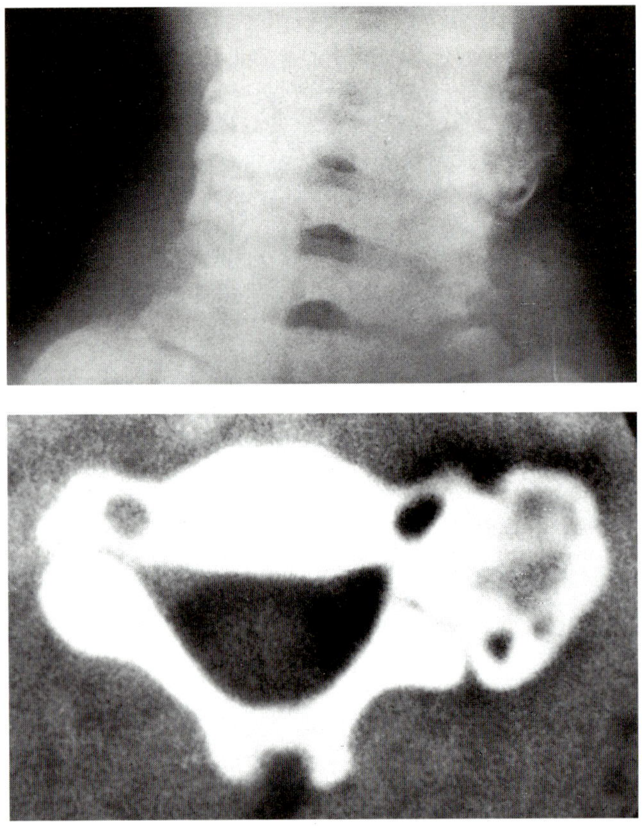

Figure 13.25 AP radiograph *(top)* of the lower cervical spine showing a well-corticated bubbly expansile lesion lateral to the lateral masses of C-4 and C-5. A CT section *(bottom)* through C-4 shows an expansile lesion extending from the left lateral mass. The cortex is thick and continuous with that of the pedicle. The neural foramina and spinal canal are uninvolved. The matrix is similar to that of a medullary cavity with coarse trabeculations. There is no evidence of calcified cartilage within the matrix and no associated surrounding soft-tissue component. (From Novick GS, Pavlov H, Bullough PG: Osteochondroma of the cervical spine: Report of two cases in preadolescent males. *Skeletal Radiol* 8:13–15, 1982)

Osteoid Osteoma

Although osteoid osteoma is considered to be a relatively common benign tumor in bone, only about 5% occur in the spine, most of them involving the vertebral arch. Because of the small size of the lesion, diagnosis may be difficult. The most important and indeed the most typical clinical complaint is that of persistent night pain relieved by aspirin. Rigidity of the spine and muscle spasm are found almost always. When the lesion is in the lumbar spine, scoliosis may be present in varying degrees, with the lesion being located in the concavity of the curve (Fig. 13.26). The resulting scoliotic curve has neither a

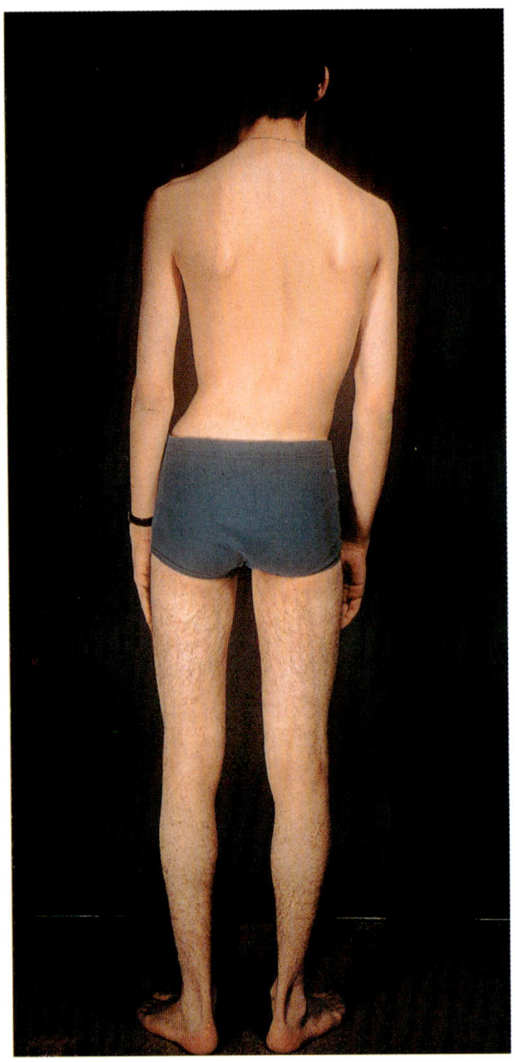

Figure 13.26 Clinical photograph demonstrating mild scoliosis in a teenage boy with an osteoid osteoma in the lumbar spine. (Courtesy of Dr. David Levine)

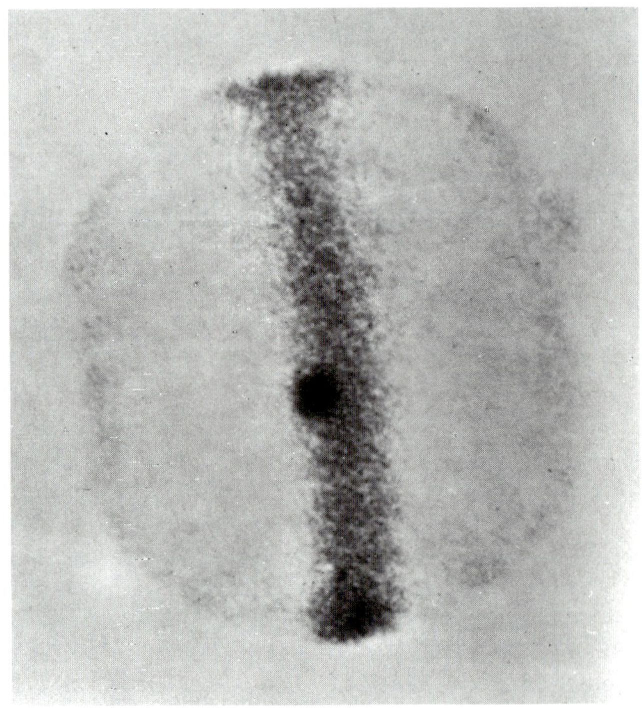

Figure 13.27 Technetium scan of the thoracic spine in a patient complaining of severe localized pain, occasionally present at night and relieved by aspirin. The localized area of high uptake, as seen here, is typical of osteoid osteoma.

rotational component nor a compensatory curve. Nerve root irritation may be present. In general, following treatment, there is regression of the associated scoliosis. Technetium scanning is the most useful method of diagnostic study, as it offers the best chance of localizing the lesion (Fig. 13.27). The lesion then may be visualized by plain laminography or by CT scan (Fig. 13.28). On gross examination, the lesion is characterized by a dark red appearance and gritty consistency, with a nidus that is generally extremely small (Fig. 13.29). Histologic examination reveals a vascular stroma, with trabeculae of immature woven bone characteristically showing a lining of plump osteoblasts; marked osteoclastic resorption indicates a high turnover rate (Fig. 13.30). In some lesions, the nidus may be compact and heavily calcified, with few cells.

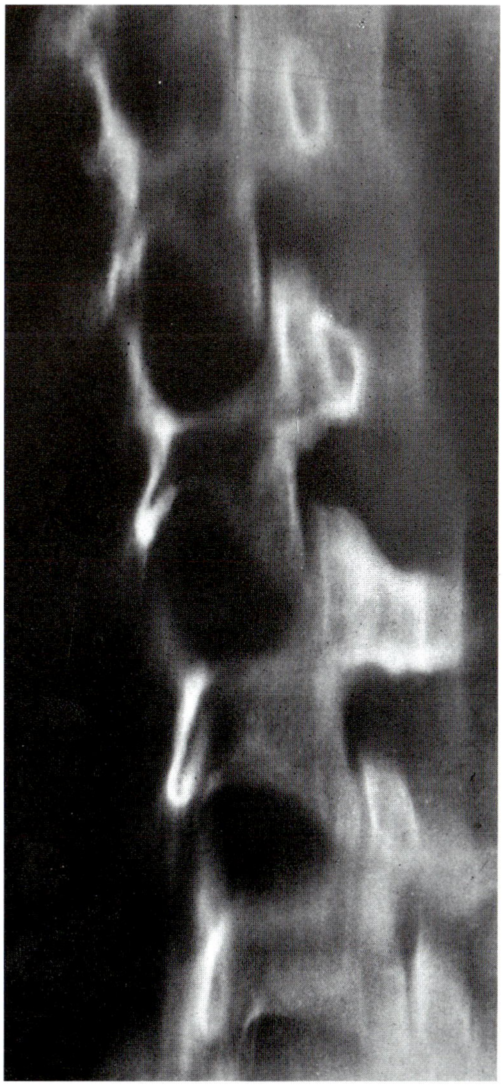

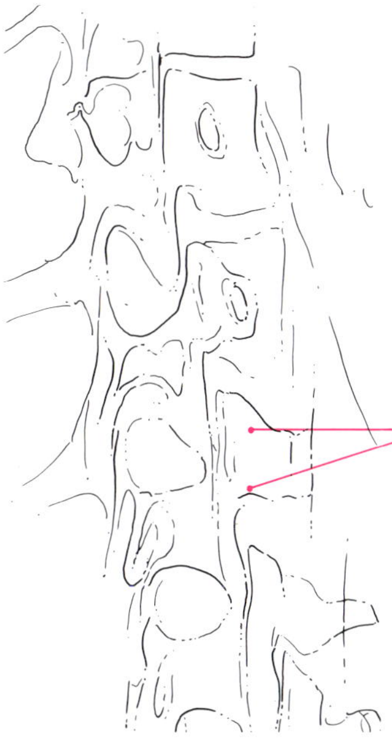

Figure 13.28 Laminogram to demonstrate a lesion in the pedicle of a thoracic vertebra. Note that there is some sclerosis of the bone but that no clearly defined nidus is recognized in this picture. In such a case, it is useful to inject the patient with radioactive technetium diphosphonate, prior to surgery. The increased uptake can be recognized intraoperatively with use of a radioactive detecting device; with this technique, it is much easier to be certain that one has in fact removed the nidus without excessive compromise of the surrounding bone.

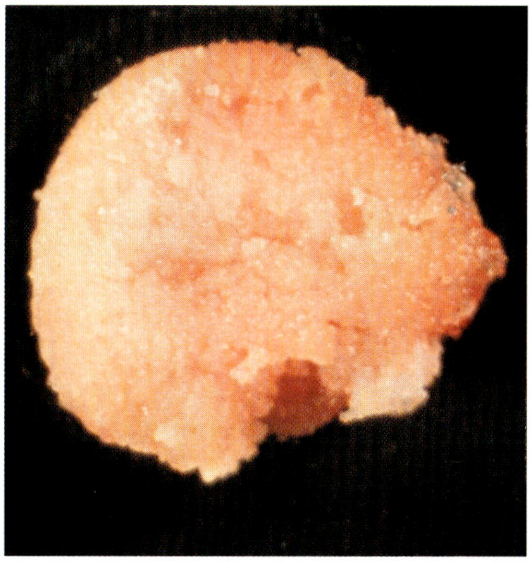

Figure 13.29 Photograph of the specimen removed from a patient with an osteoid osteoma in the spine. A small, round gritty lesion, approximately ½ cm in diameter, is seen. At one margin, a thin rim of sclerotic but normal bone is seen. (Courtesy of Dr. Krishnan K. Unni)

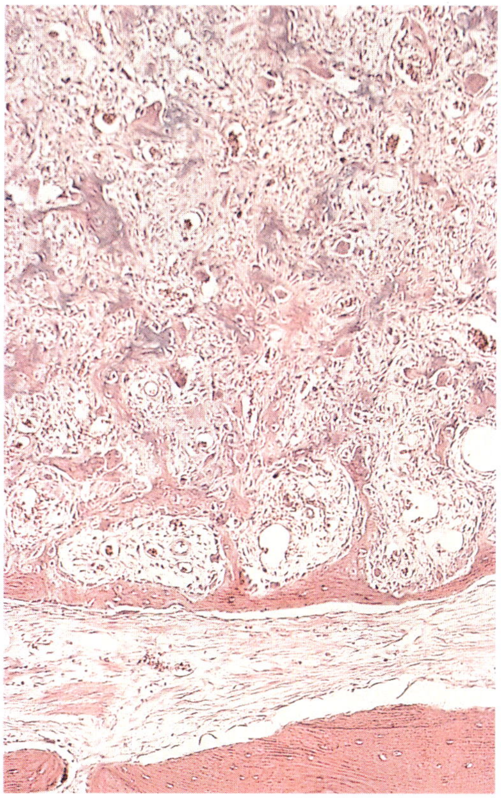

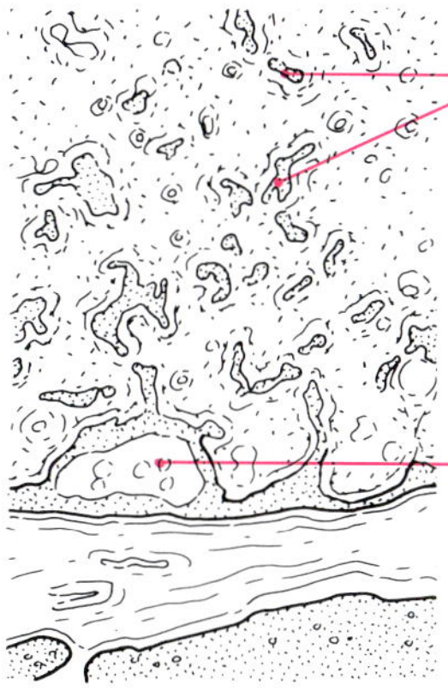

Figure 13.30 Photomicrograph to show a portion of an osteoid osteoma nidus and a part of the normal bone at the edge of the lesion. The nidus is composed of a vascular fibrous tissue in which there are small, irregular, but connected trabeculae of woven bone, demonstrating both prominent osteoblasts and prominent osteoclasts. (H & E, × 10 objective)

Eosinophilic Granuloma

Eosinophilic granuloma is a self-limiting, benign histiocytic lesion found in children, which in the spine generally presents as vertebra plana. In vertebra plana, also known as Calvé's disease, the vertebral body is reduced to a thin homogeneous lamina that is thinner than the discs on either side. Spontaneous recovery usually follows, and so a biopsy is not generally performed (Fig. 13.31). Since frequently there is more than one site of involvement, a bone scan should be performed.

Not all cases of eosinophilic granuloma present as vertebra plana. A lytic lesion of the vertebral body may occur and thus present diagnostic problems, and in such a case a biopsy may be necessary (Fig. 13.32). On gross examination, the tissue curetted away is likely to be scant and friable, with little granules of dense yellowish material scattered throughout a hemorrhagic stroma. However, in the early stages of the disease, it may be composed of soft tan tissue (Fig. 13.33). Histologically, the characteristic features are a background of vacuolated histiocytes with occasional giant cells, focal collections of eosinophils, and scattered

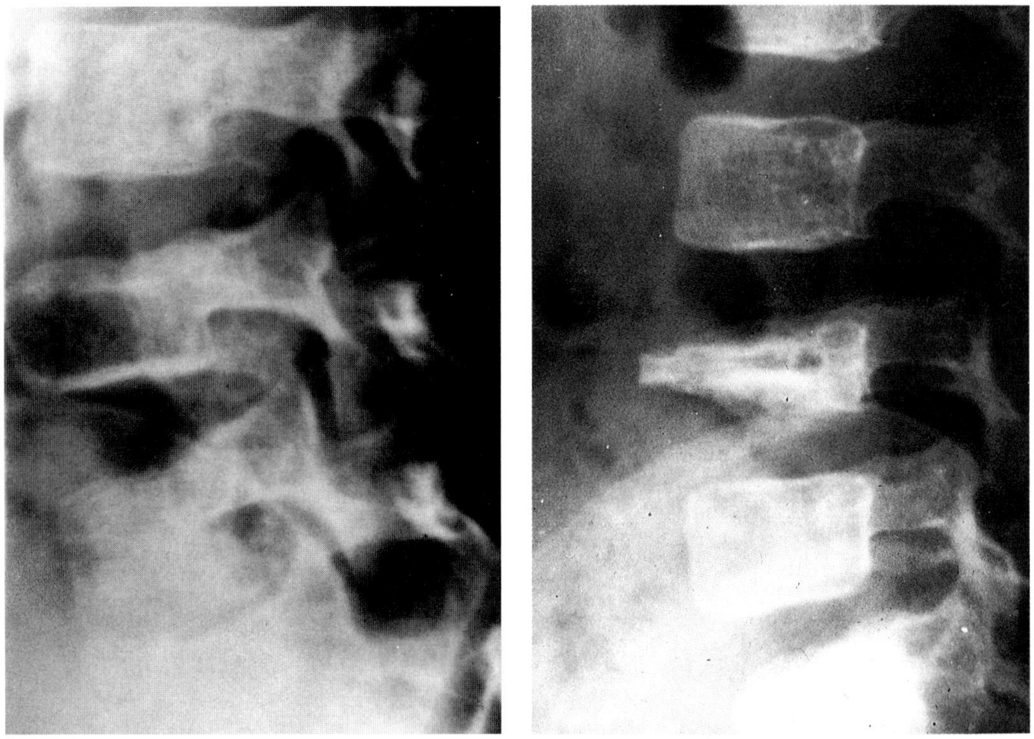

Figure 13.31 Lateral radiograph *(left)* of the lumbar spine in an 8-year-old child, showing a lytic lesion of L-3, with partial collapse. A lateral radiograph *(right)* of the same patient, one month later, shows that the vertebral body has now collapsed down to a thin sclerotic wafer, which is somewhat increased in AP diameter. This appearance is characteristic for Calvé's disease.

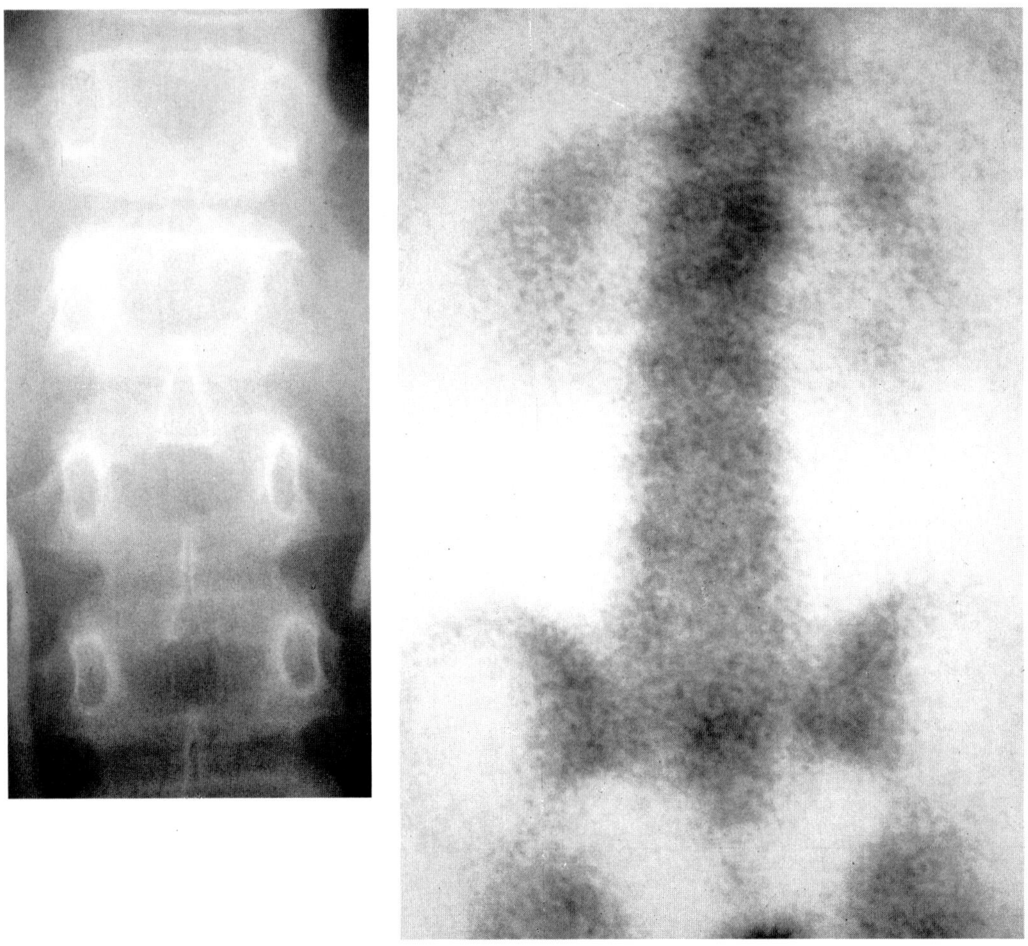

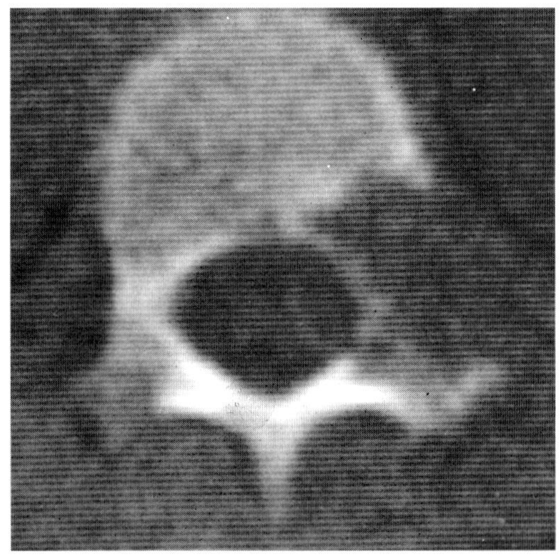

Figure 13.32 AP radiograph *(left)*, with contrast material in the kidneys, shows partial destruction of the pedicle of L-1, with loss of visualization of the lateral margin. A technetium scan *(center)* of the same patient shows increased uptake in the region of the pedicle of L-1. A CT scan *(right)* through the same lesion shows a lytic lesion involving the pedicle and the posterior portion of the vertebral body, as well as the anterior portion of the transverse process. There is very little evidence of reactive bone around this lesion.

chronic inflammatory cells. Involutional areas are associated with the presence of lipid-laden histiocytes and fibrosis (Fig. 13.34). Occasionally, with an atypical radiograph, the histologic differential diagnosis from Hodgkin's disease may be difficult; the absence of the Reed-Sternberg cells and atypical mononuclear cells, together with the usual lack of reactive fibrosis in eosinophilic granuloma, should differentiate these two conditions (Fig. 13.35).

Although other benign tumors including chondroblastoma and benign fibrous histiocytomas also occur in the spine, they are exceedingly rare.

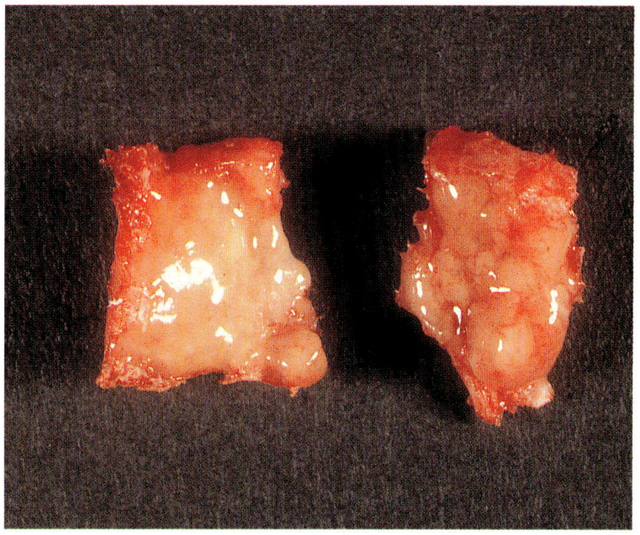

Figure 13.33 Photograph of the gross specimen resected from the patient seen in Figure 13.32. The soft, tan tissue seen here is typical of an eosinophilic granuloma in its early stages. In the later stages, flecks of opaque yellow tissue, together with more extensive hemorrhage, may be seen in the lesion.

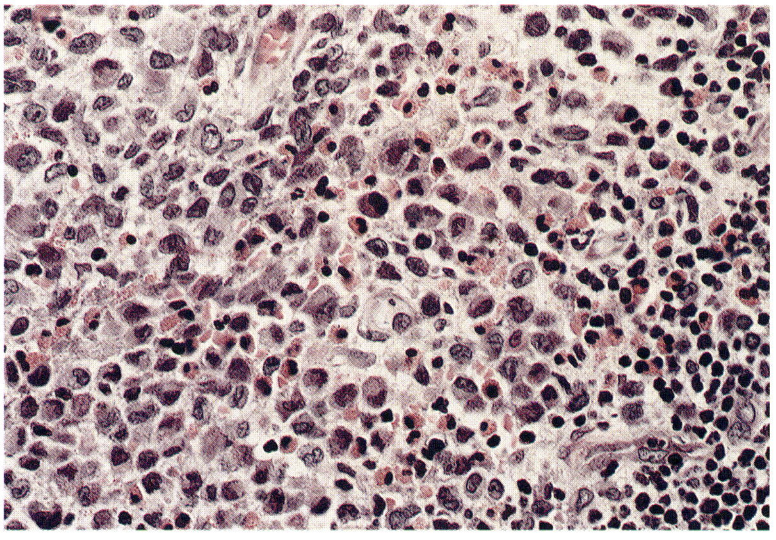

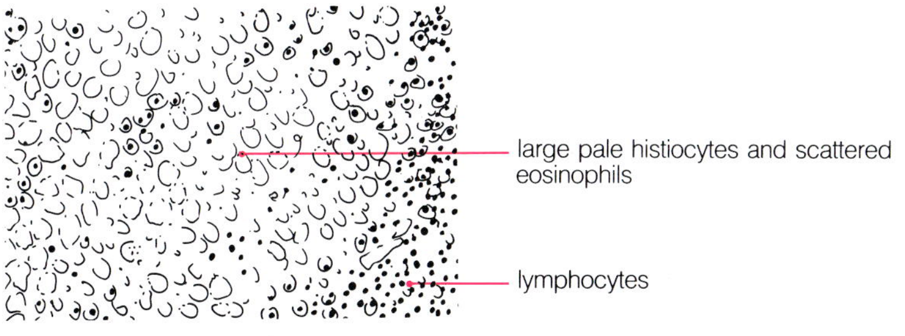

Figure 13.34 Photomicrograph of an eosinophilic granuloma to demonstrate the typical mixed cellular pattern, with the predominant cell type being the large histiocytes. Lymphocytes, plasma cells, and eosinophils also are present. (H & E, × 25 objective)

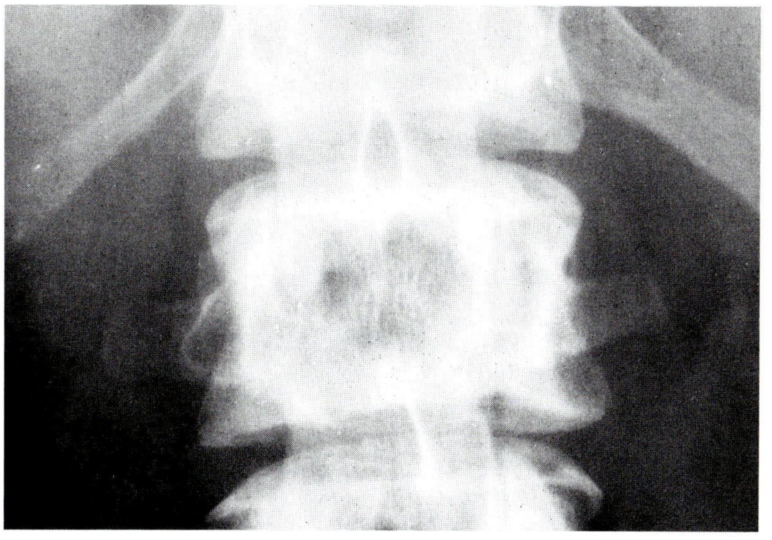

Figure 13.35 AP radiograph of L-1 in a patient with proven eosinophilic granuloma, showing increased density throughout the vertebral body suggestive of lymphoma, especially Hodgkin's disease. In such a case, correct identification of the tissue curetted away is obviously extremely important.

14 CHAPTER

SPINAL TUMORS: MALIGNANT

Metastatic Tumors

The most common malignant tumor encountered in the spine is metastatic cancer. In adults, most spinal metastases will be from the breast, prostate, lung, kidney, thyroid, or colon; in children, from neuroblastoma (Fig. 14.1), rhabdomyosarcoma, or retinoblastoma. Metastatic tumor may be limited to one vertebra or it may involve the entire vertebral column (Fig. 14.2); however, multiple involvement occurs more commonly. Metastasis occurs via the bloodstream, either through the systemic circulation or by way of the vertebral venous plexus (Batson's plexus). Only rarely will the spine be involved by direct extension, as may occur for example with rectal carcinoma. External pressure from an aortic aneurysm also may result in extensive bone loss simulating a tumor (Fig. 14.3), in some radiographic views.

Metastases are designated as either osteoblastic or osteolytic; in the former, there is an increase in bone density, while in the latter, there is bone destruction and demineralization, which is likely to lead to subsequent deformity (Figs. 14.4 and 14.5). Both may exist in the same bone or either may predominate in one vertebral body and be less conspicuous in another. Osteoblastic metastases usually are seen in association with prostatic and breast carcinoma, where-

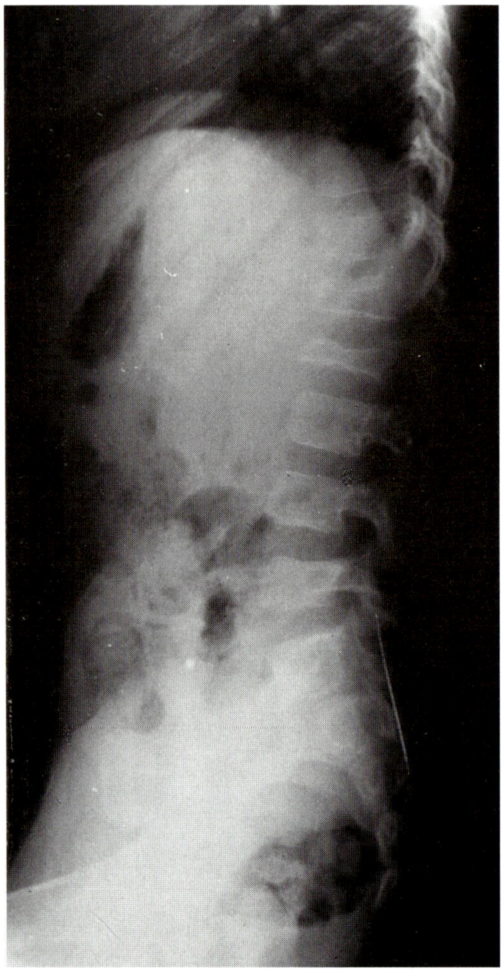

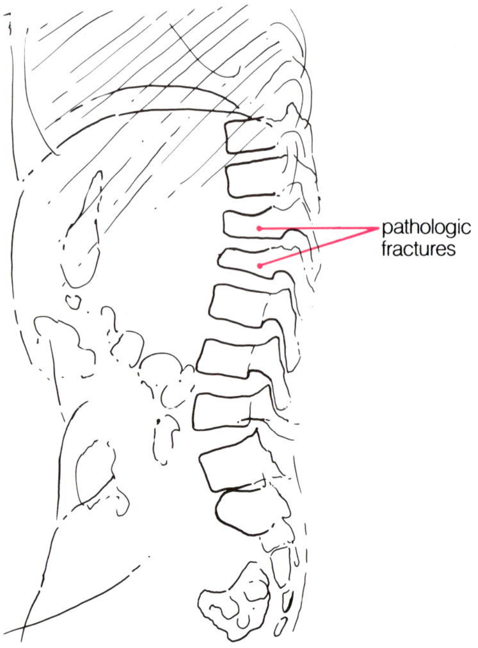

Figure 14.1 Lateral radiograph of the spine of a young child with a neuroblastoma, demonstrating multiple metastases in the spine, with compression fractures.

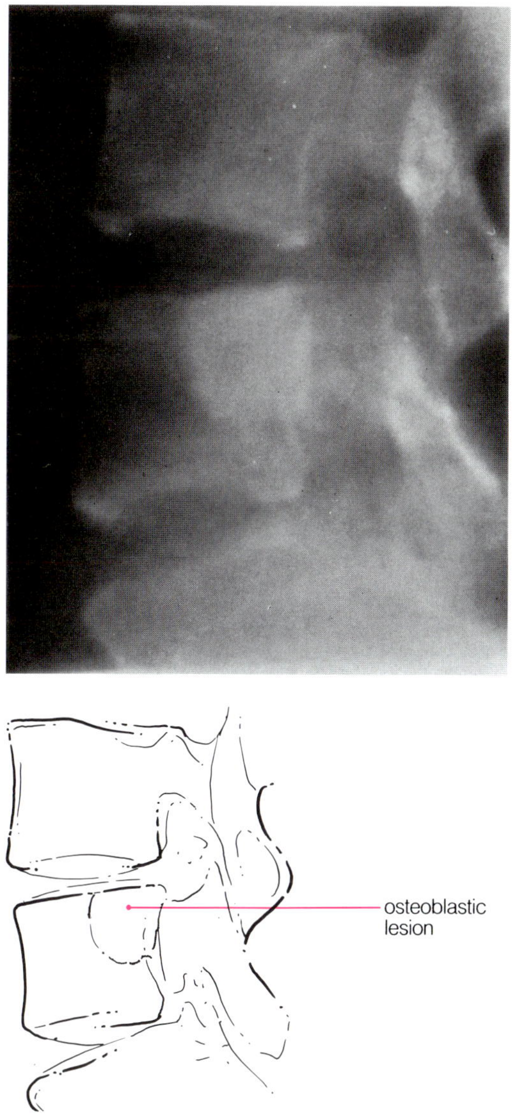

Figure 14.2 Lateral tomogram of a portion of lumbar spine from an adolescent male with a primary osteogenic sarcoma of the tibia. A solitary metastasis was found in L-4, and is seen to involve the posterior portion of the vertebral body. Like the original tumor, it is densely sclerotic. No other metastases to bone were found on radiographic examination.

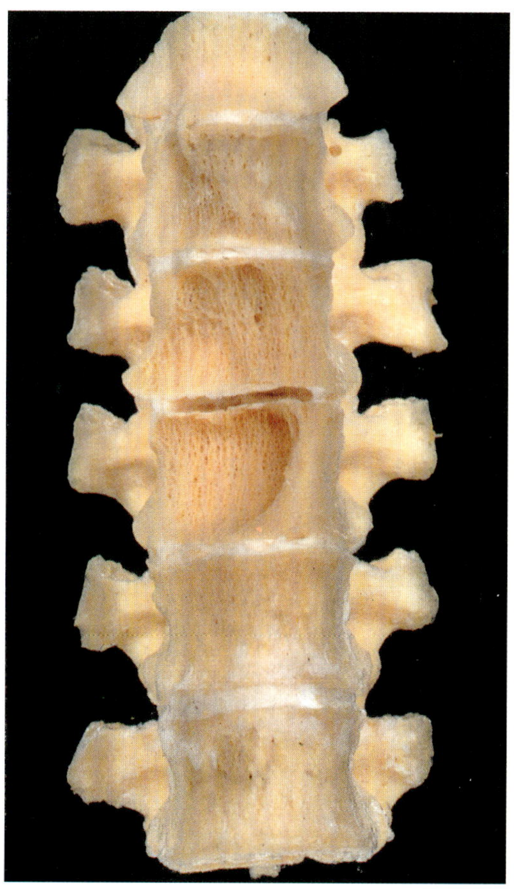

Figure 14.3 Photograph of a segment of thoracic spine from a 37-year-old male, who at autopsy was found to have a large aneurysm of the ascending aorta. The aneurysm has resulted in extensive erosion of the bodies of three of the thoracic vertebrae. (Courtesy of The Royal College of Surgeons of England)

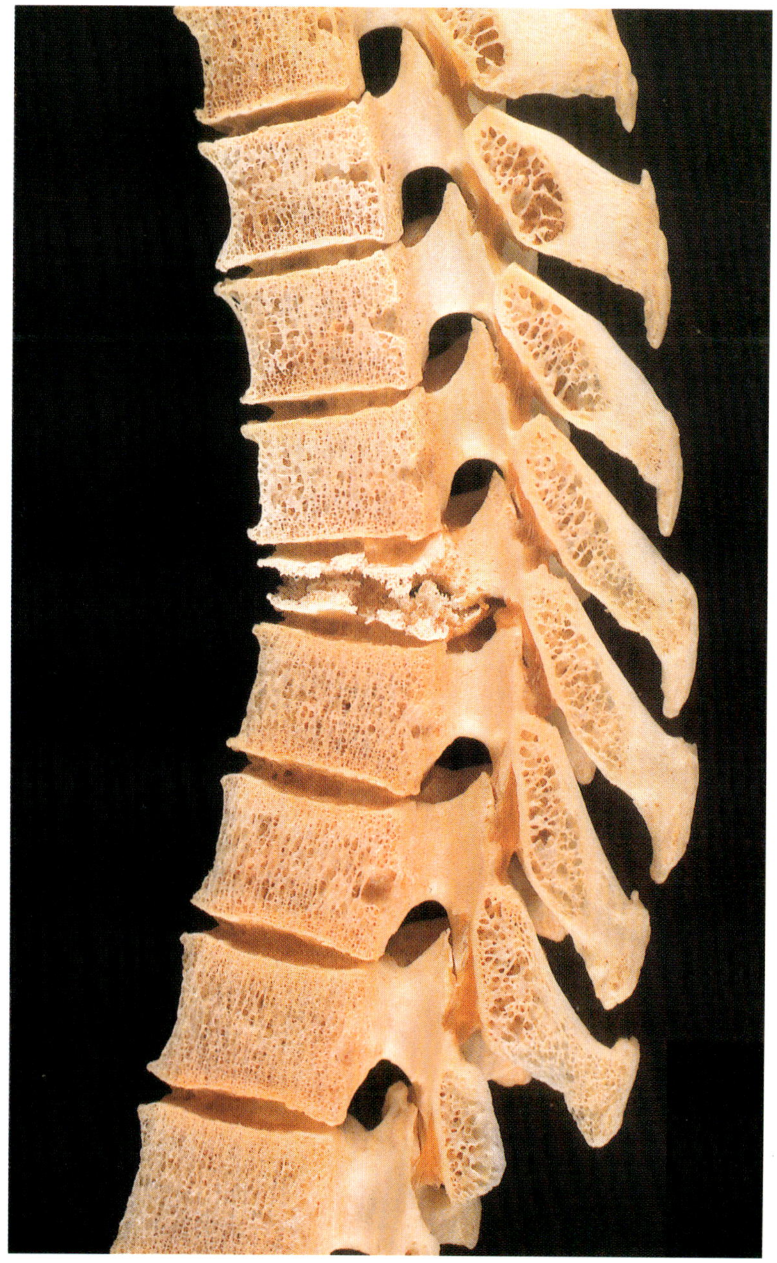

Figure 14.4 Photograph of a macerated sagittal section through the spine of a 60-year-old male with a primary carcinoma of the colon, showing total collapse of the body of T-9 without significant deformity of the spine. This photograph should be compared with Figure 14.5.

as osteolytic metastases are characteristic of the thyroid or kidney. However, these are not hard and fast rules (Figs. 14.6 through 14.9).

Tumors involving the vertebrae may extend into the epidural space, but the dura itself is generally resistant to invasion even in

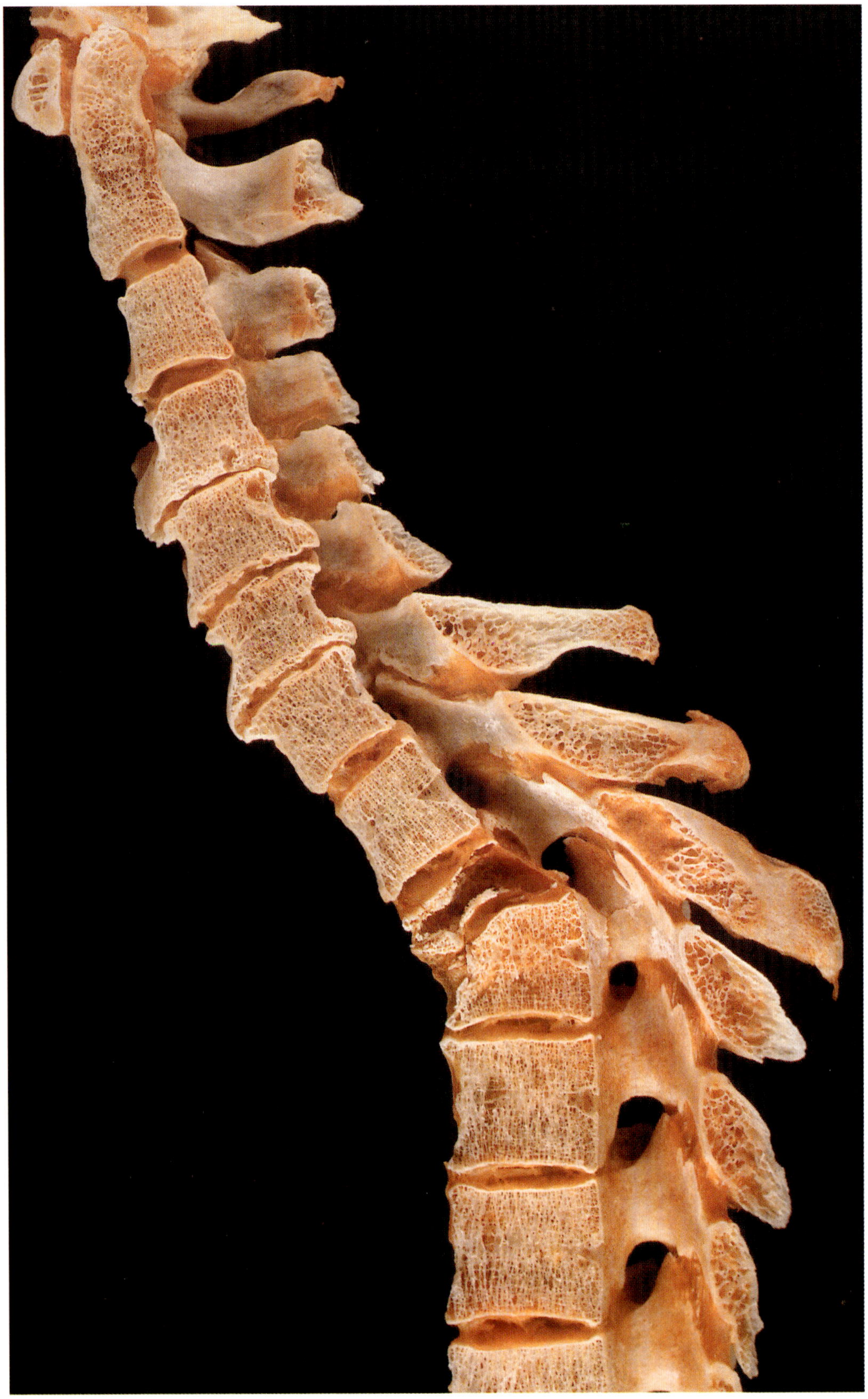

Figure 14.5 Photograph of a sagittal section of the macerated spine of a 58-year-old male with a lung carcinoma, who shortly before death developed paraplegia. The specimen shows a complete collapse of T-2, with forward subluxation of T-2 on T-3, and a kyphotic deformity.

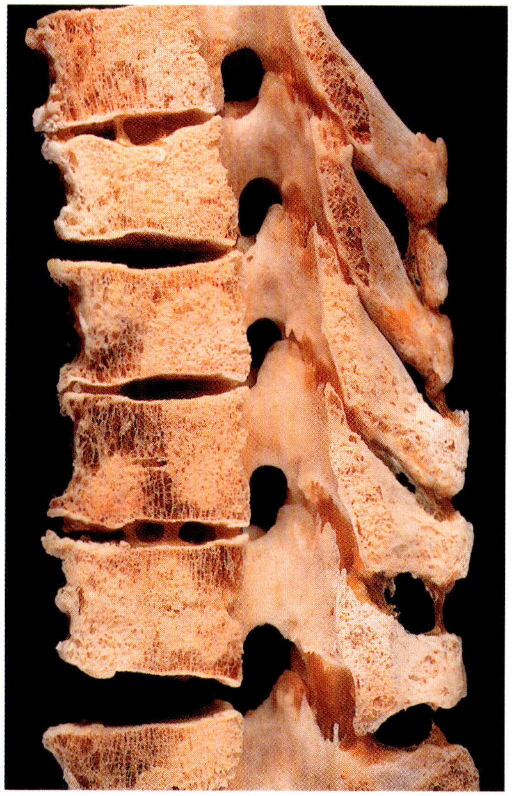

Figure 14.6 Photograph of a segment of thoracic spine, sagittally sectioned and macerated, which demonstrates multiple osteoblastic metastases involving not only the vertebral bodies but also portions of the neural arch. Areas of normal bone are seen interspersed between the areas of metastatic disease. The specimen was obtained from a 67-year-old male who died of lung cancer.

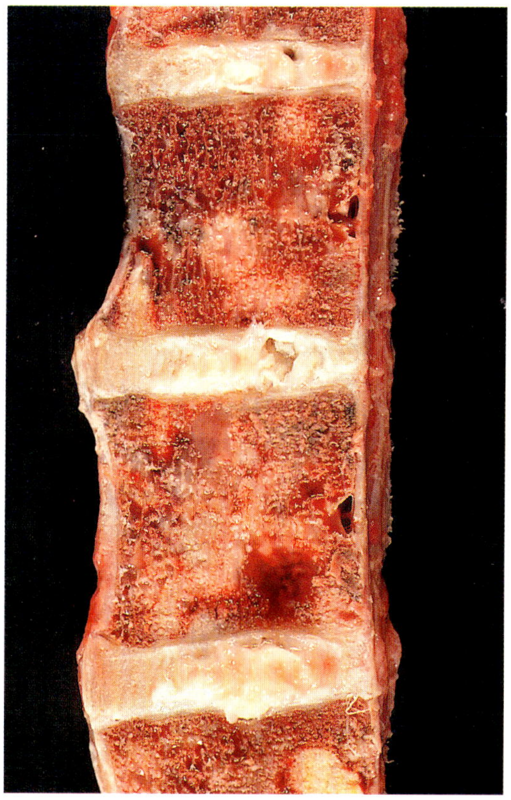

Figure 14.7 Photograph of a sagittal section through a portion of lumbar spine, which demonstrates mixed lytic and blastic areas. The blastic areas are pale while the lytic areas have a red, glistening appearance.

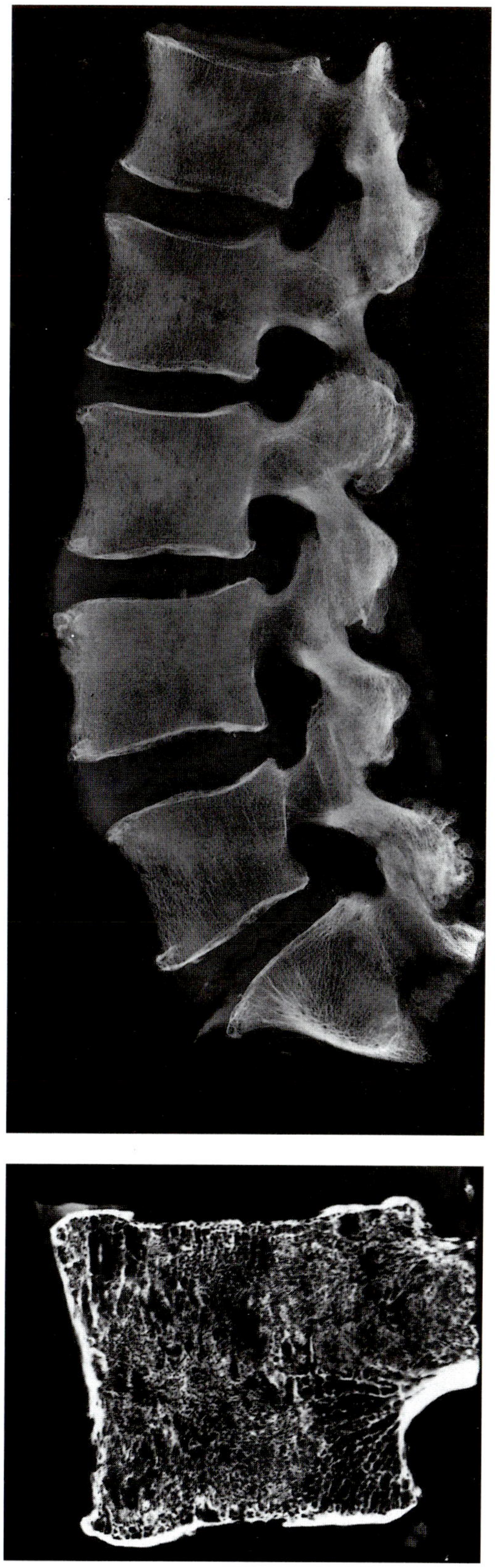

Figure 14.8 Lateral specimen radiograph *(top)* of the lumbar spine from a 70-year-old male who died of prostatic cancer with widespread metastases. In all of the vertebral bodies there is a rather diffuse increased sclerosis, which is due to new bone having been deposited in the marrow spaces. In a fine-grain radiograph *(bottom)* of a 2-mm slice of one of the vertebral bodies, the fine irregular trabeculae of new bone can be distinguished clearly from the original bone trabeculae of the vertebral body.

the presence of extensive epidural spread (Fig. 14.10).

The radiographic identification of spinal metastasis depends on the extent of bone destruction; at autopsy, one frequently will find metastases in the spine that were undetected during life (Fig. 14.11). However, with the introduction of radioisotopic scanning most metastases can now be detected.

Multiple Myeloma

Multiple myeloma is the most common primary tumor of bone, and the spine is almost always involved. It usually affects individuals over the age of 50, but occasionally it is seen at a younger age. The usual clinical picture is one in which pain predominates. Anemia is common, the ESR generally is elevated, and occasionally, especially in association with bed rest, there may be hypercalcemia. The most important diagnostic test is the identification of a monoclonal protein by serum electrophoresis (see Fig. 14.13).

Multiple myeloma is characterized radiographically by the presence of round lytic defects in the bone, without any significant sclerotic reaction around them (Fig. 14.12). Occasionally however, lytic defects may not be apparent and the radiographic picture will suggest a diffuse osteopenia. In such a case, the differential diagnosis from osteoporosis must be made by laboratory examination (Fig. 14.13). Very rarely, multiple myeloma will produce sclerotic lesions, such that the correct diagnosis may not at first

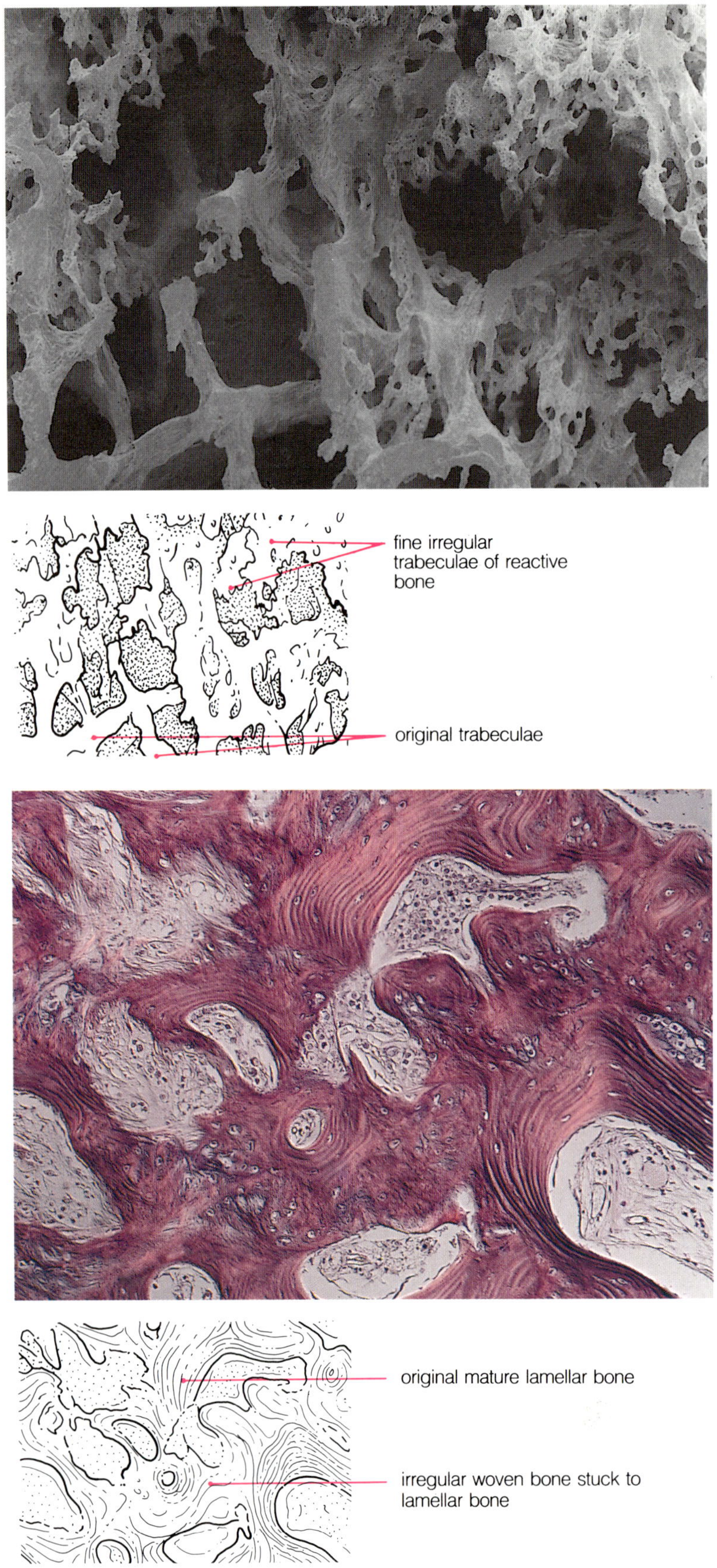

Figure 14.9 Scanning electron micrograph *(top)* of a portion of bone obtained from the specimen shown in Figure 14.8. (× 15 magnification) Here again, the fine trabeculae of bone produced in response to the tumor are apparent. Photomicrograph *(bottom)* of the same specimen shows the woven character of the new bone, which is seen to be firmly applied to the surface of the lamellar bone of the vertebral body. The spaces in between are filled with fibrous tissue and malignant cells. (H & E, × 4 objective)

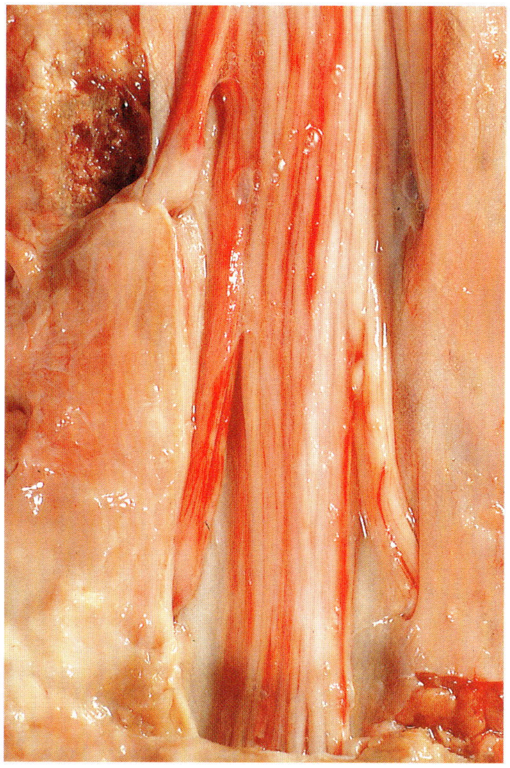

Figure 14.10 Photograph of the spinal canal in the lower lumbar region of a patient with carcinoma of the breast, who developed sciatica. There is extensive tumor involving the region of the foramina, but no tumor has broken through into the subarachnoid space.

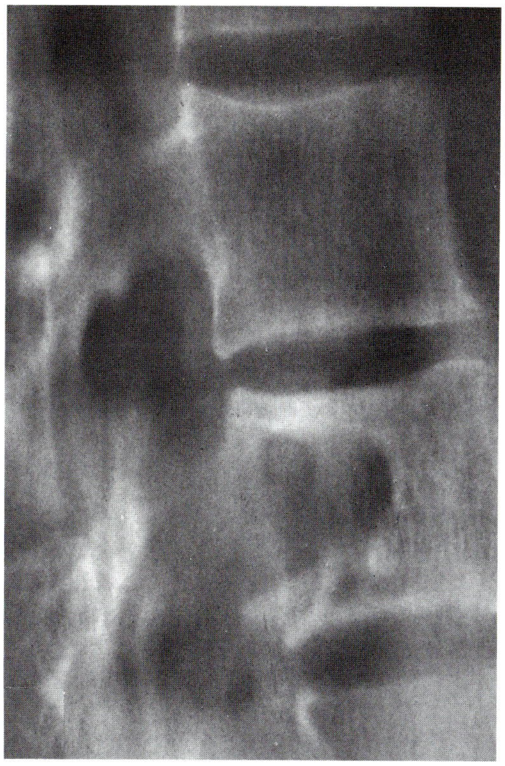

Figure 14.12 Lateral tomogram of L-2, with parts of L-1 and L-3, in a 55-year-old male with multiple myeloma to demonstrate the well-defined lytic lesions devoid of significant sclerosis, which are characteristic of this disease.

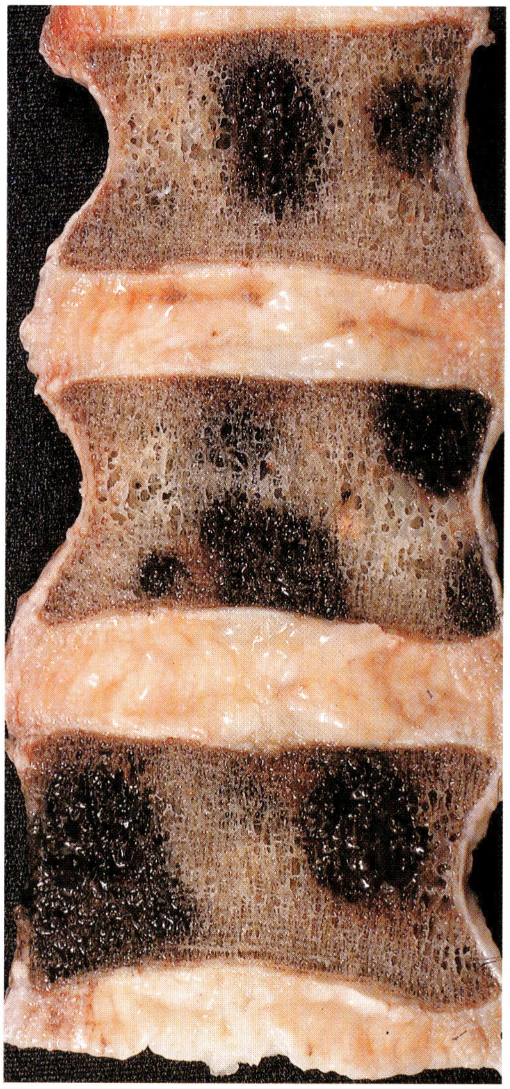

Figure 14.11 Photograph to demonstrate multiple metastases in the vertebral bodies of a patient who died with malignant melanoma. The dark color of the metastases gives a clue to the primary tumor. These metastases were not recognized on clinical radiographs of the spine obtained shortly before death. In the absence of marked bone production or bone destruction, extensive metastatic disease may be present without any obvious radiographic changes.

Serum Protein Electrophoresis

	%	NORMAL RANGE
ALBUMIN	32.3	56.4–71.6
ALPHA 1	3.6	1.9–4.5
ALPHA 2	5.3	7.3–15.0
BETA	6.8	6.2–11.5
GAMMA	52.0	7.8–18.2

Quantitative Immunoglobulin

	mg/dL	NORMAL RANGE
IgG	275	600–1450
IgA	2964	60–340
IgM	10.4	25–200

Immunofixation Electrophoresis Gel

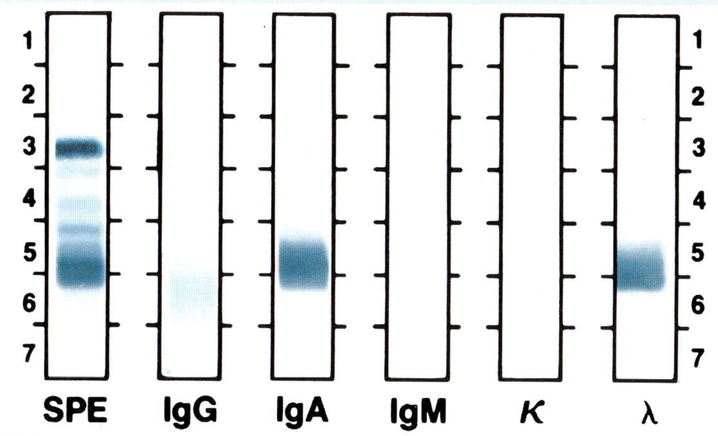

INCREASED IgA LAMBDA PRESENT

Figure 14.13 Immunoelectropherogram of the serum from a patient with myeloma. Note that there is an excess of gammaglobulin, which is overwhelmingly IgA (λ).

be considered (Fig. 14.14). In more than half of patients, pathologic fractures result in an overall loss of vertebral body height, with swelling of the adjacent intervertebral discs into the affected bodies. A fish-mouth appearance then results.

Gross examination of the affected bones will show either a diffuse gelatinous red infiltration of the marrow on the one hand, or, on the other hand, tan tumor nodules (Fig. 14.15). Microscopic examination will reveal sheets of plasma cells, which may show varying degrees of differentiation; in multiple myeloma however, no prognostic significance can be given to atypicality of the cells (Fig. 14.16). In approximately 10% of patients with myeloma, amyloidosis occurs as a complication, and amyloid deposits may be found within the bone.

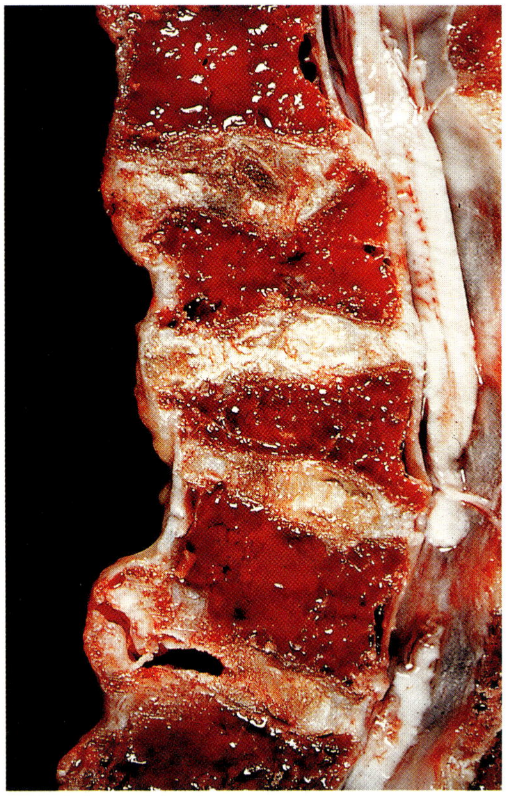

Figure 14.14 Photograph of a segment of the lower thoracic spine from a patient with multiple myeloma shows extensive replacement of the bone and marrow by a red gelatinous tissue. The resultant osteoporosis has resulted in multiple compression fractures. (Courtesy of Dr. Howard Dorfman)

SOLITARY MYELOMA

Very occasionally, patients may present with solitary lesions (plasmacytomas) and in the spine they are quite likely to present with rapidly developing paraplegia and gibbus deformity, as a result of vertebral collapse (Fig. 14.17). In fact, paraplegia is found much more frequently with solitary myeloma than with multiple myeloma, probably because the patients with multiple myeloma die before paraplegia can develop. About 70% of patients who present with an apparently solitary focus of myeloma will develop multiple myelomatosis and will usually die within five years. The remaining patients may be cured following radiation therapy, or in other cases may develop generalized disease only after many years. For the diagnosis of solitary myeloma, a skeletal survey should be done to exclude other sites of involvement; aspirate of sternal or iliac crest marrow should show no evidence of myeloma. If serum electrophoresis shows a monoclonal globulin spike, this will disappear following treatment of the solitary lesion, which usually responds well to radiation therapy.

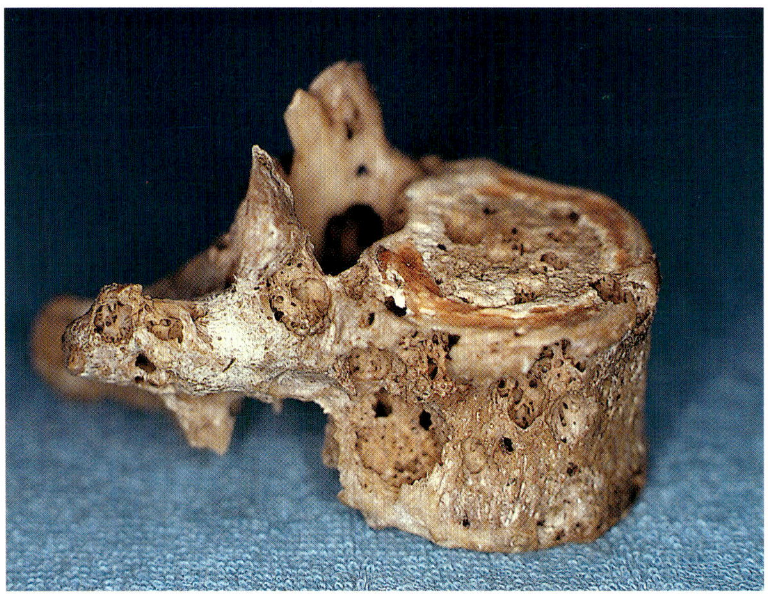

Figure 14.15 Photograph of a macerated vertebral body from a patient with multiple myeloma, showing numerous destructive round defects throughout the bone. (Specimen from the collection of the Smithsonian Institute; courtesy of Dr. Donald J. Ortner)

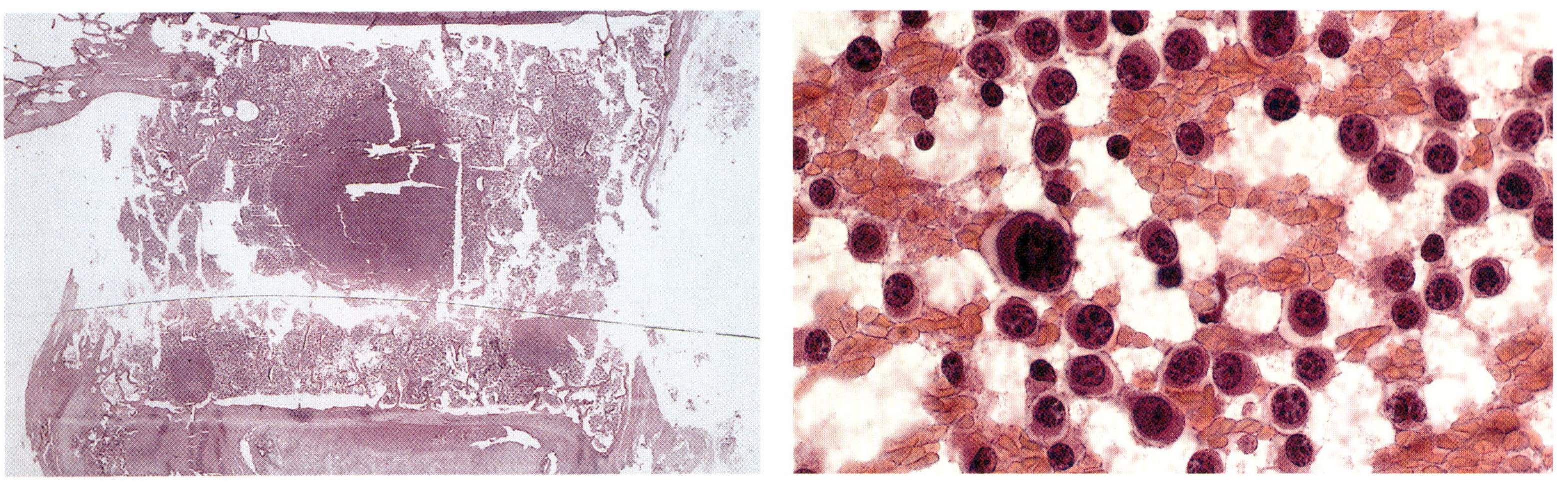

Figure 14.16 Photomicrograph *(left)* showing a section through a vertebral body affected by multiple myeloma, in which discrete nodules of tumor replace both bone and bone marrow. The structure of the vertebral bodies is maintained. In this patient there was associated DISH, as can be seen from the sclerotic bone on the anterior cortex, which is extending in front of the anulus fibrosus. A photomicrograph *(right)* of a smear obtained from a vertebral lesion in a patient with multiple myeloma. Note that there is some variation in the size of the plasma cells. However, it should be noted that the degree of cellular differentiation in multiple myeloma has no prognostic significance.

Chordoma

Chordoma is a neoplasm that arises from remnants of the notochord, and therefore occurs in the midline of the axial skeleton (see Section 1, Chapter 4 for a discussion of the notochord). About half of cases are seen in the sacrococcygeal region (Fig. 14.18), whereas one-third are present at the base of the skull. The remaining cases are seen at different sites along the vertebral column but most commonly in the cervical region. Chordoma is a slow-growing neoplasm, whose clinical symptoms depend on the site. Cranial lesions generally are smaller than sacrococcygeal lesions at the time of initial presentation. Males are affected more frequently than are females, and the average age at diagnosis is approximately 55 years.

Bone destruction is the radiographic hallmark of chordoma; however, about half of patients will show focal calcifications within the lesion (Fig. 14.19). Localization of the le-

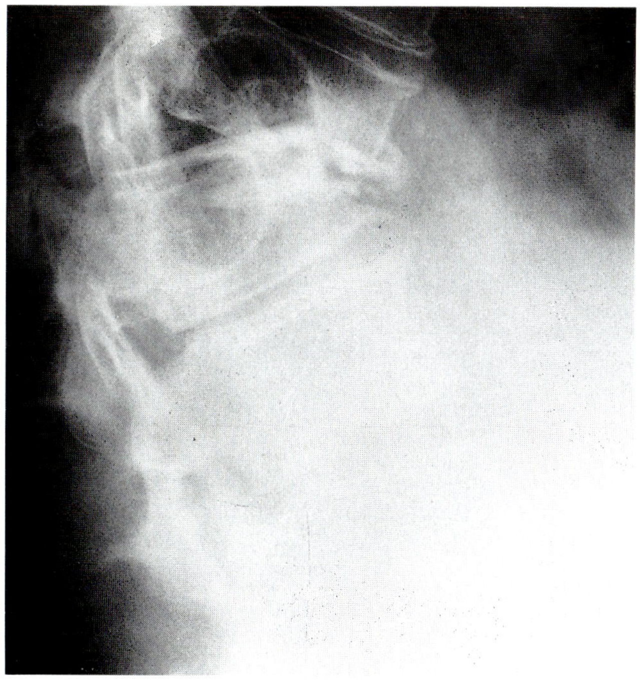

Figure 14.17 Lateral radiograph of a 45-year-old male who presented with severe thoracolumbar pain following a fall. A fracture-dislocation of T-10 and T-12 is demonstrated with virtual absence of T-11. Biopsy of the area showed a myeloma. No other sites of myeloma were demonstrated on radiographic survey. The patient received local radiation therapy and a 10-year follow-up showed no evidence of local or generalized disease.

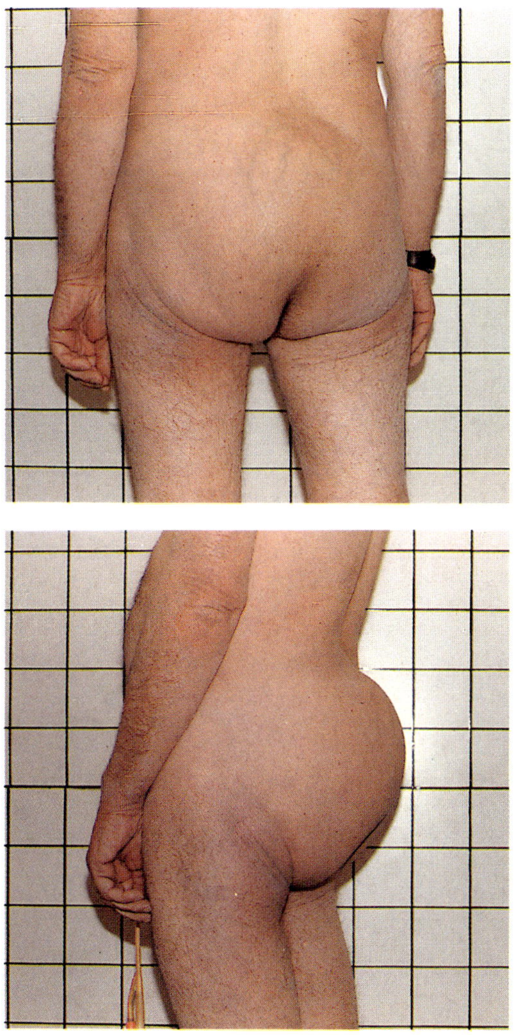

Figure 14.18 Clinical photographs *(top* and *bottom)* of a middle-aged male in posterior and lateral views to demonstrate a large posterior pelvic tumor, which proved on further study to be a chordoma. Most of the posterior part of the sacrum was involved. The tumor was resected en bloc. (Courtesy of Dr. Zdenek Matejovsky)

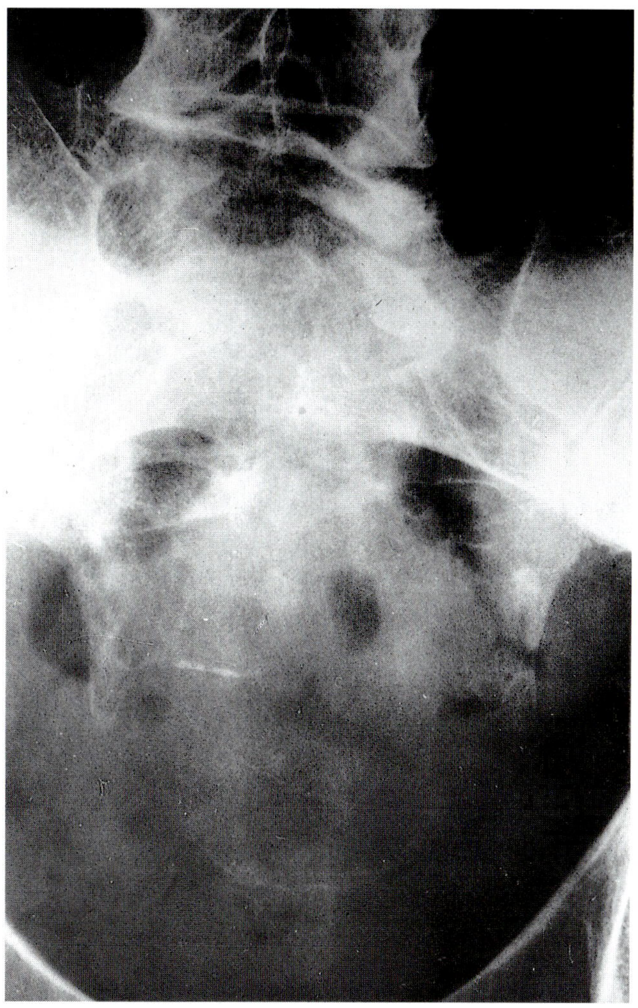

Figure 14.19 AP radiograph of a sacral chordoma shows a large destructive lesion, which extends into the soft tissues laterally and inferiorly. There is focal calcification within the lesion.

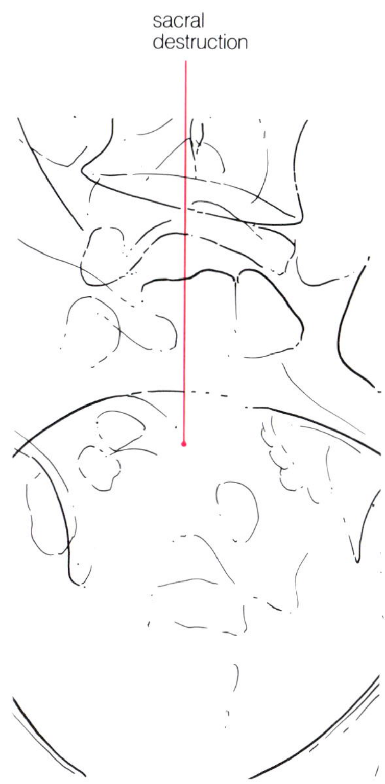

sion is aided greatly by the use of newer imaging techniques, particularly in cases of intracranial chordomas. When chordomas affect areas of the spine other than the two common ones, the lesions are likely to be seen as lytic ones, which are located centrally within the vertebral body and are slowly expansile. When the cervical vertebrae are affected, extension anteriorly into the soft tissues may result in dysphagia (Fig. 14.20) whereas posterior extension may result in neurologic complications. Systemic metastases to the regional lymph nodes, lung, liver, and bone have been reported in about half of cases.

On gross examination, chordomas are generally soft, and appear well encapsulated. Lobulations will become apparent on cut section, and the tumor will usually have a bluish-gray color with extensive gelatinous translucent areas that are focally cystic and hemorrhagic (Figs. 14.21 and 14.22). Grossly, the tissue may suggest a chondrosarcoma or even a mucinous carcinoma. Histologic examination, however, shows a characteristic arrangement of lobules of tumors separated by fibrous septa of different thicknesses. The tumor cells are of varying sizes and shapes, arranged in both cords and sheets, with an eosinophilic cytoplasm associated with intracellular mucinous vacuoles that may be minimal or abundant (Fig. 14.23). The vacuoles may be very prominent and so displace the nucleus to one edge, producing the so-called physaliphorous cell (Fig. 14.24); pools of mucin also are seen in the extracellular space.

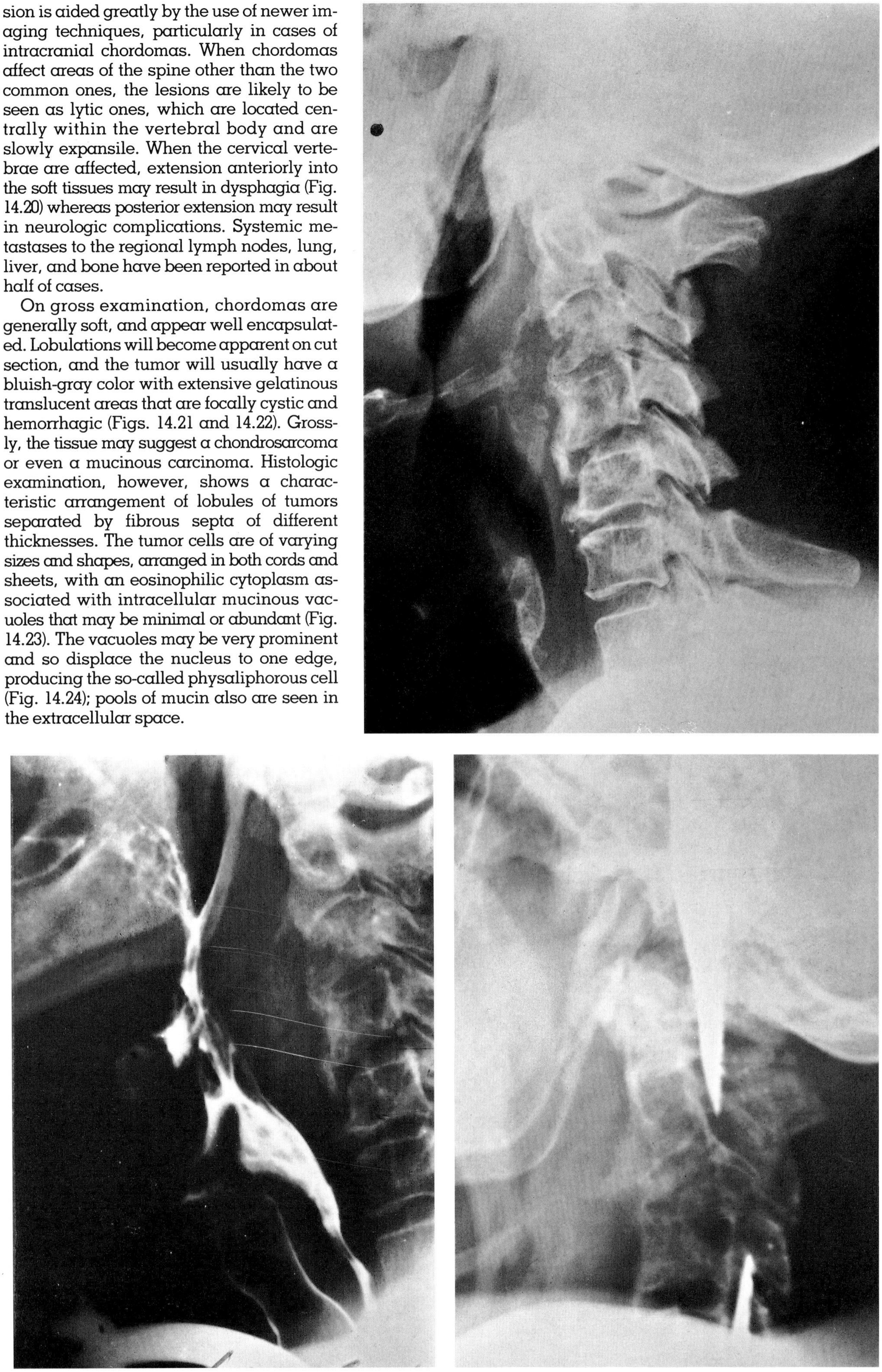

Figure 14.20 Lateral radiograph *(top)* of a 40-year-old male, who presented with dysphagia and myelopathy. There is a destructive lesion involving C-3 and C-4, with an anterior soft-tissue extension that can be seen to occlude the airway partially. A barium swallow *(bottom left)* shows both anterior displacement of the esophagus as well as partial occlusion. A cervical myelogram *(bottom right)* shows a block from C-2 to C-4, with partial collapse of C-3. Biopsy proved this to be a chordoma.

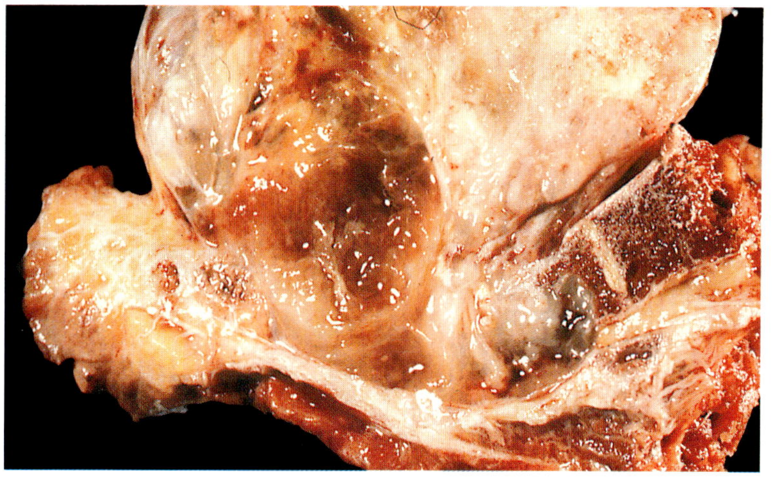

Figure 14.21 Photograph of a sagittal section obtained at autopsy, through the lower lumbar spine and sacrum of a patient with chordoma. The tumor has largely destroyed the sacrum and is involving L-5. A large anterior component is present. The tumor tissue shows a characteristic lobulated blue-gray firm tissue mass, with focal hemorrhage and cystification. (Courtesy of Dr. Mario Campanacci)

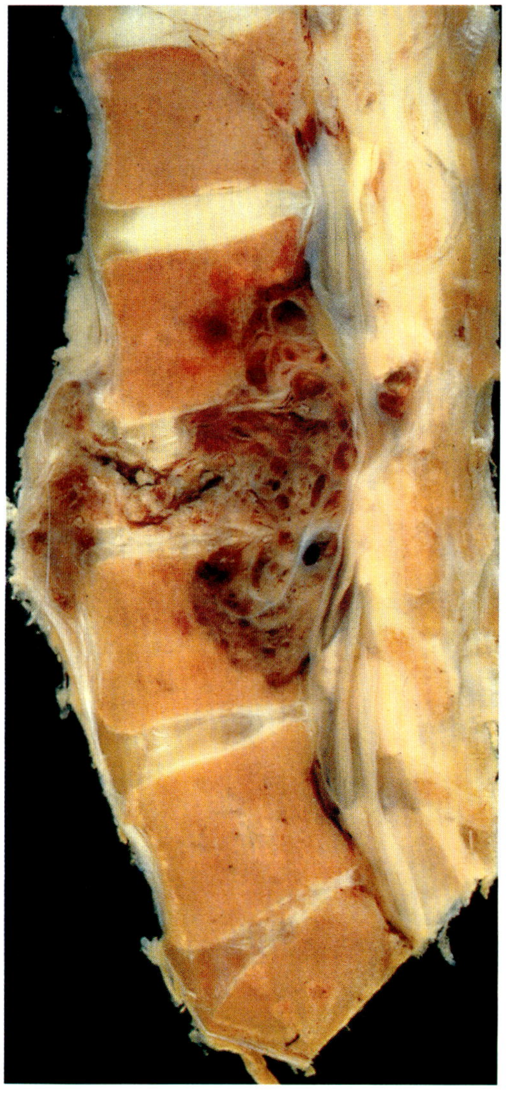

Figure 14.22 Photograph of a sagittal section through the lumbar spine from a 70-year-old male, who clinically was thought to have metastatic disease. He died with paraplegia and an intractable urinary infection. There is a destructive hemorrhagic lesion in L-3 that involves the bodies of L-2 and L-4. The lesion has extended posteriorly, and is compressing the cauda equina. Histology revealed a typical chordoma. The lumbar spine is rarely involved in this condition, and most lesions in the vertebral bodies are found in the cervical portions of the spine. (Courtesy of The Royal College of Surgeons of England)

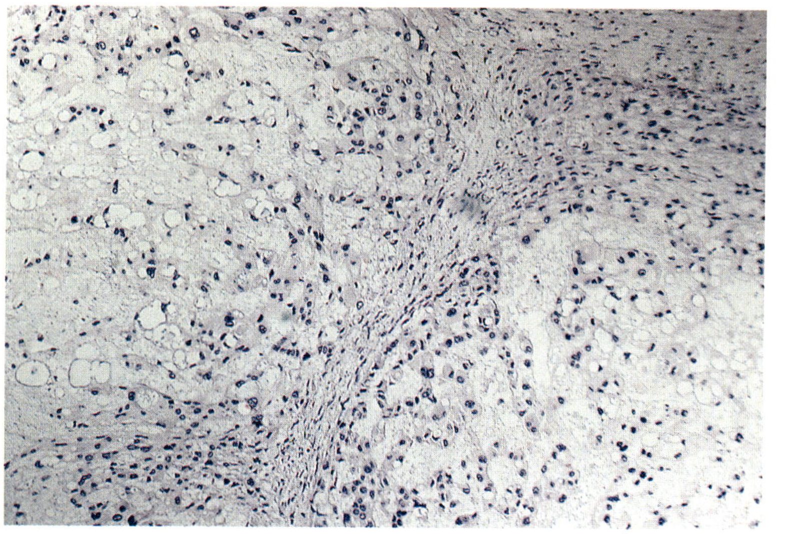

Figure 14.23 Photomicrograph of a chordoma to illustrate the lobulated pattern and the cords and nests of vacuolated and eosinophilic cells in a mucoid stroma. (H & E, × 4 objective)

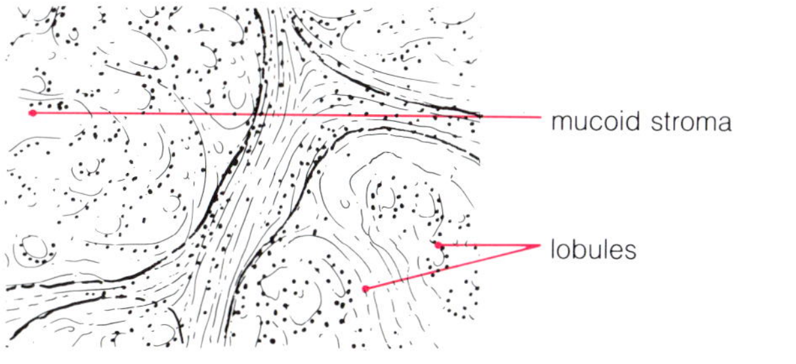

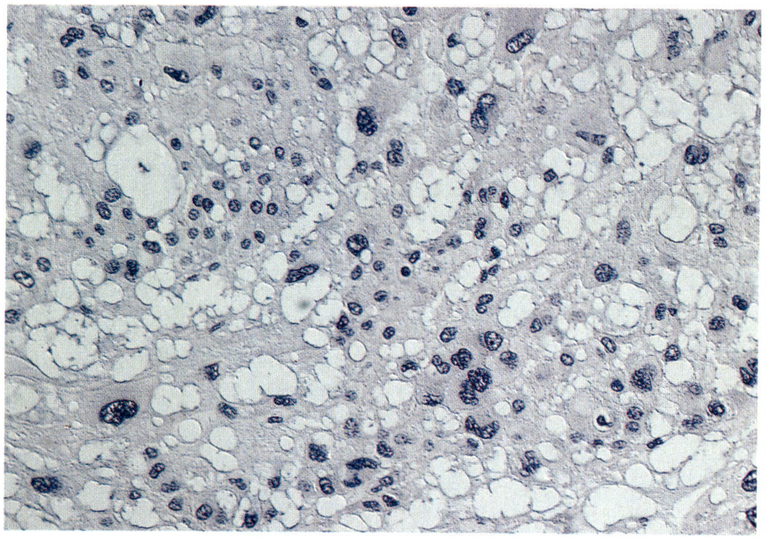

Figure 14.24 Photomicrograph of a chordoma at a higher power to show the typical vacuolated (physaliphorous) cells. Note also the variation in nuclear size. (H & E, × 25 objective)

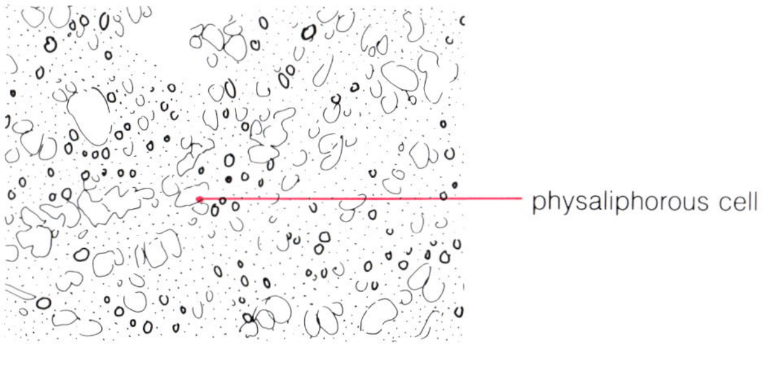

Approximately one-third of sphenooccipital chordomas contain a significant chondroid component, and these lesions may easily be confused with chondrosarcomas, especially chondrosarcomas having a predominantly myxoid structure (Fig. 14.25). Rarely in a chordoma there may be an associated malignant mesenchymal tumor, either a malignant fibrous histiocytoma or another poorly differentiated sarcoma (Figs. 14.26 and 14.27); at least some of these cases will be associated with a history of radiation therapy.

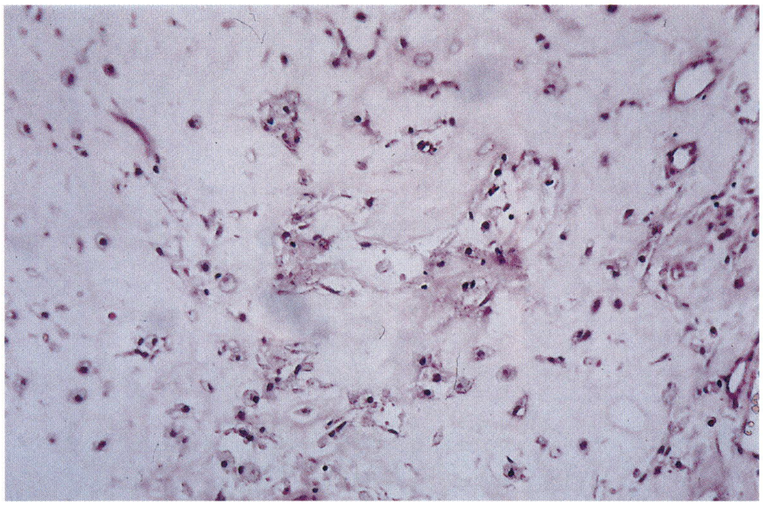

Figure 14.25 Photomicrograph of a portion of a chordoma, which had a predominantly cartilaginous appearance, as seen here. However, in other areas of the tumor, a classic appearance of chordoma was seen. (H & E)

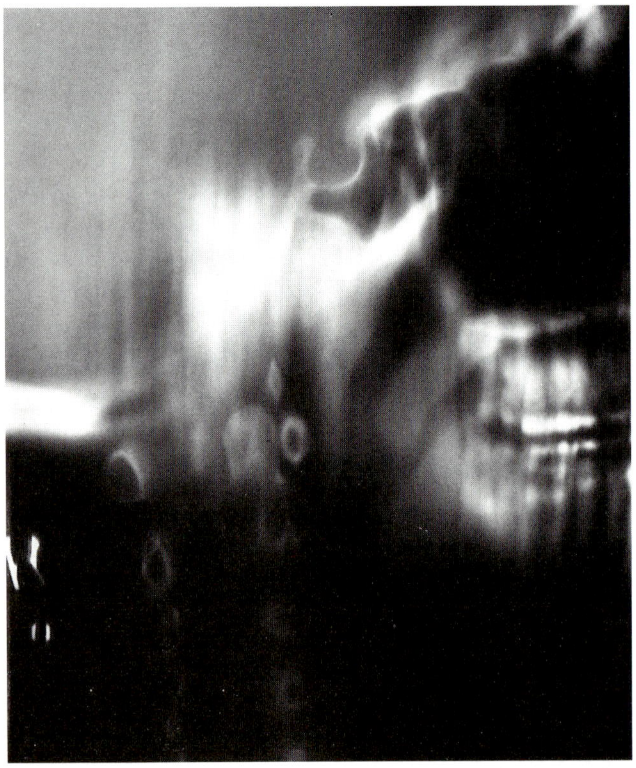

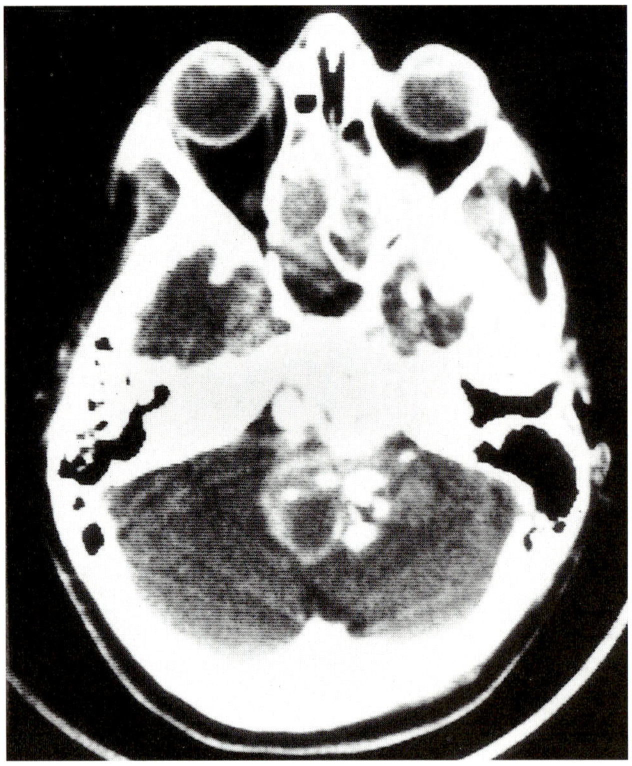

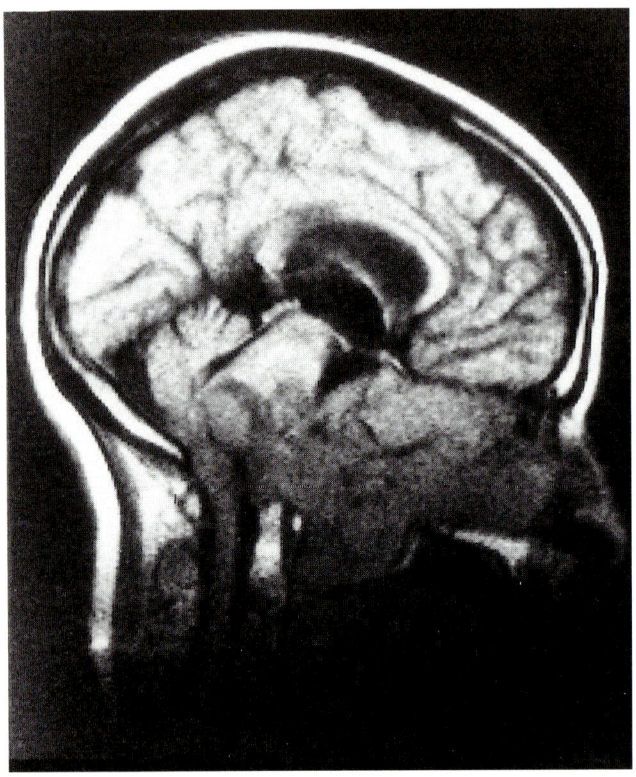

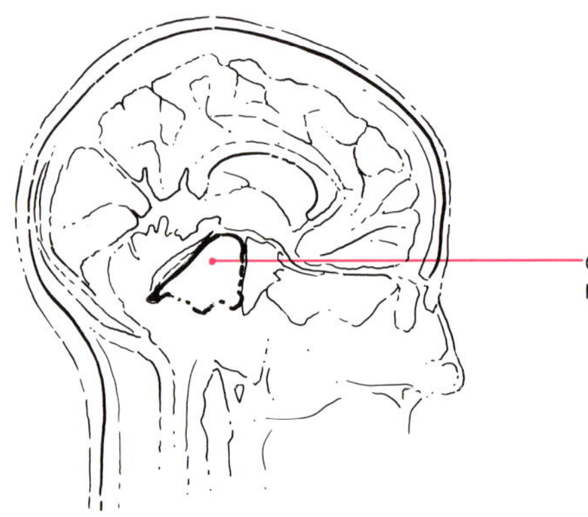

Figure 14.26 Lateral tomographic view *(top left)* of the skull of a woman with a chordoma of the clivus, which was partially removed two years previously. A large dense midline mass, which extended anteriorly into the nasopharynx and posteriorly into the posterior fossa, is seen destroying the inferior clivus. In a contrast-enhanced CT scan *(top right)*, several areas of calcification are seen within the posterior fossa and a large mass occupies the region where the brainstem is normally seen. A sagittal spin echo MRI *(bottom left)* shows an enormous mass filling the nasal cavity and ethmoid sinus anteriorly. It has obliterated the nasopharynx, extending inferiorly into the hypopharynx. Rostral to the odontoid process, it extends into the cranial cavity, completely destroying the clivus. It has invaded or displaced the brainstem, extending directly to the anterior aspect of the fourth ventricle.

Chondrosarcoma

Chondrosarcomas of the spine constitute about 15% of all chondrosarcomas. They may be either central or peripheral and occur either in the vertebral body or the neural arch, or in some cases in both elements. Often, more than one spinal level is involved. Peripheral chondrosarcomas may develop from preexisting osteochondromas (Fig. 14.28). Generally, on radiographic examination, the central lesions are destructive and demonstrate focal irregular calcification within their matrix. The initial symptoms are likely to be either myelopathic or radiculopathic. Grossly, chondrosarcomas have a lobulated glassy appearance and usually

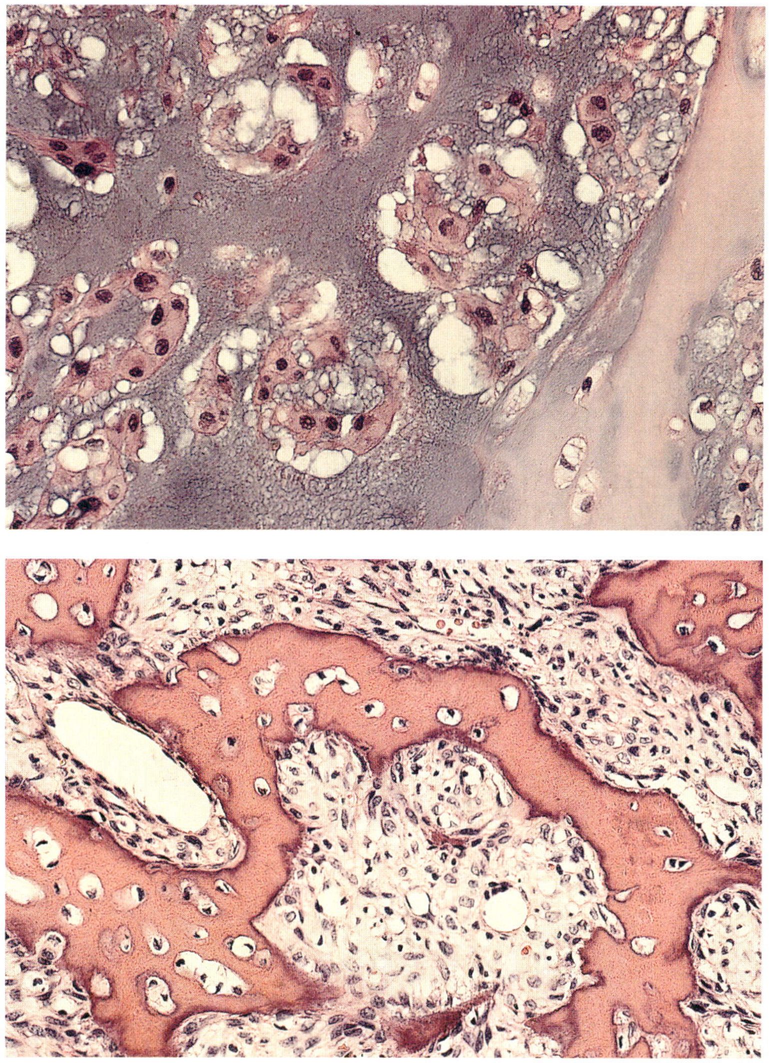

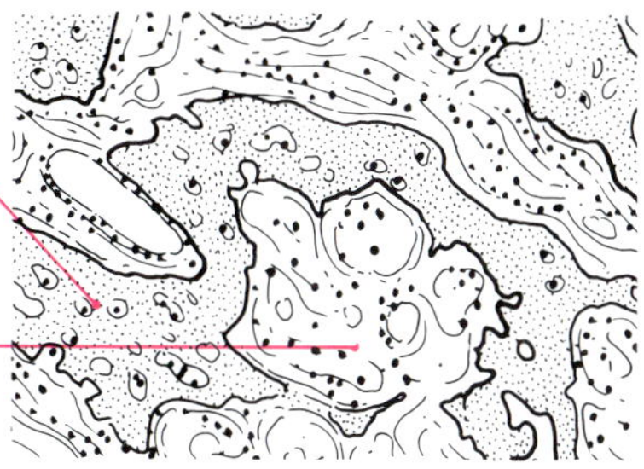

Figure 14.27 Photomicrograph *(top)* of the nasopharyngeal mass from the patient in Figure 14.26, resected at the first intervention. Cords of cells with basophilic round nuclei and abundant focally vacuolated cytoplasm are seen. They were set in a basophilic matrix, which was focally vacuolated but in many areas had a more uniform chondroid appearance. The lesion was diagnosed as a chondroid chordoma. At the second intervention, similar tissue was resected *(bottom)*, but also present were areas that showed neoplastic osteoid surrounded by malignant spindle cells diagnosed as osteosarcoma.

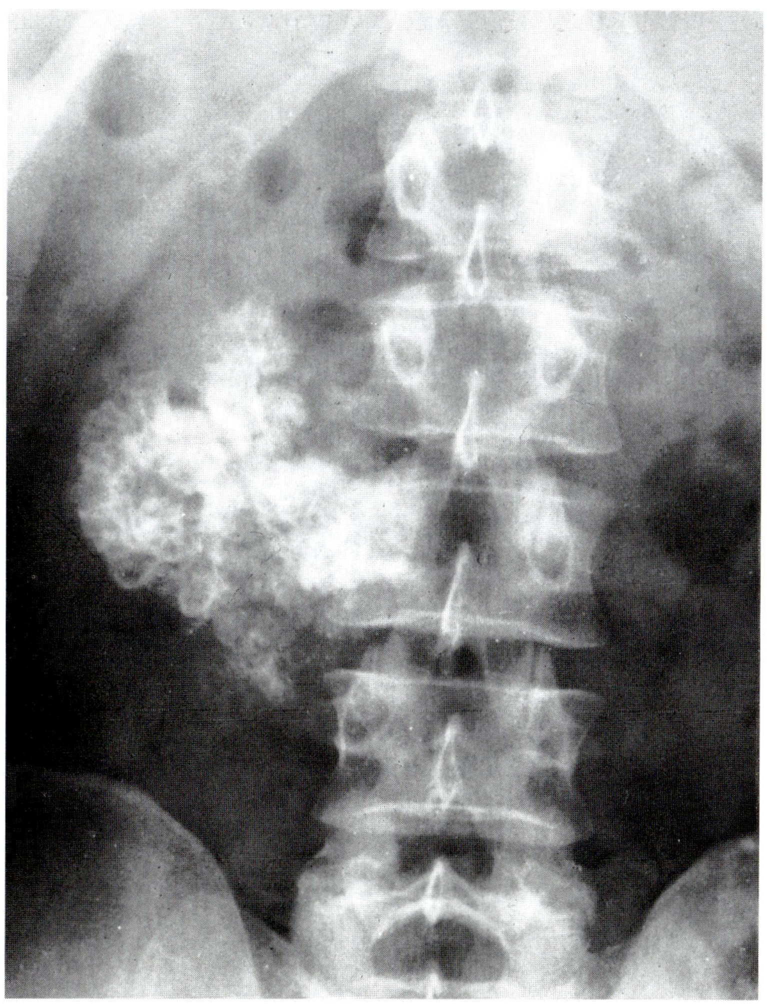

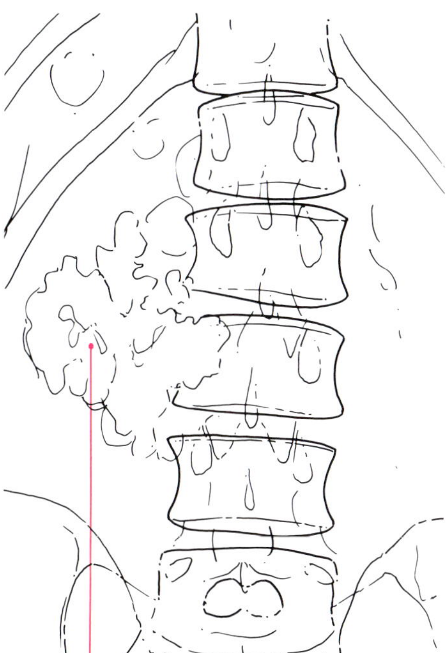

Figure 14.28 AP radiograph demonstrating a large calcified mass arising from the body of L-3, as well as from the adjacent vertebrae. This lesion, which proved on biopsy to be a chondrosarcoma, was later resected.

have focal calcification within (Fig. 14.29). Histologically, both low-grade and high-grade lesions are found; the former tend to be slow growing and expansile, while the latter tend to demonstrate early metastasis and to follow a malignant course (Fig. 14.30).

Approximately 10% of all chondrosarcomas undergo focal dedifferentiation into a malignant spindle cell tumor, often with the pattern of a malignant fibrous histiocytoma. These dedifferentiated tumors have a poor prognosis.

OSTEOSARCOMA

After myeloma, osteosarcoma is the most common primary tumor of bone. The majority of cases are seen in young people; however, the spine generally is not involved. Osteosarcomas in the spine are more likely to be associated with Paget's disease or are secondary to radiation therapy. Even so, only about one in 50 cases of osteosarcoma presents in the spine.

Osteosarcoma in the spine may affect either the body or the vertebral arches (Fig. 14.31). The radiographic pattern is not characteristic and unless there is an associated Paget's disease the diagnosis is not likely to be made radiographically. Histologically, osteosarcoma is characterized by the production of a malignant osseous matrix, although areas of malignant cartilage, in addition to undifferentiated areas, also may

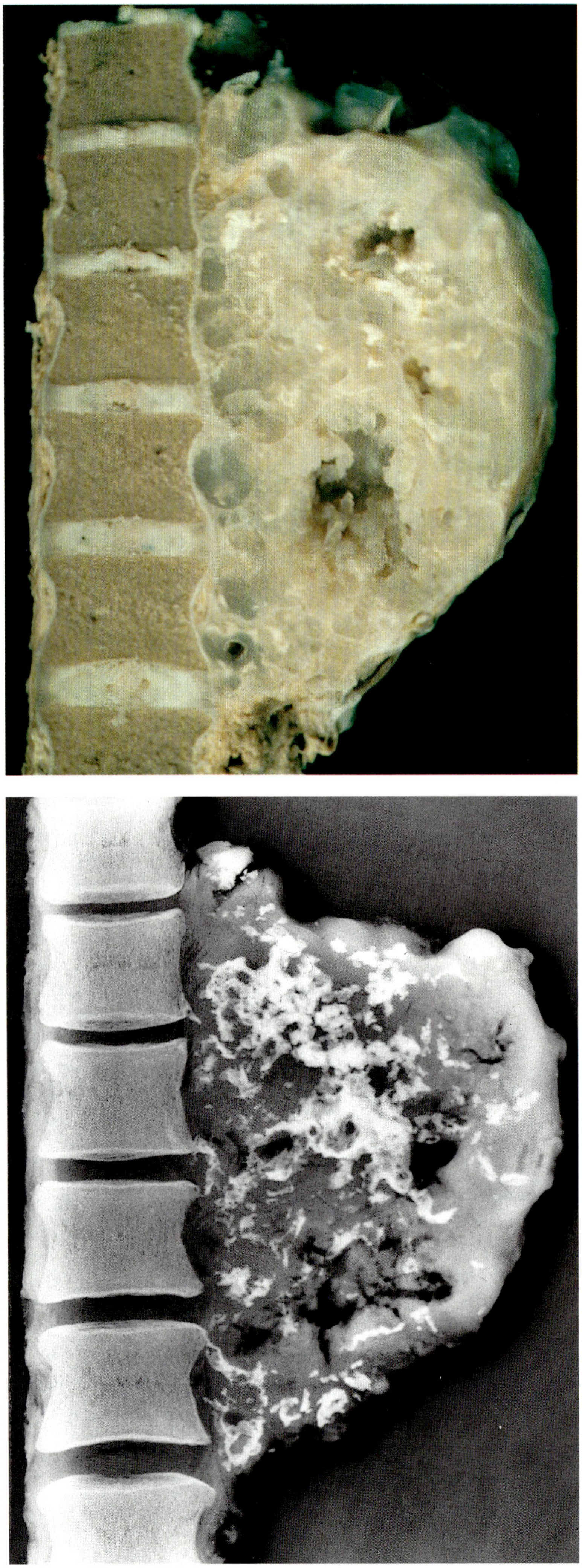

Figure 14.29 Photograph *(top)* of a coronal section of the thoracolumbar spine to demonstrate a large peripheral chondrosarcoma extending over five vertebral bodies. Grossly, focal calcification can be appreciated. The lobulated glassy appearance is typical of a cartilage tumor. A radiograph *(bottom)* of the same specimen demonstrates extensive irregular areas of calcification present within the lesion.

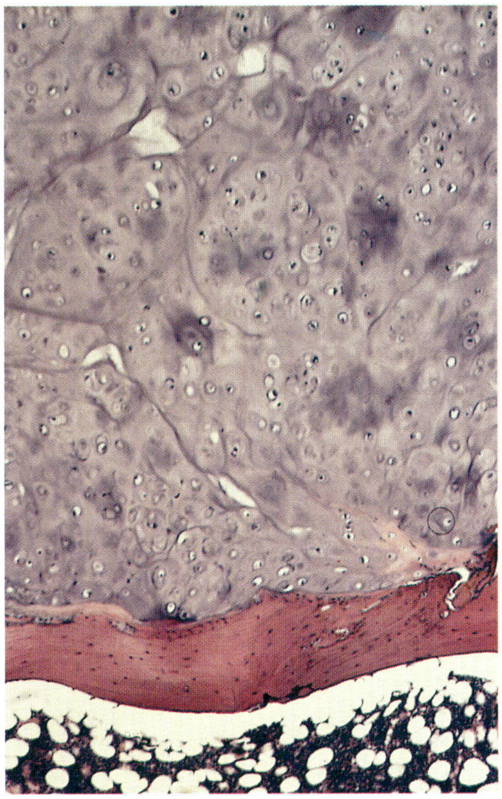

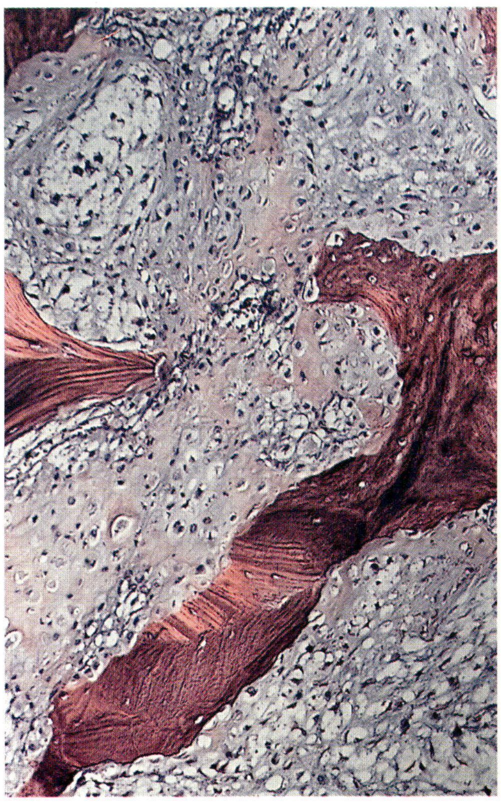

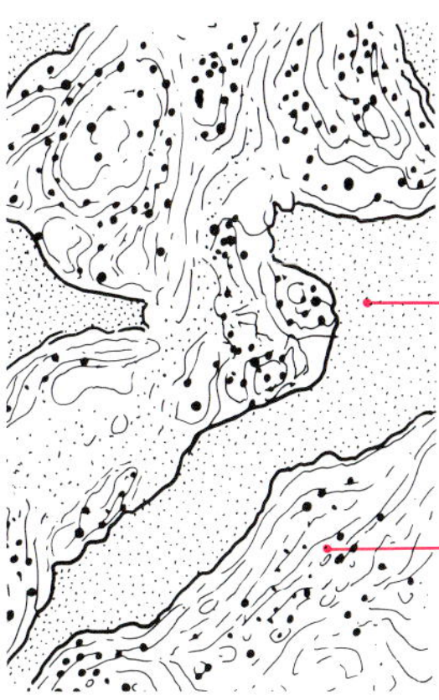

Figure 14.30 Photomicrograph *(top)* of a low-grade chondrosarcoma. The chondrocytes, though somewhat crowded, are not particularly atypical. Though this tumor is frequently edged by bone, as seen here, it does not particularly invade through the marrow spaces. (H & E, × 4 objective) In a fully malignant high-grade chondrosarcoma, however, the hallmark of the lesion is that the tumor invades between the bone spicules, as illustrated here *(bottom)*. In addition, when compared to the low-grade lesion, there is much more crowding and atypicality of the chondrocytes. (H & E, × 10 objective)

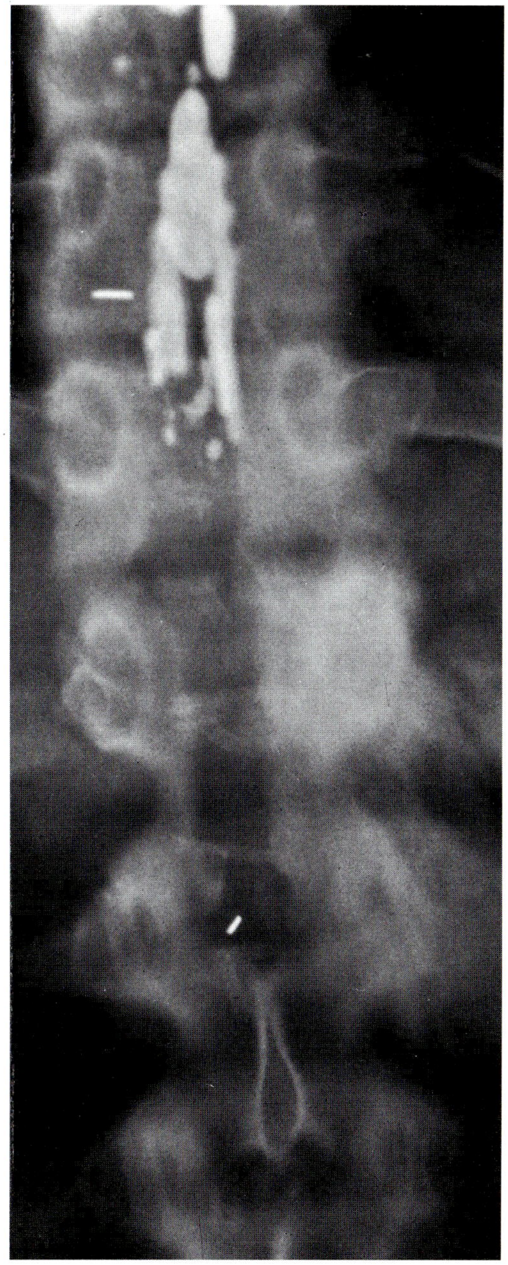

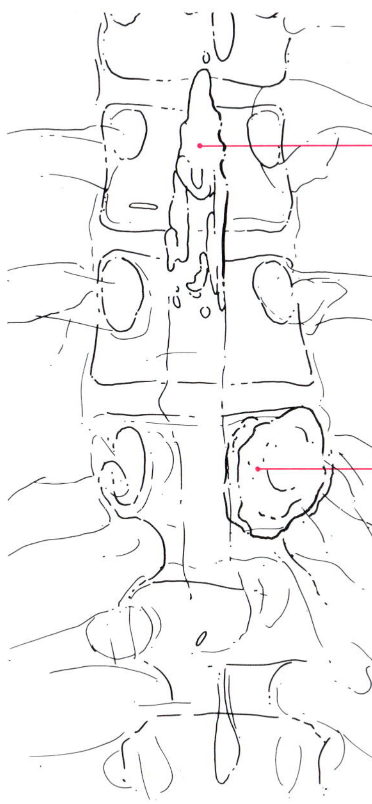

Figure 14.31 AP tomogram of a 20-year-old male, who presented at the hospital with paraplegia. A decompression laminectomy was performed. There was a large, inoperable tumor present on the right side, the residual of which can be seen in this post-laminectomy film. The posterior elements of T-12 and L-1 are involved. A large, soft-tissue extension of the tumor is producing a bony matrix, which at L-1 can be seen to have a "sunburst" appearance. Biopsy proved this to be an osteosarcoma.

be present, and for this reason adequate sampling of the tumor may be essential for proper diagnosis (Figs. 14.32 and 14.33).

Malignant Lymphoma

The spine frequently is involved in generalized lymphoma, which presents as a generalized osteopenia of the spine often with focal collapse of individual vertebrae (Fig. 14.34). Occasionally, lymphomas may present first in the spine, with initial confinement to only one vertebral body of the vertebral column. In such a case, the histologic diagnosis is likely to be either a large cell lymphoma or Hodgkin's disease (Fig. 14.35). Radiographi-

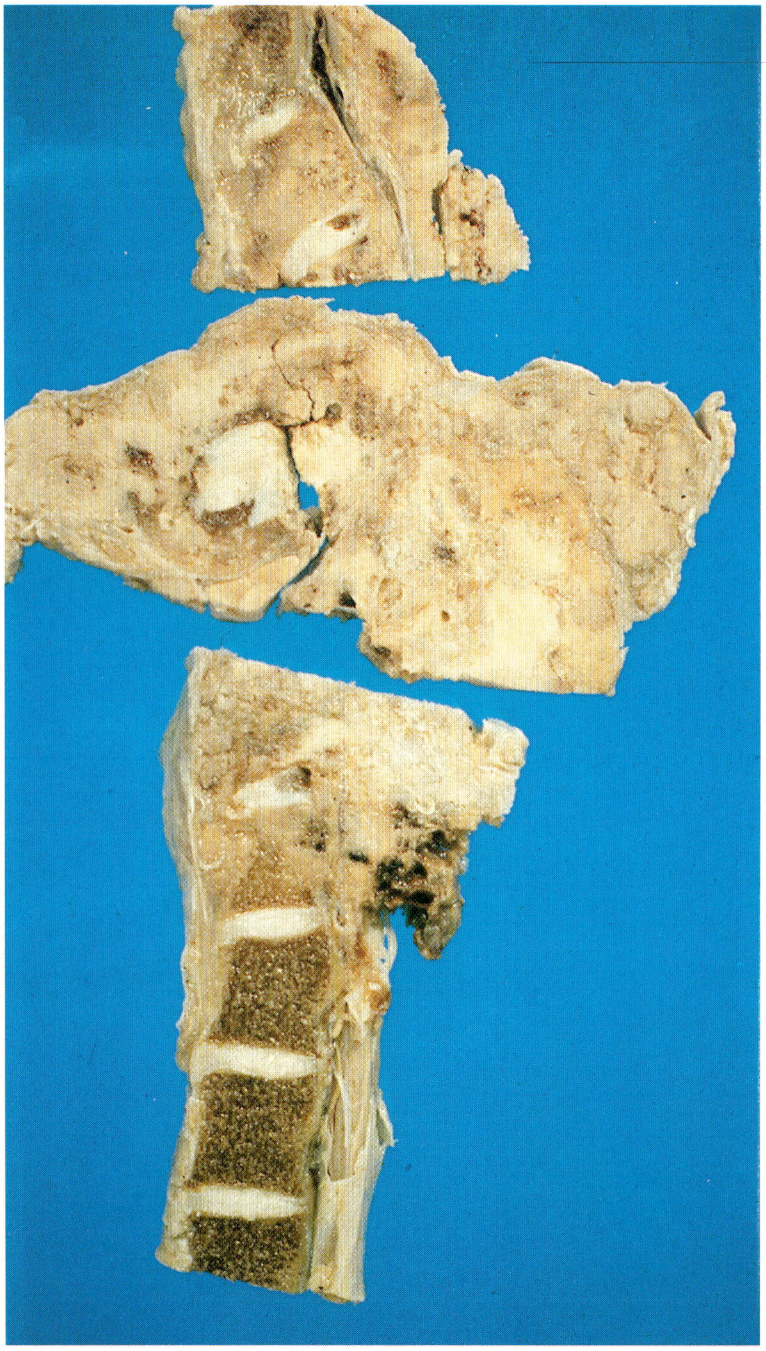

Figure 14.32 Photograph of a sagittal section through the cervical and upper thoracic spine of a 37-year-old male who died with a large osteosarcoma arising in C-4, C-5, and C-6. Before the sagittal section was obtained, a horizontal slice of tissue was taken through the level of C-5, with a portion of disc embedded in the middle. Extensive soft-tissue involvement by the osteosarcoma is seen. Much of the tissue has a dense bony appearance, although fossae of cartilaginous matrix are visible in this section. (Courtesy of Dr. Rikuo Machinami)

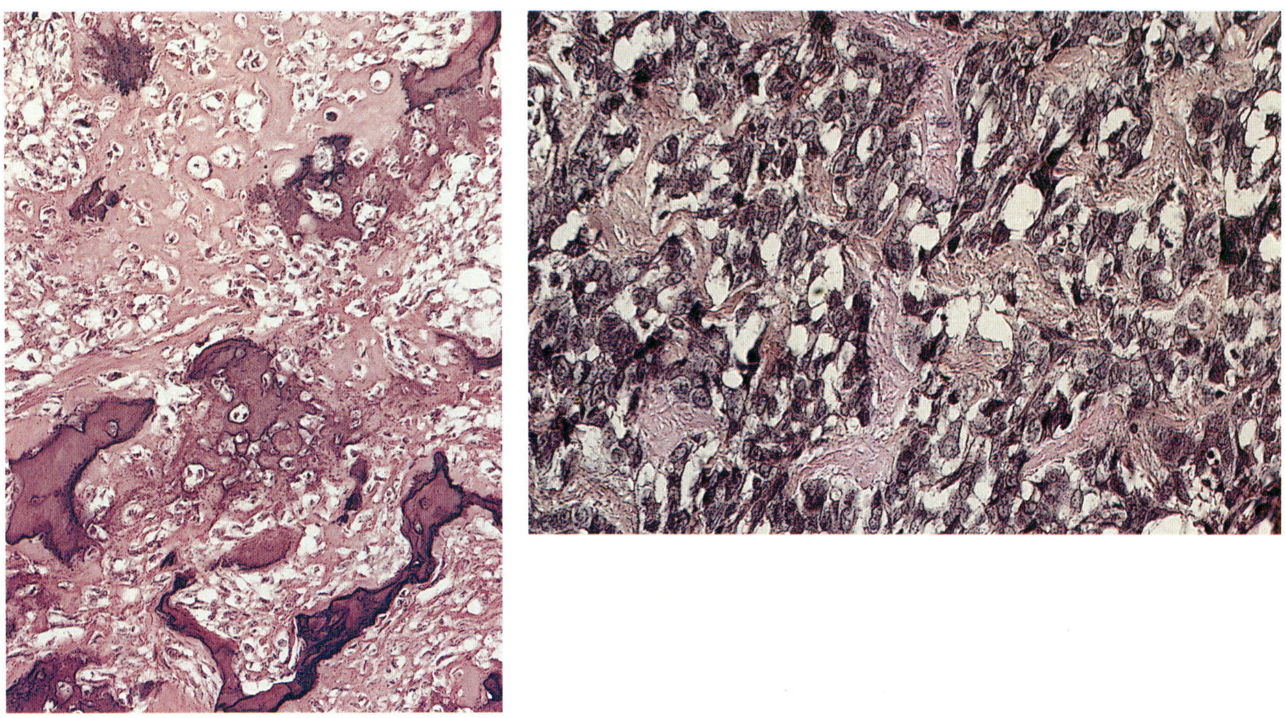

Figure 14.33 Photomicrograph *(left)* of an osteosarcoma with extensive extracellular matrix formation that is focally calcified. In a higher power photomicrograph *(right)* of a cellular osteosarcoma, the cells are producing only fine strands of collagenous matrix, as is typical of the more cellular areas in an osteosarcoma.

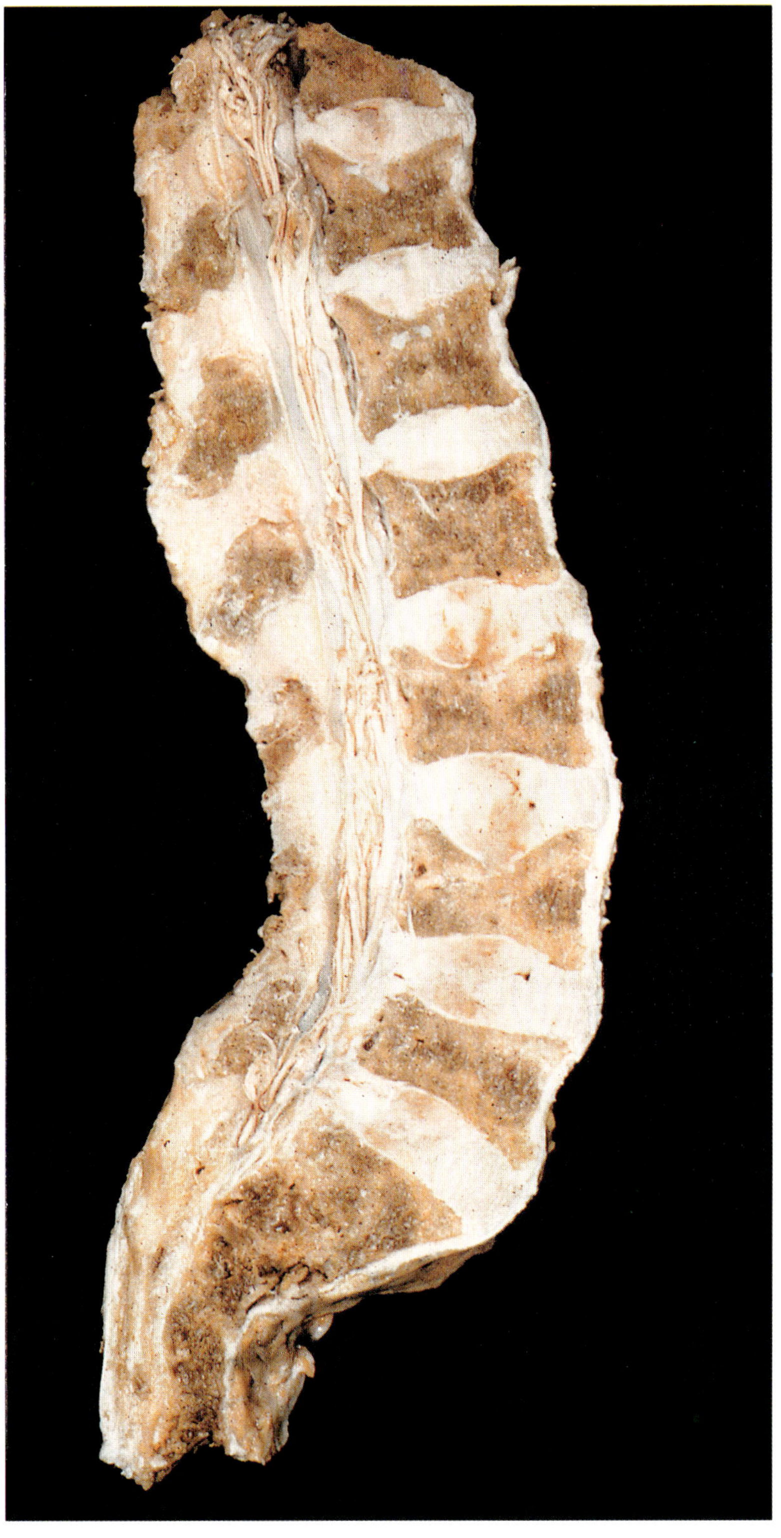

Figure 14.34 Photograph of a sagittal section through the lumbar spine of a man with diffuse lymphoma. Histologically, the bone marrow was replaced largely by lymphomatous tissue. This patient had received large doses of steroids, and the collapse of the spine is probably the result of a combination of osteoporosis resulting from the lymphomatous infiltration, with osteoporosis resulting from steroid therapy. (Courtesy of Dr. Howard Dorfman)

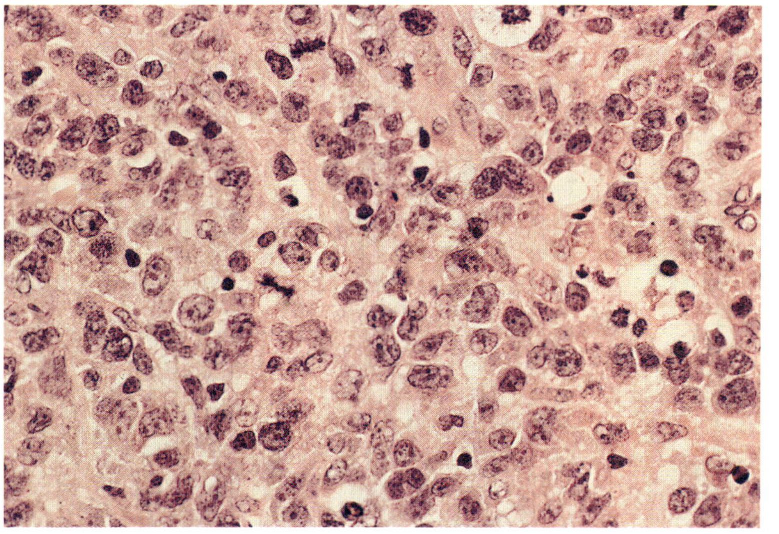

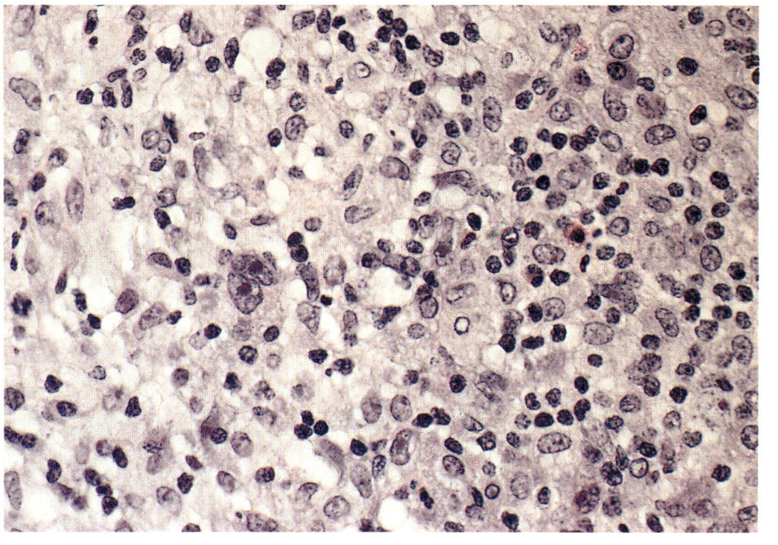

Figure 14.35 Photomicrograph *(top)* of a large cell lymphoma. Note the irregular vesicular nuclei, with prominent nucleoli and scant cytoplasm. Several mitoses are present in this field. Photomicrograph *(bottom)* of Hodgkin's disease showing a mixed cellular pattern, with a background of histiocytic cells admixed with lymphocytes, plasma cells, and eosinophils. Note the Reed-Sternberg cell, with double nuclei and large prominent eosinophilic nucleoli.

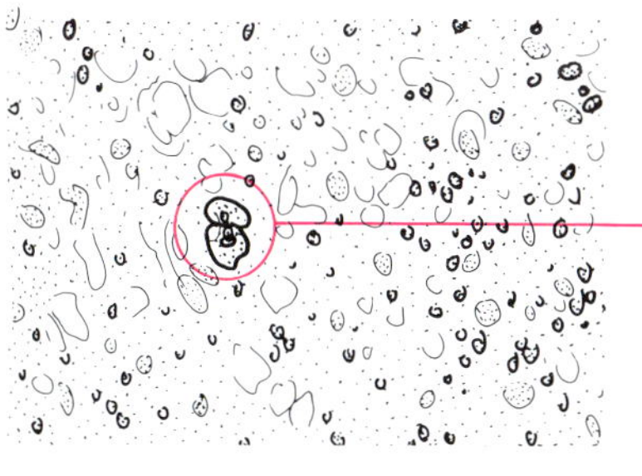

cally, one of two appearances may be seen: either localized osteolysis with collapse of the vertebral body (Fig. 14.36), or localized proliferation of reactive bone, giving rise to a dense so-called ivory vertebra (Fig. 14.37). This latter appearance is encountered most commonly in association with Hodgkin's disease, and radiographically must be distinguished from localized Paget's disease. However, in Paget's disease, one generally sees an increase in the transverse diameter of the vertebral body, with a classic picture-frame appearance around the affected vertebrae. This is not seen in lymphoma. The lymphomatous tissue may extend into the soft tissues as well as into the spinal canal, giving rise to neurologic symptoms. In cases where the disease initially appears to be confined to the vertebral column, careful investigation often will show that lymph node involvement already has occurred.

In acute leukemia of young individuals, bone changes are a frequent finding. A characteristic finding in children is that of a radiolucent band in the metaphysis of the long bones; similar bands may be found in the vertebral bodies just beneath the end plates. However, the radiographic finding that is most common in the spine is a diffuse demineralization, with compression fractures most commonly seen as anterior wedging. Epidural extension of the tumor is not uncommon in leukemia, and may on occasion constitute the presenting symptoms. In addition, the replacement of bone marrow by leukemic tissue may result in ischemic necrosis of the affected bone and bone marrow (Fig. 14.38).

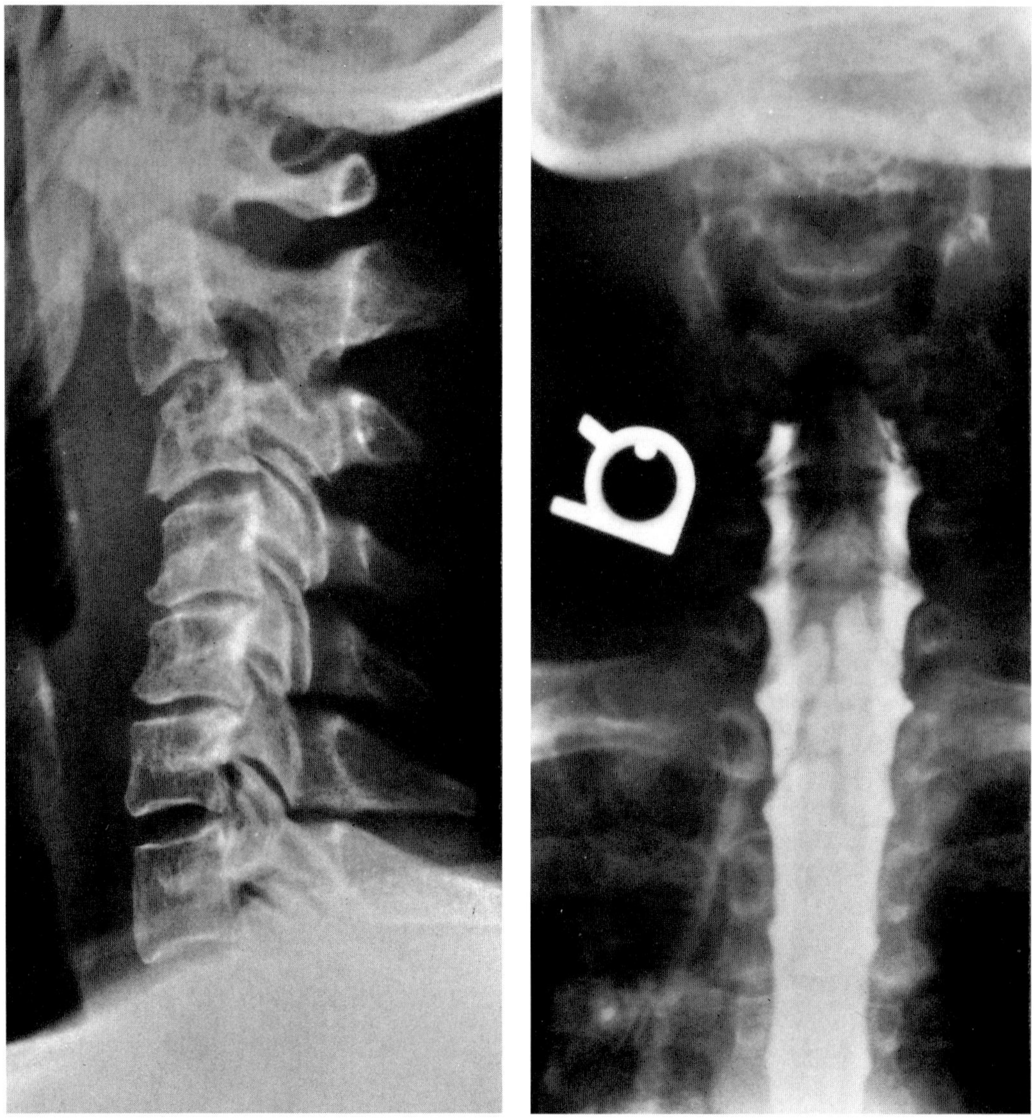

Figure 14.36 Lateral radiograph *(left)* of the neck of a middle-aged woman who presented with acute onset of pain in the upper part of the cervical spine and rapidly progressive weakness of the lower limbs. On the radiograph, note destruction of the upper third of C-3, with loss of the vertebral end plate and partial collapse. Biopsy proved this to be a large cell lymphoma. The accompanying myelogram *(right)* shows a complete block at the upper margin of C-4. In this case, at the time of presentation no other sign of lymphoma was apparent.

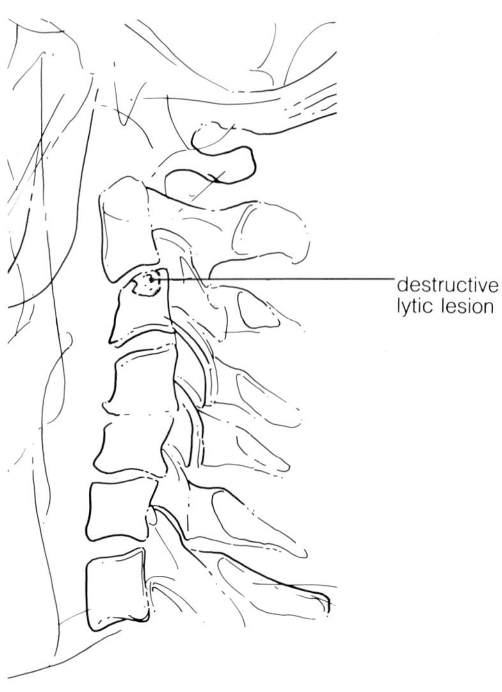

Ewing's Sarcoma

Although metastatic involvement of the vertebral column is fairly common in Ewing's sarcoma (Fig. 14.39), primary involvement of the spine is decidedly rare, occurring in perhaps 5% of cases. It has been reported to occur most frequently in the sacrococcygeal region. Extension into the paravertebral soft tissue is common. The clinical picture may be relatively acute, and may simulate infection since a moderate fever and an elevated ESR are common findings in Ewing's sarcoma. In young children, it is important to differentiate the lesion from a metastatic neuroblastoma; the latter generally is seen in children under the age of 5. Histologically the tumor is characterized by uniform small cells, with scant lacy cytoplasm that usually contains abundant glycogen demonstrated by positive PAS staining (Fig. 14.40). Extensive necrosis is common.

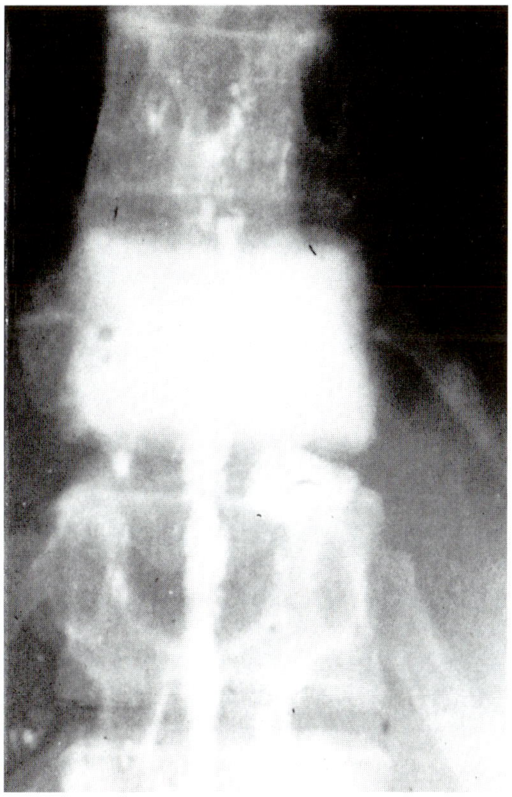

Figure 14.37 AP radiograph of a 35-year-old male who presented with vague back pain. A single dense sclerotic vertebra is seen in the lower thoracic spine, which, on biopsy, proved to be Hodgkin's disease. In Hodgkin's disease in the bone, one frequently sees considerable marrow fibrosis and reactive bone formation, which may be of such severity as to obscure the lymphomatous tissue.

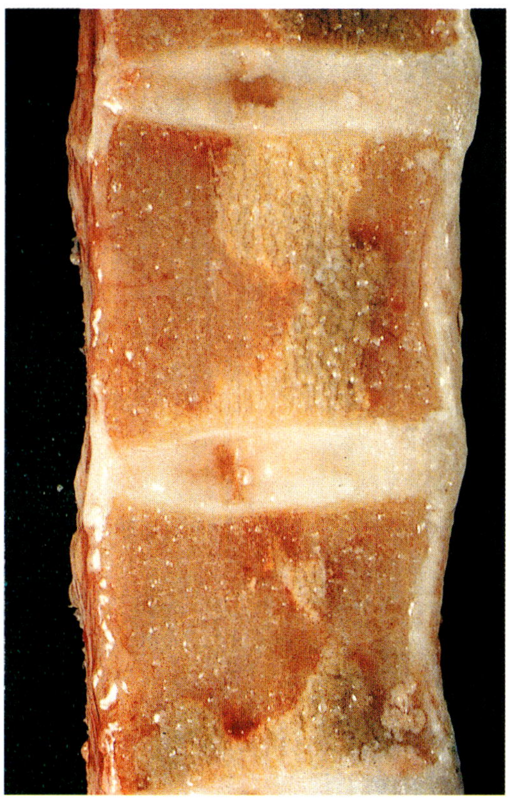

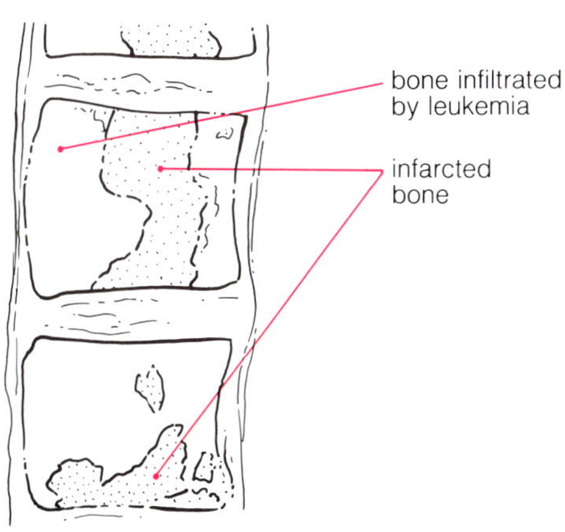

Figure 14.38 Photograph of a segment of the spine from a child who died with leukemia. Within the vertebral bodies, there are geographic areas of necrosis identified as yellow opacification of the bone and marrow. These are surrounded by a thin rim of hyperemic tissue. Note that the viable bone marrow has a fleshy tan color reflecting the leukemia infiltrate.

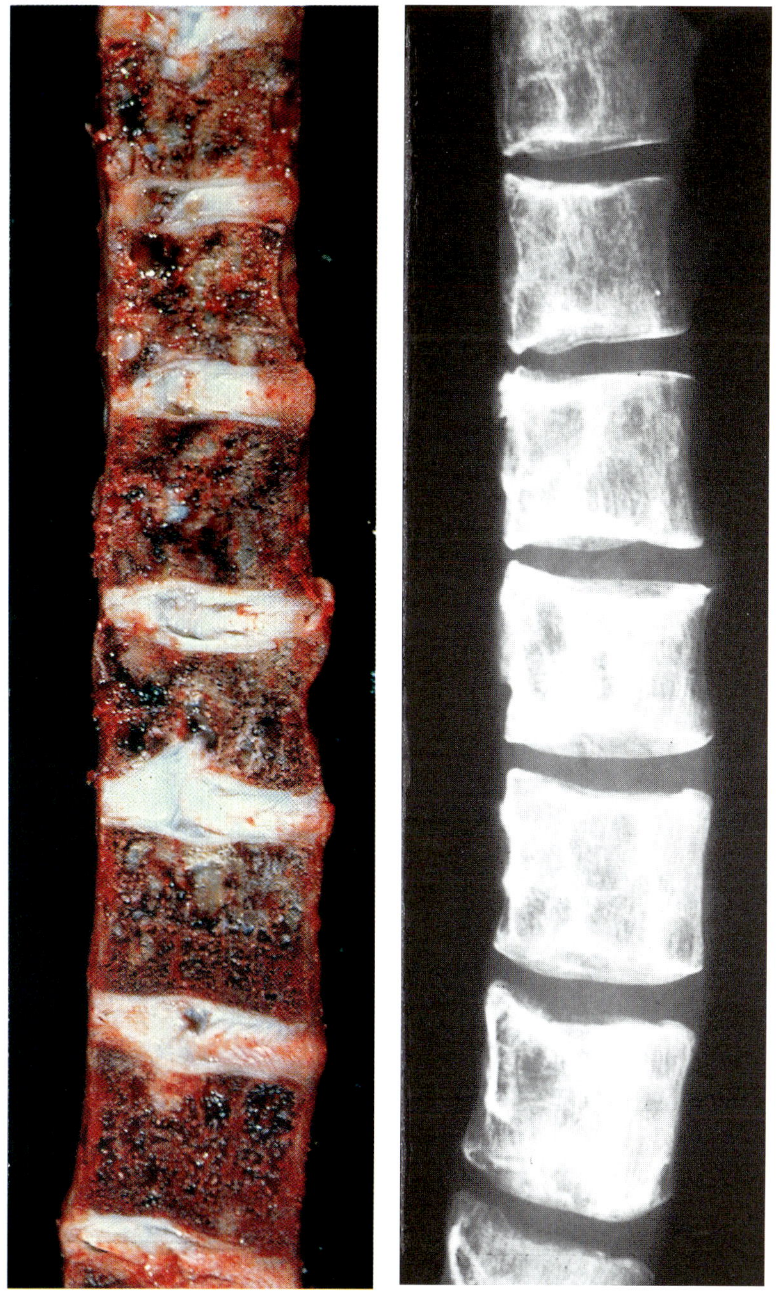

Figure 14.39 Photograph of a sagittal section of spine *(left)*, together with a specimen radiograph *(right)*, from a patient with widespread metastatic Ewing's sarcoma. Note the lytic lesions on the radiograph, which are seen grossly as masses of gray tissue, with hemorrhagic areas. (Courtesy of Dr. Krishnan K. Unni)

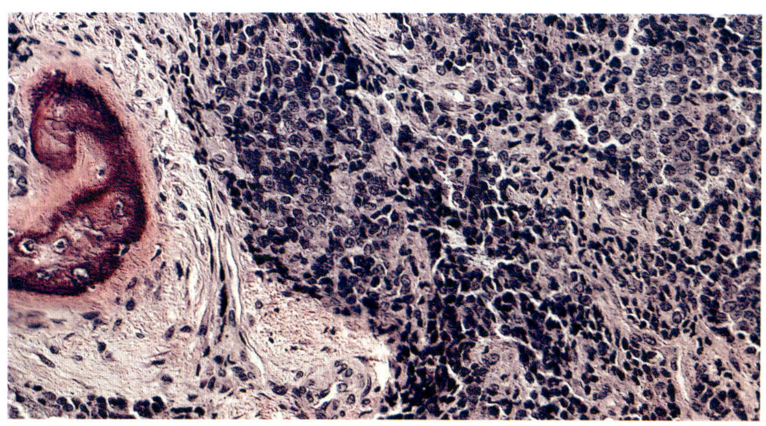

Figure 14.40 Photomicrograph of Ewing's sarcoma showing the typical small vesicular nuclei with scant, poorly defined cytoplasm and scattered foci of pyknotic nuclei throughout.

Intraspinal Neoplasms

Intraspinal neoplasms may be intramedullary (i.e., within the substance of the spinal cord) such as ependymoma, astrocytoma and glioblastoma, or, more commonly, they may be extramedullary, such as solitary meningioma, schwannoma, or neurofibroma (Fig. 14.41). Any of these lesions, which normally are intradural, may perforate the dura to become extradural.

Intraspinal lesions cause widening of the spinal canal if they have been present for a long time. More rapidly growing tumors may actually result in localized bone destruction (Fig. 14.42). Occasionally, extrinsic pressure from primary bone tumors, usually benign tumors such as osteoblastoma, aneurysmal bone cyst, and osteochondroma, may simulate intraspinal tumors because of intrusion into the canal with cord compression. Myelography and CT scanning should help in the differential diagnosis (Fig. 14.43).

In addition to the changes that may occur with solitary neurofibromas, multiple intraspinal neurofibromatosis leads to structural changes in the vertebral column, usually severe kyphoscoliosis, with a rotational deformity (Fig. 14.44). This deformity,

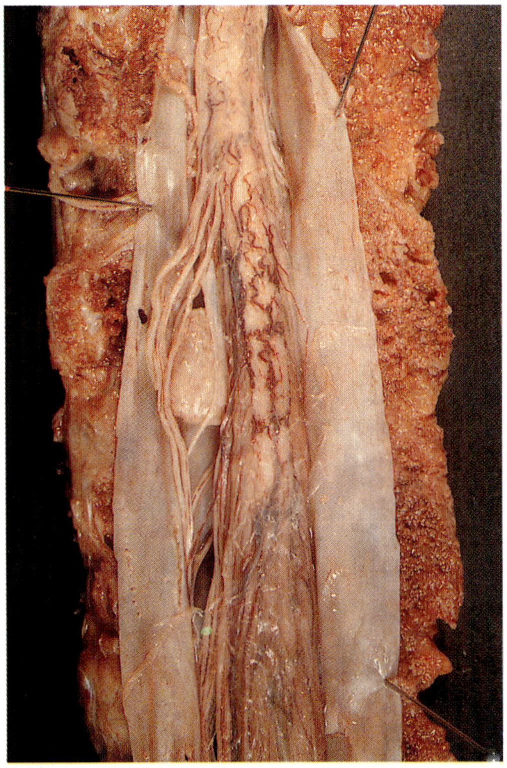

Figure 14.41 Photograph of the spinal canal in the region of the lower thoracic and upper lumbar vertebrae. The dura has been reflected to reveal on olive-sized, firm fibrous tumor lying within the dura and displacing the spinal nerves. On sectioning, this tumor proved to be a meningioma. A patient with this type of lesion might be expected to have radiculopathy or signs of spinal cord compression.

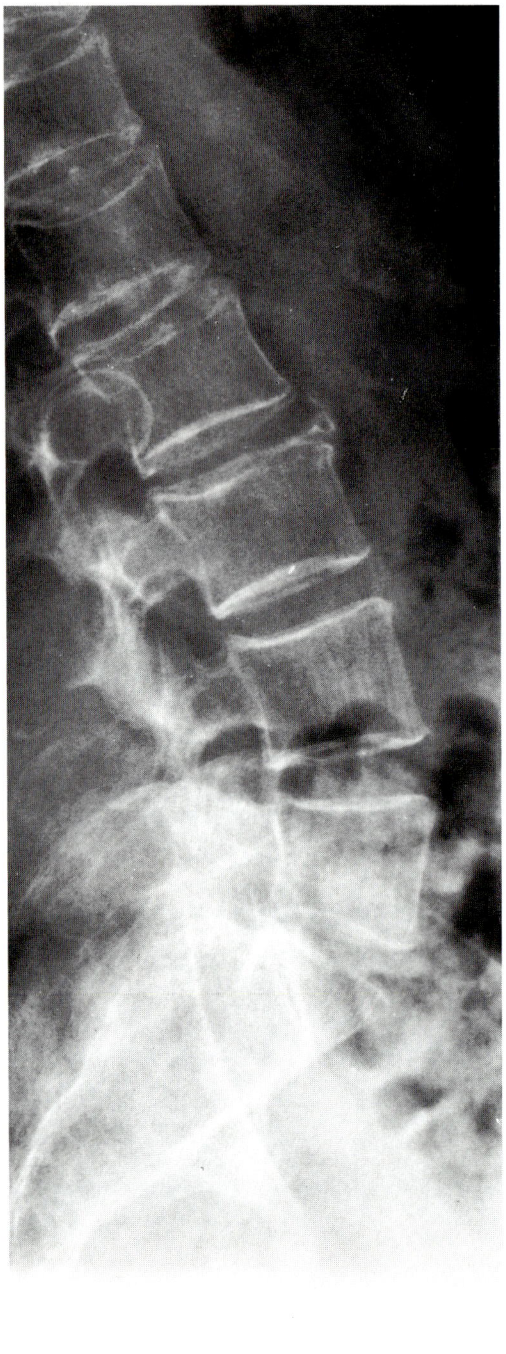

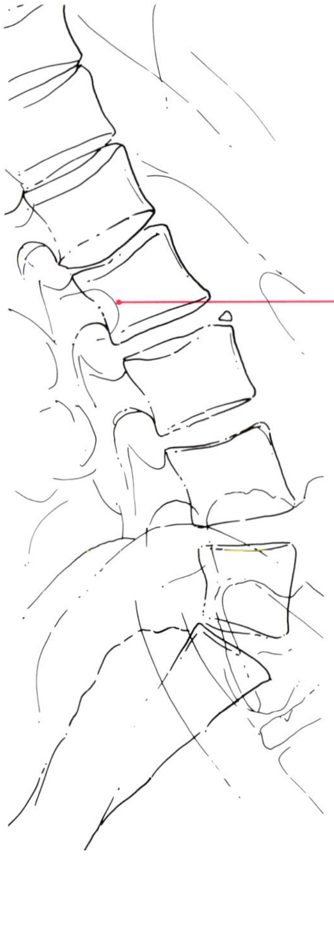

Figure 14.42 Lateral radiograph of the spine of a 55-year-old female who presented with severe night pain and symptoms of nerve-root involvement. A well-defined lytic lesion is seen behind the body of L-2, which has eroded the bone to produce a sclerotic margin around it. On exploration, this proved to be an intradural schwannoma.

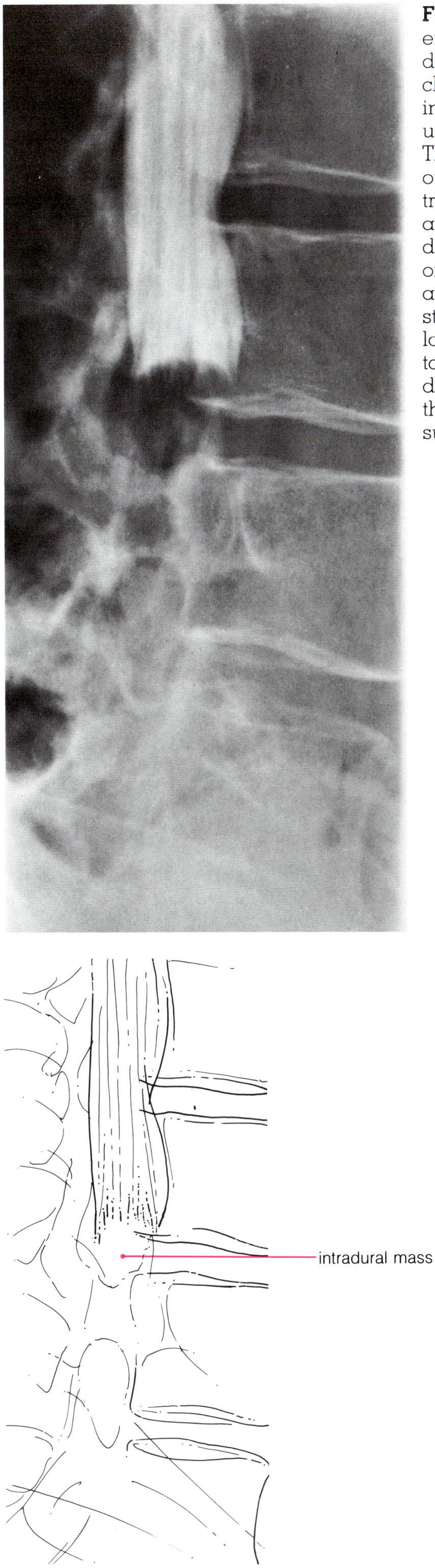

Figure 14.43 Lateral myelogram to demonstrate the characteristic findings in an intradural obstruction. The dye is seen outlining the intradural tumor and extending down the margins of the lesion. With an extradural obstruction, the myelogram shows a tapering of the dye column from the external pressure.

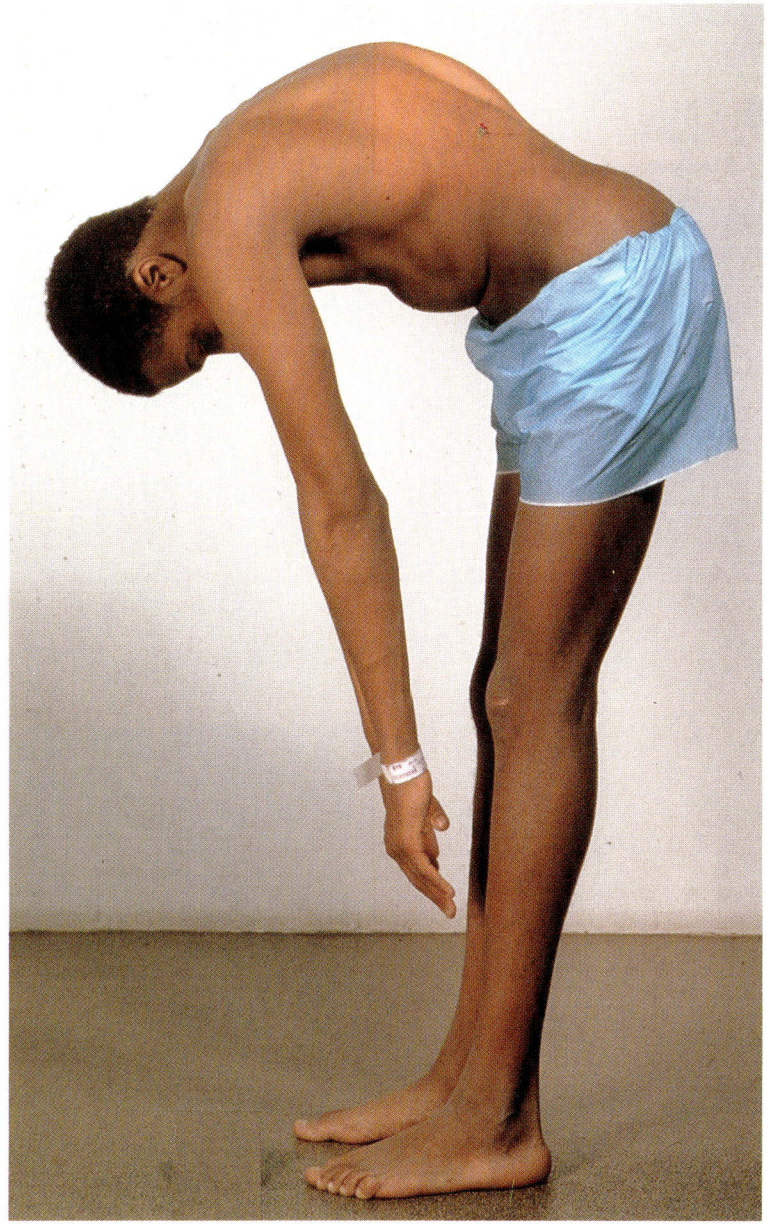

Figure 14.44 Lateral clinical photograph of a patient with von Recklinghausen's disease. The marked scoliotic deformity and the marked rotational component are prominent features of the disease. (Courtesy of Dr. David Levine)

which is seen in approximately 25% of patients with multiple neurofibromatosis (von Recklinghausen's disease), has a high morbidity (Figs. 14.45 through 14.47) and also a high mortality, from associated cardiopulmonary decompensation and paraplegia or quadriplegia, resulting perhaps from the extreme deformity or from segmental instability following erosion by the tumors. Other complications include pseudarthrosis following attempted fusion, and malignant degeneration.

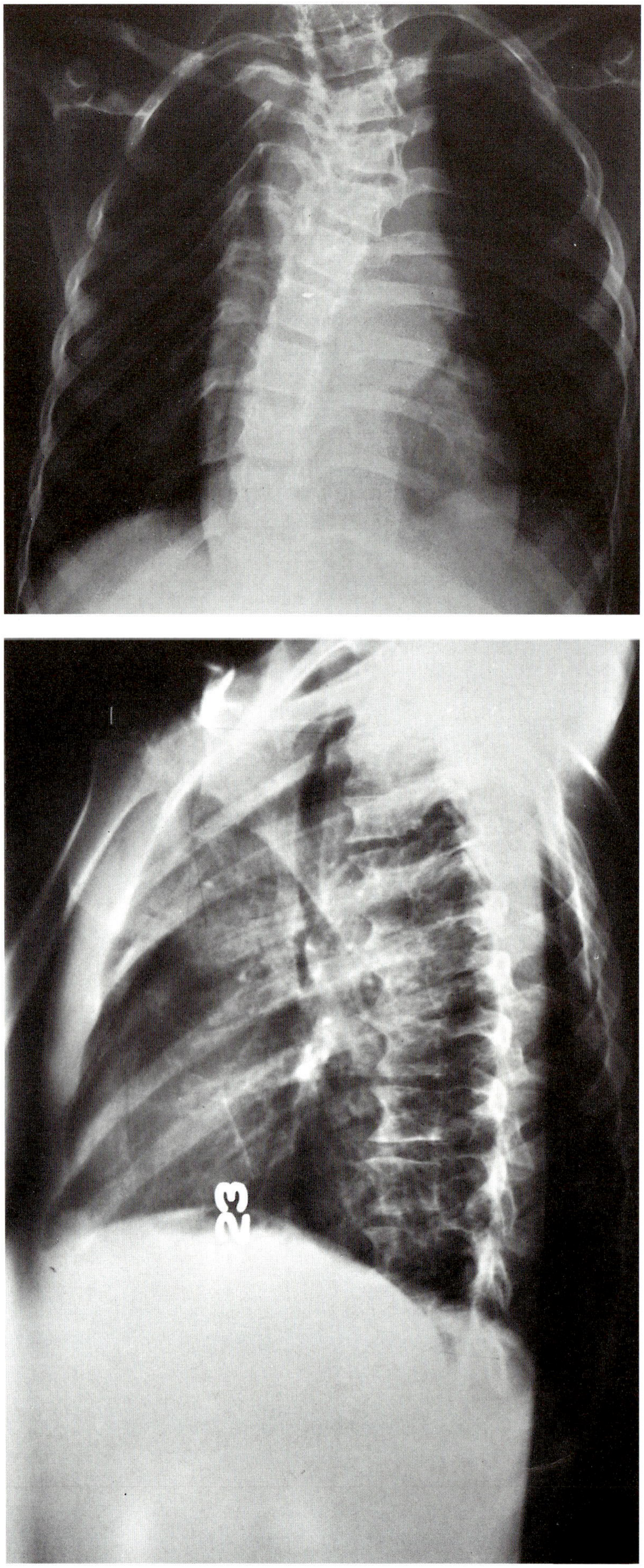

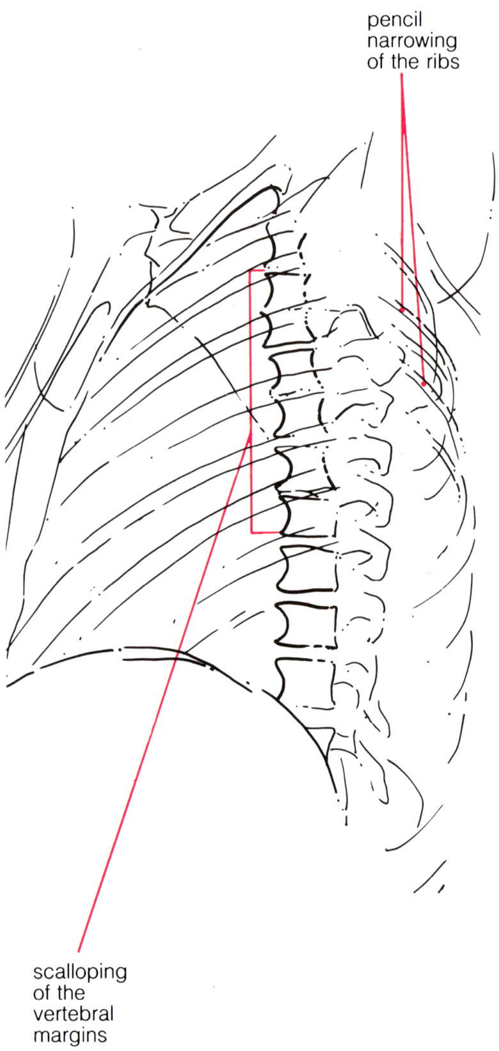

Figure 14.45 AP radiograph *(top)* of the thoracic spine in an 8-year-old with severe neurofibromatosis. A scoliotic deformity of the thoracic spine is seen together with a soft-tissue mass extending along much of the thoracic spine. On the right side, the ribs show bony attrition, with a narrowing that has been likened to a sharpened pencil. Lateral radiograph *(bottom)* of the thoracic spine two months later. Scalloping of the vertebral bodies, one of the hallmarks of the disease, is prominently seen.

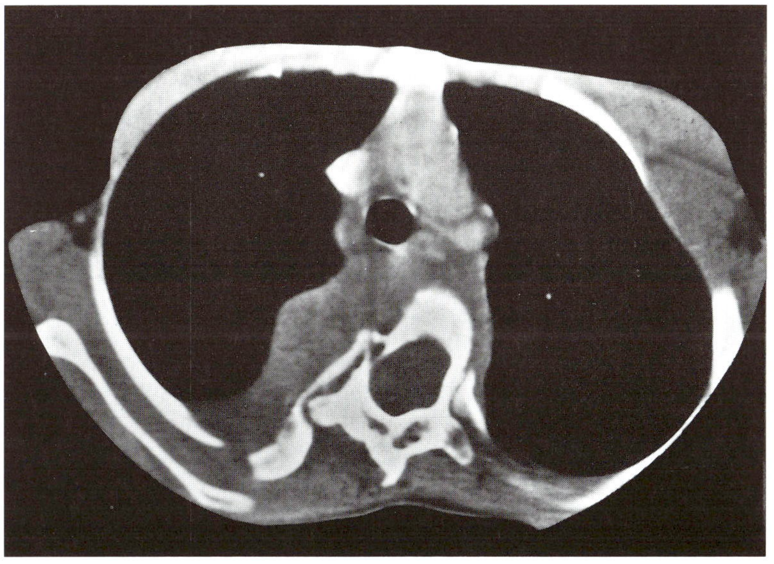

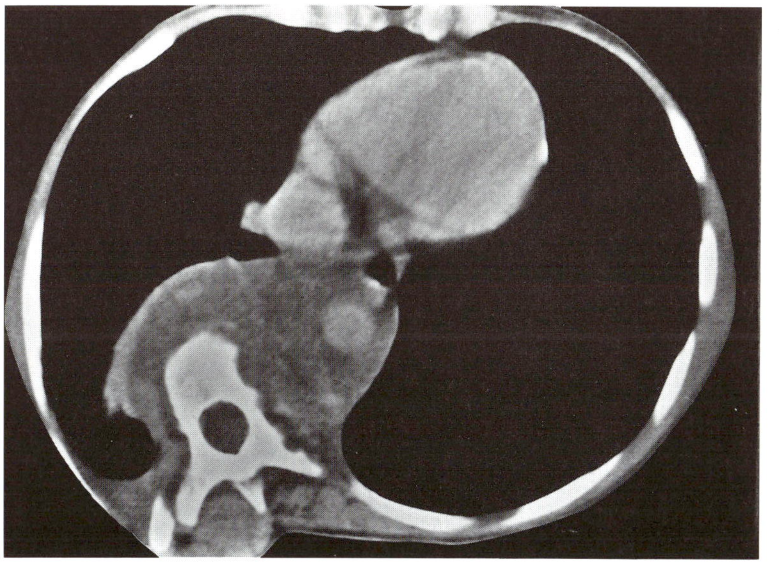

Figure 14.46 CT scan *(left)* at the level of T-5, of the same patient with neurofibromatosis seen in Figure 14.45. Here it is possible to appreciate the large soft-tissue mass surrounding the vertebral body, eroding the bone, and distorting the attachment of the rib, particularly on the right side. There is a marked increase in the diameter of the spinal canal due to bone erosion from within the canal. Rotation of the vertebral body toward the left is apparent in this cut, and posteriorly, on the right side, there is a soft-tissue mass eroding the lamina and transverse process. A cut through the lower thoracic spine *(right)* shows a large soft-tissue mass surrounding the vertebral body and parts of the neural arch anteriorly, and, on the left side, markedly eroding the bone to leave a scalloped appearance. Within this mass of neurofibromatous tissue, the aorta is embedded. When this slice is compared to the previous view, one sees that the vertebral body is rotated toward the right.

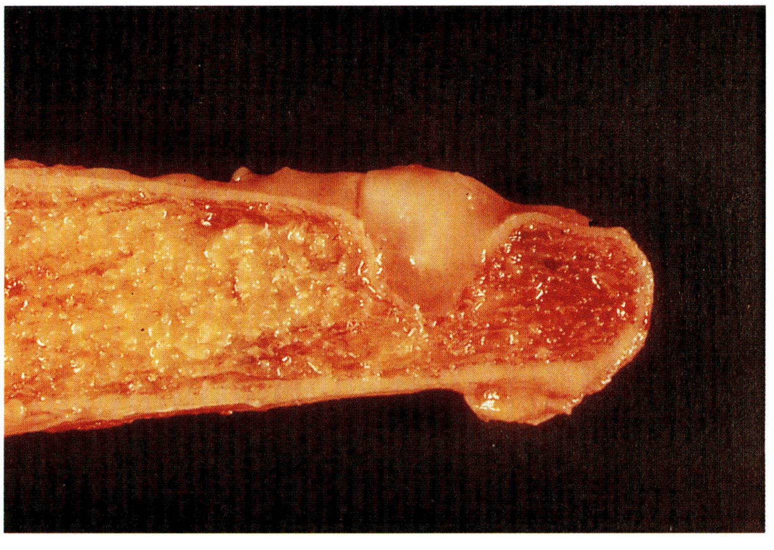

Figure 14.47 Photograph demonstrating bone erosion by a neurofibroma.

BIBLIOGRAPHY

General Readings

Brookes M: *The Blood Supply of Bone*. London, Butterworth, 1971.

Crock HV: *Practice of Spinal Surgery*. Vienna, Springer-Verlag, 1983, pp 1–134.

Crock HV, Yoshizawa H: *The Blood Supply of the Vertebral Column and Spinal Cord in Man*. New York, Springer-Verlag, 1977.

Dahlin DC, Unni KK: *Bone Tumors: General Aspects and Data on 8,542 Cases*, ed 4. Springfield, Ill, Charles C Thomas Publisher, 1986.

Jaffe HL: *Metabolic, Degenerative, and Inflammatory Diseases of Bones and Joints*. Philadelphia, Lea & Febiger, 1972.

Resnick D, Niwayama G: *Diagnosis of Bone and Joint Disorders*. Philadelphia, WB Saunders Co., 1981.

Rothman RH, Simeone FA: *The Spine*. Philadelphia, WB Saunders Co., 1982, pp 508–646.

Schajowicz F: *Tumors and Tumorlike Lesions of Bone and Joints*. New York, Springer-Verlag, 1981.

Schmorl G, Junghanns H: *The Human Spine in Health and Disease*, ed 2. Besemann EF (trans.). New York, Grune & Stratton, 1971.

White AA, Panjabi MM: *Clinical Biomechanics of the Spine*. Philadelphia, JB Lippincott, 1978.

Section 1: Normal Anatomy and Development

CHAPTER 1: METHODS OF EXAMINATION

Chafetz N, Genant HK: Computed tomography of the lumbar spine. *Orthop Clin North Am* 14:147, 1983.

Modic MT, Weinstein MA, Pavlicek W, Starnes DL, Duchesneau PM, Boumphrey F, Hardy RJ Jr: Nuclear magnetic resonance imaging of the spine. *Radiology* 148:757, 1983.

Park WM: Radiological investigation of the intervertebral disc, in Jayson MIV (ed.): *The Lumbar Spine and Back Pain*. London, Sector Publishing Ltd., 1976.

Williams PL, Warwick R: *Gray's Anatomy*, ed 36. Philadelphia, WB Saunders Co., 1980, pp 270–286.

CHAPTER 2: DESCRIPTIVE ANATOMY: GROSS AND MICROSCOPIC

Batson DV: The function of the vertebral veins and their role in the spread of metastasis. *Ann Surg* 112:138, 1940.

Bushell GR, Ghosh P, Taylor TFK, Akeson WH: Proteoglycan chemistry of the intervertebral disks. *Clin Orthop* 129:115, 1977.

Coventry MB: Anatomy of the intervertebral disc. *Clin Orthop* 67:9, 1969.

Coventry MB, Ghormley RK, Kernohan JW: The intervertebral disc: Its microscopic anatomy and pathology: I. Anatomy, development, and physiology. *J Bone Joint Surg* 28:105, 1945.

Coventry MB, Ghormley RK, Kernohan JW: The intervertebral disc: Its microscopic anatomy and pathology: II. Changes in the intervertebral disc concomitant with age. *J Bone Joint Surg* 28:233, 1945.

Coventry MB, Ghormley RK, Kernohan JW: The intervertebral disc: Its microscopic anatomy and pathology: III. Pathological changes in the intervertebral disc. *J Bone Joint Surg* 28:460, 1945.

Dommisse GF: The blood supply of the spinal cord: A critical vascular zone in spinal surgery. *J Bone Joint Surg* 56B:225, 1974.

Eyre DR: Biochemistry of the intervertebral disc, review. *Int Rev Connect Tissue Res* 8:227, 1979.

Eyre DR, Muier H: Types I and II collagens in intervertebral discs: Interchanging radial distributions in annulus fibrosus. *Biochem J* 157:267, 1976.

Krämer J: *Intervertebral Disk Diseases: Causes, Diagnosis, Treatment, and Prophylaxis*. Chicago, Year Book Medical Publishers, 1981.

Nachemson A: The load on lumbar discs in different positions of the body. *Clin Orthop* 45:107, 1966

Urban JPG, Holm S, Maroudas A, Nachemson A: Nutrition of the intervertebral disc: Effect of fluid flow on solute transport. *Clin Orthop* 170:296, 1982.

CHAPTER 3: FUNCTIONAL ANATOMY AND BIOMECHANICS

Adams MA, Hutton WC: The mechanical function of the lumbar apophyseal joints. *Spine* 8:327, 1983.

Anderson GJ: The biomechanics of the posterior elements of the lumbar spine. *Spine* 8:326, 1983.

Broberg KB: On the mechanical behavior of intervertebral discs. *Spine* 8:151, 1983.

Gracovetsky S, Farfan HF, Lamy C: The mechanism of the lumbar spine. *Spine* 6:249, 1981.

Hickey DS, Hukins DWL: Relation between the structure of the annulus fibrosis and the function and failure of the intervertebral disc. *Spine* 5:106, 1980.

Klein JA, Hukins DWL: Relocation of the bending axis during flexion-extension of lumbar intervertebral discs and its implications for prolapse. *Spine* 8:659, 1983.

Koreska J, Robertson D, Mills RH, Gibson DA, Albisser AM: Biomechanics of the lumbar spine and its clinical significance. *Orthop Clin North Am* 8:121, 1977.

Nachemson A, Morris JM: In vivo measurements of intradiscal pressure. *J Bone Joint Surg* 46A:1077, 1964.

O'Leary PF, Camins MB, Polifroni NV, Floman Y: Thoracic disc disease: Clinical manifestations and surgical treatment. *Bull Hosp Joint Dis* 44:27, 1984.

Panjabi MM, Takata K, Goel V: Kinematics of lumbar intervertebral foramen. *Spine* 8:348, 1983.

Panjabi MM, White AA III: Basic biomechanics of the spine. *Neurosurgery* 7:76, 1980.

Yang KH, King AI: The mechanism of facet load transmission as a hypothesis for low back pain. *Spine* 9:557, 1984.

CHAPTER 4: DEVELOPMENTAL ANATOMY

Angevine JB: Clinically relevant embryology of the vertebral column and spinal cord. *Clin Neurosurg* 20:95, 1973.

LaRoca H: Embryology of the musculoskeletal system, in Lovell WW, Winter RB (eds.): *Pediatric Orthopaedics*, ed 2. Philadelphia, JB Lippincott, 1986, pp 1–24.

Noback CR, Robertson GC: Sequence of appearance of ossification centers: The human skeleton during the first five prenatal months. *Am J Anat* 89:1, 1951.

Patten BN: *Human Embryology*, ed 3. New York, McGraw-Hill Book Co., 1968.

Sensenig EC: Early development of the human vertebral column. *Contrib Embryol* 33:21, 1949.

Tanaka T, Uhthoff HK: Significance in resegmentation in the pathogenesis of ver-

tebral body malformation. *Acta Orthop Scand* 52:331, 1981.
Taylor JR: Growth of human intervertebral discs and vertebral bodies. *J Anat* 120:49, 1975.
Taylor JR: Persistence of the notochordal canal in vertebrae. *J Anat* 111:211, 1972.
Taylor JR, Twomey LT: Vertebral column development and its relation to adult pathology. *Aust J Physiother* 31:83, 1985.
Williams PL, Warwick R: *Gray's Anatomy*, ed 36. Philadelphia, WB Saunders Co., 1980, pp 112–118.

SECTION 2: DEGENERATIVE DISC DISEASE AND SPINAL ARTHRITIS

CHAPTER 5: DISC TISSUE DISPLACEMENT

Adams MA, Hutton WC: Gradual disc prolapse. *Spine* 10:524, 1985.
Arseni C, Nash F: Protrusion of thoracic intervertebral discs. *Acta Neurochir* 11:3, 1963.
Bick EM: Vertebral osteophytosis: Pathologic basis of its roentgenology. *Am J Roentgenol* 73:979, 1955.
Bradford DS, Garcia A: Herniations of the lumbar intervertebral disk in children and adolescents: A review of 30 surgically treated cases. *JAMA* 210:2045, 1969.
Brown MD, Tompkins JS: Chemonucleolysis (discolysis) with collagenase. *Spine* 11:123, 1986.
Clarke NM, Cleak DK: Intervertebral lumbar disc prolapse in children and adolescents. *J Pediatr Orthop* 3:202, 1983.
Cloward R: Anterior herniation of a ruptured lumbar intervertebral disk: Comments on the diagnostic value of the discogram. *Arch Surg* 64:457, 1952.
Ghelman B, Freiberger RH: The limbus vertebra: An anterior disc herniation demonstrated by discography. *Am J Roentgenol* 127:854, 1976.
Goulub BS, Rovit RL, Mankin HJ: Cervical and lumbar disc disease: A review. *Bull Rheum Dis* 21:635, 1971.
Grobler LJ, Simmons EH, Barrington TW: Intervertebral disc herniation in the adolescent. *Spine* 4:267, 1979.
Hansson T, Roos B: The amount of bone mineral and Schmorl's nodes in lumbar vertebrae. *Spine* 8:266, 1983.
Hilton RC, Ball J, Benn RT: Annular tears in the dorsolumbar spine. *Ann Rheum Dis* 39:533, 1980.
Hilton RC, Ball J, Benn RT: Vertebral endplate lesions (Schmorl's nodes) in the dorsolumbar spine. *Ann Rheum Dis* 35:127, 1976.
Klein JA, Hukins DWL: Relocation of the bending axis during flexion-extension of lumbar intervertebral discs and its implications for prolapse. *Spine* 8:659, 1983.
Kozlowski K: Anterior intervertebral disc herniations (report of six cases). *Fortschr Röntgenstr* 129:47, 1978.
Kurobane Y, Takahashi T, Tajima T, Yamakawa H, Sakamoto T, Sawaumi A, Kikuchi I: Extraforaminal disc herniation. *Spine* 11:260, 1986.
Nathan HA, Schwartz A: Inverted pattern of development of thoracic vertebral osteophysosis in situs inversus and in other instances of right descending aorta. *Radiol Clin* 31:150, 1962.
Porter RW, Hibbert CS, Wicks M: The spinal canal in symptomatic lumbar disc lesions. *J Bone Joint Surg* 60B:485, 1978.
Quinnell RC, Stockdale HR: An investigation of artifacts in lumbar discography. *Br J Radiol* 53:831, 1980.
Resnick D, Miwayama G: Intervertebral disk herniations: Cartilaginous (Schmorl's) nodes. *Radiology* 126:57, 1978.
Stevens RL, Ryvar R, Robertson WR, O'Brien JP, Beard HK: Biological changes in the annulus fibrosis in patients with low-back pain. *Spine* 7:223, 1982.
Taylor TKF, Akeson WH: Intervertebral disc prolapse: A review of morphologic and biochemic knowledge concerning the nature of prolapse. *Clin Orthop* 76:54, 1971.
Weber H: Lumbar disc herniation: A controlled, prospective study with ten years of observation. *Spine* 8:131, 1983.

CHAPTER 6: DEPOSITION DISEASES AFFECTING THE SPINE

Calcific Deposits

Bywaters EGL, Hamilton EBD, Williams R: The spine in idiopathic haemochromatosis. *Ann Rheum Dis* 30:453, 1971.
Calvé J, Galland M: Sur une affection particuliere de la colonne vertebrale simulante le mal de potte. *J Radiol Electrol Med Nucl* 6:21, 1922.
Coventry MB: Calcification in a cervical disc with anterior protrusion and dysphagia: A case report. *J Bone Joint Surg* 52A:1463, 1970.
Dodds WJ, Steinbach HL: Gout associated with calcification of cartilage. *N Engl J Med* 275:745, 1966.
Ellman MH, Vazquez LT, Brown NL, Mandel N: Calcium pyrophosphate dihydrate deposition in lumbar disc fibrocartilage. *J Rheumatol* 8:955, 1981.
Ferrer-Roca O, Brancos MA, Franco M, Sabate C, Querol JR: Massive articular chondrocalcinosis: Its occurrence with calcium pyrophosphate crystal deposits in nucleus pulposus. *Arch Pathol Lab Med* 106:352, 1982.
Lagier R, MacGee W: Erosive intervertebral osteochondrosis in association with generalized osteoarthritis and chondrocalcinosis: Anatomicoradiological study of a case. *Z Rheumatol* 38:405, 1979.
Rechtman AM, Hermel MB, Albert SM, Boreadis AG: Calcification of the intervertebral disk: Disappearing, dormant and silent. *Clin Orthop* 7:218, 1956.
Smith DM: Acute back pain associated with a calcified Schmorl's node: A case report. *Clin Orthop* 117:193, 1976.
Sonnabend DH, Taylor TKF, Chapman GK: Intervertebral disc calcification syndromes in children. *J Bone Joint Surg* 64B:25, 1982.
Swick HM: Calcification of intervertebral discs in childhood. *J Pediatr* 86:364, 1975.
Taylor TK, Little K: Calcification in the intervertebral disc. *Nature* 199:612, 1963.
Weinberger A, Myers AR: Intervertebral disc calcification in adults: A review. *Semin Arthritis Rheum* 8:69, 1978.

Gout

Hall MC, Selin G: Spinal involvement in gout: A case report with autopsy. *J Bone Joint Surg* 42A:341, 1960.
Litvak J, Briney W: Extradural spinal depositions of urates producing paraplegia: Case report. *J Neurosurg* 39:656, 1973.
Tkach S: Gouty arthritis of the spine. *Clin Orthop* 71:81, 1970.
Vinstein AL, Cockerill EM: Involvement of the spine in gout: A case report. *Radiology* 103:311, 1972.

Ochronosis

Cervenansky J, Sitaj S, Urbanek T: Alkaptonuria and ochronosis. *J Bone Joint Surg* 41A:1169, 1959.

Lagier R, Sitaj S: Vertebral changes in ochronosis: Anatomical and radiological study of one case. *Ann Rheum Dis* 33:86, 1974.

Pomeranz MM, Friedman LJ, Tunick IS: Roentgen findings in alkaptonuric ochronosis. *Radiology* 37:295, 1941.

CHAPTER 7: AGE-RELATED CHANGES AND DEGENERATIVE DISC DISEASE (OSTEOCHONDROSIS)

General Features

Lyons G, Eisenstein SM, Sweet MBE: Biochemical changes in intervertebral disc degeneration. *Biochim Biophys Acta* 673:443, 1981.

Age-Related Changes of the Intervertebral Disc

Bernick S, Cailliet R: Vertebral end-plate changes with aging of human vertebrae. *Spine* 7:97, 1982.

Kieffer A, Stadian EM, Mohandas A, Peterson HO: Discographic-anatomical correlation of developmental changes with age in the intervertebral disc. *Acta Radiol Diagn* 9:733, 1969.

Pritzker KPH: Aging and degeneration in the lumbar intervertebral disc. *Orthop Clin North Am* 8:65, 1977.

Osteochondrosis

Adams MA, Dolan P, Hutton WC: The stages of disc degeneration as revealed by discograms. *J Bone Joint Surg* 68B:36, 1986.

Farfan HF, Cossette JW, Robertson GH, Wells RV, Kraus H: The effects of torsion on the lumbar intervertebral joints: The role of torsion in the production of disc degeneration. *J Bone Joint Surg* 52A:468, 1970.

Knutsson F: The vacuum phenomenon in the intervertebral discs. *Acta Radiol* 23:173, 1942.

Lyons E: Uncovertebral osteophytes and osteochondrosis of the cervical spine. *J Bone Joint Surg* 27A:248,1945.

Milgram JW: Osteoarthritic changes at the severely degenerative disc in humans. *Spine* 7:498, 1982.

CHAPTER 8: DEGENERATIVE ARTHRITIS OF THE SPINE

Spondylosis

Epstein BS, Epstein JA, Jones MD: Cervical spinal stenosis. *Radiol Clin North Am* 15:215, 1977.

Govoni AF: Developmental stenosis of a thoracic vertebra resulting in narrowing of the spinal canal. *Am J Roentgenol* 112:401, 1971.

Kirkaldy-Willis WH, Paine KWE, Cauchioix J, McIvor G: Lumbar spinal stenosis. *Clin Orthop* 99:30, 1974.

Kirkaldy-Willis WH, Wedge JH, Yong-Hing K, Reilly J: Pathology and pathogenesis of lumbar spondylosis and stenosis. *Spine* 3:319, 1978.

Macnab I: Cervical spondylosis. *Clin Orthop* 109:69, 1975.

Nelson MA: Lumbar spinal stenosis. *J Bone Joint Surg* 55B:506, 1973.

Payne EE, Spillane JD: The cervical spine: An anatomico-pathological study of seventy specimens (using a special technique) with particular reference to the problem of cervical spondylosis. *Brain* 80:571, 1957.

Schatzker J, Pennal GF: Spinal stenosis, a cause of cauda equina compression. *J Bone Joint Surg* 50B:606, 1968.

Stoltmann HF, Blackwood W: The role of the ligamenta flava in the pathogenesis of myelopathy in cervical spondylosis. *Brain* 87:45, 1964.

Facet Joint Arthrosis

Adams MA, Hutton WC: The mechanical function of the lumbar apophyseal joints. *Spine* 8:327, 1983.

Anderson GJ: The biomechanics of the posterior elements of the lumbar spine. *Spine* 8:326, 1983.

Dunlop RB, Adams MA, Hutton WC: Disc space narrowing and the lumbar facet joints. *J Bone Joint Surg* 66B:706, 1984.

Giles LGF: Lumbo-sacral zygapophyseal joint tropism and its effect on hyaline cartilage. *Clin Biomechanics* 2:2, 1987.

Lewin T: Osteoarthritis in lumbar synovial joints: A morphologic study. *Acta Orthop Scand Suppl* 73:1, 1964.

Lippitt AB: The facet joint and its role in spine pain: Management with facet joint injections. *Spine* 9:746, 1984.

Quinet RJ, Hadler NM: Diagnosis and treatment of backache. *Semin Arthritis Rheum* 8:261, 1979.

Taylor JR, Twomey LT: Age changes in lumbar zygapophyseal joints: Observations on structure and function. *Spine* 11:739, 1986.

Yang KH, King AI: The mechanism of facet load transmission as a hypothesis for low back pain. *Spine* 9:557, 1984.

Degenerative Spondylolisthesis

Blackburne JS, Velikas EP: Spondylolisthesis in children and adolescents. *J Bone Joint Surg* 59B:490, 1977.

Cauchoix J, Benoist M, Chassaing V: Degenerative spondylolisthesis. *Clin Orthop* 115:122, 1976.

Fisk JR, Moe JH, Winter RB: Scoliosis, spondylolysis, and spondylolisthesis: Their relationship as reviewed in 539 patients. *Spine* 3:234, 1978.

Fitzgerald JA, Newman PH: Degenerative spondylolisthesis. *J Bone Joint Surg* 58B:184, 1976.

Krenz J, Troup JDG: The structure of the pars interarticularis of the lower lumbar vertebrae and its relation to the etiology of spondylolysis. *J Bone Joint Surg* 55B:735, 1973.

Macnab I: Spondylolisthesis with an intact neural arch—the so-called pseudospondylolisthesis. *J Bone Joint Surg* 32B:325, 1950.

Newman PH: Spondylolisthesis, its cause and effect. *Ann R Coll Surg Engl* 16:305, 1955.

Newman PH, Stone KH: The etiology of spondylolisthesis. *J Bone Joint Surg* 45B:39, 1963.

Rosenberg NJ: Degenerative spondylolisthesis: Predisposing factors. *J Bone Joint Surg* 57A:467, 1975.

Wiltse LL, Newman PH, Macnab I: Classification of spondylolysis and spondylolisthesis. *Clin Orthop* 117:23, 1976.

Spinal Stenosis

Dorwart RH: Fundamentals of the computed tomographic assessment of spinal stenosis, in Genant HK (ed.): *Spine Update 1984*. San Francisco, Radiology Research and Education Foundation, 1984, p 181.

Sutro CJ: Lumbar facets–Spinal stenosis and intermittent claudication: A mini review. *Bull Hosp Joint Dis* 40:13, 1979.

Weisz GM: Lumbar spinal canal stenosis in Paget's disease. *Spine* 8:192, 1983.

Neuropathic (Charcot) Spine

Eichenholtz SN: *Charcot Joints*. Springfield, Ill., Charles C. Thomas, 1966.

CHAPTER 9: INFLAMMATORY AND ANKYLOSING SPONDYLOARTHROPATHIES

General Features

Jacobs JC: Spondyloarthritis and enthesopathy: Current concepts in rheumatology. *Arch Intern Med* 143:103, 1983.

Inflammatory Spondylitis

Ball J: The Heberden oration, 1970: Enthesopathy of rheumatoid and ankylosing spondylitis. *Ann Rheum Dis* 30:213, 1971.

Bywaters EGL: Rheumatoid and other diseases of the cervical interspinous bursae, and changes in the spinous processes. *Ann Rheum Dis* 41:360, 1982.

Bywaters EGL: Thoracic intervertebral discitis in rheumatoid arthritis due to costovertebral joint involvement. *Rheumatol Int* 1:83, 1981.

Detenbeck LC: Rheumatoid arthritis of the spinal column: Pathologic aspects and treatment. *Orthop Clin North Am* 2:679, 1971.

Eulderink F, Meijers KAE: Pathology of the cervical spine in rheumatoid arthritis: A controlled study of 44 spines. *J Pathol* 120:91, 1976.

Sims-Williams H, Jayson MIV, Baddeley H: Rheumatoid involvement of the lumbar spine. *Ann Rheum Dis* 36:524, 1977.

Ankylosing Spondyloarthropathies

Blasingame JP, Resnick D, Coutts RD, Danzig LA: Extensive spinal osteophytosis as a risk factor for heterotopic bone formation after total hip arthroplasty. *Clin Orthop* 161:191, 1981.

Calabro JJ, Maltz BA: Current concepts: Ankylosing spondylitis. *N Engl J Med* 282:606, 1970.

Carette S, Graham D, Little H, Rubenstein J, Rosen P: The natural disease course of ankylosing spondylitis. *Arthritis Rheum* 26:981, 1983.

Cruickshank B: Lesions of cartilaginous joints in ankylosing spondylitis. *J Pathol Bacteriol* 71:73, 1956.

Engleman EG, Engleman EP: Ankylosing spondylitis: Recent advances in diagnosis and treatment. *Med Clin North Am* 61:347, 1977.

Forestier J, Lagier R: Ankylosing hyperostosis of the spine. *Clin Orthop* 74:65, 1971.

Forestier J, Rotes-Querol J: Senile ankylosing hyperostosis of the spine. *Ann Rheum Dis* 9:321, 1950.

Julkinen H, Heinonen OP, Pyorala K: Hyperostosis of the spine in an adult population: Its relationship to hyperglycemia and obesity. *Ann Rheum Dis* 30:65, 1971.

Murakami N, Muroga T, Sobue J: Cervical myelopathy due to ossification of the posterior longitudinal ligament: A clinicopathologic study. *Arch Neurol* 35:33, 1978.

Ono M, Russell WJ, Kudo S, Kuroiwa Y, Takamori M, Motomura S, Murakami J: Ossification of the thoracic posterior longitudinal ligament in a fixed population: Radiological and neurological manifestations. *Radiology* 143:469, 1982.

Perry JD, Wolf H, Festenstein H, Storey GO: Ankylosing hyperostosis: A study of HLA, A, B, and C antigens. *Ann Rheum Dis* 38:72, 1979.

Resnick D, Niwayama G: Radiographic and pathologic features of spinal involvement in diffuse idiopathic skeletal hyperostosis (DISH). *Radiology* 119:559, 1976.

Resnick D, Shapiro RF, Wiesner KB, Niwayama G, Utsinger PD, Shaul SR: Diffuse idiopathic skeletal hyperostosis (DISH) (ankylosing hyperostosis of Forestier and Rotes-Querol). *Semin Arthritis Rheum* 7:153, 1978.

Singh A, Dass R, Hajreh SS, Jolly SS: Skeletal changes in endemic fluorosis. *J Bone Joint Surg* 44B:806, 1961.

Vernon-Roberts B, Pirie CJ, Trenwith V: Pathology of the dorsal spine in ankylosing hyperostosis. *Ann Rheum Dis* 33:281, 1974.

SECTION 3: DISEASES OF THE BONY ELEMENTS

CHAPTER 10: DEVELOPMENTAL AND ACQUIRED MALFORMATIONS

Segmental Malformations

Dounis E: Sacrococcygeal agenesis: A report of four new cases. *Acta Orthop Scand* 49:475, 1978.

Hensinger RN, Lang JE, MacEwen GD: Klippel-Feil syndrome: A constellation of associated anomalies. *J Bone Joint Surg* 56A:1246, 1974.

Lee CK, Weiss AB: Isolated congenital cervical block vertebrae below the axis with neurological symptoms. *Spine* 6:118, 1981.

Vertebral Body Malformations

Gjorup PA: Dorsal hemivertebra. *Acta Orthop Scand* 35:117, 1964.

Goldberg C, Fenelon G, Blake NS, Dowling F, Regan BF: Diastematomyelia: A critical review of the natural history and treatment. *Spine* 9:367, 1984.

Hood RW, Riseborough EJ, Nehme AM, Micheli LJ, Strand RD, Neuhauser EBD: Diastematomyelia and structural spinal deformities. *J Bone Joint Surg* 62A:520, 1980.

Mink JH: Case report 313. *Skeletal Radiol* 13:314, 1985.

Tanaka T, Uhthoff HK: The pathogenesis of congenital vertebral malformations: A study based on observations made in 11 human embryos and fetuses. *Acta Orthop Scand* 52:413, 1981.

Vertebral Arch Malformation

Cowell MJ, Cowell HR: The incidence of spina bifida occulta in idiopathic scoliosis. *Clin Orthop* 118:16, 1976.

Lorber J: Spina bifida cystica: Results of treatment of 270 consecutive cases with criteria for selection for the future. *Arch Dis Child* 47:854, 1972.

Developmental Abnormalities in the Cartilaginous End Plate

Bethem D, Winter RB, Lutter L, Moe JH, Bradford DS, Lonstein JE, Langer LO: Spinal disorders of dwarfism: Review of the literature and report of eighty cases. *J Bone Joint Surg* 63A:1412, 1981.

Bradford DS, Brown DM, Moe JH, Winter RB, Jowsey J: Scheuermann's kyphosis: A form of osteoporosis? *Clin Orthop* 118:10, 1976.

Ryan MD, Taylor TKF: Acute spinal cord compression in Scheuermann's disease. *J Bone Joint Surg* 64B:409, 1982.

Wynne-Davies R, Walsh WK, Gormley J: Achondroplasia and hypochondroplasia: Clinical variation and spinal stenosis. *J Bone Joint Surg* 63B:508, 1981.

Defects of the Pars Interarticularis

Eisenstein S: Spondylosis: A skeletal investigation of two population groups. *J Bone Joint Surg* 60B:488, 1978.

Strauss ED, Kahanovitz N, Ghelman B: Congenital absence of the thoracic pedicle: A case report. *Spine* 8:48, 1983.

Wiltse LL, Newman PH, Macnab I: Classification of spondylolysis and spondylolisthesis. *Clin Orthop* 117:23, 1976.

CHAPTER 11: METABOLIC AND HEMATOLOGIC DISEASES OF THE SPINE

Diseases Resulting from a Structurally Defective Matrix

Beighton P, Horan F: Orthopaedic aspects of the Ehlers-Danlos syndrome. *J Bone Joint Surg* 51B:444, 1969.

Cristofaro RL, Hoek KJ, Bonnett CA, Brown JC: Treatment of spine deformity in osteogenesis imperfecta. *Clin Orthop* 139:40, 1979.

Lipson SJ: Dysplasia of the odontoid process in Morquio's syndrome causing quadriparesis. *J Bone Joint Surg* 59A:340, 1977.

Nelson JD: The Marfan syndrome, with special reference to congenital enlargement of the spinal canal. *Br J Radiol* 31:561, 1958.

Nelson AM, Riggs BL, Jowsey JO: Atypical axial osteomalacia: Report of four cases with two having features of ankylosing spondylitis. *Arthritis Rheum* 21:715, 1978.

Renshaw TS, Cook RS, Albright JA: Scoliosis in osteogenesis imperfecta. *Clin Orthop* 145:163, 1979.

Diseases Resulting from Disturbances in Bone Remodeling

Amstutz HC, Sissons HA: The structure of the vertebral spongiosa. *J Bone Joint Surg* 51B:540, 1969.

Atkinson PJ: Variation in trabecular structure of vertebrae with age. *Calcif Tissue Res* 1:24, 1967.

Dauphine RT, Riggs BL, Scholz DA: Back pain and vertebral crush fractures: An unemphasized mode of presentation for primary hyperparathyroidism. *Ann Intern Med* 83:365, 1975.

Hansson T, Roos B: Microcalluses of the trabeculae in lumbar vertebrae and their relation to the bone mineral content. *Spine* 6:375, 1981.

Hartman JT, Dohn DF: Paget's disease of the spine with cord or nerve-root compression: A report of six cases. *J Bone Joint Surg* 48A:1079, 1966.

Horensten ML, Boner G, Rosenfeld JB: The shrinking man: A manifestation of severe renal osteodystrophy. *JAMA* 244:267, 1980.

Huang TL, Cohen NJ, Sahgal S, Tseng CH: Osteosarcoma complicating Paget's disease of the spine with neurologic complications. *Clin Orthop* 141:260, 1979.

Milgram JW, Jasty M: Osteopetrosis: A morphological study of twenty-one cases. *J Bone Joint Surg* 64A:912, 1982.

Diseases Resulting from Hematologic Disturbances

Amstutz HC, Carey EJ: Skeletal manifestations and treatment of Gaucher's disease: Review of twenty cases. *J Bone Joint Surg* 48A:670, 1966.

Cassady JR, Berdon WE, Baker DH: The "typical" spine changes of sickle-cell anemia in a patient with thalassemia major (Cooley's anemia). *Radiology* 89:1065, 1967.

Diggs LW: Bone and joint lesions in sickle-cell disease. *Clin Orthop* 52:119, 1967.

Greenfield GB: Bone changes in chronic adult Gaucher's disease. *Am J Roentgenol Radium Ther Nucl Med* 110:800, 1970.

Henkin WA: Collapse of the vertebral bodies in sickle-cell anemia. *Am J Roentgenol* 62(3):395, 1949.

Reynolds J: A re-evaluation of the "fish vertebra" sign in sickle cell hemoglobinopathy. *Am J Roentgenol* 97:693, 1966.

CHAPTER 12: SPINAL INFECTIONS

Pyogenic Spondylitis

Griffiths HED, Jones DM: Pyogenic infection of the spine: A review of twenty-eight cases. *J Bone Joint Surg* 53B:383, 1971.

Spiegel PG, Kengla KW, Isaacson AS, Wilson JC: Intervertebral disc-space inflammation in children. *J Bone Joint Surg* 54A:284, 1972.

Stauffer RN: Pyogenic vertebral osteomyelitis. *Orthop Clin North Am* 6:1015, 1975.

Wiley AM, Trueta J: The vascular anatomy of the spine and its relationship to pyogenic vertebral osteomyelitis. *J Bone Joint Surg* 41B:796, 1959.

Tuberculosis Spondylitis (Pott's Disease)

Forienza SW, Axelrod JL, Grieco MH: Pott's disease in heroin addicts. *JAMA* 241:379, 1979.

Walker AN, Fechner RE: Granulomatous inflammation of bones and joints, in Joachim HL (ed.): *Pathology of Granulomas*. New York, Raven Press 1983, p 421.

CHAPTER 13: SPINAL TUMORS: BENIGN

General Features of Spinal Tumors

Fornasier VL, Czitrom AA: Collapsed vertebrae: A review of 659 autopsies. *Clin Orthop* 131:261, 1978.

Sim FH, Dahlin DC, Stauffer RN, Laws ER: Primary bone tumors simulating lumbar disc syndrome. *Spine* 2:65, 1977.

Giant Cell Tumor

Lubicky JP, Patel NS, DeWald RL: Two-stage spondylectomy for giant cell tumor of L4: A case report. *Spine* 8:112, 1983.

Jacobs TP, Michelsen J, Polay JS, D'Adamo AC, Canfield RE: Giant cell tumor in Paget's disease of bone: Familial and geographic clustering. *Cancer* 44:742, 1979.

Aneurysmal Bone Cyst

Hay MC, Paterson D, Taylor TKF: Aneurysmal bone cysts of the spine. *J Bone Joint Surg* 60B:406, 1978.

Benign Osteoblastoma

Griffin JB: Benign osteoblastoma of the thoracic spine: Case report with fifteen-year follow up. *J Bone Joint Surg* 60A:833, 1978.

Marsh BW, Bonfiglio M, Brady LP, Enneking WF: Benign osteoblastoma: Range of manifestations. *J Bone Joint Surg* 57A:1, 1975.

Hemangioma

Bell RL: Hemangioma of a dorsal vertebra with collapse and compression myelopathy. *J Neurosurg* 12:570, 1955.

Bergstrand A, Hook O, Lidvall H: Vertebral haemangiomas compressing the spinal cord. *Acta Neurol Scand* 39:59, 1963.

Julien L, Riemens V, Vital C, Lagueny A, Miet G: Cervical cord compression by solitary osteochondroma of the atlas. *J Neurol Neurosurg Psychiatry* 41:479, 1978.

Osteochondroma

Novick GS, Pavlov H, Bullough PG: Osteochondroma of the cervical spine. *Skeletal Radiol* 8:13, 1982.

Osteoid Osteoma

Keim HA, Reina EG: Osteoid osteoma as a cause of scoliosis. *J Bone Joint Surg* 57A:159, 1975.

Eosinophilic Granuloma

Compere EL, Johnson WE, Coventry MB: Vertebra plana (Calvé's disease) due to eosinophilic granuloma. *J Bone Joint Surg* 36A:969, 1954.

CHAPTER 14: SPINAL TUMORS: MALIGNANT

Metastatic Tumors

Boland PJ, Lane JM, Sundaresan N: Metastatic disease of the spine. *Clin Orthop* 169:95, 1982.

Multiple Myeloma

Griffiths DL: Orthopaedic aspects of myelomatosis. *J Bone Joint Surg* 48B:703, 1966.

Solitary Myeloma

Valderrama JAF, Bullough PG: Solitary myeloma of the spine. *J Bone Joint Surg* 50B:82, 1968.

Chordoma

Ulich TR, Mirra JM: Ecchordrosis physaliphora vertebralis. *Clin Orthop* 163:282, 1982.

Volpe R, Mazabraud A: A clinicopathologic review of 25 cases of chordoma (a pleomorphic and metastasizing neoplasm). *Am J Surg Pathol* 7:161, 1983.

Chondrosarcoma

Camins MB, Duncan AW, Smith J, Marcove RC: Chondrosarcoma of the spine. *Spine* 3:202, 1978.

Wronski J, Byrc S, Kaminski J, Chibowski D: Chondrosarcoma of cervical spine causing compression of the cord. *J Neurosurg* 21:419, 1964.

Osteosarcoma

Barwick KW, Huvos AG, Smith J: Primary osteogenic sarcoma of the vertebral column: A clinicopathologic correlation of ten patients. *Cancer* 46:595, 1980.

Malignant Lymphoma

Epstein BS: Vertebral changes in childhood leukemia. *Radiology* 68:65, 1957.

Irvine RA, Robertson WB: Spinal cord compression in the malignant lymphomas. *Br Med J* 5394:1354, 1964.

Solgaard S, Kristiansen B: Vertebra plana due to a malignant lymphoma. *Acta Orthop Scand* 51:267, 1980.

Ewing's Sarcoma

Russin LA, Robinson MJ, Engle HA, Sonni A: Ewing's sarcoma of the lumbar spine: A case report of long-term survival. *Clin Orthop* 164:126, 1982.

Intraspinal Neoplasms

DaRoza AC: Primary intraspinal tumors: Their clinical presentation and diagnosis; an analysis of ninety-five cases. *J Bone Joint Surg* 46B:8, 1964.

Davis RA, Washburn PL: Spinal cord meningiomas. *Surg Gynecol Obstet* 131:15, 1970.

Wiesel SW, Ignatius P, Marvel JP, Rothman RH: Intradural neurofibroma simulating lumbar-disc disease: Report of six cases. *J Bone Joint Surg* 58A:1040, 1976.

Winter RB, Moe JH, Bradford DS, Lonstein JE, Pedras CV, Weber AH: Spine deformity in neurofibromatosis: A review of one hundred and two patients. *J Bone Joint Surg* 61A:677, 1979.

INDEX

Note: Numbers in **boldface** refer to Figure numbers.

A

B

C

D

M

N

O

P

R

S

T

U

V

W

Z